Noninvasive Imaging of Myocardial Ischemia

Constantinos D. Anagnostopoulos,
Jeroen J. Bax, Petros Nihoyannopoulos
and Ernst van der Wall (Eds)

Noninvasive Imaging of Myocardial Ischemia

With 129 Figures
Including 45 Color Plates

Springer

Constantinos D Anagnostopoulos, MD, PhD, FRCR, FESC
Royal Brompton Hospital *and*
Chelsea & Westminster Hospital, London, UK, *and*
National Heart and Lung Institute, Imperial College School of Medicine, London, UK

Petros Nihoyannopoulos, MD, FRCP, FACC, FESC
Imperial College, Hammersmith Hospital, London, UK

Jeroen J. Bax, MD, PhD
Leiden University Medical Center, Leiden, The Netherlands

Ernst van der Wall, MD, FESC, FACC
Leiden University Medical Center, Leiden, The Netherlands

British Library Cataloguing in Publication Data
Noninvasive imaging of myocardial ischemia
1. Coronary heart disease – Imaging 2. Diagnostic imaging
I. Anagnostopoulos, Constantinos D.
616.1′23′0754
ISBN-10: 1846280273

ISBN-10: 1-84628-027-3 ISBN: 1-84628-156-3 (eBook)
ISBN-13: 978-1-4471-7121-8
DOI: 10.1007/1-84628-027-3
Printed on acid-free paper

Softcover re-print of the Hardcover 1st edition 2006

Printed in Singapore (BS/KYO)

9 8 7 6 5 4 3 2 1

Springer Science+Business Media
springer.com

To those who have devoted their lives to
their patients and the art of medicine

"... And if you find her poor, Ithake won't have fooled you. Wise as you will have become, so full of experience, you will have understood by then what these Ithakes mean."

Konstantinos Kavafis, Ithake, 1910

Foreword I

Noninvasive cardiac imaging is an integral part of the practice of current clinical cardiology. During the past three decades a number of distinctly different noninvasive imaging techniques of the heart, such as radionuclide imaging, echocardiography, magnetic resonance imaging, and X-ray computed tomography have been developed. Remarkable progress has been made by each of these technologies in terms of technical advances, clinical procedures, and clinical applications/indications. Each technique was propelled by a devoted group of talented and dedicated investigators who explored the potential value of each technique for making clinical diagnoses and for defining clinical characteristics of heart disease that might be most useful in the management of patients. Thus far, most of these clinical investigations using various non-invasive cardiac imaging techniques were conducted largely in isolation from each other, often pursuing similar clinical goals. There now exists an embarrassment of riches of available imaging techniques and the potential for redundant imaging data. However, as each noninvasive cardiac imaging technique matured, it became clear that they were not necessarily competitive but rather complementary, each offering unique information under unique clinical conditions.

The development of each technique in isolation resulted in different clinical subcultures, each with its separate clinical and scientific meetings and medical literature. Such a narrow focus and concentration on one technology may be very beneficial during the development stage of a technology, but once the basic practical principles have been worked out and clinical applications are established, isolation contains the danger of duplication of pursuits and scientific staleness when technology limits are reached. It should be obvious that each technique provides different pathophysiologic and/or anatomic information. Coming out of the isolation and cross-fertilization is the next logical step to evolve to a higher and more sophisticated level of cardiac imaging. Patients would benefit tremendously if each technique were to be used judiciously and discriminately, and provided just those imaging data needed to manage a specific clinical scenario. I anticipate that in the future a new type of cardiac imaging specialist will emerge. Rather than one-dimensional subspecialists, such as (I apologize) nuclear cardiologists or echocardiographers, multimodality cardiac imagers will be trained who have in-depth knowledge and experience of all available non-invasive cardiac imaging techniques. These imaging specialists will fully understand the value and limitations of each technique and will be able to apply each of them discriminately and optimally to the benefit of cardiac patients.

In *Noninvasive Imaging in Myocardial Ischemia*, the editors Drs. Anagnostopoulos, Nihoyannopolos, Bax, and Van der Wall, provide a wealth of information on the clinical value of various noninvasive cardiac imaging techniques. The editors collaborated with a distinguished group of authors – each recognized experts in their particular area of cardiac imaging. This book not only provides the reader with the present state of the art of currently available noninvasive cardiac imaging techniques, but also the comparative value (as far as information is available) of various techniques in different clinical conditions and in different patient groups. After a general introduction to the pathophysiology of coronary artery disease as it relates to cardiac imaging, the first six chapters discuss the basic principles and technology of echocardiography, cardiac magnetic resonance imaging, radionuclide myocardial perfusion imaging, and computed X-ray tomography. Subsequent chapters deal with specific clinical conditions for which noninvasive cardiac imaging may be used. Unique to this book is that in each chapter the available evidence by alternative imaging techniques is discussed. In some chapters (Chapters 9–12), this consists merely of a comparison of stress radionuclide imaging and stress echocardiography, since no data are available for other imaging techniques. In other chapters (Chapters 7, 8, 13–15) data from the full spectrum of noninvasive cardiac imaging is available, and the authors discuss how it may be utilized to obtain optimal anatomic and pathophysiologic information relevant for patient management. Several chapters propose practical algorithms for stepwise testing by various imaging techniques in different patient cohorts. The editors and authors are to be applauded for their effort to come to grips with the difficult task of sorting out the relative and complementary value of each imaging technique. It is clear that much is not (yet) known and much work is still to be done. This well-illustrated and well-referenced book is a first step to clinical multimodality cardiac imaging and should be an invaluable resource for anyone interested in cardiac imaging. This book will be an important aid to cardiology fellows, nuclear medicine and radiology residents, cardiologists, radiologists, and nuclear medicine physicians who wish to take the step to multimodality, noninvasive cardiac imaging.

Frans J. Th. Wackers, MD
Professor of Diagnostic Radiology
and Medicine
Director, Cardiovascular Nuclear Imaging and Stress Laboratories
Yale University School of Medicine
New Haven, CT
USA

Foreword II

Noninvasive Imaging of Myocardial Ischemia provides a comprehensive discussion and review of the noninvasive myocardial imaging techniques that are currently available to detect myocardial ischemia and infarction. Topics covered include echocardiography, cardiac magnetic resonance imaging, myocardial perfusion scintigraphy, positron emission tomography, and computed tomography. There are also chapters on myocardial imaging techniques in the evaluation of asymptomatic individuals, prognostic assessments of patients with CAD by noninvasive imaging techniques, and imaging in the Emergency Department in patients with chest pain. Risk stratification in patients with coronary heart disease, imaging techniques used to distinguish hibernating from irreversibly injured myocardium, and myocardial imaging in non-coronary and congenital heart disease causes of myocardial ischemia are also discussed in the book. The chapters are comprehensive, informative, and written by experts in imaging of the myocardium.

This will be a very useful book for everyone interested in noninvasive myocardial imaging of ischemic heart disease. However, it will need to be updated with some frequency as one anticipates future advances with multidetector CT imaging, magnetic resonance imaging, detection of vulnerable atherosclerotic plaques, stem cell therapies, and the addition of nanotechnology methods to the evaluation and treatment of patients with coronary artery disease. Hopefully, the Editors will be able to provide periodic updates of the information available in this book, as well as of the new developments one anticipates.

James T. Willerson, MD
President, The University of Texas Health Science Center
President-Elect and Medical Director, Texas Heart Institute
Houston, TX 77030
USA

Preface

Noninvasive cardiac imaging covers a broad spectrum of investigations including echocardiography, radionuclide imaging, computed tomography (CT), and magnetic resonance imaging (MRI). Major developments have occurred in this field recently and imaging data are now utilized almost on a daily basis for clinical decision making.

This book tries to capture the important advances and new directions in which the field is heading. It provides a forum for a fertile discussion on the strengths and limitations of the various imaging modalities in different clinical settings offering also practical recommendations for their appropriate use. It focuses on the interrelations and complimentary roles of different techniques thus reflecting the multifaceted manifestations of myocardial ischemia.

It is our belief that the field of noninvasive cardiac imaging can only advance and strengthen its role in the decision-making process when comprehensive evidence-based information is used. We are very privileged that the contributors to this volume are international opinion leaders in their field. They have made every effort not only to provide state of the art information on their respective topics but also to keep alive the discussion on imaging as a whole. We hope that the book will be a very helpful reference for practitioners from different background and disciplines including cardiologists, general physicians and imagers.

The first section (Chapters 1 to 6) discusses principles of pathophysiology relevant to noninvasive cardiac imaging and provides up to date information on the technical aspects of different imaging modalities. The second section (Chapters 7 to 15) focuses on the role of imaging in the assessment of myocardial ischemia offering valuable information on diagnostic and management issues, both within the stable and acute clinical setting. The accompanying CD contains 10 clinical cases and is designed to provide examples illustrating the clinical usefulness of noninvasive cardiac imaging in every day practice.

In a multi-authored book covering topics which are related to each other, a degree of overlap is inevitable. Every effort has been made to keep that to a minimum whilst maintaining at the same time the autonomy and completeness of each chapter.

We are indebted to all the contributors for their hard work and commitment to achieve this delicate balance and we wish to thank all of them for their superb chapters. We are very grateful to the staff of our departments for their contribution to the presentation of the images and cases of this book, to all those who supported our work and to the staff of Springer for their assistance and editorial advice.

C. Anagnostopoulos
J.J. Bax
P. Nihoyannopoulos
E. Van der Wall

Contents

List of Contributors

Constantinos D. Anagnostopoulos, MD, PhD, FRCR, FESC
Royal Brompton Hospital
and Chelsea & Westminster Hospital
and Imperial College School of Medicine
London, UK

A. Anagnostopoulos-Tzifa M.D, MRCPCH
Guy's & St Thomas' Hospital
London, UK

Jeroen J. Bax, MD, PhD
Leiden University Medical Center
Leiden, The Netherlands

George A. Beller, MD
University of Virginia Health System
Charlottesville, VA, USA

Frank M. Bengel, MD
Nuklearmedizinische Klinik der TU München
München, Germany

Daniel S. Berman, MD, FACC
Cedars-Sinai Medical Center
Los Angeles, CA, USA

Nicholas Bunce MD, MRCP
St. Georges' Hospital
London, UK

Filippo Cademartiri, MD, PhD
Erasmus Medical Center
Rotterdam, The Netherlands

Ignasi Carrió, MD
Autonomous University of Barcelona
Hospital de la Santa Creu i Sant Pau
Barcelona, Spain

P.J. de Feyter, MD, PhD
Erasmus Medical Center
Rotterdam, The Netherlands

Vijay Anand Dhakshinamurthy, MBBS, MRCP
Wellington Hospital
London, UK

Abdou Elhendy MD, PhD
Nebraska Medical Center
Omaha, NE, USA

Albert Flotats, MD
Autonomous University of Barcelona
Hospital de la Santa Creu i Sant Pau
Barcelona, Spain

Michael A. Gatzoulis, MD, PhD
Royal Brompton Hospital
London, UK

Mark Harbinson, MD, FRCP
Queen's University Belfast
Belfast, Northern Ireland

Rory Hachamovitch, MD, MSc
Keck School of Medicine, U.S.C.
Los Angeles, CA, USA

Miklos D. Kertai, MD
Erasmus Medical Centre
Rotterdam, The Netherlands

Philip J. Kilner, MD, PhD
Royal Brompton Hospital
London, UK

Avijit Lahiri, BS, MB, MSc, MRCP
Wellington Hospital
London, UK

W. Li, MD, PhD
Royal Brompton Hospital
London, UK

Eric Tien Siang Lim, MRCP, MA Cantab
Wellington Hospital
London, UK

C.Y. Loong, MBBS, MRCP
Royal Brompton Hospital
London, UK

Thomas H. Marwick, MBBS, PhD, FRACP, FACC
University of Queensland
Princess Alexandra Hospital
Brisbane, Australia

Tarun K. Mittal, MBBS
Royal Brompton & Harefield Hospital NHS Trust
London, UK

Niko R. Mollet, MD
Erasmus Medical Center
Rotterdam, The Netherlands

Eike Nagel, MD
German Heart Institute Berlin
Berlin, Germany

K. Nieman, MD, PhD
Erasmus Medical Center – Thoraxcenter
Rotterdam, The Netherlands

Petros Nihoyannopoulos, MD, FRCP, FACC, FESC
Imperial College London
Hammersmith Hospital, NHLI
London, UK

Roderic I. Pettigrew, PhD, MD
National Institute of Biomedical Engineering and Biological Imaging
National Institutes of Health
Bethesda, MD, USA

Don Poldermans, MD, PhD
Erasmus Medical Centre
Rotterdam, The Netherlands

Frank E. Rademakers, MD, PhD
University Hospitals Leuven
Catholic University Leuven
Leuven, Belgium

Dhrubo Rakhit, MD
University of Queensland
Princess Alexandra Hospital
Brisbane, Australia

Eliana Reyes, MD
National Heart and Lung Institute
Imperial College
London, UK

Michael B. Rubens, MBBS, DMRD, FRCR
Royal Brompton & Harefield Hospital NHS Trust
London, UK

Arend F.L. Schinkel, MD
Thoraxcentre
Erasmus Medical Centre
Rotterdam, The Netherlands

Olaf Schouten, MD
Erasmus Medical Centre
Rotterdam, The Netherlands

Roxy Senior, MD, DM, FRCP, FESC, FACC
Northwick Park Hospital and Institute for Medical Research
Harrow, Middlesex, UK

Leslee J. Shaw, PhD
Cedars-Sinai Medical Center
Los Angeles, CA, USA

Prem Soman, MD, PhD, MRCP
Tufts-New England Medical Center
and Tufts University School of Medicine
Boston, MA, USA

Ju-Le Tan, MBBS, MRCP
Royal Brompton Hospital
London, UK

James E. Udelson, MD
Tufts-New England Medical Center
and Tufts University School of Medicine
Boston, MA, USA

1

Principles of Pathophysiology Related to Noninvasive Cardiac Imaging

Mark Harbinson and Constantinos D. Anagnostopoulos

This chapter considers the principal mechanisms involved in regulating myocardial blood flow, and reviews the pathophysiologic changes observed during myocardial ischemia. A detailed discussion of the precise biochemical and cellular mechanisms involved is beyond the scope of this review, but the basic mechanisms by which cardiac stress techniques allow interrogation of the many changes occurring during ischemia are presented. Although we focus on myocardial ischemia, strictly speaking, imaging techniques do not always detect ischemia itself. Changes in local perfusion accompany ischemia, and may indeed be induced without frank ischemia actually developing. It should be recognized, therefore, that many of the stress techniques discussed actually precipitate changes in myocardial blood flow as their primary effect.

Hypoxia is frequently defined in terms of a reduction in tissue oxygen supply despite adequate perfusion, whereas ischemia additionally implies reduced removal of metabolites (for example, lactate) attributed to failure of an appropriate level of perfusion. Hypoxia may therefore be seen with chronic lung disease or carbon monoxide poisoning, for example. The most frequent cause of myocardial ischemia in humans is coronary atherosclerosis. As well as being a chronic process associated with coronary luminal narrowing and impaired endothelial function, atherosclerosis is associated with acute episodes of plaque rupture, coronary vasospasm, and thrombosis causing acute coronary syndromes. This chapter deals mainly with the pathophysiologic effects of chronic atherosclerosis, which results in chronic ischemic syndromes such as angina pectoris. Myocardial ischemia for other reasons or as a result of nonatheromatous disease processes is not discussed in detail, although the underlying physiology is similar.

1. Causes of Myocardial Ischemia

In humans, atherosclerosis is by far the most common cause of acute and chronic ischemic syndromes. Atherosclerosis, and its imaging, are briefly reviewed, and, finally, nonatheromatous causes of myocardial ischemia are discussed.

1.1 Atherosclerosis

Atherosclerosis is a chronic condition characterized by deposition of cholesterol-laden plaques and inflammatory cells in the vascular wall. The chronic expansion of plaques can lead to the development of flow-limiting coronary stenoses, which are associated with angina pectoris. It is therefore the main disease process underlying angina and hence the main target for imaging. It is punctuated with acute episodes of plaque instability leading to acute coronary syndromes including myocardial infarction.

It is thought that lipid accumulation in the arterial wall is one of the first stages in the development of atherosclerotic lesions. Low density lipoprotein molecules have been identified in the arterial wall and once bound there are susceptible to modification, with oxidation believed to be particularly important.[1] Leukocytes are then recruited to the area and enter the intima. Monocytes accumulate the lipid deposited in the intima and become characteristic "foam cells."[2] The earliest macroscopic change in atherosclerosis, the "fatty streak," consists largely of lipid-laden foam cells. After the formation of this basic lesion, atheroma then progresses chronically over some time period, with an increase in vascular smooth muscle and extracellular matrix. At first, the artery expands outward rather than inward, i.e., the whole cross-sectional area of the vessel increases and the lumen is little changed.[3] As the vessel continues to enlarge, however, the lumen then begins to be compromised. This may lead to chronic stable angina, and demonstration of coronary flow limitation related to such stenotic plaques is central to noninvasive assessment of ischemic heart disease.

Besides this chronic progressive increase, sudden changes in plaque size and morphology have been noted, and may occur silently or be manifest as an acute coronary syndrome. The main processes are acute plaque rupture[4] or acute plaque erosion,[5] and then subsequent thrombosis. It has been suggested that plaques mainly composed of lipid with a thin fibrous cap ("soft plaques") are more liable to rupture and hence precipitate acute coronary syndromes, whereas plaques with less lipid and better-formed fibrous caps are more stable and tend to cause chronic angina rather than acute vessel occlusion.[6]

Atherosclerotic plaques are ubiquitous as age advances, but several risk factors for earlier development of atheromatous coronary artery disease have been identified. Nonmodifiable risk factors include advancing age, male gender, and genetic factors, often described in terms of family history of premature onset disease. Modifiable risk factors include hyperlipidemia, hypertension, cigarette smoking, and diabetes mellitus.

1.2 Imaging Atherosclerosis

Beyond the more conventional imaging strategies assessing myocardial perfusion, that is, the functional consequence of coronary stenosis, several techniques are now available to image atheroma itself. These are briefly described below.

Intravascular ultrasound catheters can be delivered directly into the coronary arteries and an ultrasound image of the circumferential extent and composition of plaques can be obtained. This can be useful in assessing the anatomy before and after percutaneous coronary intervention and may be helpful in defining the extent and severity of lesions noted on X-ray coronary arteriography. Doppler ultrasound can also be used to measure the velocity of blood flow in the coronary arteries. This can then be measured before and after areas of stenosis, compared with proximal blood flow, and with blood flow after maximum pharmacologic vasodilatation. Hence, the functional significance of lesions can be assessed. A similar technique uses pressure rather than Doppler velocity measurement.[7]

More recently, magnetic resonance imaging (MRI) has been used to assess atheromatous plaques including those in coronary arteries. The use of different sequences, including contrast agents, has demonstrated plaque morphology including the lipid pool. This has led to the suggestion that similar methods might be able to characterize plaque composition and differentiate "vulnerable" from stable lesions.[8] Multislice computed tomographic images of the coronary arteries are now almost of a similar standard to X-ray angiography in many patients.[9] Similarly, early reports on the application of 18-fluorodeoxyglucose have been presented.[10] This tracer localizes to areas of metabolic activity, and can be detected with positron emission tomographic (PET) technology. Using coregistration with anatomic images, it is possible that active or vulnerable plaques may be identified and differentiated from more metabolically quiescent plaques with in theory a lower propensity to rupture. Several other approaches to imaging the pathophysiologic processes underlying atherosclerosis are currently being investigated.[11] These include imaging of vascular smooth muscle cells (using the labeled antibody Z_2D_3) and of the inflammatory processes within the vessel wall (for example, using radiolabeled matrix metalloproteinase). Similarly, apoptosis, the process of programmed cell death, can be imaged using 99m-technetium-labeled annexin V. Apoptosis of macrophages is seen in active atherosclerotic plaques, and also in the myocardium in acute myocardial infarction; annexin V uptake has been demonstrated in human myocardial infarction.[12]

1.3 Other Causes of Myocardial Ischemia

Although the vast majority of patients with angina have coronary atherosclerosis, other etiologies are recognized (see also Chapters 14 and 15). Problems with blood oxygen-carrying capacity, and with increased demand as a result of ventricular hypertrophy, may cause ischemia in the absence of what would normally be considered severe flow-limiting coronary stenoses (see below). The most common causes of ischemia beyond the atheromatous coronary disease are discussed in Chapters 14 and 15.

Syndrome X is a clinical entity characterized by anginal chest pain but unobstructed epicardial coronary arteries at angiography. This group of patients is rather heterogeneous, but, in some cases, ischemia has been demonstrated.[13] In these cases, dysfunction of the microvascular circulation has been identified.[14] Indeed, assessment of myocardial perfusion using magnetic resonance techniques has shown that an abnormal gradient develops between subepicardial and subendocardial perfusion during vasodilator stress with adenosine.[15] Not all patients with putative syndrome X have evidence of ischemia, however, and the group may also include patients with alternative causes for chest pain or with abnormal sensitivity to pain.

Coronary spasm may also cause chest pain similar to angina. Spasm may occur on atherosclerotic plaques in the coronary vessels, but also in patients without apparent atherosclerotic coronary disease. Variant or Prinzmetal's angina causes chest pain at rest and may be associated with ST segment elevation on the 12-lead electrocardiogram (ECG).[16] Coronary arteriography has demonstrated coronary artery spasm in these patients, and perfusion defects have been reported.[17] Abnormal resting coronary tone and abnormalities of resting sympathetic coronary innervation have also been suggested as possible etiologic factors.

It should be clear, therefore, that the finding of a perfusion defect during cardiac stress should not always lead to the conclusion that atherosclerotic coronary disease is the underlying cause.

2. The Coronary Circulation

Blood is delivered to the heart by the right and left coronary arteries, which arise normally from the aortic sinuses immediately above the aortic valve. The heart is a very active metabolic organ and requires a high level of oxygen delivery. Furthermore, oxygen extraction from delivered blood is high even at rest. Any increase in oxygen demand, therefore, must be met by increasing coronary blood flow, because there is little scope to increase oxygen extraction. To meet this level of oxygen demand, resting coronary blood flow is relatively high compared with other arteries, resting oxygen extraction is high, and the distribution of capillaries in the myocardium is dense. In addition, the coronary vessels are essentially end-arteries. Taken together with this high metabolic demand, these factors mean that the heart is relatively susceptible to ischemia and infarction.

3. Physiology of Myocardial Oxygen Supply and Oxygen Demand

The balance between myocardial oxygen requirements, and oxygen delivery, is central to understanding the mechanisms by which ischemia may occur. This balance is upset spontaneously during attacks of angina and other clinical manifestations of ischemia, and can be manipulated by various maneuvers during cardiac stress. An unmet increase in oxygen demand, a reduction in oxygen supply, or a combination of both can cause myocardial ischemia.

3.1 Myocardial Oxygen Demand

Cardiac oxygen requirements depend on a variety of parameters.[18] In the acute situation, it is mainly cardiac work that is important. This is determined by both heart rate and blood pressure, and their overall effect may be assessed as the rate-pressure product (RPP).[19] This is strongly correlated with myocardial oxygen consumption; therefore, an increase in RPP causes an increase in oxygen demand which, if not met by compensatory mechanisms, leads to myocardial ischemia. This is the parameter most frequently targeted by cardiac stress, with dynamic exercise and also to some extent with dobutamine stress, acting to increase RPP and hence to precipitate myocardial ischemia.

Myocardial wall tension may also change fairly rapidly and is an important determinant of myocardial oxygen demand. An increase in ventricular volume will be associated with an increase in wall tension and then usually increased velocity of contraction. This extra work requires additional oxygen supply.

Other significant determinants of myocardial oxygen requirements are of less importance in the context of this chapter because they usually are not amenable to direct manipulation during cardiac stress. The inotropic status of the myocardium and overall cardiac mass are the other parameters of significance. As the inotropic status of the heart is augmented, the energy requirements for this active process increase, and hence oxygen demand increases.

Table 1.1. Important factors in the control of myocardial oxygen supply and myocardial perfusion

1. Oxygen-carrying capacity of blood
2. Overall driving pressure (aortic diastolic pressure)
3. Coronary vascular tone/resistance
Metabolic regulation
Endothelium-dependent factors
Autoregulation of blood flow
Autonomic nerves
Circulating hormones
Extravascular compressive forces

Although cardiac mass does not change acutely, patients with ventricular hypertrophy are predisposed to myocardial ischemia because of increased oxygen demand of the additional myocyte mass.

3.2 Myocardial Oxygen Supply

Oxygen delivery depends on adequately oxygenated hemoglobin reaching the myocyte. The main determinants of myocardial oxygen supply are therefore the oxygen-carrying capacity of the blood and coronary blood flow. The former largely depends on the hemoglobin concentration, and anemia may precipitate angina in susceptible patients. Other situations in which blood oxygen delivery or extraction is inadequate, such as CO poisoning, are rare. The latter, namely, coronary blood flow, depends on two parameters: the driving pressure from the aorta, and control of coronary vascular tone (resistance). Aortic diastolic pressure is usually sufficient to perfuse the coronary artery ostia at most normal levels of blood pressure and is not generally a cause of myocardial ischemia. From the standpoint of stress testing for assessment of myocardial ischemia in patients, coronary blood flow, and its relationship to coronary tone, is the most important parameter to understand. These factors are briefly summarized in Table 1.1.

4. Coronary Blood Flow

The arterioles and pre-arteriolar vessels constitute the major resistance vessels in the coronary system. Vasodilatation in this bed increases coronary blood flow and is the main method for increasing myocardial perfusion. The balance between vasodilator and vasoconstrictor tone in this arteriolar bed therefore determines coronary blood flow. Several factors are involved in this balance (Table 1.1) and are discussed in turn. Many noninvasive methods, therefore, interrogate the perfusion system rather than induce ischemia itself.

4.1 Metabolic Regulation of Coronary Blood Flow

An important local method for regulating coronary blood flow is termed metabolic hyperemia. Any increase in metabolic activity, for example, exercise, leads to a release of chemical substances into the local interstitial fluid. These substances cause a vasodilatation of the arterioles and therefore an increase in local blood flow to match the increase in metabolic activity. This metabolic hyperemia is carefully controlled and studies have shown that blood flow increases almost linearly with the local tissue metabolic rate or myocardial oxygen consumption.[18] Several substances may be involved in the process; some of these are briefly mentioned below.

Adenosine is a potent vasodilator and is produced by hypoxic myocytes. It is probably the most important effector molecule in coronary metabolic regulation.[20] During hypoxia and ischemia, adenosine monophosphate is formed by the degradation of the high-energy phosphate adenosine triphosphate (ATP). Adenosine is then generated by the action of the enzyme 5′ nucleotidase on adenosine monophosphate. Adenosine acts as a powerful vasodilator. Adenosine therefore seems to be linked to the vasodilatation and reduction in coronary vascular tone observed during ischemia.[21] Because of this strong vasodilatory effect, exogenous adenosine may be administered as a pharmacologic stress agent. It causes an increase in blood flow in normal vessels of at least four-fold.[22] Because areas subtended by a resting stenosis already have utilized these metabolic mechanisms to maintain a normal blood flow at rest, further dilatation is substantially less or even absent, and flow heterogeneity is generated.

Although adenosine is believed to be the most important mediator of metabolic flow regulation, other substances may have a part. The potent vasodilator nitric oxide (NO) increases blood flow during metabolic activity, and is released during hypoxia.[23] This is discussed in more detail later. The ATP-dependent potassium channel is also activated during ischemia and causes a local compensatory vasodilatation, as well as having other effects.

4.2 Endothelial-dependent Modulation of Coronary Blood Flow

The coronary endothelial lining is metabolically active and secretes a variety of vasoactive substances. The balance between dilator and constrictor molecules helps to determine overall coronary tone. Some of these substances are briefly discussed below.

The substance endothelium-derived relaxing factor is most important among the vasodilators, and has been identified as the NO radical.[24] NO is synthesized from the amino acid L-arginine by the enzyme NO synthase. NO is produced continuously by the epithelium and acts as a potent vasodilator locally. The main stimulus to local NO secretion is shear stress, that is, the force exerted on the endothelial wall by the sliding action of flowing blood. Under resting circumstances, this maintains a low basal NO level. In the nonresting state, this shear stress-induced NO release is also important. During exercise, distal arterioles dilate by a metabolic hyperemia mechanism (see above). This leads to blood flow changes in the feeding artery, and to activation of the shear stress-mediated NO pathway. In this way, the feeding vessel can dilate to increase blood delivery to the arteriolar system. This is an example of flow-mediated vasodilatation.

Prostacyclin (PGI2) is also a potent vasodilator agent, and has some role in flow-mediated vasodilatation and metabolic regulation.[25] It is produced from arachidonic acid by the enzyme cyclooxygenase. It has a relatively short duration of action and is not believed to be as important as NO.

The endothelium also produces vasoconstrictor molecules. One such group is the endothelin family of molecules. The most relevant of the three forms is endothelin 1. It is synthesized and released continuously, causing a persistent and relatively long-acting vasoconstriction.[26] Endothelin 1 therefore counteracts the effects of NO on basal resting tone.

Endothelial control of coronary vasodilator tone has received considerable attention because there is a large body of evidence to suggest that it is compromised in patients with atherosclerotic vascular disease, or indeed with significant risk factors for it. Indeed, many patients with atheroma tend to exhibit a relatively vasoconstrictor basal coronary tone.

4.3 Autoregulation of Coronary Blood Flow

It has been noted that despite significant variations in the driving (diastolic) aortic perfusion pressure, there is little or only very transient change in myocardial perfusion. This is termed autoregulation.[27] It is important as a compensation for minute-to-minute variations in diastolic blood pressure, and also in patients with epicardial coronary stenoses. In the latter, coronary perfusion is maintained partly because of adaptation (namely, vasodilatation) in the resistance vessels. This explains why patients with significant coronary stenoses do not usually experience angina at rest and do not have evidence of perfusion abnormalities during resting myocardial perfusion (e.g., nuclear) studies. During stress or increased metabolic demand, however, this is not the case. The relative increase in blood flow in stenotic arteries with exercise is greatly reduced compared with normal arteries, which have not yet exhausted this compensatory mechanism. The difference between coronary blood flow at rest and after maximal vasodilatation is termed coronary flow reserve.[28] The mechanisms that underlie coronary autoregulation are unclear but may again involve NO. It has recently been shown that autoregulatory changes in arteriolar blood volume can be measured by myocardial contrast echocardiography.[29]

4.4 Autonomic Nervous Control

Overall neural control of coronary tone is probably not as important as the factors discussed above. Vasoactive nerves are autonomic and have sympathetic or parasympathetic effects.[30] Activation of parasympathetic nerves results in vasodilatation. Sympathetic nerve activity may produce either a dilating (beta-2 receptor) or constricting (alpha receptor) effect. Although these are significant effectors, they have relatively little part in the pathophysiology of noninvasive imaging, except perhaps during exercise and dobutamine stress, and are not discussed in detail.

4.5 Circulating Hormones

General control mechanisms, which have widespread effects throughout the body, can still exert a significant influence on coronary blood flow. Various circulating hormones exert a generalized effect on arteriolar tone, and therefore coronary tone in addition. Catecholamine secretion has been well studied. Noradrenaline has a vasoconstrictive effect largely mediated via alpha receptors. Adrenaline has high affinity for beta-2 receptors and often therefore causes predominantly a vasodilatation. Of course, catecholamines have other effects on heart rate and inotropy that are relevant in the development of ischemia. Other circulating hormones, including vasopressin and angiotensin II, are vasoconstrictors.

4.6 Extravascular Compressive Forces

Coronary blood flow is predominant during diastole. This is because, during left ventricular contraction (i.e., systole), intramyocardial vessels are compressed and deformed, and consequently blood flow is compromised and often halted completely. In addition, the intraventricular systolic pressure exerts an adverse effect on subendocardial blood flow.

5. Events During Ischemia

The pathophysiologic events underlying ischemia have been described in terms of a "cascade."[31] This is a useful concept because it allows the various imaging and stress modalities to be correlated with the pathophysiologic mechanisms. A brief summary is given in Table 1.2.

5.1 Metabolic and Blood Flow Changes, and Imaging Findings

As alluded to above, as myocardial oxygen demand increases or coronary blood flow decreases, autoregulatory and metabolic regulatory mechanisms become active to try to maintain myocardial perfusion at a normal level.

Table 1.2. Pathophysiologic events in ischemia and their correlates in imaging and noninvasive testing

Event	Frequently used stress correlates	Imaging method
Reduced local perfusion/perfusion mismatches	Dynamic exercise	Usually SPECT
	Vasodilator stress, e.g., adenosine will unmask areas of flow heterogeneity	SPECT or PET
		Contrast echo
		MRI with contrast
Regional contractile abnormality	Dobutamine-induced wall motion abnormality	2D echocardiography
		Novel echo methods, e.g., TDI
		Cardiovascular MRI
	Dynamic exercise	2D echocardiography
Electrocardiographic changes	Exercise	Exercise stress testing
	Changes noted with other modalities but not primary abnormality being sought	
Chest pain/angina	Exercise	Exercise stress testing
	Dobutamine pharmacologic stress	Stress echo or MRI

The various pathophysiologic changes occurring during ischemia are listed in the left-hand column. Frequently used stress techniques that rely on this mechanism or are related to it are given in the middle column. The right-hand column indicates the imaging method used for each type of stress.

Metabolic and blood flow changes are therefore intimately linked.

During myocardial ischemia, multiple complex events occur at a local cellular level. High-energy ATP is gradually utilized resulting in an increase in its metabolites, and hence in adenosine. This subsequently acts as a vasodilator in an attempt to compensate for the reduced perfusion. The reduction in high-energy phosphates also impairs several energy-requiring metabolic processes in myocardial cells. Intracellular calcium overload occurs because of an impairment of active metabolic processes that regulate sodium and calcium gradients.[32] This may lead to cell injury and death. ATP-dependent potassium channels are also active during ischemia and result in potassium efflux and a shortening in local action potential duration. This could potentially predispose to arrhythmias. Various catabolites such as lactate and hydrogen ions accumulate, and these can also cause coronary vasodilatation.[33]

These compensatory changes (including autoregulation and metabolic regulation) become exhausted and ischemia finally results as myocardial blood flow decreases.[31] In patients with atherosclerotic heart disease, compensatory mechanisms to maintain myocardial perfusion in the face of significant epicardial stenoses are already active. Vasodilatation of the distal vascular bed occurs and pressure gradient across the stenosis increases. The exhaustion of compensatory mechanisms in patients with coronary disease is also compounded by abnormal endothelial function and impaired endothelium-derived vasodilator mechanisms. The first abnormality to be apparent during ischemia is therefore reduced perfusion to the affected territory. It is not until a diameter stenosis of approximately 80% that resting perfusion is finally reduced, and certainly any stenosis less than 50% diameter is unlikely to have any hemodynamic consequences even during maximum coronary dilatation (see Figure 1.1).[34]

Patients with reduced perfusion at rest caused by severe stenotic plaques may present acutely

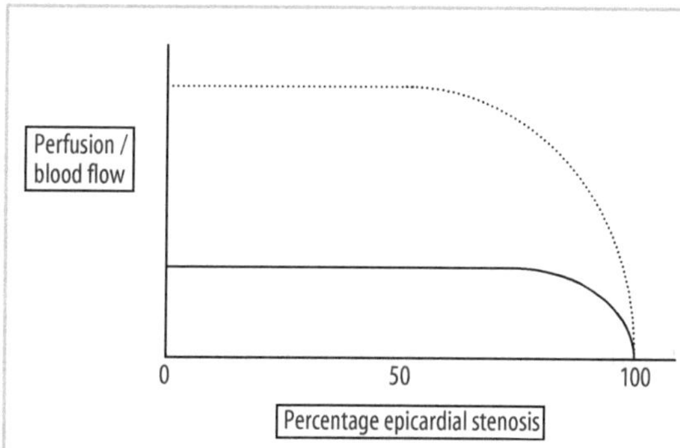

Figure 1.1. The effects of epicardial coronary artery stenosis (*x* axis) on myocardial blood flow (*y* axis). Blood flow at rest (solid line) is little altered until there is an obstruction of at least 80%. This is due to compensatory mechanisms which result in dilatation of the coronary resistance vessels, ensuring blood delivery is maintained even in the face of significant stenosis. Blood flow increases dramatically during exercise or pharmacological vasodilatation (dashed line). It is noted that the maximal blood flow gradually falls once there is an epicardial stenosis of around 50%. In patients with coronary disease these vasodilator compensatory mechanisms are already active at rest and the large increase in blood flow with exercise or pharmacological stress cannot occur. A large difference in blood flow at peak stress can therefore be noted between areas subtended by normal and stenotic arteries. For detailed discussion see text (Based on Gould 33).

with an acute coronary syndrome. In such patients, resting perfusion abnormalities can be demonstrated by nuclear cardiology techniques. A radiotracer is injected during symptoms and subsequently a myocardial perfusion scan is obtained using a gamma camera. A single photon emission computed tomographic (SPECT) study is usually performed instead of planar imaging. This method can accurately demonstrate active ischemia in patients presenting acutely, and has been studied in the emergency department setting.[35]

In patients with stenotic plaques but no reduction in flow at rest attributed to the above compensatory mechanisms, perfusion abnormalities can be induced by stressing the perfusion system. Any further increase in myocardial oxygen demand will result in ischemia, because compensatory mechanisms are already maximally activated. These phenomena are displayed in Figure 1.1. Exercise stress, combined with tomographic myocardial perfusion scan, is the most common way of demonstrating this in clinical practice. The radionuclide involved (either 99m-technetium-labeled tracers or 201-thallium) is extracted into the myocardium in a flow-dependent way. During exercise, myocardial blood flow increases in areas supplied by relatively normal coronary vessels, but there is no increase in the areas supplied by stenotic arteries. Tracer uptake in ischemic areas is therefore reduced compared with areas of normal perfusion. These differences in regional tracer uptake on the perfusion scan images reflect this in a semiquantitative way.[36]

Perfusion abnormalities secondary to stenotic coronary plaques can also be demonstrated using pharmacologic stress agents. As discussed earlier, vasodilators such as adenosine are important in determining myocardial blood flow during ischemia and at rest. Adenosine can be infused intravenously and will cause a significant increase (at least four-fold) in coronary blood flow in normal arteries. Because endogenous vasodilators are already active to compensate for coronary stenoses, in affected territories, there will not be such a significant increase in flow, creating flow heterogeneity between areas with normal and impaired blood delivery. Dipyridamole acts via the adenosine pathway and has similar effects. The flow heterogeneity that results from these agents may cause ischemia, possibly via coronary steal mechanisms, but this is not universal. It is important, therefore, to appreciate that these techniques demonstrate flow heterogeneity rather than ischemia, although the latter may accompany the blood flow changes, usually if collateral circulation is present. Injection of a suitable tracer during pharmacologic stress will therefore allow the identification of territories subtended by stenotic arteries, in a similar way to exercise stress. As with exercise, both 99m-technetium and 201-thallium radiotracers are in common usage for this indication.[36] Technetium agents have the advantage that they are fixed in the myocardium after injection, giving a "snapshot" of perfusion at the time of injection. This is convenient for subsequent imaging. (These techniques are discussed in great detail in Chapters 4 and 8.)

Less commonly, positron-emitting tracers can be injected and imaged using PET systems. Agents such as $H_2{}^{15}O$, ${}^{13}NH_3$, or Rubidium 82 are used for this purpose.[37] These are mainly used for research purposes because they require generation in a cyclotron and have very short half-lives.

More recently, other imaging methods have been combined with pharmacologic stress to assess coronary perfusion. Transpulmonary bubble contrast agents have been developed for use with echocardiography. These microbubbles are injected intravenously and are small enough to pass through the pulmonary circulation without significant degradation and eventually appear on the left side of the heart. They can be visualized as they appear in the myocardial capillaries. Several protocols can be used. The most common is to measure how long it takes for contrast agent to appear in the myocardium at rest and during pharmacologic stress with, for example, adenosine. This is a function of myocardial perfusion. One method is to intermittently destroy the bubbles by disrupting them with a high-power (large mechanical index) ultrasound pulse.[38] The time taken for fresh contrast to wash in to the myocardium can be measured and perfusion assessed. This technique, for example with dipyridamole stress, has identified coronary artery disease with good sensitivity and specificity in patients with heart failure.[39]

Cardiovascular MRI can also be used to assess myocardial perfusion using the same underlying principles. Most techniques are based on first-pass perfusion analogous to the echocardiographic method outlined above. Vasodilator stress is usually performed with adenosine, and the contrast agent gadolinium given intravenously.[40] In most sequences, an inversion recovery pulse is used to null the myocardium and the wash-in of gadolinium is then observed. The first-pass perfusion images obtained can be observed qualitatively, or semiquantitatively by examining the wash-in curves and peak signal intensity.[41] (See also Chapters 2 and 3, respectively.)

5.2 Contractile Dysfunction and Imaging Findings

The second main event to occur during ischemia is contractile dysfunction.[42] Again, there is a temporal progression in the abnormality. Initially the changes occur in a regional manner in the territory involved, but, as the insult worsens, there is global impairment of left ventricular function. Both diastolic and systolic abnormalities occur during ischemia. Calcium is required for myocardial contraction, and, as indicated above, intracellular calcium handling may be impaired during ischemia; this may partially explain the contractile abnormalities observed.

Ischemia results in a regional reduction in systolic contraction. Contractile function requires adequate oxygen delivery, and clearly this is impaired as perfusion is compromised. Hypokinesia, akinesia, and eventually dyskinesia can be observed in the myocardial segments in the ischemic territories.[43] Subendocardial myocardial fibers are more sensitive to ischemia than epicardial fibers, because they lie further from the epicardial coronary vessels. The subendocardial fibers generally lie in a longitudinal (or long axis) orientation, and therefore contractile dysfunction may first be observed in this axis. Subsequently, as the ischemia spreads to involve the transmural extent of the myocardium, contractile dysfunction spreads to involve the transverse or short axis fibers. As the extent of the ischemic territory increases, global ventricular dysfunction results. Stroke volume, cardiac out-put, and left ventricular ejection fraction all decrease.[44] Left ventricular failure or cardiogenic shock result in severe cases. Global systolic dysfunction is therefore a late sign of myocardial ischemia and reflects involvement of a large proportion of the myocardium.

Diastolic dysfunction also occurs during ischemia, but clinically is rarely targeted for specific assessment. Ischemia shifts the ventricular end-diastolic pressure-volume relationship to the left; in other words, for any specific ventricular volume, the end-diastolic pressure is higher. Ventricular relaxation is also impaired. These abnormalities together predispose to pulmonary edema.

Although considered separately, the diastolic and systolic abnormalities rarely occur as isolated events in clinical practice. The clinical picture is therefore usually a combination of increased ventricular pressure with contractile dysfunction, presenting as pulmonary congestion or edema if the extent of ischemia is sufficient.

The contractile abnormalities described frequently do not return to normal immediately after ischemia is abolished, and may remain for several hours. This period of prolonged, but reversible, contractile dysfunction after a period of significant ischemia has been termed myocardial stunning.[45] It can be observed after prolonged ischemia as a result of stable or unstable angina, after myocardial infarction, and after percutaneous coronary intervention.[46]

These contractile images can be imaged clinically using cardiac ultrasound.

Echocardiography may be utilized in patients with acute coronary syndromes. Regional wall abnormalities demonstrated during chest pain may help in the diagnosis of ischemia, ventricular function can be assessed, and complications such as ischemic mitral regurgitation can be detected. Echocardiography also allows visualization of the development of regional wall motion abnormalities with stress and detects ischemia in this way; this is the basis of stress echocardiography. The development of hypokinesia in a normally contracting segment, or worsening of function in an already hypokinetic segment, implies stress-induced ischemia. Compensatory hyperkinesis in nonischemic segments or ventricular dilation may also be observed during the stress test; the latter suggests multivessel coronary artery disease. Echocardiography can be performed with exercise,[47] but usually is performed after dobutamine infusion.[48] Dobutamine increases myocardial oxygen demand by increasing heart rate and blood pressure and hence RPP. Atropine may be added to increase the tachycardia further if no contractile changes are noted or the increase in heart rate is insufficient at a dobutamine dose of 40 μg/kg/min. In general, each myocardial segment is assessed using the standard echo views. Some authors have suggested that this is a rather late sign of ischemia, and that long axis function should be investigated. M mode examination of the amplitude of long axis contraction, and its rate of change, can be measured and in some series correlates relatively well with ischemia detected using more traditional techniques.[49] An alternative is to use vasodilator stress, typically with dipyridamole, and attempt to demonstrate ischemia-related regional wall changes secondary to changes in coronary blood flow.[50] As alluded to above, perfusion may now be assessed by echocardiography and may replace or complement this traditional strategy. Currently, the newer technologies such as tissue Doppler imaging (TDI) are being applied to the detection of ischemia.[51] TDI measures changes in regional velocities in different myocardial segments and may therefore be more sensitive than observing hypokinesia by traditional methods. One potential hazard in interpretation of wall motion abnormalities is the traction of akinetic segments by normally contracting neighboring ones. This may be overcome with TDI by measuring the differences in regional velocities, and assessing the changes in velocities between two points (strain and strain rate imaging).[52] Recently, TDI studies have suggested that post-systolic motion may be an accurate indicator of ischemia.[53]

Nuclear techniques can also be used to measure regional and global changes in left ventricular function related to ischemia. Radionuclide ventriculography is a technique for assessing the left ventricular blood pool. An injection of technetium-radiolabeled red cells is given and the counts from the left ventricular blood pool are obtained using gamma camera imaging. The use of ECG gating allows determination of ventricular volume throughout the cardiac cycle. Both systolic and diastolic characteristics can therefore be measured and quantified. Radionuclide ventriculography imaging can be performed at rest or in combination with dynamic exercise.[54] Changes in regional and global function with stress can therefore be demonstrated.

Alternatively, assessment of regional wall changes can be performed using gated SPECT-PET imaging. As discussed above, these studies are a powerful tools for assessment of myocardial perfusion. If, however, the images are obtained with ECG gating, additional information about regional contractile function can be obtained. Hence, ischemia-induced functional abnormalities can be obtained from the same study as perfusion, with relatively little extra time or cost.[55] In addition, global systolic and diastolic volumes and ejection fraction at rest and with stress, can be added to the perfusion data.[56] Stress-induced chamber dilatation and impairment of systolic function with stress can also be noted, particularly with exercise stress.[57] Increased lung uptake of tracer with stress can sometimes be observed, mainly with 201-thallium.[58] This may well reflect the increased ventricular pressures, in particular end-diastolic pressure or pulmonary wedge pressure (effectively left atrial pressure) alluded to above. Regional wall abnormalities can also be sought using dobutamine gated SPECT, rather than after exercise.

Magnetic resonance techniques again image regional wall abnormalities induced by stress.[59,60] It is similar to traditional two-dimensional (2D) echocardiography in this respect. However, the spatial resolution is excellent, and there are no limitations of image plane, and poor nondiagnostic images because of patient physical factors are rare. The contrast between endocardium and blood pool in general is also excellent. Dobutamine stress is mainly used because of the limitations of physical exercise in the magnet, although the latter has been used in some centers. A brief summary of frequently performed tests is given in Table 1.2.

5.3 Electrocardiographic Changes and Imaging Findings

Electrocardiographic abnormalities occur late in the ischemic cascade, and in general are related to electrical changes in the ischemic myocardium. The mechanisms by which these phenomena occur are currently incompletely understood. During ischemia, the action potential duration in the ischemic territory is reduced. Ion channels, such as the ATP-sensitive potassium channel, are activated. As a result, various electrical gradients are created, and ST segment change is observed. This results in ST segment depression, which is the ECG hallmark of acute myocardial ischemia. Other ECG manifestations of acute ischemia include T wave changes (which are not specific) and alterations in R wave amplitude.

During acute coronary occlusion, the ST segment usually becomes increased. There are at least two postulated mechanisms for this.[61] The diastolic injury current theory supposes that the regional injury is associated with a flow of current from the uninjured to the affected area. This causes depression of the TQ segment, which after correction for the resulting baseline change on the ECG, appears as ST segment elevation. The systolic injury current theory supposes that the injured area undergoes early repolarization. Current therefore flows from the injured to the uninjured area during the period of the ST segment, causing its increase. Because of the electrical characteristics of the ECG record, ischemic ST segment depression and elevation may be seen at the same time in different leads, or in a reciprocal manner.

Ischemia may also cause arrhythmias. Ventricular arrhythmias may be precipitated by the electrochemical changes that occur during ischemia. Activation of ATP-sensitive potassium channels during ischemia shortens action potential duration and therefore may promote re-entrant arrhythmias such as ventricular tachycardia.

From the above discussion, it is apparent that ST segment changes will be the diagnostic hallmark of ischemia to be observed during noninvasive testing. The classical test used is the exercise stress test.[62] During dynamic physical exercise on a treadmill or bicycle ergometer, heart rate and blood pressure increase as cardiac work increases. Ischemia is precipitated as discussed earlier in this chapter. The 12-lead ECG is continuously monitored for ST segment depression. In addition to ST segment depression, other changes may occur during exercise that are indicative of myocardial ischemia and may aid interpretation of the test. A decrease in systolic blood pressure, or a failure to increase as expected, may indicate widespread myocardial ischemia. Chest pain may also occur, thus reproducing the clinical manifestation of angina.

Whereas induction of angina and ST segment depression are the main diagnostic elements of the exercise stress test, these are relatively late events in the ischemic cascade. This has two implications. First, the stress test may fail to diagnose ischemia because of the relative insensitivity of these abnormalities compared with earlier changes such as abnormalities in regional function or perfusion. This may explain disparate results between tests. Second, other noninvasive tests may be positive without necessarily reproducing chest pain or ST depression, but when they do occur, they often suggest significant disease.

6. Consequences of Ischemia

The discussion above has mainly centered on the findings during acute ischemia or on patients with chronic angina. Other ischemic syndromes have been recognized in recent years and are briefly reviewed in this section.

6.1 Myocardial Hibernation and Stunning

The phenomenon of myocardial stunning is described as transient ventricular systolic dysfunction persisting for some time after ischemia. It is discussed above (section 5.2). Myocardial hibernation is a chronic ischemic syndrome. It is identified as resting left ventricular contractile dysfunction, associated with significant coronary artery disease, which can be reversed by revascularization; the definition is therefore retrospective. The time of functional recovery after revascularization is very variable with improvement noted even some months after intervention.[63] The pathophysiology of chronic myocardial hibernation is not completely known. Some studies have noted reduced resting coronary blood flow to hibernating segments[64]; this suggests that myocardial contractile function is "downgraded" to match the reduced perfusion supply. Other studies have found that the reduction in blood flow is minimal, although there may be exhausted coronary flow reserve.[65] In this situation, it is postulated that recurrent episodes of ischemia result in hibernation by causing repetitive myocardial stunning. Certain characteristics of potentially hibernating myocardium have been targeted by imaging methods and will be considered in more detail in Chapter 13. In general, it is mandatory to demonstrate regional contractile dysfunction and evidence that the area concerned is alive or "viable" and ischemic. This is frequently assessed by nuclear cardiology techniques,[66] although other methods are available. Resting 201-thallium, 99m-technetium (using SPECT imaging), or 18-fluordeoxyglucose uptake (using PET imaging) usually identifies viable myocardium. Reduced blood flow may be demonstrated by PET using flow tracers, and a mismatch between reduced resting flow, but intact or even increased metabolic activity detected by 18-fluordeoxyglucose is said to be a sensitive finding. Improvement in contractile function with low-dose dobutamine ("contractile reserve") followed by worsening of function at a higher dose (biphasic response) also predicts improvement after revascularization. Dobutamine can be combined with either echocardiography or MRI. Each method has its own characteristics[67,68] and will be reviewed in Chapter 13.

6.2 Ischemic Preconditioning

As discussed above, a prolonged and severe episode of myocardial ischemia leads to mechanical dysfunction, which can continue for some time after blood flow is restored, i.e., myocardial stunning. However, after a single, relatively short episode of ischemia with reperfusion, or after infrequent attacks of ischemia, a different phenomenon may be observed. Initially there is contractile dysfunction as expected. However, after recovery, the myocardium seems to adapt to the metabolic consequences of ischemia, and a further episode will not cause such significant dysfunction, and may be associated with enhanced protection against infarction. This phenomenon is termed ischemic preconditioning.[69] There appear to be two temporal "windows" during which ischemic preconditioning is observed. The first occurs in the immediate period after the first ischemic episode. The mechanism for this is not entirely clear but seems to involve activation of the ATP-sensitive potassium channel. During ischemia, ATP levels decrease, as discussed previously. This activates the channel leading to loss of potassium from the cell, and reduced calcium influx. This in turn leads to reduced contractile activity and therefore preservation of energy stores.[70] There is a second delayed window when the protection of ischemic preconditioning may be observed. The mechanism for this is less certain but may again involve the ATP-sensitive potassium channel.[70]

There is some evidence in patients that these phenomena may be important. It has been noted that those patients experiencing preinfarction angina have greater recovery in left ventricular systolic function after myocardial infarction than those without prior symptoms.[71] Such findings also have importance as pointers to potential strategies to protect the heart during ischemia and in reduction of infarct size.

6.3 Ischemia-reperfusion Injury and No-reflow Phenomenon

Restoration of blood flow to myocardium subtended by an occluded coronary vessel is the aim of treatment for acute myocardial infarction. Although this clearly is highly desirable, certain problems may be associated with the process. Sudden restoration of blood flow may cause reperfusion injury. This is a syndrome characterized by myocardial stunning, arrhythmias, and microvascular injury. The mechanical systolic dysfunction resulting from myocardial stunning is discussed elsewhere in this chapter. Ventricular tachycardia or fibrillation may occur in close temporal relationship to reperfusion in patients with acute myocardial infarction; the former may be self-terminating.

Microvascular injury and no-reflow may be related to several phenomena. The no-reflow phenomenon describes circumstances when, after the coronary occlusion is removed and the vessel is patent, antegrade blood flow is not restored. Microvascular injury has been implicated. Activated lymphocytes may be attracted to areas of myocardial injury and cause plugging of the microvasculature[72]; this causes no-reflow. A number of studies with MRI or contrast echocardiography have shown that microvascular obstruction is a predictor of adverse prognosis. The reasons are not well understood but may relate to greater postinfarction remodeling. Furthermore, severely ischemic myocytes are exposed suddenly to oxygen, calcium, and other molecules on restoration of blood flow; the consequent generation of oxygen free radicals has been implicated in reperfusion injury and stunning also.[73]

In the infarct zone, there is clearly cell necrosis; however, further myocytes also die by the process of apoptosis, or programmed cell death. This has been detected in the ischemic zone and in fact has been demonstrated in human myocardial infarction using the tracer annexin V (see section 1.2). Annexin V is labeled with 99m-technetium and binds to membrane-bound phosphatidyl serine, which is expressed on apoptotic cells.

7. Clinical Phenomena and Their Relation to Imaging

Angina is chest pain caused by myocardial ischemia. In many patients, it may present as discomfort rather than pain. Various sites apart from the classical central chest location have been described. Precipitation by exertion and emotion and relief by rest and nitrates are characteristic of stable exertional angina.[74]

Reproduction of anginal symptoms during any noninvasive test is always helpful in confirming a positive result. Induction of ischemia is the object of many noninvasive tests such as exercise testing and dobutamine stress methods. Chest pain is therefore relatively common during these procedures. Vasodilator stress with adenosine is primarily designed to demonstrate flow heterogeneity and therefore ischemia does not always result. Angina may occur as a result of coronary steal phenomena and chest pain may result from adenosine receptor stimulation attributed to the agent itself. Chest pain is reported in approximately a third of patients receiving adenosine or dobutamine.[75,76]

Other clinical manifestations of ischemia may include dyspnea, caused by ischemic left ventricular dysfunction or increased ventricular pressures. This may be suspected in patients with normal left ventricular function at rest who develop dyspnea on exertion ("angina equivalent"). Other clinical effects that may be observed are induction of arrhythmias secondary to ischemia, and hypotension caused by marked systolic impairment. The mechanism for these is discussed above.

8. Conclusions

The pathophysiology of myocardial ischemia involves a series of progressive changes from the cellular level through perfusion abnormalities, contractile dysfunction, electrocardiographic abnormalities, and finally symptoms. In clinical practice, it has multiple potential manifestations, with atherosclerotic coronary disease being the most important underlying etiology. Uncovering these abnormalities or their underlying causes requires selection of the most appropriate stress method depending on the question being asked, and the clinical status of the patient. A sound understanding of the principles of imaging will contribute to informed interpretation of test results. Only by integrating knowledge of the pathophysiology of myocardial ischemia, the role of the various stress modalities, and the strengths and weaknesses of the available imaging technologies will the best possible test be selected for each patient.

References

The following references are chosen mainly as useful reviews of the subjects discussed in this chapter, and should prove a useful starting point for those wishing to study the topic in more detail.

1. Rong JX, Rangaswamy S, Shen L, et al. Arterial injury by cholesterol oxidation products causes endothelial dysfunction and arterial wall cholesterol accumulation. Arterioscler Thromb Vasc Biol 1998; 18:1885–1894.
2. Faggiotto A, Ross R, Harker L. Studies of hypercholesterolemia in the non human primate. I. Changes that lead to fatty streak formation. Arteriosclerosis 1984;4: 323–340.
3. Glagov S, Weisenberg E, Zarins C, et al. Compensatory enlargement of human atherosclerotic coronary arteries. N Engl J Med 1987;316:371–375.
4. Falk E, Shah P, Fuster V. Coronary plaque disruption. Circulation 1995;92:657–671.
5. Farb A, Burke A, Tang A, et al. Coronary plaque erosion without rupture into a lipid core: a frequent cause of coronary thrombosis in sudden coronary death. Circulation 1996;93:1354–1363.
6. Libby P. Molecular bases of the acute coronary syndromes. Circulation 1995;91:2844–2850.
7. Pijls NH, De Bruyne B, Peels K, et al. Measurement of fractional flow reserve to assess the functional severity of coronary artery stenoses. N Engl J Med 1996;334: 1703–1708.
8. Sirol M, Itskovich VV, Mani V, et al. Lipid-rich atherosclerotic plaques detected by gadofluorine-enhanced in vivo magnetic resonance imaging. Circulation 2004; 109:2890–2896.
9. Morgan-Hughes GJ, Roobotham CA, Owen PE, et al. Highly accurate non-invasive coronary angiography using sub-millimetre multislice computed tomography. Heart 2004;90(suppl II):A56.
10. Rudd JHF, Warburton EA, Fryer TD, et al. Imaging atherosclerotic plaque inflammation with [^{18}F]-fluorodeoxyglucose positron emission tomography. Circulation 2002;105:2708–2711.
11. Zaret BL. Second Annual Mario S. Verani, MD, Memorial Lecture: nuclear cardiology, the next 10 years. J Nucl Cardiol 2004;11:393–407.
12. Hofstra L, Liem IH, Dumont E, et al. Visualization of cell death in vivo in patients with acute myocardial infarction. Lancet 2000;356:209–212.
13. Camici PG, Marraccini P, Lorenzoni R, et al. Coronary haemodynamics and myocardial metabolism in patients with syndrome X: response to pacing stress. J Am Coll Cardiol 1991;17:1461.
14. Mohri M, Koyanagi M, Egashira K, et al. Angina pectoris caused by coronary microvascular spasm. Lancet 1998;351:1165.
15. Panting JR, Gatehouse PD, Yang G-Z, et al. Abnormal subendocardial perfusion in cardiac syndrome X detected by cardiovascular magnetic resonance imaging. N Engl J Med 2002;346:1948–1953.
16. Prinzmetal M, Kennamer R, Merliss R, et al. Angina pectoris. I. A variant form of angina pectoris: preliminary report. Am J Med 1959;27:375.
17. Berman ND, McLaughlin PR, Huckell VF, et al. Prinzmetal's angina with coronary artery spasm. Angiographic, pharmacologic, metabolic and radionuclide perfusion studies. Am J Med 1976;60:727.
18. Braunwald E. Control of myocardial oxygen consumption. Am J Cardiol 1971;27:416–432.

19. Rooke GA, Feigl EO. Work as a correlate of canine left ventricular oxygen consumption, and the problem of catecholamine wasting. Circ Res 1982;50:273–286.
20. Berne RM. The role of adenosine in the regulation of coronary blood flow. Circ Res 1980;47:807–813.
21. Belardinelli L, Linden J, Berne RM. The cardiac effects of adenosine. Prog Cardiovasc Dis 1989;32:73–97.
22. Wilson RF, Wyche K, Christensen BV, et al. Effects of adenosine on human arterial circulation. Circulation 1990;82:1595–1606.
23. Brown IP, Thompson CI, Belloni FL, et al. Role of nitric oxide in hypoxic coronary vasodilatation in isolated perfused guinea pig heart. Am J Physiol 1993;264: H821–H829.
24. Jones CJ, Kuo L, Davis MJ, et al. Role of nitric oxide in the coronary microvascular responses to adenosine and increased metabolic demand. Circulation 1995;91: 1807–1813.
25. Duffy SJ, Castle SF, Harper RW, et al. Contribution of vasodilator prostanoids and nitric oxide to resting flow, metabolic vasodilation, and flow-mediated dilation in human coronary circulation. Circulation 1999;100: 1951–1957.
26. Haynes WG, Webb DJ. Endothelin as a regulator of cardiovascular function in health and disease. J Hypertens 1998;16:1081–1098.
27. Johnson PC. Autoregulation of blood flow. Circ Res 1986:59:483–495.
28. Uren NG, Melin JA, De Bruyne B, et al. Relation between myocardial blood flow and the severity of coronary artery stenosis. N Engl J Med 1994;330:1782–1788.
29. Wei W, Tong KL, Belcik T, et al. Detection of coronary stenoses at rest with myocardial contrast echocardiography. Circulation 2005;112:1154–1160.
30. Feigl EO. Neural control of coronary blood flow. J Vasc Res 1998;35:85–92.
31. Leong-Poi H, Rim S, Le E, et al. Perfusion versus function: the ischaemic cascade in demand ischaemia. Circulation 2002;105:987–992.
32. Marban E, Koretsune Y, Corretti M, et al. Calcium and its role in myocardial cell injury during ischaemia and reperfusion. Circulation 1989;80(Suppl 4):80.
33. Ishizaka H, Kuo L. Acidosis-induced coronary arteriolar dilation is mediated by ATP-sensitive potassium channels in vascular smooth muscle. Circ Res 1996; 78:50–57.
34. Gould KL, Lipscomb K. Effects of coronary stenoses on coronary flow reserve and resistance. Am J Cardiol 1974;34:48–55.
35. Hilton TC, Thompson RC, Williams H, et al. Technetium 99m sestamibi myocardial perfusion imaging in the emergency room evaluation of chest pain. J Am Coll Cardiol 1994;23:1016–1022.
36. Coyne EP, Belvedere DA, Vande Streek PR, et al. Thallium-201 scintigraphy after intravenous infusion of adenosine compared with exercise thallium testing in the diagnosis of coronary artery disease. J Am Coll Cardiol 1991;17:1289.
37. Bol A, Melin A, Vanoverschelde L, et al. Direct comparison of ^{13}N ammonia and ^{15}O water estimates of perfusion with quantification of regional myocardial flow by microspheres. Circulation 1993;87:512–525.
38. Monaghan MJ. Stress myocardial contrast echocardiography. Heart 2003;89:1391–1393.
39. Senior R, Janardhanan R, Jeetly P, et al. Myocardial contrast echocardiography for distinguishing ischemic from nonischemic first-onset acute heart failure. Insights into the mechanism of acute heart failure. Circulation 2005;112:1587–1593.
40. Giang TH, Nanz D, Coulden R, et al. Detection of coronary artery disease by magnetic resonance myocardial perfusion imaging with various contrast medium doses: first European multicentre experience. Eur Heart J 2004;25:1657–1665.
41. Manning WJ, Atkinson DJ, Grossman W, et al. First pass nuclear magnetic resonance imaging studies using gadolinium-DPTA in patients with coronary artery disease. J Am Coll Cardiol 1991;18:959–965.
42. Theroux P, Franklin D, Ross J Jr, et al. Regional myocardial function during acute coronary artery occlusion and its modification by pharmacological agents in the dog. Circ Res 1974;35:896–908.
43. Herman MV, Heinle RA, Klein MD, et al. Localised disorders in myocardial contraction. N Engl J Med 1967;227:222.
44. Forrester JS, Wyatt HL, Daluz PL, et al. Functional significance of regional ischaemic contraction abnormalities. Circulation 1976;54:64–70.
45. Braunwald E, Kloner RA. The stunned myocardium: prolonged postischemic ventricular dysfunction. Circulation 1982;66:1146–1149.
46. Bolli R, Marban E. Molecular and cellular mechanisms of myocardial stunning. Physiol Rev 1999;79:609–634.
47. Roger VL, Pellikka PA, Oh JK, et al. Identification of multivessel coronary artery disease by exercise echocardiography. J Am Coll Cardiol 1994;24:109.
48. Beleslin BD, Ostojic M, Stepanovic J, et al. Stress echocardiography in the detection of myocardial ischaemia. Circulation 1994;90:1168–1176.
49. Henein MY, Anagnostopoulos C, Das SK, et al. Left ventricular long axis disturbances as predictors for thallium perfusion defects in patients with known peripheral vascular disease. Heart 1998;79:295–300.
50. Severi S, Picano E, Michelassi C, et al. Diagnostic and prognostic value of dipyridamole echocardiography in patients with suspected coronary artery disease. Circulation 1994;89:1160–1173.
51. Cain P, Baglin T, Case C, et al. Application of tissue Doppler to interpretation of dobutamine echocardiography: comparison with quantitative angiography. Am J Cardiol 2001;87:525–531.
52. Marwick TH. Clinical applications of tissue Doppler imaging: a promise fulfilled. Heart 2003;89:1377–1378.
53. Celutkiene J, Sutherland GR, Laucevicius A, et al. Is post-systolic motion the optimal ultrasound parameter to detect induced ischaemia during dobutamine stress echocardiography? Eur Heart J 2004;25:932–942.
54. Gibbons RJ, Fyke FE, Clements IP, et al. Noninvasive identification of severe coronary artery disease using exercise radionuclide angiography. J Am Coll Cardiol 1988;11:28.
55. Chua T, Kiat H, Germano G, et al. Gated technetium-99m sestamibi for simultaneous assessment of stress myocardial perfusion, postexercise regional ventricular function and myocardial viability. Correlation with echocardiography and thallium-201 scintigraphy. J Am Coll Cardiol 1994;23:1107–1114.
56. Germano G, Kiat H, Kavanaugh PB, et al. Automatic quantification of ejection fraction from gated myocardial perfusion SPECT. J Nucl Med 1995;36:2138–2147.

57. Weiss AT, Berman DS, Law AS, et al. Transient ischemic dilation of the left ventricle on stress thallium-201 scintigraphy: a marker of severe and extensive coronary artery disease. J Am Coll Cardiol 1987;9:752–759.
58. Levy R, Rosanski A, Berman DS, et al. Analysis of the degree of pulmonary thallium washout after exercise in patients with coronary artery disease. J Am Coll Cardiol 1983;2:719–728.
59. Pennell DJ, Underwood SR, Manzara CC, et al. Magnetic resonance imaging during dobutamine stress in coronary artery disease. Am J Cardiol 1992;70:34.
60. Wahl A, Paetsch I, Gollesch A, et al. Safety and feasibility of high-dose dobutamine-atropine stress cardiovascular magnetic resonance for diagnosis of myocardial ischaemia in 1000 consecutive cases. Eur Heart J 2004; 25:1230–1236.
61. Vincent GM, Abildskov JA, Burgess MJ, et al. Mechanisms of ischaemic ST-segment displacement. Evaluation by direct current recordings. Circulation 1977;56: 559–566.
62. Gibbons RJ, Balady GJ, Brocker JT, et al. ACC/AHA 2002 guideline update for exercise testing: a report of the American College of Cardiology/American Heart Association Task Force on Practice Guidelines (Committee on Exercise Testing). Available at www.acc.org/clinical/guidelines/exercise/dirIndex.htm. 2002.
63. Camici PG, Wijns W, Borgers M, et al. Pathophysiological mechanisms of chronic reversible left ventricular dysfunction due to coronary artery disease (hibernating myocardium). Circulation 1997;96:3205–3214.
64. Tawakol A, Skopici HA, Abrahmam SA, et al. Evidence of reduced resting blood flow in viable myocardial regions with resting asynchrony. J Am Coll Cardiol 2000;36:2146–2153.
65. Vanoverschelde JLJ, Wijns W, Depre C, et al. Mechanisms of chronic regional postischaemic dysfunction in humans. New insights from the study of noninfarcted collateral-dependent myocardium. Circulation 1993; 87:1513–1523.
66. Bax JJ, van der Wall EE, Harbinson MT. Radionuclide techniques for the assessment of myocardial viability and hibernation. Heart 2004;90(suppl V):v26–v33.
67. Bax JJ, Poldermans D, Elhendy A, et al. Sensitivity, specificity and predictive accuracies of various noninvasive techniques for detecting hibernating myocardium. Curr Probl Cardiol 2001;26:141–186.
68. Underwood SR, Bax JJ, vom Dahl J, et al. Imaging techniques for the assessment of patients with chronic ischaemic heart failure. Eur Heart J 2004;25:815–836.
69. Murry CE, Jennings RB, Reimer KA. Preconditioning with ischaemia: a delay of lethal cell injury in ischemic myocardium. Circulation 1986;74:1124–1136.
70. Sato T. Signaling in late ischaemic preconditioning: involvement of mitochondrial K (ATP) channels. Circ Res 1999;85:1113–1114.
71. Nado T, Minatoguchi S, Fujii K, et al. Evidence for the delayed effect in human ischemic preconditioning: prospective multicenter study for preconditioning in acute myocardial infarction. J Am Coll Cardiol 1999; 34:166–174.
72. Meisel SR, Shapiro H, Radnay J, et al. Increased expression of neutrophil and monocyte adhesion molecules LFA-1 and Mac-1 and their ligand ICAM-1 and VLA-4 throughout the acute phase of myocardial infarction: possible implications for leukocyte aggregation and microvascular plugging. J Am Coll Cardiol 1998; 31:120–125.
73. Bolli R. Oxygen derived free radicals and postischemic myocardial dysfunction ("stunned myocardium"). J Am Coll Cardiol 1988;12:239–249.
74. Douglas PS, Ginsburg GS. The evaluation of chest pain in women. N Engl J Med 1996;333:1311–1315.
75. Cerqueira M, Verani M, Schwaiger M, et al. Safety profile of adenosine stress perfusion imaging: results from the Adenoscan multicentre trial registry. J Am Coll Cardiol 1994;23:384–389.
76. Hays JT, Mahmarian JJ, Cochran AJ, et al. Dobutamine thallium-201 tomography for evaluating patients with suspected coronary disease unable to undergo exercise or vasodilator pharmacologic stress testing. J Am Coll Cardiol 1993;21:1583–1590.

2

Echocardiography in Coronary Artery Disease

Petros Nihoyannopoulos

Echocardiography is a noninvasive procedure that describes the anatomy of the heart, including valves and valve motion, chamber size, wall motion, and thickness. Doppler echocardiography assesses the cardiac hemodynamics such as volumes, severity of valvular regurgitation and gradients across the stenotic valves or between cardiac chambers, and the detection of intracardiac shunts.

Echocardiography has seen a rapid evolution from single-crystal M mode to two-dimensional (2D) echocardiography, Doppler, and now color flow imaging. Clinical use of echocardiography now extends from the operating room, as its utility in both transesophageal and intraoperative echocardiography, to the community. In patients with known or suspected coronary artery disease (CAD), echocardiography has become a pivotal first line investigation for the differential diagnosis of acute chest pain syndromes, assessing global and regional left ventricular (LV) function at rest and during stress as well as evaluating complications of myocardial infarction.

1. Imaging Techniques

1.1 Two-dimensional Echocardiography

Cardiac ultrasound is a tomographic imaging modality of the heart. Unlike computed tomography, echocardiography produces sequential sections of the heart using ultrasound. Therefore, its greatest advantage is the total absence of radiation involved while realizing the highest frame rates among all other imaging modalities.

Two-dimensional echocardiography is today the standard ultrasound imaging technique and has evolved from the original single-crystal M mode echocardiography. When electric impulses are applied to the crystal, it vibrates at a frequency determined by its mechanical dimensions. Transducers used for echocardiography typically generate frequencies in the range 1.5–7 MHz. Whereas the original M mode echocardiography used a single crystal, 2D echocardiography uses up to approximately 256 crystals in one transducer. This produces a cross-sectional section (slice) of the heart of less than 1-mL thickness (Figure 2.1). By using several such sections and from different positions and orientations from the chest wall, the entire heart can be visualized.

1.2 Three-dimensional Echocardiography

The clinical use of 3D echocardiography has been previously hindered by the prolonged and tedious nature of data acquisition. The recent introduction of real-time 3D echocardiographic imaging techniques has revolutionized echocardiography, because images are obtained in just one beat. This has been achieved by the development of a full-matrix array transducer (X4; Phillips Medical Systems, Andover, MA), which uses 3000 elements. This leads into a volume of data acquisition from a single projection in the shape of a pyramid (Figure 2.2). This has resulted in:

1. Improved image resolution
2. Higher penetration

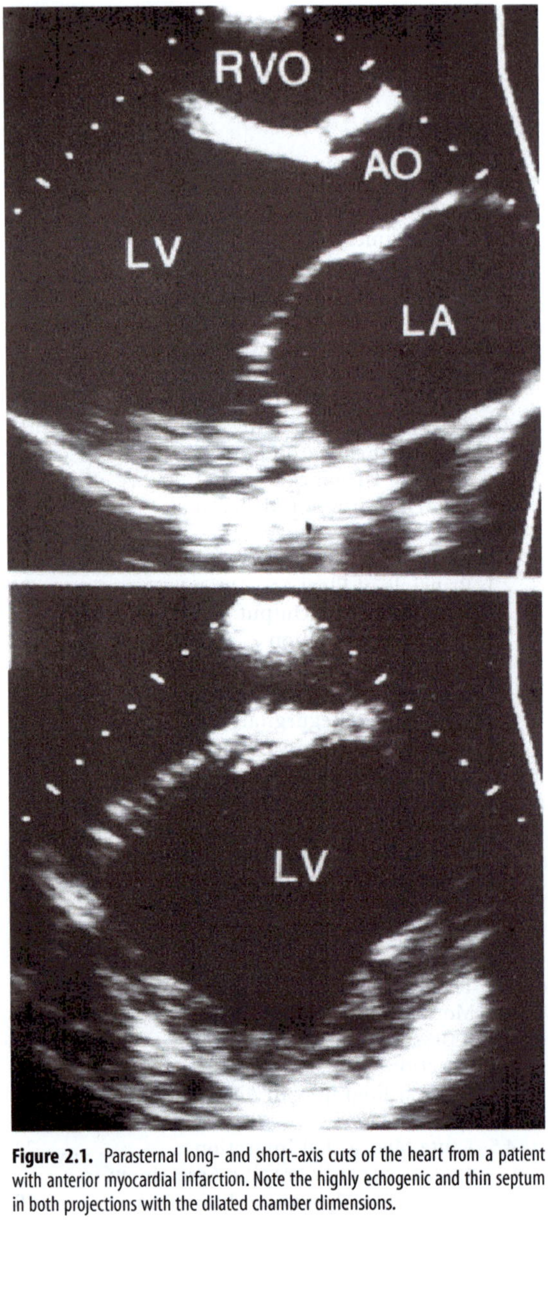

Figure 2.1. Parasternal long- and short-axis cuts of the heart from a patient with anterior myocardial infarction. Note the highly echogenic and thin septum in both projections with the dilated chamber dimensions.

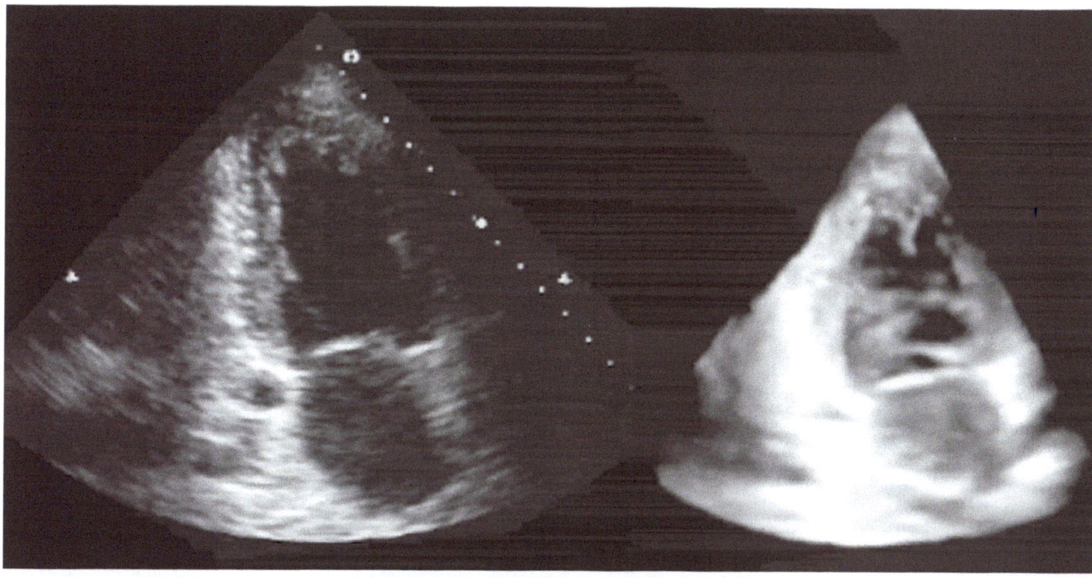

Figure 2.2. Apical projection demonstrating the two-dimensional long-axis cut of the left ventricle (left) with the simultaneous three-dimensional acquisition (right). Notice the depth of the image with the left ventricular trabeculations clearly captured in the three-dimensional picture.

3. Harmonic capabilities, which may be used for both gray-scale and contrast imaging. In addition, this transducer displays "on-line" 3D volume-rendered images and is also capable of displaying two simultaneous orthogonal 2D imaging planes (i.e., biplane imaging).

One of the most important requests in cardiac imaging is the simple and accurate assessment of LV function. With real-time 3D imaging, LV volumes may be obtained quickly and accurately. The left ventricle (apical four-, three-, and two-chamber views) is usually acquired from apical projections using a wide-angled acquisition. Images are displayed either using orthogonal parasternal views (Figure 2.3), or using multiple short-axis views, obtained at the level of the LV apex, papillary muscles, and the base.

The major advantage of real-time 3D echocardiography is that, for the first time, volumetric analysis does not rely on geometric assumptions, as has been the case with 2D echocardiography. Quantification of LV volumes and mass using real-time 3D echocardiography can be performed from an apical wide-angled acquisition using different methods. Currently, data analysis is performed on a desktop or laptop computer with dedicated 3D software (4D LV analysis; TomTec GMBH, Munich, Germany). Because a data set comprises the entire LV volume, multiple slices may be obtained from the base to the apex of the heart to evaluate wall motion. This acquisition can then be combined with the use of an infusion of contrast agents, particularly in patients with difficult acoustic window in whom it might be of benefit to improve the delineation of the endocardial border.

1.3 Transesophageal Imaging

Two-dimensional imaging from a transducer positioned in the esophagus has been commercially available since the late 1980s. A miniature transducer is mounted at the tip of a gastroscope, which can be rotated in 180 degrees. This currently has 64 elements, compared with 128 or 256 for transthoracic transducers, but because there is no attenuation from the chest wall, it operates at higher frequencies (up to 7.5 MHz) and produces excellent image quality. Because limited manipulation is possible within the esophagus, the complete transducer array can be rotated by a small electric motor controlled by the operator to provide image planes that correspond to the orthogonal axes of the heart. The

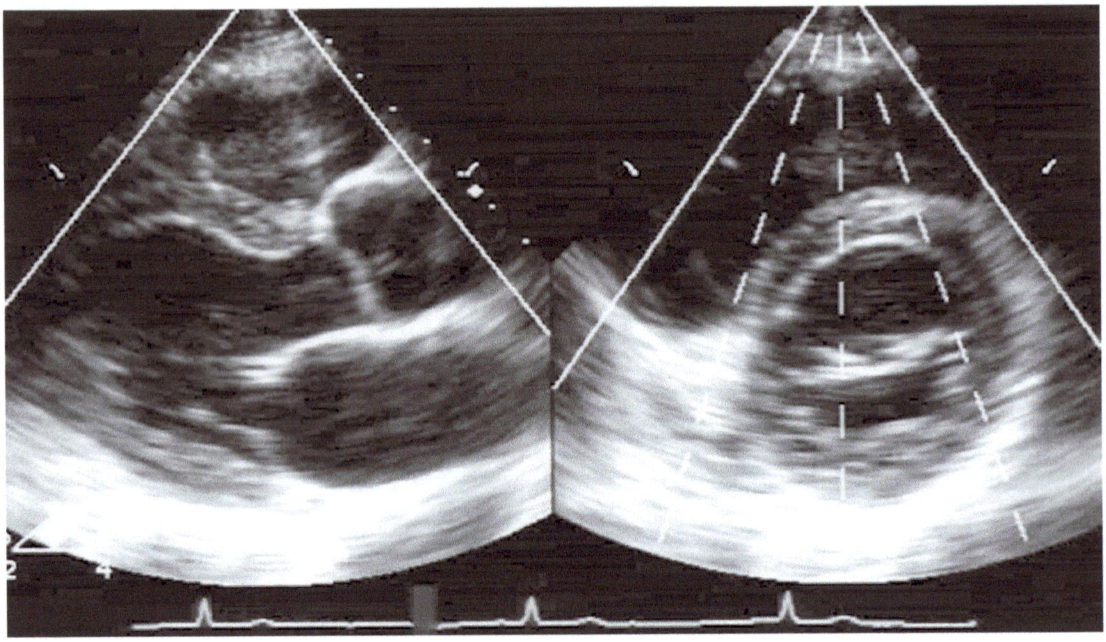

Figure 2.3. Simultaneous parasternal projections displaying two orthogonal to each other views using real-time three-dimensional imaging.

main advantage of transesophageal imaging of the heart is the excellent image quality of the posterior structures of the heart and thoracic aorta (Figure 2.4; see color section). It is also ideally suited for monitoring the heart during cardiac or noncardiac surgery. Because mitral surgery has now evolved toward preserving the mitral valve, transesophageal echocardiography has become an integral part of reconstructive mitral valve surgery because of its ability to describe with great detail the precise mechanisms of mitral regurgitation.

1.4 Doppler Echocardiography

Doppler echocardiography today is used for the determination of the direction and velocity of a moving blood volume, the estimation of valvular gradients, and the estimation of intracardiac pressures.

Doppler ultrasound measures the difference between the transmitted and returned frequencies. This change in frequency occurs when the ultrasound wave hits the moving blood cells. The faster the blood flow in relationship to the transducer, the greater the change in frequency. When the flow is going away from the transducer, the frequency changes from high to low. Flow moving toward the transducer results in an increase in returned frequency.

Normal blood flow is laminar; the direction and velocity of red blood cells are approximately the same. When there is disturbance to this blood flow, there is disruption to the normal laminar pattern becoming turbulent. Most of the time, turbulent blood flow indicates underlying pathology. For example, stenotic or regurgitant valves have both an increased turbulence and a marked increase in blood flow velocity.

1.4.1 Continuous Wave Doppler

Of the various Doppler systems used today, continuous wave Doppler is the oldest and easiest form to understand. The advantage of continuous wave Doppler lies in its ability to accurately record the highest intracardiac velocities. Many of the Doppler machines in current use can record velocities up to 15 m/s. This is twice what is normally considered the peak velocity found in the human body. However, the one disadvantage of continuous wave Doppler is its lack of depth discrimination. That is, the operator does not know where along the ultrasound beam this highest velocity is originating from.

1.4.2 Pulsed Wave Doppler

Pulsed wave systems allow the operator to selectively interrogate the flow velocity in a specific region of interest in the heart or great vessels. The sampling depth can easily be selected by the operator and velocities of up to about 2 m/s can readily be measured.

The main disadvantage of pulsed wave Doppler is that there is a technical limit to optimally evaluate the highest velocities. This limitation is known as “aliasing” and is represented on the spectral trace as a cutoff or limiting of the velocity in any one direction.

One of the prime uses of pulsed wave Doppler is the evaluation of the blood flow velocities originating from the flow across the mitral and tricuspid valves and pulmonary veins, which may be used to evaluate LV filling pressures and stroke volumes (SVs).

1.4.3 Color Flow Doppler

Doppler color flow imaging is a form of pulsed Doppler that displays flow data directly onto the 2D image. It allows excellent spatial information to exist together with anatomy and blood flow. The color display allows for the rapid identification of size, direction, and velocity of blood flow. It also significantly reduces the examination time for regurgitant jets.

Because color flow systems utilize the same principle as pulsed Doppler, there is a limitation to the velocity that can be recorded in any one direction based on the pulsed repetition rate. Aliasing in a color flow system results in a color shift when the mean velocity exceeds the Nyquist limit. Aliasing is easily seen because the shift occurs between the brightest reds and brightest blues.

Besides direction and velocity information, color flow systems can also detect the presence of turbulent flow. When turbulence is detected, a multitude of colors (a mosaic of red, blue, yellow, and cyan) is seen in the area of the abnormal turbulent flow such as valvular regurgitation.

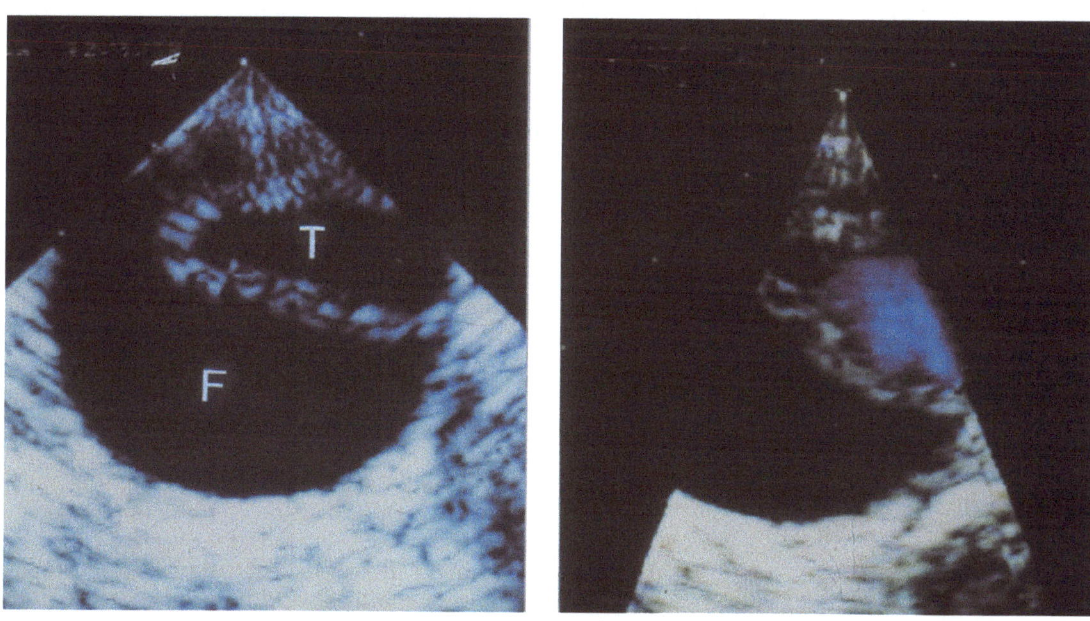

Figure 2.4. A 34-year-old patient with acute coronary syndrome. After negative troponines, he had a transesophageal echocardiographic examination, where a clear type A aortic dissection was demonstrated. T, true lumen; F, false lumen. Note the color Doppler display of aortic flow in the true lumen (left).

1.5 Tissue Doppler Imaging

All moving objects intersected by the ultrasound beam generate Doppler shifts, including the fastest-moving blood cells as well as the slower-moving structures such as valves and muscle. For study of blood flow, Doppler signals from the slower-moving heart structures such as valve leaflets are removed by selective filtering. The filtering is possible because the characteristics of Doppler signals from blood and tissue are markedly different: blood generally has high velocities, and relatively low signal amplitude because the red cell scatterers are relatively sparse. Conversely, muscle and valve tissue have much slower velocities and higher signal amplitudes because the cells are packed together.

If, instead of removing low velocities, the high velocity signals from blood are filtered out and the velocity and amplification scales suitably adjusted, Doppler signals from tissue motions can be recorded, either as pulse wave spectral displays or in color (2D or M mode).

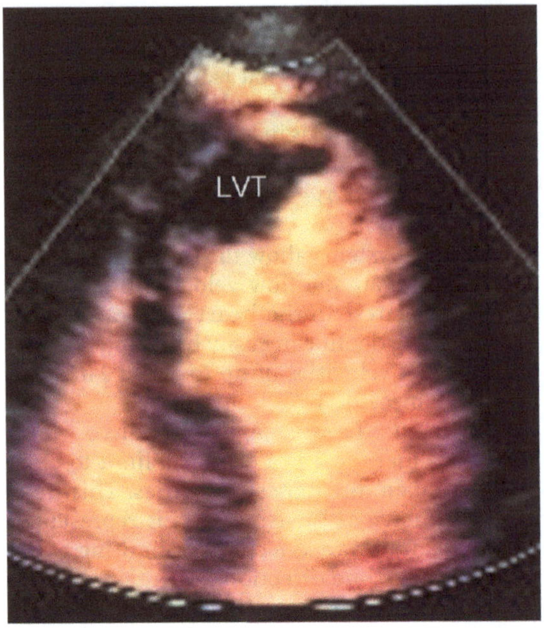

Figure 2.5. Apical four-chamber projection of the left ventricle after contrast injection demonstrating a clear endocardial border detection round the left ventricle. After contrast, it became clear that there was an organized thrombus at the apex (LVT).

1.6 Contrast Echocardiography

Contrast enhancement is used extensively in diagnostic and clinical radiology. Modalities such as X-ray, computed tomography, magnetic resonance imaging (MRI), and nuclear scintigraphy regularly rely on the introduction of foreign material into tissue in order to improve the contrast resolution in the image. The development of contrast media in echocardiography has been slow and sporadic. Only recently, transpulmonary contrast agents have become readily available for clinical use.[1] The primary indication for the use of contrast echocardiography is at present to improve endocardial border delineation in patients in whom adequate imaging is difficult. In CAD patients, in whom particular attention should be focused on regional myocardial contraction, clear endocardial definition is crucial. Intravenous contrast agents can improve endocardial delineation at rest[1] and with stress.[2]

1.6.1 LV Opacification

Despite improvement in imaging, there are still some patients whose endocardial definition remains a problem. This may be overcome by the use of intravenous ultrasound contrast agents.

Contrast agents consist of gas-filled microbubbles in a protein shell, which reflect ultrasound, generate harmonic backscatter, and, thus, enhance ultrasound information. The development of gas-filled microbubbles, which can be injected intravenously and remain stable through the pulmonary circulation into the LV cavity, has been a major advance in contrast technology.

Opacification of the left ventricle (Figure 2.5; see color section) has been shown to significantly improve endocardial border delineation in several studies and is now being used in patients with poor images in both resting and stress modalities. The use of intravenous contrast for LV opacification has also improved the rate of inter- and intraobserver variability in the assessment of regional wall motion abnormalities.[2] Importantly, the addition of contrast, both at rest and during stress, has proved to be cost effective.[3]

1.6.2 Detection of Myocardial Perfusion

The major future application of transpulmonary contrast agents is in the detection of myocardial perfusion, or lack of it. We and others proposed that this is indeed possible in patients after myocardial infarction (Figure 2.6; see color section). Intravenous injection of Sonazoid™ (Nycomed-Amersham, Oslo, Norway) consistently produced myocardial opacification in patients with previous myocardial infarction and allowed delineation of myocardial perfusion abnormalities. The anatomic location of each myocardial perfusion abnormality detected by contrast echo correlated reasonably well with that of single photon emission computed tomographic (SPECT) perfusion imaging and wall motion abnormalities. However, the results indicated also that assessment of myocardial perfusion by either SPECT or myocardial contrast is subject to attenuation artifacts that dominate in the inferior wall for SPECT and the anterior and lateral walls for echocardiography.[4]

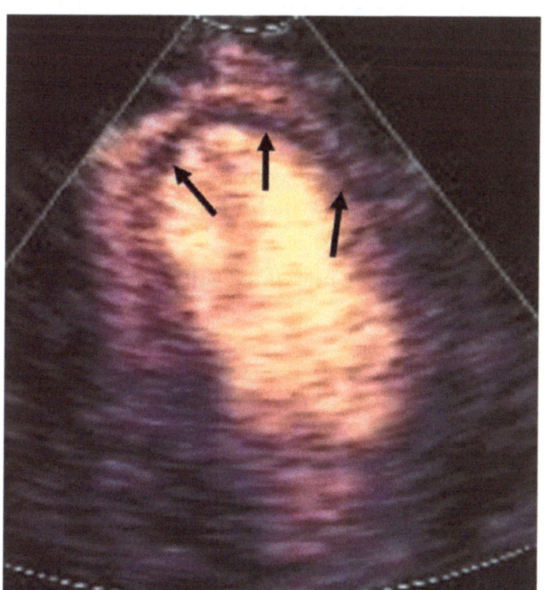

Figure 2.6. Apical four-chamber view during stress demonstrating the occurrence of a clear subendocardial perfusion defect (arrows) around the apex. Notice that the subepicardium is fully opacified with the contrast agent.

2. Hemodynamic Assessment of the Heart

2.1 Principle of Flow Assessment

Although Doppler measures velocities, blood flow through a vessel or across a valve can be calculated using the hydraulic equation. This is the product of flow velocity and cross-sectional area of the vessel at the site where velocity is measured. The area can be assumed to be circular and calculated as follows:

$$\text{Area} = \pi \times r^2,$$

where r = radius of the circular area and $\pi = 3.14$.

2.2 SV and Cardiac Output

One of the fundamental functions of the heart as a pump is to provide an adequate amount of blood flow to the entire body. In the past, the cardiac output (CO) determination required invasive comprehensive and time-consuming methods based on Fick and indicator dilution principles. Today, SV and CO may be reliably measured by 2D/Doppler noninvasively.

The forward SV may be determined by Doppler, which can be applied to any of the cardiac valves. For this, the flow through the aortic valve (or LV outflow tract) is most often used because the aortic annulus has the least change in size during the cardiac cycle. The aortic annulus diameter is measured in the parasternal long-axis view where the maximum diameter is obtained. The velocity at the annulus is obtained using the apical long-axis view and by placing the pulsed wave Doppler sample volume at the level of the aortic annulus. This velocity is then planimetered along its outer edge to obtain the time velocity integral (TVI). The SV may then be calculated as:

$$SV = \pi r^2 \times TVI.$$

CO is the product of SV and heart rate (HR) (Figure 2.7; see color section):

$$CO = SV \times HR.$$

2.3 Continuity Equation

The continuity equation is based on the principle of conservation of mass. This principle states

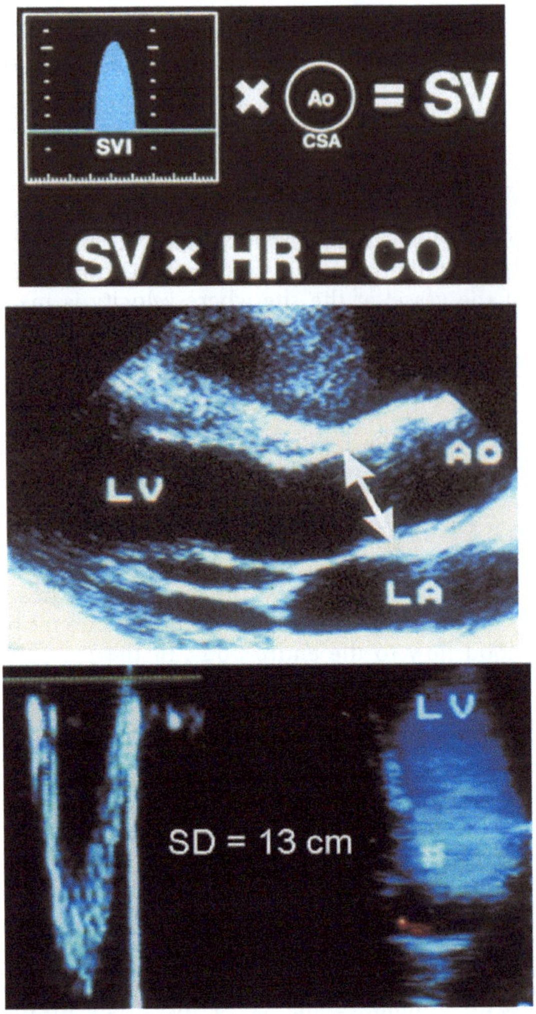

Figure 2.7. LV volume calculations, assuming that the LV outflow track is circular (top). Consequently, its area may be calculated from the LV outflow diameter as an area of a circle (left) and multiplied by the velocity measured at the same position from apical five-chamber projections (right) (see text).

that, under conditions of cardiovascular stability without any regurgitation or shunt, the net blood volume at any part of circulation must equal the net blood volume at any other part next to it (what comes in must go out). This situation is true under certain assumptions:

- The two points are directly connected.
- Blood is neither added nor removed from the system (closed circuit).

2.4 Calculation of Regurgitant Volumes

In applying the continuity equation to the blood flow in and out of the heart, the mitral valve SV is equal to the aortic valve SV provided there is no valve regurgitation. In the same way, the aortic SV is equal to pulmonic valve SV provided neither significant regurgitation is present in any of the valves nor any intracardiac shunt.

2.4.1 Mitral Regurgitation

In mitral regurgitation, the aortic SV is less than the forward mitral SV because part of the blood contained in the LV at the end of diastole is ejected back to the left atrium through the regurgitant mitral valve.

$$\text{Aortic SV} = \text{mitral SV} - \text{RV (mitral)}.$$

Therefore,

$$\begin{aligned}\text{Mitral RV} &= \text{mitral SV} - \text{aortic SV}\\ &= (0.785 \times D_{MA}^2 \times TVI_{MA})\\ &\quad - (0.785 \times D_{AA}^2 \times TVI_{AA}).\end{aligned}$$

2.4.2 Aortic Regurgitation

In aortic regurgitation, the aortic SV is more than the mitral SV because the regurgitant volume through the aortic valve will be added to the subsequent SV from the mitral valve. The same methodology described to assess the mitral valve regurgitant volume is used to assess the aortic regurgitant volume. The difference is that the aortic SV will be higher than that of mitral SV (see above).

$$\text{Aortic SV} = \text{mitral SV} + \text{RV (aortic)}.$$

Therefore,

$$\begin{aligned}\text{Aortic RV} &= \text{aortic SV} - \text{mitral SV}\\ &= (0.785 \times D_{AA}^2 \times TVI_{AA})\\ &\quad - (0.785 \times D_{MA}^2 \times TVI_{MA}).\end{aligned}$$

2.5 Transvalvular Pressure Gradient

One of the most fundamental applications of Doppler echocardiography is the determination of transvalvular pressure gradient using Bernoulli equation. This theorem states that the pressure decrease across a discrete stenosis in the heart or vasculature occurs because of energy loss attributed to three processes:

1. Acceleration of blood through the orifice (*convective acceleration*)
2. Inertial forces (*flow acceleration*)
3. Resistance to flow at the interfaces between blood and the orifice (*viscous friction*).

Therefore, the pressure decrease across any orifice can be calculated as the sum of these three variables. Although the original equation appears complex, most of its components (flow acceleration and viscous friction) are clinically insignificant and can be ignored. Furthermore, the flow velocity proximal to the fixed orifice (V^1) is usually much lower than the peak velocity through the orifice (V^2) and can also be ignored. Therefore, the simplified form of the Bernoulli equation is used in most clinical situations.

$$P1 - P2 \text{ (pressure reduced} = \Delta P) = 4\ V^2,$$

where V is the maximum instantaneous velocity and 4 is equal to ½ of the blood density.

The maximum instantaneous velocity of blood is therefore directly proportional to the peak gradient between the flow proximal and flow distal to the orifice.

It is important to remember that the maximum instantaneous pressure gradient obtained by Doppler is *different* from the peak-to-peak pressure gradient frequently measured in the catheterization laboratory. The latter is a nonphysiologic parameter because the peak LV pressure and peak aortic pressure do not occur simultaneously. The transvalvular mean gradient can also be measured by averaging all the individual velocities (TVI) over the entire flow period. This can be achieved by tracing the outer border of the spectral Doppler envelope from the continuous wave Doppler interrogation of flow through the aortic valve. In patients with normal LV systolic function, the mean gradient correlates well with the severity of aortic stenosis and aortic valve area.[5]

2.6 Right Ventricular Pressure

The TR jet velocity is the most common method used to assess the right ventricular systolic pressure (RVSP). RVSP is estimated from the peak transtricuspid pressure gradient. With the transducer at the apex, the continuous wave Doppler is used to obtain the peak tricuspid regurgitant velocity, that is, the peak instantaneous systolic pressure gradient between RV and RA. In case of weak signal, saline contrast enhancement should be performed. RVSP is calculated as follows:

$$\text{Peak trans-tricuspid pressure gradient} = \text{RVSP} - \text{RAP}.$$

$$\text{RVSP} = \text{peak trans-tricuspid pressure gradient} + \text{RAP} = 4\ (V_{TR})^2 + \text{RAP}.$$

3. New Methods in Improving Assessment of LV Function

Clear visualization of the ventricular walls and in particular the endocardial border is vital to the accurate assessment of regional wall function. Approximately 15% of patients may have poor endocardial definition on conventional echocardiographic imaging. This may be attributed to a variety of reasons, including large body habitus, lung disease, or distorted architecture of the left ventricle.

Several new methods have been developed to help overcome these limitations and improve LV delineation.

3.1 Harmonic Imaging

Conventional (or fundamental) echocardiography uses a transducer to emit and receive ultrasound waves at one frequency. However, not all signals reflected back from myocardial tissue are of the original frequency and some may reflect back in twice or even three times the original frequency. These are known as harmonic frequencies.

Harmonic imaging uses broad-band transducers that are capable of receiving reflected signals of twice (second harmonic) or three times (ultraharmonics) the original frequency and thus improve image quality. This technique reduces the number of spurious echos detected within the LV cavity and allows clearer definition of the endocardial border (Figure 2.8). Harmonic imaging is now well validated and is being used routinely.

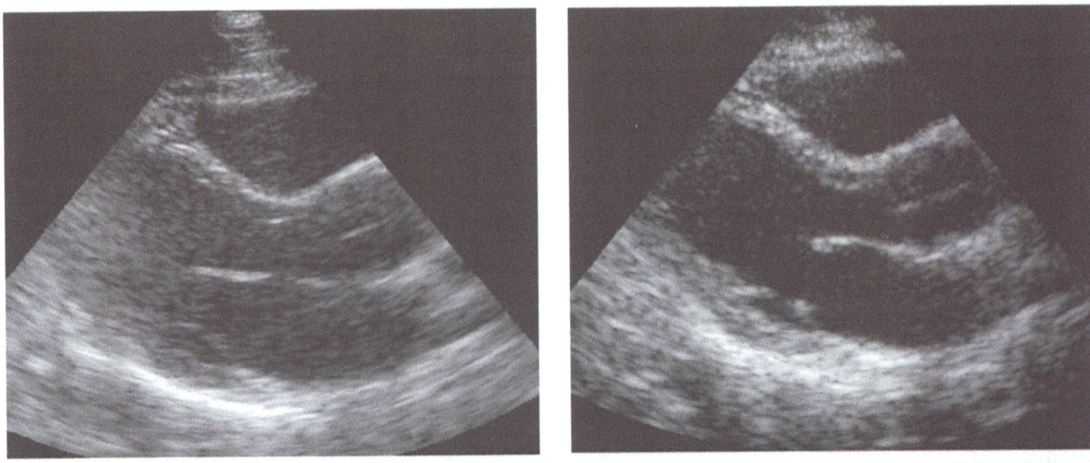

Figure 2.8. Parasternal long-axis projections demonstrating images acquired with fundamental mode (left) and second harmonic mode (right). Notice the clear difference of image quality.

3.2 Automated Endocardial Border Tracking

Analysis of 2D gray-scale images obtained during 2D imaging tend to be subjective, qualitative, and dependent on the experience of the observer as in many other imaging modalities. In an attempt to provide a less operator-dependent method of assessing wall motion, methods that automatically trace endocardial borders have been developed.

When an image is acquired, the backscatter information along the scan line is analyzed and each pixel classified as either blood or tissue. There is sufficient difference between the energy returned from the blood in the LV (low) and the endocardium (high) for this distinction to be made. Once this interface has been established along the entire endocardium, it can then be tracked and presented in a parametric display. Each pixel is color coded and is superimposed onto the 2D image. The construction is then integrated with the original scan image and all can be performed on-line. This leads to real-time tracking of the endocardial border, which is continually updated in each frame.

4. Echocardiography in CAD

4.1 Assessing LV Function

The assessment of LV function and particularly regional wall motion and thickening is of pivotal importance in determining the severity and prognosis of CAD. Echocardiography, with its high spatial and temporal resolution, is ideally suited for assessing LV function noninvasively without the use of irradiation. In acute coronary syndromes, the ability to detect regional LV dysfunction may prove useful in the early detection of myocardial ischemia, preceding electrocardiogram (ECG) changes and symptoms. Conversely, in patients presenting acutely with chest pain syndromes, the presence of normal regional wall function may exclude underlying ischemia with a pooled negative predictive accuracy of 95%.

In patients with a history of CAD, the presence of regional LV dysfunction and extent of LV wall thinning can indicate the site and severity of myocardial damage. Because of its noninvasive nature, echocardiography may be used for the reevaluation of these patients looking for any change in LV function and shape caused by treatment (remodeling).

Whereas image quality was an issue in the 1970s and 1980s, the improved image quality on modern machines, particularly with harmonic imaging and contrast enhancement, has allowed an almost 100% accuracy of regional wall function assessment and makes regional ventricular function clearly understood even by the nonexperts.

In summary, there should be no excuse for suboptimal image quality in a modern echocardiographic department, where modern equipment and transvenous ultrasound contrast agents ought to be available.

4.2 The Mechanism for Regional Wall Motion Abnormality

There is a well-established parallel relationship between regional coronary blood flow and contractile function in the corresponding territory.[6–9] In patients with normal coronary arteries, coronary perfusion is maintained even after an increase in oxygen demand. Thus, during stress, there is increased myocardial blood flow (coronary flow reserve) and hence increased wall motion thickening (contractile reserve).

In patients with a significant coronary artery stenosis (>70%), resting regional blood flow remains normal. However, when oxygen demand increases (e.g., during exercise), there is an inability to increase coronary perfusion to that area. This leads to a reduction of flow in the corresponding myocardial region leading to a reduction in wall thickening (hypokinesia). When oxygen demand is reduced, or returns to normal, there is resolution of ischemia and wall motion/thickening returns to normal.

Acute coronary artery occlusion leads to a rapid reduction in resting myocardial blood flow and hence cessation of muscular contraction in the area supplied. Relief of the occlusion, either spontaneously or by treatment (such as thrombolysis) resolves to recovery of regional wall function eventually. The duration and severity of myocardial ischemia determines the degree of wall motion abnormality and indeed wall motion may not return to normal for several hours after the acute episode ("stunned myocardium").

In chronic CAD, progressive reduction in myocardial blood flow caused by the progression of CAD may result in down-regulation of myocardial contractile function with preserved metabolic activity ("hibernating myocardium"). When the myocardial blood flow is restored through revascularization of the stenotic arteries, contractile function is usually gradually restored.

The detection of such regional LV dysfunction is important because it occurs early in the "ischemic cascade" preceding ECG changes and symptoms.

It is important to remember that myocardial ischemia is not the only cause of regional myocardial dysfunction. Abnormal septal motion can also occur in several conditions (Table 2.1). Generally, however, in these conditions, endocardial excursion is abnormal but regional wall thickening remains normal. This distinction permits the separation of nonischemic etiology from reversible ischemia.

4.3 Assessment of Regional Wall Function

The usual method of assessing LV wall function by echocardiography is the use of standard apical four-, two-, three-chamber apical and parasternal long- and short-axis views. This allows complete visualization of all the LV walls and hence all three vascular territories, although care must be taken to ensure that endocardial border definition is clear. It is also important to obtain different views of the same region to make an accurate assessment of regional wall function. This is usually done by combining the use of the standard apical views with the parasternal projections, particularly in the short axis, where different levels of function from base through papillary muscle down to apex may be visualized.

Whereas in normal subjects regional systolic wall thickening is increased during stress by 50%–100%, during myocardial ischemia, there is a reduction of the amplitude of wall thickening, often barely appreciable (akinesia). This can best be appreciated when compared with adjacent normally contracting myocardial regions.

Although assessing regional myocardial function is qualitative, it is possible to semiquantitate this using a four-point scale:

1. Normal thickening
2. Hypokinetic – reduced endocardial excursion and wall thickening

Table 2.1. Causes of abnormal regional wall motion abnormalities

1. Right ventricular volume/pressure overload
2. Left bundle branch block
3. Wolf-Parkinson-White
4. Permanent pacing (ventricular septum)
5. Post-cardiac surgery
6. Cardiac sarcoidosis
7. Focal myocarditis
8. Aortic regurgitation

3. Akinetic – absent wall motion/thickening
4. Dyskinetic – systolic bulging of the wall with no thickening

The sum of the individual segment scores gives a wall motion score (WMS), which can be used to give an indication of the severity of ischemia; a WMS index can also be used (WMS divided by the number of segments assessed) and has been shown to be an important prognostic indicator in patients with CAD.

4.4 Echocardiography in Acute Coronary Syndromes

Acute coronary syndromes encompass a spectrum of conditions ranging form unstable angina through to non-Q wave infarction with or without ST segment elevation and Q wave myocardial infarction. The pathologic process remains the same, however. An atherosclerotic plaque in an epicardial artery undergoes rupture leading to thrombus formation.

After acute coronary thrombosis, there is reduction of myocardial blood flow with concomitant reduction of wall thickening, which parallels the reduction of blood flow. If the duration of ischemia is brief, reduced regional wall thickening will recover. The longer the ischemic burden, however, the longer the duration of myocardial dysfunction eventually leading to myocardial necrosis and scar tissue formation.

In the emergency department, echocardiography may be useful in detecting the presence and extent of regional myocardial dysfunction. If the patient, however, complains of chest pain but the ECG is equivocal, and there is no regional wall motion abnormality, then the presence of acute ischemia is unlikely. The use of echocardiography for diagnosis of acute myocardial infarction is most helpful when the clinical history and ECG findings are nondiagnostic. Table 2.2 describes the current indications for the use of echocardiography in patients presenting with chest pain.

Once the diagnosis of an acute coronary syndrome has been established with the help of biomarkers, echocardiographic assessment of LV function becomes important for the assessment of the precise site and extent of jeopardized myocardium.

Table 2.2. Indications for echocardiography in patients with chest pain

	Class
1. Diagnosis of underlying cardiac disease in patients with chest pain and clinical evidence of valvular, pericardial, or primary myocardial disease.	I
2. Evaluation of chest pain in patients with suspected acute myocardial ischemia, when baseline ECG is nondiagnostic and when study can be obtained during pain or soon after its abatement.	I
3. Evaluation of chest pain in patients with suspected aortic dissection.	I
4. Chest pain in patients with severe hemodynamic instability.	I
5. Evaluation of chest pain for which a noncardiac etiology is apparent.	III
6. Diagnosis of chest pain in a patient with electrocardiographic changes diagnostic of myocardial ischemia/infarction.	III

Source: Modified from the AHA/ACC/ASE recommendation. Circulation 1997.

4.5 Acute Myocardial Infarction

The degree of myocardial damage seen after infarction is directly related to the duration of artery occlusion supplying that area, the extent of the myocardium at risk, and the degree of collateral circulation. Pathologic studies have demonstrated that if 20% undergoes infarction, there is a reduction in wall thickening during systole of >50%.

4.5.1 Echocardiographic Assessment in Acute Myocardial Infarction

Because both myocardial ischemia and infarction produce regional wall thickening abnormalities, it is difficult to differentiate between the two in patients presenting acutely with chest pain. However, because 90%–100% of patients presenting with acute myocardial infarction have regional wall motion abnormalities, echocardiography may be helpful in excluding ischemia in patients presenting with chest pain with equivocal ECGs. Assessment of regional wall function allows localization of the infarct-related artery. An occlusion of the left anterior descending (LAD) often leads to anterior septal, anterior ventricular wall and apical akinesia.

Left circumflex stenosis often involves the lateral and posterior LV walls. Identification of a posterior wall motion abnormality (using the apical three-chamber and parasternal long-axis view) may be helpful in the acute setting, because 12-lead ECG diagnosis of a posterior myocardial infarct is often missed.

Right coronary artery occlusion involves the inferior wall and inferior septum. This is clearly seen in the apical two-chamber view. The right coronary artery also commonly supplies the right ventricle leading to significant RV dysfunction. Echocardiography is probably the best bedside method to assess RV function, particularly when patients present with symptoms of heart failure and increased jugular venous pressure. It may also have important management implications. RV function can be assessed from the apical four-chamber view as well as parasternal inflow and outflow track projections.

The presence of a wall motion abnormality after acute ischemia may be the result of myocardial necrosis, stunned or hibernating myocardium, or, more frequently, combinations of the above. After acute myocardial infarction, the extent and severity of wall motion abnormality lead to unfavorable outcome. Between 2–4 weeks after acute myocardial infarction, akinetic segments become thinned and scarred. Because of the sheer and pressure changes that occur in the LV, these areas can change the shape and size of the ventricle (remodeling), and may become aneurysmal, representing the final stages in the infarct expansion process.

Areas that remain severely hypokinetic or akinetic, but do not demonstrate any other changes, may be stunned or hibernating. Myocardial hibernation occurs when there is prolonged wall motion abnormality caused by repetitive stunning. To distinguish necrotic from viable myocardium (i.e., stunned or hibernating), techniques assessing contractile reserve (dobutamine stress echocardiography), the microcirculation (myocardial contrast echocardiography), or metabolism (radionuclide techniques) are useful. If these studies demonstrate lack of significant myocardial necrosis, these areas are considered viable and contractile function in these segments may improve if revascularization is undertaken.

4.5.2 Complications of Myocardial Infarction

These are associated with increased morbidity and mortality. Echocardiography can be used to evaluate virtually any complication of acute myocardial infarction at the bedside.

4.5.2.1 Congestive Heart Failure. After acute myocardial infarction, the infarct territory expands with wall thinning and compensatory ventricular hypertrophy in the noninfarcted territory. This ventricular remodeling may lead to heart failure, particularly when the LAD territory is involved. This process can be followed by regular echocardiographic assessment at the bedside. Perhaps one of the most important contributions of echocardiography is the description of the extent of LV damage or jeopardized myocardium. If there is a large LAD territory that is jeopardized, urgent revascularization may be recommended in an attempt to salvage myocardium. The presence of LV thrombus can also be identified.

4.5.2.2 Right Ventricular Infarction. This can cause a similar clinical picture to heart failure and hypotension, necessitating fluid administration rather than inotropic agents and this is very difficult to diagnose clinically or by ECG alone. Conversely, the right ventricle can easily be described using echocardiography and, as with LV dysfunction, right ventricular asynergy is a sensitive marker of myocardial infarction.

4.5.2.3 Ventricular Septal Rupture. Ventricular septal rupture or papillary muscle dysfunction may easily be identified with 2D and color flow imaging in a patient who develops a heart murmur, heart failure, or cardiogenic shock. Papillary muscle dysfunction and rupture can cause severe mitral regurgitation with pulmonary edema and decrease in blood pressure. Echocardiography with its fine spatial resolution can detect the underlying cardiac abnormality and assess the severity of mitral regurgitation.

A cruciat differential diagnosis for a patient with a new systolic murmur after myocardial infarction is the development of a ventricular septal defect, usually at the apex, after acute anterior myocardial infarction. Usually they develop between day 1 and day 7 post-myocardial infarction and may be difficult to differentiate from acute mitral regurgitation clinically, particularly in a patient with heart failure. Again, echocardiography is ideally suited for the differential diagnosis at the bedside (Figure 2.9; see color section).

Occasionally, the free wall may rupture into the pericardial sac and lead to a pseudoaneurysm. This needs to be distinguished from

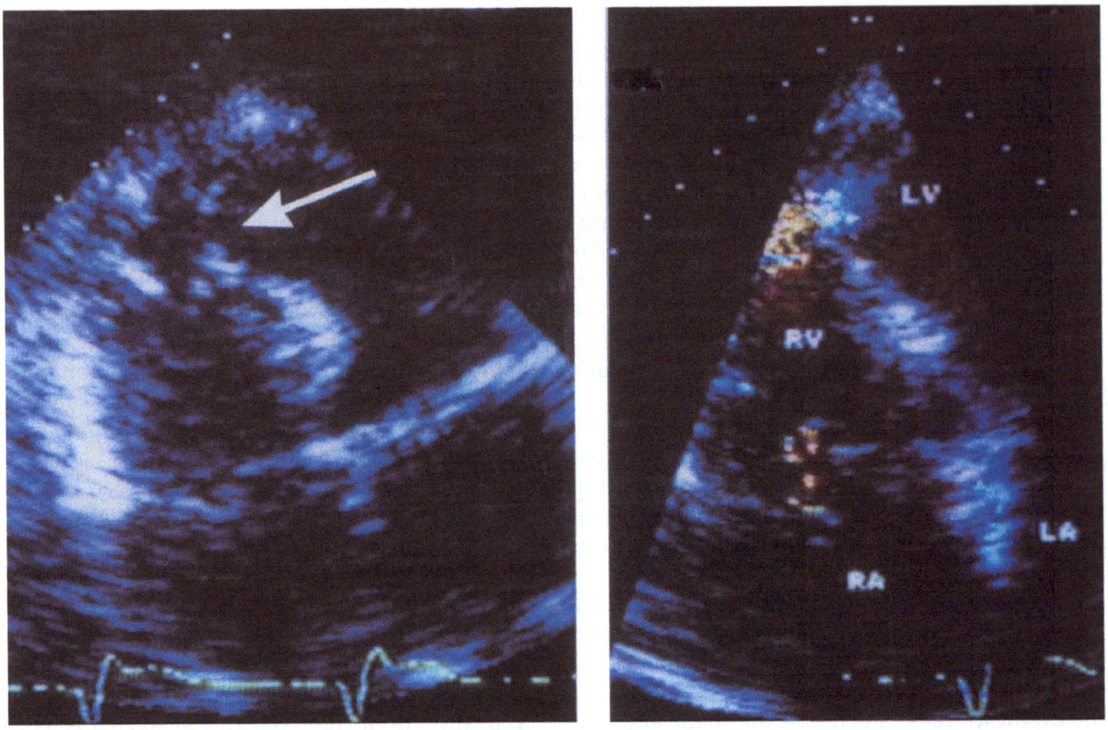

Figure 2.9. Apical projections demonstrating a discontinuation of the ventricular septal continuity near the apex (left, arrow) suggestive of a ventricular septal defect. On the right, this has been confirmed with the addition of color Doppler, which clearly demonstrates an abnormal flow through the septal "drop out."

the more stable true aneurysm, because it may rupture suddenly with catastrophic consequences.

4.6 Stress Echocardiography

Myocardial ischemia is accompanied by characteristic mechanical, electrical, and perfusional abnormalities, each of which has been used to detect CAD. Although coronary angiography is the gold standard for the diagnosis of CAD, the anatomic description alone does not indicate the physiologic significance of stenosis. Exercise ECG, perfusion defects on SPECT or PET studies, or abnormalities of myocardial contraction detected by stress echocardiography, all permit assessment of the functional severity of coronary stenoses. Echocardiography has a better spatial resolution (2 mm) than SPECT (10 mm) or PET (4 mm at best) imaging (see also Chapter 8). Because of this, every single myocardial region corresponding to each coronary vascular bed can be visualized from several projections such as the parasternal long-axis, short-axis, or apical four- and two-chamber views.

What makes echocardiography unique over other imaging modalities, perhaps with the exception of MRI, is its ability to visualize the whole of myocardium (including the right ventricle so often ignored) from several projections so that one segment can be visualized from more than one view. The advantage of this is that if one region is not seen sufficiently well from one projection there will be an alternative. Consequently, the success rate of stress echocardiography (often misquoted as a limitation of the technique) should be 100% for an experienced laboratory. As a result, stress echocardiography has acquired an unquestioned clinical role as an accurate and inexpensive stress imaging technique.[10–13]

4.6.1 The Importance of Bayes' Theorem

In using any testing method, it is important to consider the pretest likelihood of the disorder being sought. The diagnostic value of stress echocardiography is greatest in patients with an intermediate pretest probability of clinical CAD. Such patients would include symptomatic middle-aged women with typical angina, patients with coronary risk factors and abnormal ECG findings at baseline, and patients with risk factors and/or atypical angina. In such patients, stress echocardiography would be expected to have the greatest value in increasing (based on a positive result) or lowering (based on a negative result) the likelihood of CAD. In patients with a very low pretest likelihood for CAD (such as patients with no risk factors or those with highly atypical or nonanginal chest pain), positive stress echocardiography results may often be false-positive. In patients with a very high pretest likelihood of CAD (such as middle-aged or elderly men with multiple coronary risk factors and classic angina pectoris), negative stress echocardiography results are often false-negative.

4.6.2 Rationale of Stress Echocardiography

As early as 1935, Tennant and Wiggers[6] described the loss of regional myocardial contraction during coronary artery occlusion. Studies at rest in which progressive coronary stenosis is produced in the conscious dog have shown a linear correlation between regional wall motion and subendocardial blood flow in contrast with a poor correlation with subepicardial blood flow. A 20% decrease in blood flow produces a corresponding small reduction in systolic wall thickening.[7] This close coupling between the level of ischemia as assessed by reduced regional blood flow and regional contraction suggests in the strongest possible way that regional wall motion is a sensitive and meaningful marker of acute ischemic events.

4.6.3 Methods of Stress Echocardiography

The use of stress testing to unveil LV contractile abnormalities is based on the concept of myocardial metabolic supply and demand. The demand side of the equation is highly dependent on many factors including LV pressure, volume, wall stress, HR, and contractility. All of these parameters relate to myocardial oxygen consumption mainly through their combined effect on LV wall forces linked together by the Marquee de La Place's equation (product of intracavitary pressure and radius of curvature of the myocardial segment divided by wall thickness).

4.6.3.1 Exercise Echocardiography. The fundamental advantage of exercise, particularly that of treadmill, over pharmacologic stress testing is that it provides excellent natural physiologic cardiovascular stress, physician's familiarity with ECG changes and symptoms, and allows these to be analyzed in combination with cross-sectional echocardiography to detect ischemia-induced wall motion abnormalities. With exercise, there is an overall LV fiber shortening resulting from both the preload-dependent stretching of the myocardial fibers (Starling effect) as well as from elevated contractility caused by catecholamine-induced acceleration of intracellular phosphorylation and metabolism. Its diagnostic accuracy has previously been documented in atherosclerotic CAD producing regional myocardial dysfunction in patients with angina in contrast to patients with syndrome X in whom no regional wall motion abnormalities are identified.[14]

The main disadvantage of using treadmill exercise with echocardiography is that imaging cannot be obtained throughout the stress test and can only be performed immediately after cessation of exercise. The second disadvantage is that the high respiratory and HRs preclude optimal echocardiographic imaging when this is recorded on videotapes. For this reason, digital technology must be used with this type of stress echocardiography.

Digital acquisition allows ECG-triggered automatic acquisition of a preselected number of consecutive images starting from the R wave. Images can be captured speedily immediately after exercise while the patient still breathes heavily with deep inspiratory and expiratory cycles. Selecting only the images captured during deep expiration (therefore the best) whereas discarding the poor images in deep inspiration results in excellent imaging immediately after exercise, often even better than the resting images. In this way, the disadvantage of heavy respiration immediately after exercise turns to an advantage with improved imaging.

4.6.3.2 Dobutamine Stress Echocardiography. Pharmacologic stress testing is also important, particularly when patients are unable to exercise. The two leading categories of pharmacologic stress testing are those producing vasodilation, such as dipyridamole and adenosine and those producing inotropic stimulation such as dobutamine and isoprenaline. Although the vasodilators were the first pharmacologic agents to be used in combination with echocardiography by mimicking the nuclear stress testing rationale, they proved to be inefficient in triggering wall motion abnormalities in a satisfactory way to be clinically useful.[15–17]

Dobutamine stress has now emerged as the best alternative to exercise with very similar diagnostic accuracy. Dobutamine is a catecholamine with selective β_1-adrenoreceptor agonist activity and a relatively week action on α and β_2-adrenoreceptors. Given intravenously, its half-life is 2.37 ± 0.7 minutes. It increases myocardial contractility with consequent increase in SV and CO. It also decreases central venous pressure, pulmonary arterial, and capillary wedge pressures reducing LV filling pressures and volume. Reduction of ventricular size is particular responsible for a decrease in wall stress. During stress, echocardiography it is given intravenously starting from 5 to 40 mg/kg/min in increments of 5 or 10 mg/kg/min for 3–5 minutes each. At these doses, myocardial oxygen demand increases through an increase in HR, systolic blood pressure, and contractility.

The main disadvantage of dobutamine stress testing is the occurrence of "paradoxical" hypotension occurring in approximately 20% of patients.[18] The precise mechanism of this paradoxical hypotension remains unclear. However, it is likely that this is the result of a cardiovascular vasodepressor reflex. Dobutamine stress testing is easier to perform than exercise echocardiography because the operator has time to optimize imaging in each projection while continuously recording every myocardial region throughout the infusion. However, it is preferentially used in patients unable to exercise as an alternative test but also for the detection of myocardial viability. The latter has made dobutamine stress echocardiography the single most popular myocardial stressor to be used in combination with echocardiography.

4.6.3.3 Feasibility of Stress Echocardiography. The perceived disadvantage of stress echocardiography is its inability to obtain meaningful information in all patients with suspected CAD. Several studies from a variety of institutions, including our own, have clearly demonstrated that the success rate of stress echocardiography is or approaching 100%. This is similar to either exercise or dobutamine stress.

It is common that a number of myocardial regions may not be adequately seen from one or the other view. The advantage of being able to image one coronary vascular bed from more than one projection should allow diagnostic information to be obtained for all or at least 70% of myocardium in each patient in established laboratories. Proper training and experience is therefore pivotal. Automatic schemes for analysis and interpretation are not widely available at present and, as in every echocardiographic technique, require substantial expert input. Every imaging modality, however, is expert dependent, whether it is nuclear testing or MRI, and local expertise is widely variable, very similar to echocardiography.

4.6.4 Assessing Myocardial Ischemia

Stress echocardiography is frequently used for the detection of CAD. In reality, however, it is the presence of myocardial ischemia that is demonstrated because it usually requires a 40%–60% narrowing of the coronary vessel to obtain a measurable reduction in maximal flow.

Stress echocardiography not only detects the presence of ischemia but also can assess its magnitude. The severity of ischemia can be ascertained by the degree of motion impairment from minimal (hypokinesia) to severe (akinesia), up to paradoxical systolic expansion (dyskinesia). The greater the wall thickening reduction, the greater the magnitude of ischemia. On the horizontal axis, the extent of ischemia can also be ascertained. The number of ischemic zones can easily be depicted by utilizing imaging of all 16 segments. In the presence of single ischemic zone, the number of ischemic segments along one coronary vascular territory would be expected to become akinetic. The greater the number of akinetic segments, the more proximal the stenosis would be. If more than one vascular bed becomes ischemic, a multivessel CAD should be expected. Finally, the timing of the wall motion abnormality being detected will also reflect the magnitude of ischemia. The earlier the hypokinesia, the more severe the ischemic burden would be. This grading, however, is valid mainly in patients undergoing continuous echocardiographic imaging such as during dobutamine infusion, whereas for postexercise echocardiography this may not be applicable.

The diagnostic accuracy of stress echocardiography relies mostly on the arbitrary angiographic cut-off value to define "significant" stenosis. This is often performed visually. The purely anatomic-functional approach of comparing myocardial ischemia in CAD patients may itself be insufficient and wrongly estimate sensitivities and specificities of the test when only the presence of stenosis is considered. The value of careful quantification of stenosis severity in the prediction of a positive stress echocardiography test should be emphasized. The best cut-off point for predicting wall motion abnormalities during bicycle ergometry seems to be in the region of 52% stenosis with a minimal lumen diameter of 1.13 mm in patients with single vessel CAD. Complex coronary stenotic lesions with irregular borders and/or multiple irregularities, however, are more likely to be associated with a positive stress test than patients with symmetric lesions.[19]

Contrast echocardiography is now implemented during stress echocardiography with increased sensitivities and specificities. Whereas contrast may improve endocardial border detection, perhaps the most important application of transvenous contrast agents is to detect myocardial perfusion. According to the ischemic cascade, perfusion deficits precede contractile dysfunction during stress. This means that the sensitivity of perfusion modalities would be higher than functional tests such as echocardiography or MRI. However, with the combination of intravenous contrast injection during dobutamine stress echocardiography, the sensitivity of stress echocardiography can increase without the loss of specificity.[20]

4.6.5 Clinical Settings

Stress echocardiography is appropriate where exercise ECG is unlikely to provide satisfactory answers to the clinical questions being posed and should improve the selection of patients for tertiary referral. Speed and convenience strengthen the economic argument in favor of this technique, the reliability of which was emphasized early on by results that were comparably concordant with those obtained by SPECT perfusion imaging.

Stress echocardiography emerges as a vital modality for screening high-risk patients before major peripheral vascular surgery,[21] orthopedic surgery, or in patients with chronic renal failure.[22] Others[23] emphasized the value of exercise echocardiography after coronary artery bypass surgery in predicting compromised vascular supply.

Assessment of patients' prognosis is important in an era when clinical decision-making must be rendered in a cost-effective manner. A number of studies have demonstrated that the 1- and 2-year prognosis after a normal exercise or dobutamine stress echocardiogram is excellent and similar to that seen after a normal thallium scintigraphy.[24]

4.6.6 Assessing Myocardial Viability

In the setting of ischemia, loss of myocardial contractile function may be attributed to myocardial necrosis, stunning, or hibernation. Whereas myocardial necrosis usually alludes to irreversible myocardial dysfunction, stunning and hibernation reflect reversibility of myocardial function. It is therefore important to be able to differentiate the potential reversibility of such myocardial dysfunction. A variety of noninvasive methods are undergoing investigation and validation for detecting viability in akinetic or severely hypokinetic myocardial regions including SPECT with ^{201}Tl, ^{99m}Tc sestamibi, positron emission tomography imaging of regional flow, and F-labeled ^{18}FDG uptake as well as assessment of inotropic contractile reserve with dobutamine stress echocardiography. A recent meta-analysis has shown that the average positive predictive values are 84% for echocardiography and 75% for nuclear imaging and the negative predictive values 69% and 80%, respectively.[25] A more detailed discussion on this topic can be found in Chapter 13.

4.6.7 Stress Echocardiography Laboratory

Echocardiography has dramatically expanded over recent years with more and more physicians requesting studies. Its major advantages of being safe and inexpensive have become a disadvantage as more and more people use it, many inappropriately trained and therefore with progressively increasing chance of inaccurate reports. Recently, the British Society of Echocardiography has issued guidelines for training, which are essential for those performing and interpreting echocardiography.[26] Stress echocardiography is steadily going down a similar road except that it is more difficult to perform and even more difficult to interpret. Because of the radiation hazards, nuclear stress testing is confined to experts generally, thus somewhat avoiding the potential for irresponsible use of stress testing with radioisotopes. There is no such protective net with stress echocardiography, which is open to wide use (or abuse). It is therefore of pivotal importance to increase individual expertise steadily and cautiously in a protected center before using it as a decision-making investigation.

Generally, a center becomes expert when it performs at least five stress echocardiographic examinations a week with the appropriate exposure and feedback. To do this, echocardiography laboratories are in increasing need for space, time, equipment, and personnel.

5. Conclusions

Echocardiography is an important tool for patients with CAD. It can be used to differentiate regional myocardial ischemia from other etiologies of chest pain, can be used to evaluate the extent of myocardial dysfunction, at rest and with stress, and to ascertain the presence of complications in patients with acute myocardial infarction. With the prospect of identifying myocardial perfusion defects, echocardiography is clearly an approach that can provide a "one-stop" strategy for assessing cardiac anatomy, function, and perfusion.

References

1. Crouse LJ, Cheirif J, Hanly DE, et al. Opacification and border delineation improvement in patients with suboptimal endocardial border definition in routine echocardiography: results of phase III Albunex multicenter trial. J Am Coll Cardiol 1993;22:1494–1500.
2. Ikonomidis I, Holmes E, Narbuvold H, Bolstad B, Muan B, Nihoyannopoulos P. Left venticular wall motion assesment and endocardial border delineation after intravenous injection of Infoson™ during dobutamine stress echocardiography. Coron Artery Dis 1998;9: 567–576.
3. Shaw LJ, Monaghan MJ, Nihoyannopoulos P. Clinical and economic outcomes assessment with myocardial contrast echocardiography. Heart 1999;82(suppl 3): 16–21.
4. Jucquois I, Nihoyannopoulos P, D'Hontdt A-M, et al. Comparison of myocardial contrast echocrdiography with NC100100 and Tc-99m sestamibi single photon emission computed tomography for detection of resting myocardial perfusion abnormalities in patients with previous myocardial infarction. Heart 2000;83: 518–524.
5. Zoghbi WA, Farmer KL, Soto JG, Nelson JG, Quinones MA. Accurate noninvasive quantification of stenotic aortic valve area by Doppler echocardiography. Circulation 1986;73:452–459.
6. Tennant R, Wiggers CJ The effect of coronary artery occlusion on myocardial contraction Am J Physiol 1935; 12:351.
7. Gallagher KP, Matsuzaki M, Osakada G, Kemper S, Ross J Jr. Effect of exercise on the relationship between myocardial blood flow and systolic wall thickening in dogs with acute coronary stenosis. Circ Res 1983;52: 716–729.
8. Leighton RF, Nelson D, Brewster P. Subtle left ventricular asynergy with completely obstructed coronary arteries. Am J Cardiol 1983;52:693.
9. Lima JAC, Becker LC, Melin JA, et al. Impaired thickening of nonischaemic myocardium during acute regional ischaemia in the dog. Circulation 1985;71:1048–1059.
10. Marwick TH, Nemec JJ, Pashkow FJ, Stewart WJ, Salcedo EE. Accuracy and limitations of exercise echocardiography in a routine clinical setting. J Am Coll Cardiol 1992;19:74–81.
11. Armstrong WF. Exercise echocardiography: ready, willing and able. J Am Coll Cardiol 1988;11:1359–1361.
12. Limacher MC, Quinones MA, Poliner LR, Nelson JG, Winters WL Jr, Waggoner AD. Detection of coronary artery disease with exercise two-dimensional echocardiography. Circulation 1983;67:1211–1218.
13. Armstrong WF, O'Donnell J, Dillon JC, et al. Complementary value of two dimensional exercise echocardiography to routine treadmill exercise testing. Ann Intern Med 1986;105:829–835.
14. Nihoyannopoulos P, Kaski JC, Crake T, Maseri A. Absence of myocardial dysfunction during stress in patients with syndrome X. J Am Coll Cardiol 1991; 18:1463–1470.
15. Sawada SG, Segar DS, Ryan T, et al. Echocardiographic detection of coronary artery disease during dobutamine infusion. Circulation 1991;83:1605–1614.
16. Sear DS, Brown SE, Sawada SG, Ryan T, Feigenbaum H. Dobutamine stress echocardiography: correlation with coronary lesion severity as determined by quantitative angiography. J Am Coll Cardiol 1992;19:1197–1202.
17. Marwick T, Willemart B, D'Hondt A, et al. Selection of the optimal myocardial dysfunction and malperfusion. Comparison of dobutamine and adenosine using echo-cardiography and 99mTc-MIBI single photon emission computed tomography. Circulation 1993;87: 345–354.

18. Rallidis LS, Moyssakis IE, Nihoyannopoulos P. Hypotensive response during dobutamine stress echocardiography in coronary patients: a common event of well-functioning left ventricle. Clin Cardiol 1998;21:747–752.
19. Lu C, Picano E, Pingitore A, et al. Complex coronary lesion morphology influences results of stress echocardiography. Circulation 1995;91:1669–1675.
20. Elhendy A, O'Leary EL, Xie F, MvGrain AC, Anderson JR, Porter TR. Comparative accuracy of real-time myocardial contrast perfusion imaging and all motion analysis during dobutamine stress echocardiography for the diagnosis of coronary artery disease. J Am Coll Cardiol 2004;44:2185–2191.
21. Krivokapich J, Child JS, Gerber RS, et al. Dobutamine stress echocardiography for assessment of cardiac risk before non-cardiac surgery. Am J Cardiol 1993;71:646–651.
22. Reis G, Marcovitz PA, Leichtman AB, et al. Usefulness of dobutamine stress echocardiography in detecting coronary artery disease in end-stage renal disease. Am J Cardiol 1995;75:707–710.
23. Kafka H, Leach A, Fitzgibbon GM. Exercise echocardiography after coronary artery bypass surgery: correlation with coronary angiography. J Am Coll Cardiol 1995;25:1019–1023.
24. Sawada SG, Ryan T, Conley MJ, et al. Prognostic value of a normal exercise echocardiogram. Am Heart J 1990;120:49–55.
25. Underwood SR, Bax JJ, vom Dahl J, et al. Imaging techniques for the assessment of patients with chronic ischaemic heart failure. Eur Heart J 2004;25:815–836.
26. Monaghan MJ, Anderson V, Chambers J, et al. Training in echocardiography. Br Heart J 1994;71:2–5.

3

Cardiac Magnetic Resonance

Frank E. Rademakers

Over the last decade, cardiovascular magnetic resonance (CMR) has developed from an experimental technique to a clinical tool that has become the gold standard for several cardiovascular parameters, i.e., left ventricular (LV) mass, volume, and function. Improvements in hard- and software have enhanced the quality of the images, shortened the acquisition duration, and widened the applicability of the technique. Although CMR was used primarily in congenital heart disease, the differentiation of cardiac masses and angiography of the great vessels, the introduction of faster sequences for functional assessment and the use of delayed gadolinium (Gd) enhancement have put CMR in the mainstream of the imaging modalities for ischemic heart disease.

This chapter will describe the general image sequences used in cardiovascular magnetic resonance (MR) imaging and discuss the different aspects of CMR in ischemic heart disease.

1. Basic Sequences

CMR, similar to most imaging techniques, is a cross-sectional technique but with the specific advantage of free selection of slice orientation and three-dimensional (3D) capabilities. In case of the heart, which is not aligned with any of the normal body planes (sagittal, frontal or coronal, transverse or axial), this is a major advantage.

Images usually are acquired either in one or more parallel slices or as a 3D volume (which can then be resliced or displayed as a maximal intensity projection). Because the heart moves continuously throughout the cardiac cycle and with the respiration, gating for both has to be obtained. The former is accomplished through electrocardiogram (ECG) gating, the latter through breath-holding, respiratory gating, or respiratory navigator techniques.

Although real-time CMR imaging is at present feasible, temporal resolution (in comparison to echocardiography) is poor and spatial resolution still suboptimal. Presently, the necessary data (RF signal) to reconstruct an image are usually acquired over several cardiac cycles and ECG gating is mandatory (prospective or retrospective) (Figure 3.1); the quality of the ECG trace is crucial in this respect. Although the magnetic field interferes with the electrical signal of the ECG, present vector-cardiographic techniques have all but solved this problem. ECG gating can be used either to "freeze" the cardiac cycle and to obtain very high-resolution morphologic

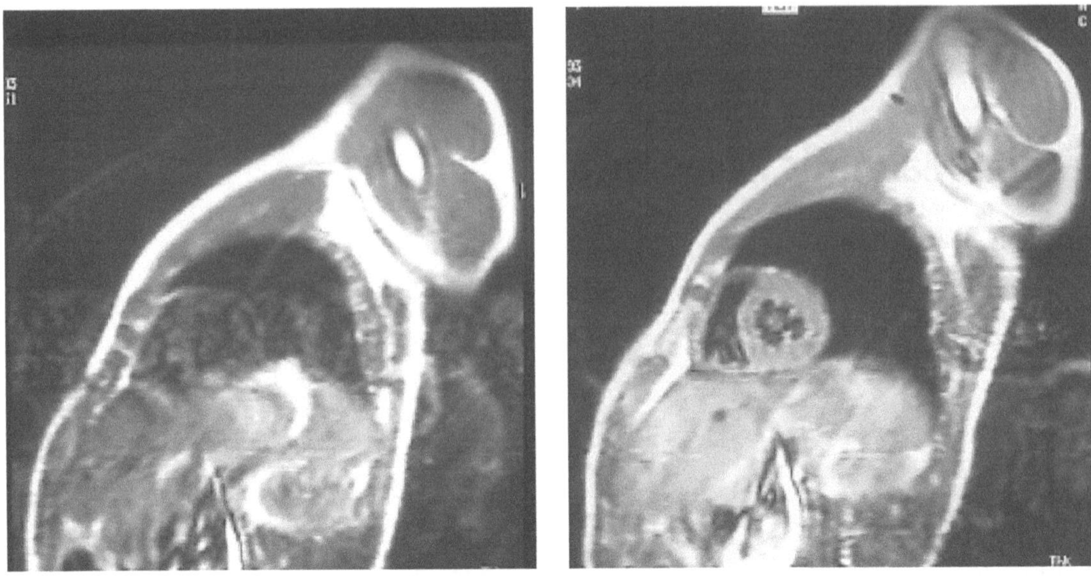

Figure 3.1. Effect of ECG triggering on image quality. Left, without ECG gating; right, with ECG gating.

images of the heart at a specific time point of the cardiac cycle or to obtain images of the same slice of the heart during the entire cycle, offering a cine mode.

With the advent of the high-resolution, high-contrast cine imaging (steady-state free precession or balanced gradient-echo, white blood), morphology and function can be analyzed using the same basic image sequence.[1,2] When morphology, however, is the primary goal (myocardial abnormalities, congenital heart disease, etc.), black blood images (breath-hold dual-inversion spin-echo) can be obtained, but with the disadvantage that one breath-hold is required for each image slice. Several adjustments have been made to these basic black and white blood image sequences to be used in perfusion, delayed enhancement, angiography, etc. (Figure 3.2).

For tissue characterization, different image sequences detailing T1, T2 (Figure 3.3), or proton density contrast can be used, often combined with the specific enhancement pattern early and late after administration of Gd contrast.

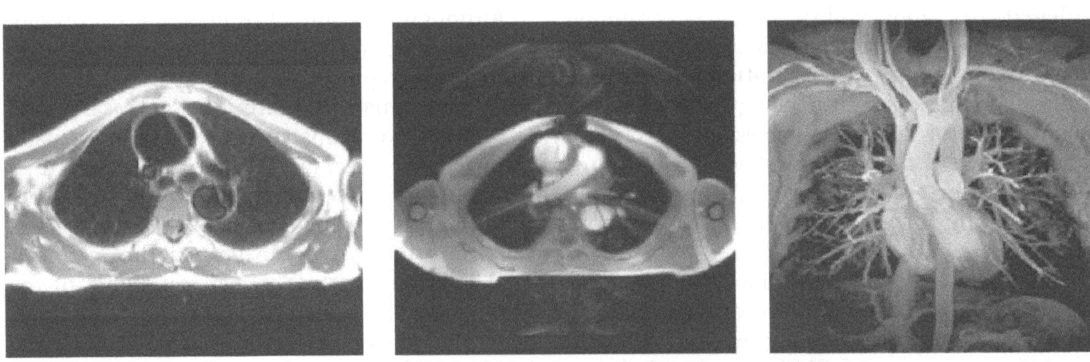

Figure 3.2. Basic image sequences: spin-echo flow void ("black") blood (left), gradient-echo inflow of relaxed spins ("bright") white blood (center), and gradient-echo contrast-enhanced 3D MR angiography (right).

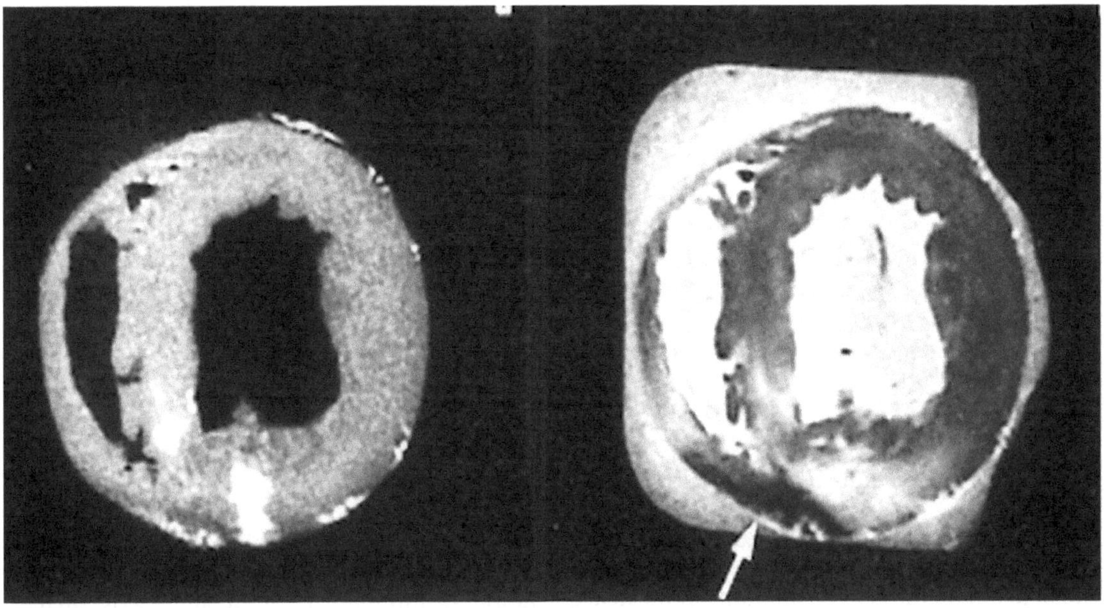

Figure 3.3. Ex vivo experimental infarction heart: T1 shows infarct area (left); T2 shows edema (right), corresponding to area at risk (notice high signal intensity of fluid in container).

Besides a map of the absolute value of MR signal (magnitude image), each MR scan also contains information about the phase of the spins in the image. Using this phase information, the velocity of the tissue in the image plane can be calculated. This can be applied to blood [yielding flow velocity (cm/s) and volume flow (mL/s), as in regular echo Doppler] (Figure 3.4)

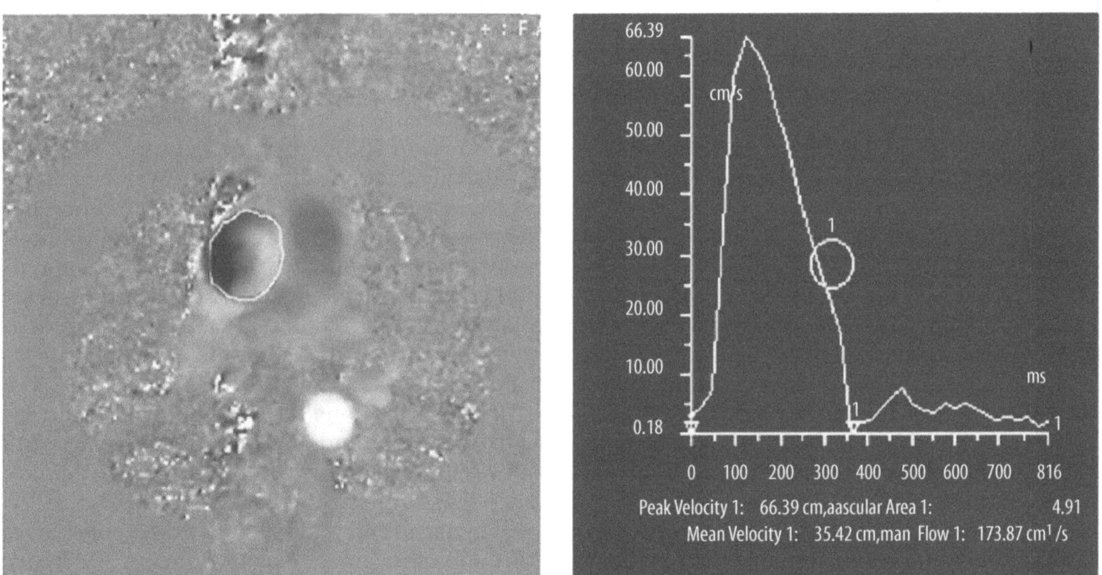

Figure 3.4. Phase image at the level of the ascending aorta (ROI indicated) with corresponding flow curve.

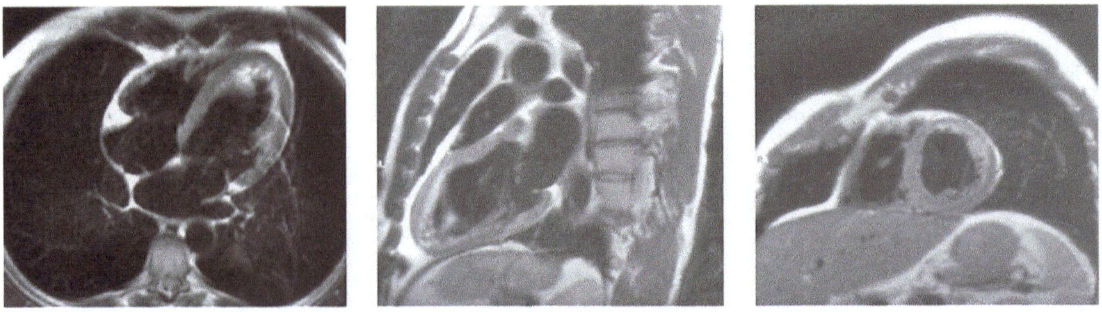

Figure 3.5. Standard images in cardiac axes: left, four-chamber view, horizontal long axis; center, atrioventricular view vertical long axis; right, biventricular view short axis.

and to the myocardium (as in tissue Doppler imaging).

A comprehensive cardiac examination will start with a localizer (in the three basic orientations) to obtain the general anatomy of the heart. From this localizer, the cardiac long axes (vertical, corresponding to the two-chamber view and horizontal, corresponding to the four-chamber view) are defined as well as the short-axis orientations (Figure 3.5), which are stacked from base to apex. Depending on the specific clinical condition or the question, any supplementary image plane can be obtained. Subsequent imaging (morphology, function, perfusion, etc.) will use these same image orientations, enabling the overlay of these different images to obtain complementary information on the same region of myocardium. A prerequisite is, however, stable breath-holding by the patient or the use of navigator techniques (acquisition of the position of the diaphragm to gate images to a narrow window of cardiac displacement with respiration).

1.1 Contraindications

A comprehensive, up-to-date list of safety issues can be obtained at Dr. Shellock's Web site (http://www.mrisafety.com/home.asp). In general, all metallic objects in the brain or eye, pacemakers, and implanted cardiac defibrillators,[3] pacing leads in the heart, are a contraindication, although patients with pacemaker have been scanned without apparent side effects.[4] Coronary stents,[5] prosthetic valves, orthopedic implants, vascular clips, sternal wires, etc., do not create problems in the acquisition and processing of the data.

2. Morphology

Morphology of the heart can be studied in great detail with CMR. Using either the black or white blood techniques, a set of short-axis images, encompassing the entire heart from above the base at the origin of the great vessels to beyond the apex, can be obtained (Figure 3.6). When acquired as a set of cine images, the end-systolic (ES) and end-diastolic (ED) time points can be identified. By contouring the endocardium of the ventricular cavities (both left and right) (Figure 3.7; see color section) and summing the different slices (taking into account slice thickness and interslice distance), the ES and ED volumes can be measured. With the excellent contrast between myocardium and blood in the cavity on balanced gradient-echo cines, this can be easily accomplished either by manual contouring or in general with computer-aided contouring. From these measurements, stroke volume (SV), ejection fraction (EF), and cardiac output (CO) are easily calculated. If also the epicardial contours of the left ventricle are obtained, the difference between the epicardial and endocardial volumes provides the myocardial volume and, when multiplied with specific myocardial density, myocardial mass. From the regional analysis of the epi- and endocardial contours, wall thickness is calculated.

Because the long axis of the heart shortens during systole and the base of the heart thus moves toward the more fixed apex, the image slice that contains the basal myocardium at ED will image the atrium at ES (the valve ring moves through the image plane during ejection). Although this is usually seen quite easily, it sometimes it is difficult to be sure which image

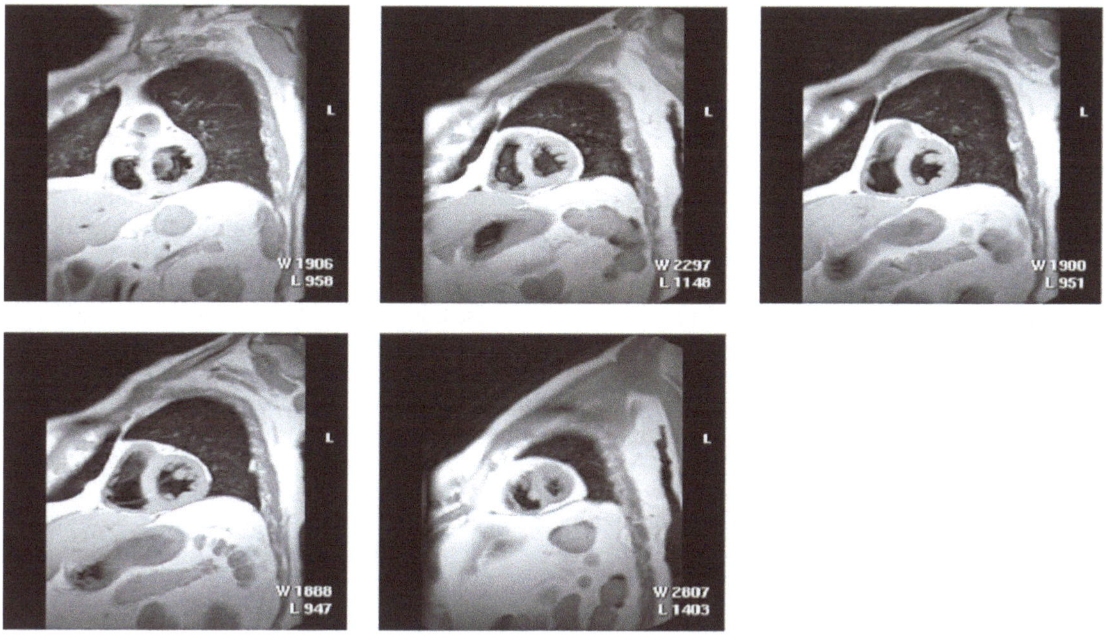

Figure 3.6. Black blood short-axis images.

planes to include and to clearly identify the mitral valve plane.[6] Near the apex, the LV wall runs obliquely to the image plane, because of the tapering of the LV apex, which can cause overestimation of myocardial wall thickness and underestimation of cavity size, secondary to the partial volume effect. To overcome both these difficulties, imaging not only the short-axis planes but also two or three long-axis planes is required; on the long-axis planes, the apical wall thickness and cavity contours are easily defined and the upper extent of the myocardium, the valve ring, and mitral or tricuspid valve itself can be identified. Although this is not yet routine clinical practice, such an integration of short- and long-axis information will further improve reliability of the morphologic and functional CMR parameters.

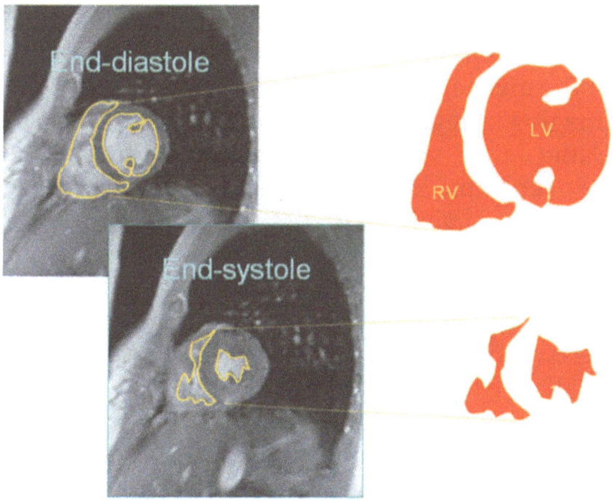

Figure 3.7. Contours of left and right ventricular cavities at end diastole and end systole.

For tissue characterization (edema,[7] infarction, scar, benign and malignant masses[8]), a combination of image sequences with and without contrast is applied. Relevant to ischemic heart disease, these make it possible to indicate the presence and extent of edema in the case of acute coronary syndromes, but also in myocarditis or related conditions, and to quantitate the presence of inflammation, acute infarction, or scar. The temporal contrast enhancement is crucial in this respect (see paragraph on perfusion and contrast enhancement). This approach has been successfully used in hypertrophic and restrictive cardiomyopathies,[9] the differentiation between ischemic and nonischemic dilated cardiomyopathies, arrhythmogenic right ventricular dysplasia, iron overload,[10,11] inflammatory syndromes (myocarditis,[12,13] sarcoidosis,[14,15] systemic lupus erythematosus, endomyocardial fibrosis, carcinoid, etc.), and cardiac transplantation.

The pericardium can be directly imaged with CMR [although calcifications are better studied with computed tomography (CT)] and the thickness measured.[16] In addition, the functional impact of pericardial disease (constrictive pericarditis) can be evaluated.

For ischemic heart disease, the overall dimensions and shape of the ventricles are important as well as regional myocardial wall thickness: a thin wall usually points to an old scar, although extensive remodeling with wall thinning can occur in hibernation with subsequent recovery of both wall thickness and function upon revascularization (infarct imaging can help with this). In addition, the presence and extent of aneurysms is easily studied; the overall dilation of the left ventricle and more spherical shape point to negative remodeling. Moreover, the excellent spatial resolution, high accuracy, and reproducibility of CMR[17,18] make it possible to use the technique for therapeutic follow-up of individual patients.[19]

Several complications of ischemic heart disease can be studied with MR: remodeling,[20,21] thrombi, rupture, pericardial effusions, valvular insufficiencies, etc.,[22] contributing to the comprehensive nature of a CMR examination for ischemic heart disease.

An experimental but possibly important application is vessel wall imaging.[23,24] Because of the small size and unpredictable motion of the coronary arteries, this is still difficult[25] but for the carotids and aorta, vessel wall characteristics as well as plaque constitution can be visualized.[26] In addition, CMR offers the potential to identify plaques and to evaluate the extent of atherosclerotic disease and more importantly to monitor the response to therapeutic interventions (diet, exercise, weight loss, statins, angiotensin-converting enzyme inhibitors, etc.).

3. Function

Global function is obtained from the morphologic studies (ED volume, ES volume, and their derived parameters, SV, EF, and CO). Regional function can be evaluated by visual assessment of regional endocardial motion or by looking at wall thickness throughout the cardiac cycle and evaluating wall thickening. In order to make a quantitative analysis of wall thickening. In order to make the papillary muscles, which were included in the myocardial mass for the morphologic examination, have to be excluded. This means that two sets of endocardial contours may be required for a combined morphologic and functional examination.[27] With the higher spatial resolution of the newer imaging techniques, the endocardial trabeculations of both left and right ventricle are clearly visible (Figure 3.8), mostly on the ED images; at ES, these trabeculations tend to converge and to fuse in a compact (thicker) ES wall. Because it is difficult to contour all these small trabeculations at ED, this can cause a small overestimation of wall thickening.

Wall thickening represents the deformation of the myocardium in the radial direction (radial strain); that is one of six different strains that completely characterize myocardial deformation. The others are circumferential and longitudinal normal strain and circumferential-radial, longitudinal-radial, and circumferential-longitudinal shear strain; the latter objectively describes the wringing or torsional motion of the LV.[28] To obtain all these different strain components, regional noninvasive markers have to be applied to the heart; this can be done with MR tagging, which puts stripes, dots, or a grid (SPAMM) (Figure 3.9) on the heart at ED so that the deformation of small regions of myocardium can subsequently be analyzed.[29,30] Although tissue doppler imaging remains the technique of choice in the assessment of heart failure patients for resynchronization therapy, the timing and extent of regional deformation as defined with MR tagging can contribute to our understanding of the mechanisms involved.[31,32] Harmonic phase imaging tagging automates the analysis.[33,34] Using the velocity information from the myocardium, deformation of the wall can also be studied,[35,36] similar to tissue Doppler imaging but in 3D.

To evaluate diastolic function, the global and regional parameters, as described above, can be measured during the diastolic phase of the cardiac cycle. Emptying volume curves, wall thinning, but also (using tagging) untwisting of the left ventricle can be studied.[37] Moreover, the different velocity and volume curves, used in echo Doppler to describe diastolic function, can

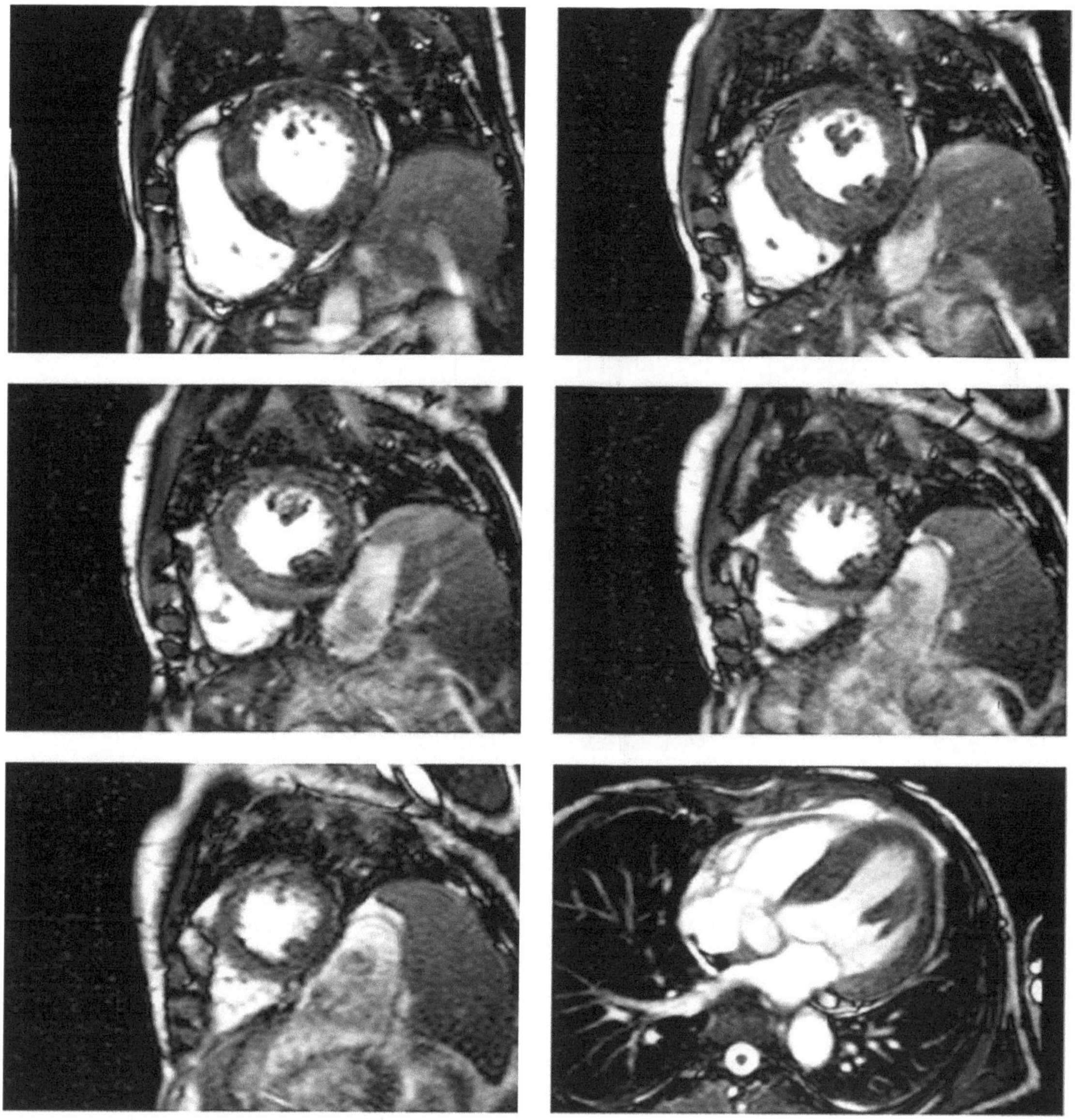

Figure 3.8. Three short-axis and one long-axis still frames illustrating the left ventricular trabeculations.

be obtained by CMR flow sequences: mitral and tricuspid inflow,[38] pulmonary vein flow, long-axis tissue velocities, etc.

All these functional parameters of myocardial performance can also be acquired during stress, either physical or pharmacologic. Because physical exercise is rather difficult in the magnet and often causes patient movement, mostly pharmacologic stress is used; just like during echo stress, increasing doses of dobutamine are applied, combined, if needed with atropine in cases of inadequate chronotropic response.[39] Because of the overall superior image quality, dobutamine stress MR (DSMR) has a better sensitivity and specificity than dobutamine ECHO studies,[40] although the use of harmonic imaging and contrast agents has improved image quality in ECHO studies. The combination with tagging offers a further advantage to quantify regional performance parameters[41] but often requires a greater experience and/or time-consuming post-processing. In general, DSMR should be used as

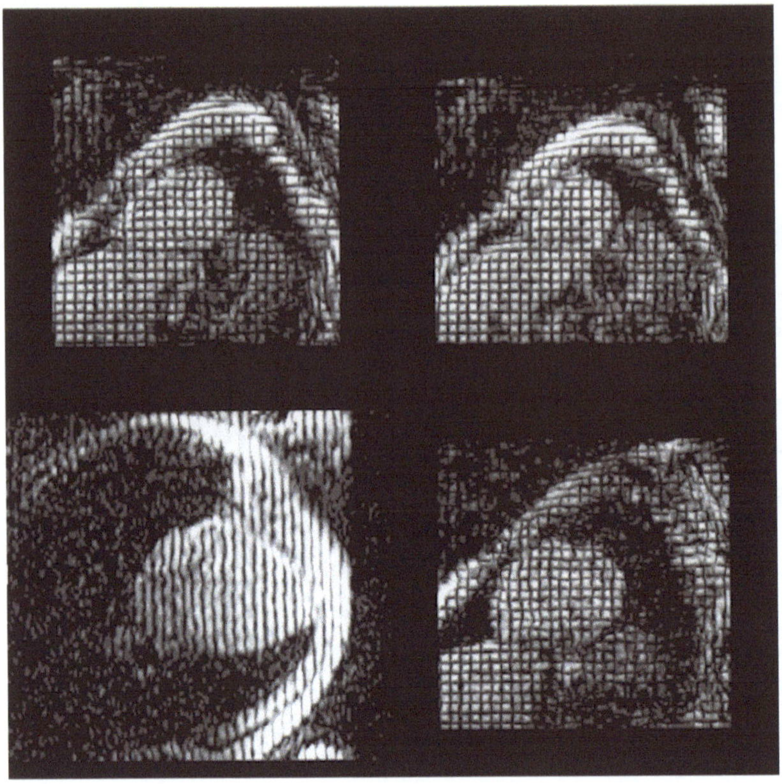

Figure 3.9. Three short-axis grid images and one long-axis line tag image of one heart.

the preferred mode of stress imaging when echo image quality is suboptimal.

The risk of complications of DSMR is similar to those of stress echo, but direct surveillance of the patient and monitoring of the ST segment on ECG are difficult. However, functional abnormalities occur earlier than ECG disturbances or angina and these functional abnormalities can be immediately seen on the CMR cine loops, which can be displayed in a quad format similar to stress echo. Personnel has to remain in the MR room during the examination to check on patient symptoms and MR-compatible equipment (monitoring: blood pressure, oxygen pulse, heart rate; first aid and defibrillator) has to be on site. Using these precautions, severe complications seldom occur.

4. Perfusion

Similar to nuclear techniques, the parameters studied with CMR contrast passage through the myocardium do not quantify perfusion, neither rate of perfusion nor capillary volume, but rather contrast content of the tissue. Special techniques or calculations are needed to obtain the true perfusion parameters as they are noninvasively studied with echo contrast imaging.

However, the intrinsic high signal-to-noise and good spatial resolution that can now be easily obtained with CMR perfusion studies, have several advantages.[42] The sequences specifically used for this purpose null the signal intensity of the myocardium before arrival of the contrast and allow the simultaneous acquisition of multiple image slices (mostly parallel short-axis images, but also long-axis images) during the first pass of the contrast through the myocardium <3 minutes. Both visual and semi-quantitative evaluation of the images is possible and differences in subendocardial versus transmural perfusion abnormalities can be seen.

To evaluate perfusion imaging, the different parameters that ultimately influence signal intensity in the image have to be understood. Contrast (Gadolinium compounds) is injected in a peripheral vein as a bolus. Because Gd is water-soluble, it readily diffuses in all tissues, including the myocardial interstitium and does not stay in the intravascular space.

4.1 First-pass Perfusion

Signal intensity (caused by shortening of T1 relaxation time by Gd) increases in the areas where Gd enters the myocardium, but this increase is not linearly related to concentration of Gd at higher doses. A low dose, 0.02–0.025 mmol kg^{-1}, is thus mandatory when quantitative analyses will be performed; a higher dose, 0.05 mmol kg^{-1}, may be more appropriate for visual interpretation (Figure 3.10).

A reason for decreased and delayed regional perfusion at rest is a severe stenosis on the cor-

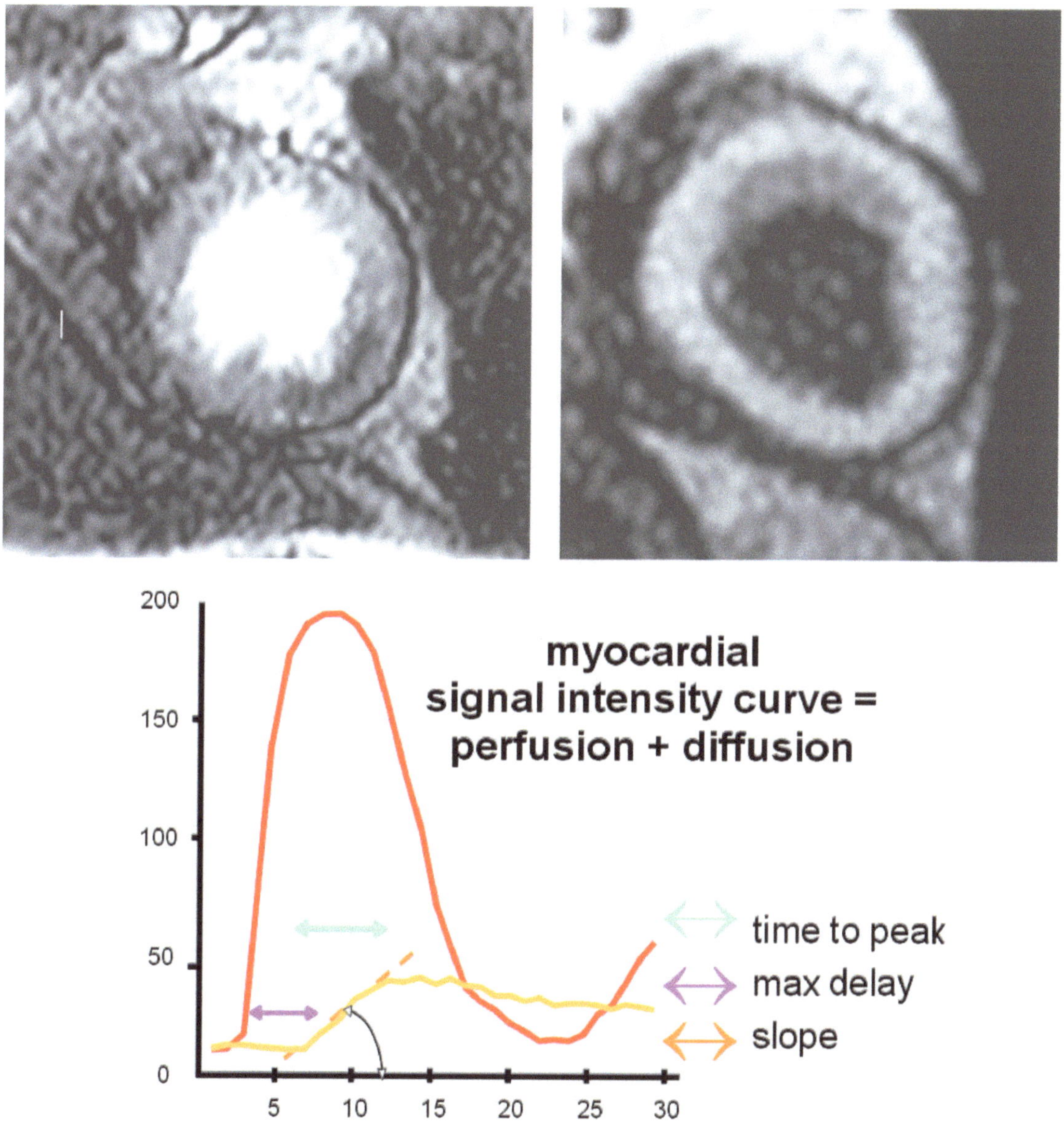

Figure 3.10. Two still frames from a first-pass perfusion study illustrating subendocardial perfusion defects in the posterior (left) and anterior (right) wall. Signal intensity (SI) curve of left ventricle (red) and myocardium (yellow). Different parameters are illustrated: time to peak SI, max SI delay of myocardial perfusion after LV, slope of inflow of contrast in myocardium.

responding coronary artery; in case of delayed perfusion alone with a later than normal but adequate peak signal intensity, a less severe stenosis is usually present. Absence of perfusion, certainly in the setting of an acute coronary syndrome points to a coronary occlusion and/or microvascular obstruction; a chronic scar after a myocardial infarction usually shows a subendocardial absence of perfusion but this is not always the case, because scar tissue may have low perfusion.

To improve interpretation, a stress study is usually required. Either adenosine or dipyridamole can be used for this purpose, but because the half-life is much shorter for adenosine this is the preferred drug in the setting of a magnet study. Infusion can best be started with the patient moved out of the magnet, because most side effects occur early. Subsequently, the patient is put back in the magnet and the perfusion study is performed during infusion of adenosine (see also Chapter 8). Normal tissue will respond to the vasodilator stimulus with a further increase in signal intensity, which can be used as a crude parameter for perfusion reserve when semiquantitative analysis is performed using the upslope of the signal intensity-time curve[43,44] or with a tracer kinetic model.[45] A moderate stenosis that has a delayed peak signal intensity at rest will show a further delay and a decrease in peak intensity during adenosine; with visual assessment, the delay is difficult to see so that the hypoenhancement during adenosine is the hallmark of a stenotic artery with decreased flow reserve. A severe stenosis, having reduced perfusion at rest without any reserve, will remain hypoenhanced during adenosine. An infarcted territory will have no perfusion at all at rest and will not change during adenosine. For the interpretation, it is also important to realize that collateral flow will contribute to the signal intensity but this will not change significantly during adenosine.

It is clear that interpretation of perfusion imaging,[46] even when image quality is very good, remains difficult and is only one piece of the puzzle to make a comprehensive interpretation using the different possibilities of CMR, including delayed infarct enhancement. Using semiquantitative analyses, parametric maps (bull's eye) can be constructed showing the areas of decreased flow reserve[47] or global abnormalities in microvascular disease.[48] Use of the difference in perfusion characteristics of subendocardium and subepicardium (where the former is more sensitive to ischemia),[49] certainly if combined with a semiquantitative analysis, further strengthens the interpretation.[50]

An alternative to contrast-based perfusion imaging is the use of blood oxygenation level-dependent (BOLD) T2* measurents.[51]

5. Delayed Contrast Enhancement

5.1 Subsequent Dynamics of Contrast

After the first pass (and diffusion) of the contrast through the myocardium, the concentration of contrast in the tissue is mainly governed by two factors: in- and outflow kinetics and the distribution volume of the contrast (Figure 3.11).

Normal (and normally perfused) tissue is characterized by a fast in- and outflow, i.e., a peak is reached early but contrast disappears relatively fast. Inflammatory myocardium (myocarditis, some systemic diseases) will show an early increase in contrast concentration, in comparison to normal tissue. In case of a stenotic artery, inflow is somewhat delayed, is slower, and removal is also slower. In case of an acute infarction, inflow is very significantly delayed and also removal is very slow. Also, the distribution volume of the contrast is higher because of cell membrane disruption. In stable infarcts (scar), the distribution volume is also higher (smaller cell/matrix volume). Finally, in the setting of an acute coronary syndrome with total occlusion of the microvasculature (often at the endocardial core of an infarct territory), hardly any contrast reaches the tissue. Using these differences in contrast kinetics and distribution volumes, typical patterns of contrast can be established.

Early after contrast administration (1–3 minutes), normal tissue has higher signal intensity than before arrival of the contrast. Inflammatory tissue is even more enhanced and depicted as white areas. Microvascular-obstructed myocardium remains black. Late after contrast administration, the contrast is washed out of the normal and inflammatory tissues but does not disappear from the acute or chronic infarct regions, which will be depicted as bright areas on a dark normal myocardium (the specific sequence used for such a delayed contrast imaging nulls the normal myocardium). In the presence of microvascular obstruction, the

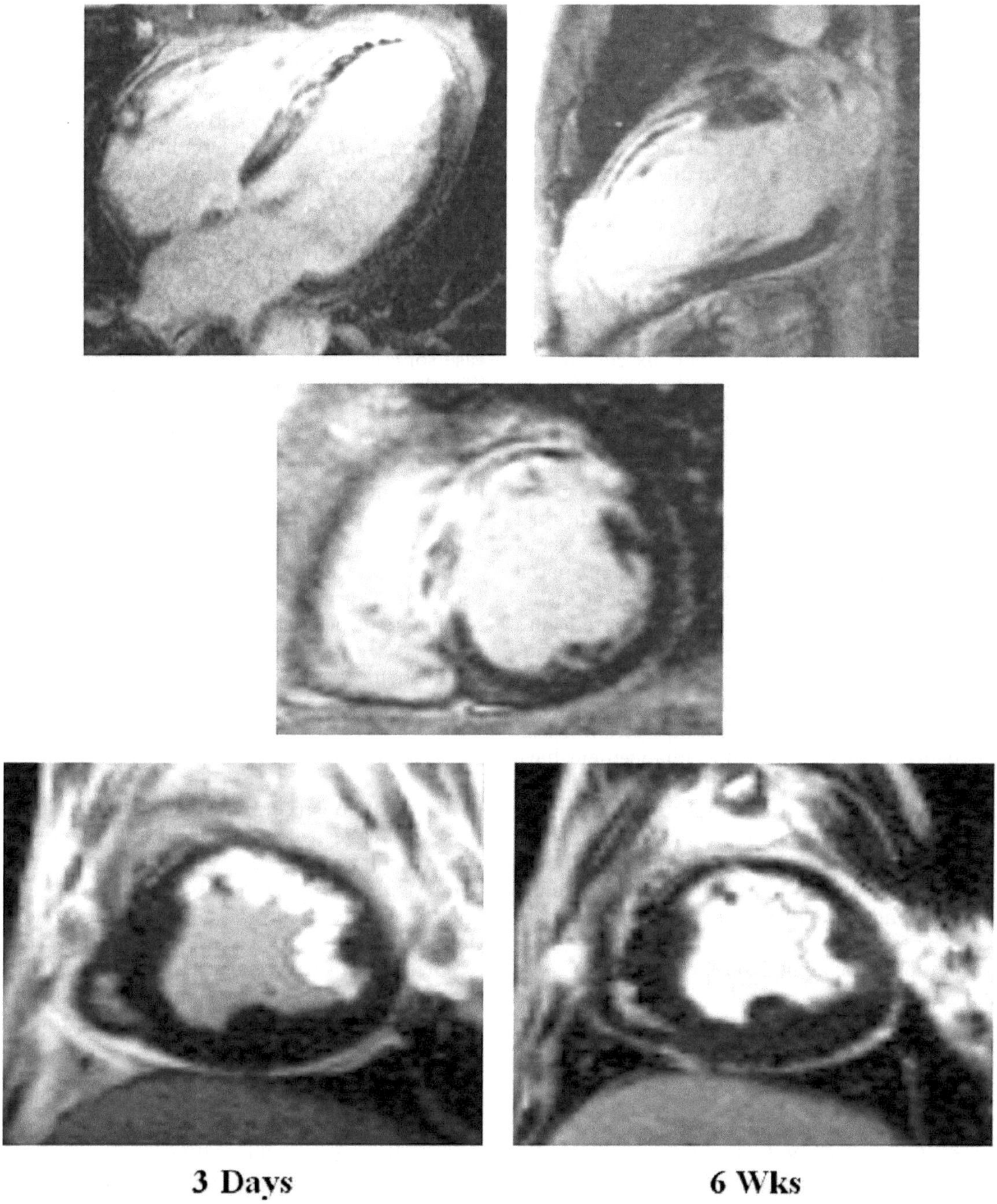

Figure 3.11. Delayed contrast enhancement of an anteroseptal infarct in the horizontal, vertical long axis and short axis (top three images). Notice dark core within region of high signal intensity corresponding to zone of microvascular obstruction in the center of the infarct. Two short-axis images illustrating the reduction of infarct size over time.

bright infarct region has a dark core that will remain darker or eventually (after 30–60 minutes) will slightly increase in signal intensity by mere diffusion of contrast. These patterns of enhancement and their correlation to pathology have been very extensively studied and validated in animal and human studies.[52–55]

This delayed contrast enhancement can thus be used to show the presence of infarcted tissue[56] (differentiating ischemic from dilated cardiomyopathy[57]) and to delineate and quantify its extent (in grams of infarcted tissue, which can be reported as a percentage of total myocardial mass).[58] By definition, all tissue that does not enhance is not dead and is therefore viable, thus making delayed enhancement a very powerful viability imaging tool.[59–61] The extent of the infarction can also be reported as a percent of the (regional) wall thickness, because of the very good spatial resolution.[62] This transmural extent is a predictor of the chances of a regional functional recovery after revascularization[63,64] or medical treatment[65] and provides additional information compared with nuclear techniques[66,67] which do not have a similar spatial resolution.[68] However, prognostic data using CMR viability are still sparse[69] compared with the wealth of information provided by radionuclide imaging.

Since the wide application of delayed enhancement with the appropriate imaging sequences, other patterns of enhancement have been described in many different disease entities, such as cardiomyopathies[70] and infiltrative disease, and probably represent an end-stage fibrotic reaction of the myocardium. Usually, the distribution and location of the enhancement (not subendocardially, crossing classic coronary territories) make it possible to differentiate these from typical ischemic infarctions.

6. Flow

Using the spin phase information, flow can be quantified with CMR. In the cardiac cavities, this can be used to measure velocities and flows at the inflow and outflow regions, to measure SV, to quantify valvular insufficiencies (regurgitant volumes and fractions) and stenoses (peak flow velocities and gradients), to quantify shunt fractions and flows in congenital heart disease,[71,72] and to analyze parameters of diastolic function.

In ischemic heart disease, the major application is the flow in the main coronary arteries, their side branches, and in bypass grafts.[73] Although technically challenging because of the small size of these vessels, the newest flow sequences are capable of quantifying flow with a reasonable temporal resolution. Systolic and diastolic flow velocities and volume flow can be measured both in basal conditions and after administration of a vasodilator-like adenosine. Coronary flow reserve can thus be calculated.

Flow can also be obtained in the coronary sinus and measured before and after vasodilatation[74] to obtain a global parameter of coronary hemodynamics which can be useful in diffuse myocardial disease, i.e., hypertensive heart disease, some cardiomyopathies, and diffuse endothelial dysfunction (normalized for myocardial mass).

Combined with myocardial perfusion, the coronary perfusion reserve can offer an insight in the status of the coronary hemodynamics. Because perfusion abnormalities are at the origin of the ischemia cascade, this could be a clinically relevant tool but this remains to be shown in larger clinical trials. Also, the relative advantage of perfusion versus functional stress studies (with dobotamiye) remains to be established.

7. Angiography

Using exogenous (Gd) contrast or the inherent contrast between flowing blood and the vessel wall, vascular structures can be imaged in great detail with CMR. This has been successfully applied to the cerebral and peripheral circulation and to the thoracic vessels.

For ischemic heart disease, however (with the exception of some abnormalities of the aorta), the clinician is interested in the coronary circulation.

The coronary arteries offer a specific challenge because of their small size, the neighboring epicardial fat, their erratic motion during the cardiac cycle which differs per coronary segment, the nature of the pathology (calcium is hypointense), and their tortuous course. Earlier attempts using repetitive 2D imaging in contiguous slices was unsatisfactory; 3D imaging using selective volumes along the course of one of the three major coronary arteries has been much more successful (Figure 3.12; see color

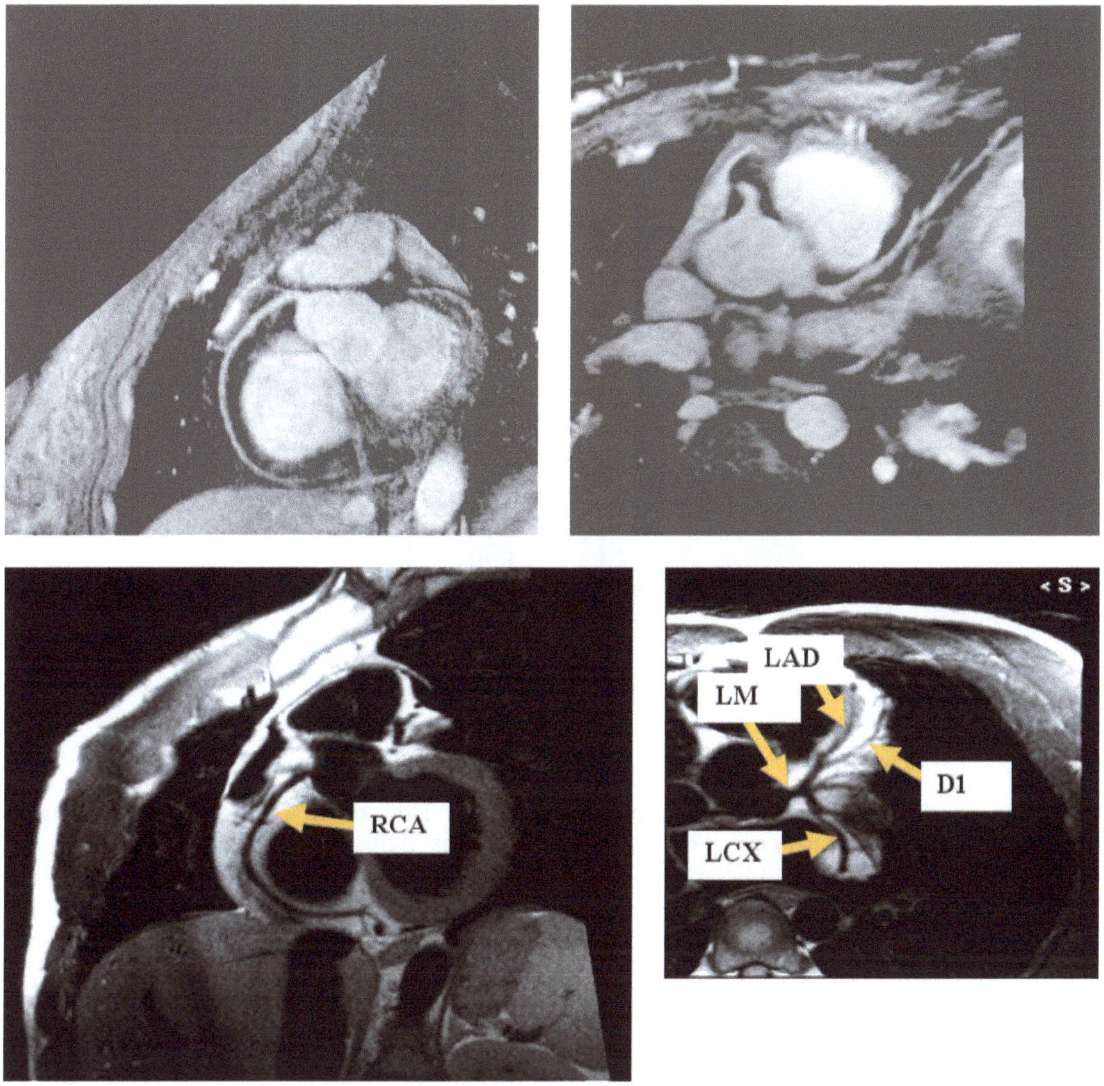

Figure 3.12. Two white (top) and two black blood (bottom) images of the right (left) and left (right) coronary arteries. LM, left main; RCA, right coronary artery; LAD, left anterior descending; LCX, left circumflex; D1, first diagonal.

section). Not only does this take care of the tortuous course of the arteries but it also makes it possible to create projection images and to postprocess the images to render the arteries in a desired format. Spatial resolution remains, however, below the resolution of X-ray angiography, and the time required for a 3D acquisition (although much shortened) still requires ECG and respiratory gating: navigator (Figure 3.13; see color section). In cases of arrhythmias and/or irregular breathing or breath-holding, image quality suffers and it remains difficult to reliably identify coronary artery stenoses and their significance. MR coronary angiography has shown a good negative predictive value in a multicenter trial but it is not yet ready for mainstream use in clinical cardiologic practice. An exception is congenital coronary abnormalities in which the 3D nature of the acquisition offers a major advantage over X-ray projection imaging to determine not only the presence of an abnormally originating artery but also its course. MR angiography is the technique of choice in this (usually) young population.[75]

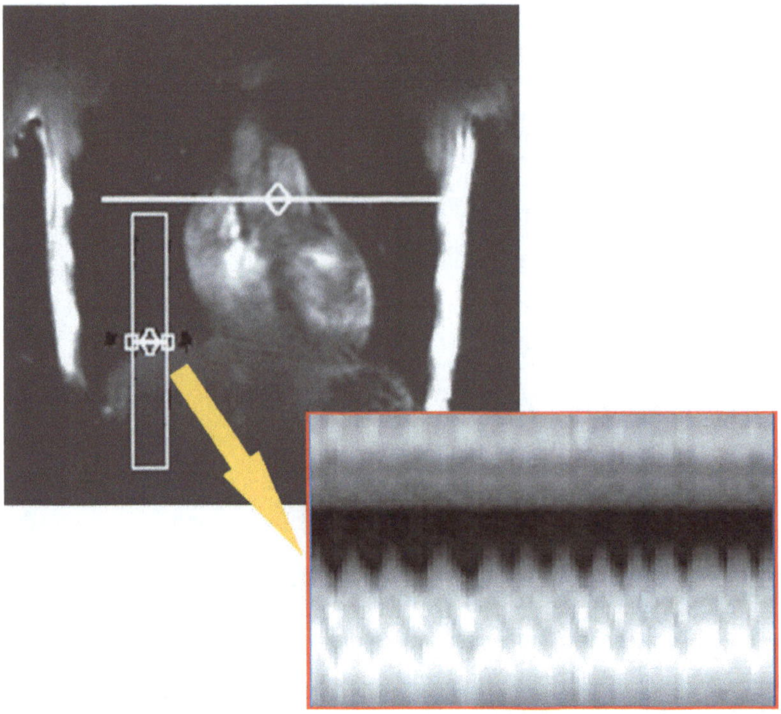

Figure 3.13. Navigator encompassing the right diaphragm and showing the respiratory motion of the diaphragm. Images are triggered to a narrow band of the diaphragmatic position to gate the respiratory motion.

Coronary artery bypass graft angiography is easier to perform[76] than native coronary imaging but its application in clinical practice where one usually also wants to visualize the native vessels, seems limited for the moment.

Whether MR coronary angiography will ever be able to compete with X-ray angiography or even CT coronary angiography remains debatable and only the future (and its evolution in hard- and software developments) will tell. It is clear, however, that a noninvasive technique that can offer not only morphologic but also functional information on the myocardium and the coronary hemodynamics could prove to be an advantage. This will require, however, a change of attitude in which showing the impact of a coronary stenosis on perfusion and function is more important for deciding to intervene than the presence and angiographic aspect of the lesion alone.

8. Spectroscopy

Although spectroscopy has the potential to give global and regional metabolic information,[77–79] its practical implementation has been very difficult. The advent of higher field strengths (3Tesla systems) with better signal-to-noise ratios and therefore better spatial resolution could overcome many of the present problems,[80] but this remains to be proven.[81]

If clinically implemented, MR spectroscopy could provide information on the energy status of the myocardium and on pH, which are important in ischemia. Further developments using other atoms[82] could provide a whole spectrum of metabolic information challenging the present possibilities offered by positron emission tomography imaging.

9. Post-processing

Because the image quality of CMR is overall excellent, information can be derived from simple visual qualitative assessment of the still frames and cines. A major advantage is also the high inter-study reproducibility which permits the follow-up of individual patients with respect to global and regional parameters of morphology and function, such as LV mass, volume, and EF. To do so, quantification of the information is necessary and most indices require the delineation of the epi- and endocardial borders of the ventricles.[83] Computer-aided contouring is presently the standard whereby the investigator identifies the cavities or roughly delineates the epi- and endocardial borders in one short-axis slice at one time point. Starting from this single slice, the information is then used to contour the other slices of the same time point and all slices of the other time points. The user can then verify the contours and, where needed, adjust them. From such a data set, a volume curve with emptying and filling parameters, LV mass, and regional wall thickening can be derived. Although the contrast between cavity and myocardium is excellent on the newer balanced gradient-echo sequences, the presence of small trabeculations, image (flow and other) artifacts, and uncertainty at the most basal and apical slices (partial volume effects and base motion) can cause some problems requiring more user interaction than hoped for. Further development in the algorithms for automated contouring and the use of both short- and long-axis information will improve this process and provide online quantification of the most important parameters.

Delineating the regions of late enhancement allows the quantification of the amount of infarcted tissue. The thickness of the image slices is crucial in this respect because thicker image slices will cause significant in-slice partial volume effects, which can lead to overestimation of infarct mass. When comparing infarct size over time in one patient or between patients, this has to be taken into account.

Perfusion analysis with the semiquantitative slope method [slope of the signal intensity of the regional myocardium during the first entrance of contrast (after passing through the left ventricle)] requires identification of the epi- and endocardial contours, which can be a challenge on some of these (lower resolution, lower contrast) images; subsequently, myocardial regions (17 segment model) have to identified as regions of interest (ROI) to measure the signal intensity over time. During the passage of contrast, however, the heart can move in and through the image plane, necessitating readjustment of the contours and ROIs at each time point (usually one per one or two cycles). Although computer-aided algorithms exist, this can require painstaking manual adjustments. From these regional perfusion analyses, parametric maps (bull's eye or other) can be constructed by comparing the patient's values with normal standards and/or by comparing rest and stress measurements (flow reserve).

A similar problem exists for flow quantification. CMR velocity encoding is presently the most accurate and reproducible noninvasive method for flow measurement, but, depending on the investigation (arterial or venous flow, valvular flow, myocardial velocities), the structure will also move in and through the image plane requiring adjustment of the ROI.

At present, a comprehensive CMR study with functional analysis, morphology, qualitative flow, and late enhancement requires about half an hour of post-processing. Adding semiquantitative perfusion, flow studies, stress examinations (dobutamine function or adenosine perfusion) will multiply this time investment, stressing the need for further automation.

10. Conclusions

CMR has become of age over the last decade and has an increasingly important role in clinical cardiology, including ischemic pathology, by the advent of faster and better sequences and by the wider use of contrast-enhanced perfusion and late-enhanced imaging.[84] The most important limiting factors for the moment are the availability of magnet time for cardiac studies both by the absolute shortage of magnets (increased use in other pathologies: neurology, gastrointestinal, orthopedics, rheumatology, etc.) and by the lack of cooperation between radiologists and cardiologists.

Because of its noninvasive nature, the absence of ionizing radiation, and side effects of the used contrast media, CMR is certainly going to have an important place among the arsenal of cardiovascular imaging modalities. Its relative importance with respect to the invasive methods, to (MS)CT, and the nuclear techniques is hard to predict but offering a comprehensive, quantifiable analysis of cardiac morphology, function, and perfusion is a major asset, which can even be applied in the setting of acute coronary syndromes.[85,86] Further automation of the post-processing is a major issue in this respect.

Future applications of CMR in ischemic heart disease involve the use of targeted CMR and interventional techniques. Binding Gd to microparticles, which can be loaded with antibodies to specific tissues or tissue components, makes it possible to selectively image these targets. Presently under investigation, clot[87]and plaque imaging are among the possible applications. Also, the selective imaging of injected stem cells is being pursued.[88,89] Interventional techniques are already being used in congenital pathologies (closure devices)[90,91] and peripheral arterial stenoses. This development requires the use of active or passive catheter tracking, the development of MR-compatible devices, and a better access to the patient in the (open or shorter bore) magnet. Drug or stem cell delivery could also be performed in the magnet but requires special sequences[92] allowing simultaneous catheter tracking, tissue, and visualization of the injected material.[93–96] Coronary interventions have also been performed mainly in animal models.[97]

Finally, the increased use of CMR on the one hand but also of pacing and defibrillator devices on the other hand should stimulate investigators and industry to develop MR-compatible stimulators and defibrillators,[98] an area presently under study.

References

1. Plein S, Bloomer TN, Ridgway JP, Jones TR, Bainbridge GJ, Sivananthan MU. Steady-state free precession magnetic resonance imaging of the heart: comparison with segmented k-space gradient-echo imaging. J Magn Reson Imaging 2001;14:230–236.
2. Thiele H, Nagel E, Paetsch I, et al. Functional cardiac MR imaging with steady-state free precession (SSFP) significantly improves endocardial border delineation without contrast agents. J Magn Reson Imaging 2001; 14:362–367.
3. Shellock FG, Tkach JA, Ruggieri PM, Masaryk TJ. Cardiac pacemakers, ICDs, and loop recorder: evaluation of translational attraction using conventional ("long-bore") and "short-bore" 1.5- and 3.0-Tesla MR systems. J Cardiovasc Magn Reson 2003;5:387–397.
4. Martin ET, Coman JA, Shellock FG, Pulling CC, Fair R, Jenkins K. Magnetic resonance imaging and cardiac pacemaker safety at 1.5-Tesla. J Am Coll Cardiol 2004; 43:1315–1324.
5. Gerber TC, Fasseas P, Lennon RJ, et al. Clinical safety of magnetic resonance imaging early after coronary artery stent placement. J Am Coll Cardiol 2003;42: 1295–1298.
6. Marcus JT, Gotte MJ, DeWaal LK, et al. The influence of through-plane motion on left ventricular volumes measured by magnetic resonance imaging: implications for image acquisition and analysis. J Cardiovasc Magn Reson 1999;1:1–6.
7. Nilsson JC, Nielsen G, Groenning BA, et al. Sustained postinfarction myocardial oedema in humans visualised by magnetic resonance imaging. Heart 2001; 85:639–642.
8. Hoffmann U, Globits S, Schima W, et al. Usefulness of magnetic resonance imaging of cardiac and paracardiac masses. Am J Cardiol 2003;92:890–895.
9. Friedrich MG. Magnetic resonance imaging in cardiomyopathies. J Cardiovasc Magn Reson 2000;2:67–82.
10. Anderson LJ, Holden S, Davis B, et al. Cardiovascular T2-star (T2*) magnetic resonance for the early diagnosis of myocardial iron overload. Eur Heart J 2001; 22:2171–2179.
11. Anderson LJ, Wonke B, Prescott E, Holden S, Walker JM, Pennell DJ. Comparison of effects of oral deferiprone and subcutaneous desferrioxamine on myocardial iron concentrations and ventricular function in beta-thalassaemia. Lancet 2002;360:516–520.
12. Friedrich MG, Strohm O, Schulz-Menger J, Marciniak H, Luft FC, Dietz R. Contrast media-enhanced magnetic resonance imaging visualizes myocardial changes in the course of viral myocarditis. Circulation 1998;97: 1802–1809.
13. Mahrholdt H, Goedecke C, Wagner A, et al. Cardiovascular magnetic resonance assessment of human myocarditis: a comparison to histology and molecular pathology. Circulation 2004;109:1250–1258.
14. Skold CM, Larsen FF, Rasmussen E, Pehrsson SK, Eklund AG. Determination of cardiac involvement in sarcoidosis by magnetic resonance imaging and Doppler echocardiography. J Intern Med 2002;252: 465–471.
15. Schulz-Menger J, Strohm O, Dietz R, Friedrich MG. Visualization of cardiac involvement in patients with systemic sarcoidosis applying contrast-enhanced magnetic resonance imaging. MAGMA 2000;11:82–83.
16. Frank H, Globits S. Magnetic resonance imaging evaluation of myocardial and pericardial disease. J Magn Reson Imaging 1999;10:617–626.
17. Bellenger NG, Burgess MI, Ray SG, et al. Comparison of left ventricular ejection fraction and volumes in heart failure by echocardiography, radionuclide ventriculography and cardiovascular magnetic resonance: are they interchangeable? Eur Heart J 2000;21:1387–1396.
18. Ioannidis JP, Trikalinos TA, Danias PG. Electrocardiogram-gated single-photon emission computed tomography versus cardiac magnetic resonance imaging for the assessment of left ventricular volumes and ejection fraction: a meta-analysis. J Am Coll Cardiol 2002;39: 2059–2068.
19. Mankad S, d'Amato TA, Reichek N, et al. Combined angiotensin II receptor antagonism and angiotensin-converting enzyme inhibition further attenuates postinfarction left ventricular remodeling. Circulation 2001;103:2845–2850.
20. Bogaert J, Bosmans H, Maes A, Suetens P, Marchal G, Rademakers FE. Remote myocardial dysfunction after acute anterior myocardial infarction: impact of left ventricular shape on regional function – a magnetic resonance myocardial tagging study. J Am Coll Cardiol 2000;35:1525–1534.
21. Groenning BA, Nilsson JC, Sondergaard L, Fritz-Hansen T, Larsson HB, Hildebrandt PR. Antiremodeling effects on the left ventricle during beta-blockade with metoprolol in the treatment of chronic heart failure. J Am Coll Cardiol 2000;36:2072–2080.
22. Mollet NR, Dymarkowski S, Volders W, et al. Visualization of ventricular thrombi with contrast-enhanced magnetic resonance imaging in patients with ischemic heart disease. Circulation 2002;106:2873–2876.

23. Worthley SG, Helft G, Fuster V, et al. Noninvasive in vivo magnetic resonance imaging of experimental coronary artery lesions in a porcine model. Circulation 2000; 101:2956–2961.
24. Botnar RM, Bucker A, Kim WY, Viohl I, Gunther RW, Spuentrup E. Initial experiences with in vivo intravascular coronary vessel wall imaging. J Magn Reson Imaging 2003;17:615–619.
25. Kim WY, Stuber M, Bornert P, Kissinger KV, Manning WJ, Botnar RM. Three-dimensional black-blood cardiac magnetic resonance coronary vessel wall imaging detects positive arterial remodeling in patients with nonsignificant coronary artery disease. Circulation 2002;106:296–299.
26. Cai JM, Hatsukami TS, Ferguson MS, Small R, Polissar NL, Yuan C. Classification of human carotid atherosclerotic lesions with in vivo multicontrast magnetic resonance imaging. Circulation 2002;106:1368–1373.
27. Sievers B, Kirchberg S, Bakan A, Franken U, Trappe HJ. Impact of papillary muscles in ventricular volume and ejection fraction assessment by cardiovascular magnetic resonance. J Cardiovasc Magn Reson 2004;6: 9–16.
28. Hees PS, Fleg JL, Dong SJ, Shapiro EP. MRI and echocardiographic assessment of the diastolic dysfunction of normal aging: altered LV pressure decline or load? Am J Physiol Heart Circ Physiol 2004;286: H782–H788.
29. Bogaert J, Maes A, Van de WF, et al. Functional recovery of subepicardial myocardial tissue in transmural myocardial infarction after successful reperfusion: an important contribution to the improvement of regional and global left ventricular function. Circulation 1999; 99:36–43.
30. Gotte MJ, van Rossum AC, Twisk JWR, Kuijer JPA, Marcus JT, Visser CA. Quantification of regional contractile function after infarction: strain analysis superior to wall thickening analysis in discriminating infarct from remote myocardium. J Am Coll Cardiol 2001;37:808–817.
31. Leclercq C, Faris O, Tunin R, et al. Systolic improvement and mechanical resynchronization does not require electrical synchrony in the dilated failing heart with left bundle-branch block. Circulation 2002;106:1760–1763.
32. Prinzen FW, Hunter WC, Wyman BT, McVeigh ER. Mapping of regional myocardial strain and work during ventricular pacing: experimental study using magnetic resonance imaging tagging. J Am Coll Cardiol 1999;33:1735–1742.
33. Garot J, Bluemke DA, Osman NF, et al. Fast determination of regional myocardial strain fields from tagged cardiac images using harmonic phase MRI. Circulation 2000;101:981–988.
34. Kraitchman DL, Sampath S, Castillo E, et al. Quantitative ischemia detection during cardiac magnetic resonance stress testing by use of FastHARP. Circulation 2003;107:2025–2030.
35. Arai AE, Gaither CC III, Epstein FH, Balaban RS, Wolff SD. Myocardial velocity gradient imaging by phase contrast MRI with application to regional function in myocardial ischemia. Magn Reson Med 1999;42: 98–109.
36. Masood S, Yang GZ, Pennell DJ, Firmin DN. Investigating intrinsic myocardial mechanics: the role of MR tagging, velocity phase mapping, and diffusion imaging. J Magn Reson Imaging 2000;12:873–883.
37. Nagel E, Stuber M, Burkhard B, et al. Cardiac rotation and relaxation in patients with aortic valve stenosis. Eur Heart J 2000;21:582–589.
38. Houlind K, Schroeder AP, Egeblad H, Pedersen EM. Age-dependent changes in spatial and temporal blood velocity distribution of early left ventricular filling. Magn Reson Imaging 1999;17:859–868.
39. Hundley WG, Hamilton CA, Thomas MS, et al. Utility of fast cine magnetic resonance imaging and display for the detection of myocardial ischemia in patients not well suited for second harmonic stress echocardiography. Circulation 1999;100:1697–1702.
40. Nagel E, Lehmkuhl HB, Bocksch W, et al. Noninvasive diagnosis of ischemia-induced wall motion abnormalities with the use of high-dose dobutamine stress MRI: comparison with dobutamine stress echocardiography. Circulation 1999;99:763–770.
41. Kuijpers D, Ho KY, van Dijkman PR, Vliegenthart R, Oudkerk M. Dobutamine cardiovascular magnetic resonance for the detection of myocardial ischemia with the use of myocardial tagging. Circulation 2003;107: 1592–1597.
42. Wilke NM, Jerosch-Herold M, Zenovich A, Stillman AE. Magnetic resonance first-pass myocardial perfusion imaging: clinical validation and future applications. J Magn Reson Imaging 1999;10:676–685.
43. al Saadi N, Nagel E, Gross M, et al. Improvement of myocardial perfusion reserve early after coronary intervention: assessment with cardiac magnetic resonance imaging. J Am Coll Cardiol 2000;36:1557–1564.
44. Doyle M, Fuisz A, Kortright E, et al. The impact of myocardial flow reserve on the detection of coronary artery disease by perfusion imaging methods: an NHLBI WISE study. J.Cardiovasc.Magn Reson 2003;5: 475–485.
45. Cullen JH, Horsfield MA, Reek CR, Cherryman GR, Barnett DB, Samani NJ. A myocardial perfusion reserve index in humans using first-pass contrast-enhanced magnetic resonance imaging. J Am Coll Cardiol 1999; 33:1386–1394.
46. Klocke FJ, Simonetti OP, Judd RM, et al. Limits of detection of regional differences in vasodilated flow in viable myocardium by first-pass magnetic resonance perfusion imaging. Circulation 2001;104:2412–2416.
47. Schwitter J, Nanz D, Kneifel S, et al. Assessment of myocardial perfusion in coronary artery disease by magnetic resonance: a comparison with positron emission tomography and coronary angiography. Circulation 2001;103:2230–2235.
48. Taskiran M, Fritz-Hansen T, Rasmussen V, Larsson HB, Hilsted J. Decreased myocardial perfusion reserve in diabetic autonomic neuropathy. Diabetes 2002;51: 3306–3310.
49. Panting JR, Gatehouse PD, Yang GZ, et al. Abnormal subendocardial perfusion in cardiac syndrome X detected by cardiovascular magnetic resonance imaging. N Engl J Med 2002;346:1948–1953.
50. Muehling OM, Wilke NM, Panse P, et al. Reduced myocardial perfusion reserve and transmural perfusion gradient in heart transplant arteriopathy assessed by magnetic resonance imaging. J Am Coll Cardiol 2003;42:1054–1060.
51. Wacker CM, Bock M, Hartlep AW, et al. BOLD-MRI in ten patients with coronary artery disease: evidence for imaging of capillary recruitment in myocardium supplied by the stenotic artery. MAGMA 1999;8:48–54.

52. Kim RJ, Fieno DS, Parrish TB, et al. Relationship of MRI delayed contrast enhancement to irreversible injury, infarct age, and contractile function. Circulation 1999; 100:1992–2002.
53. Oshinski JN, Yang Z, Jones JR, Mata JF, French BA. Imaging time after Gd-DTPA injection is critical in using delayed enhancement to determine infarct size accurately with magnetic resonance imaging. Circulation 2001;104:2838–2842.
54. Saeed M, Lund G, Wendland MF, Bremerich J, Weinmann H, Higgins CB. Magnetic resonance characterization of the peri-infarction zone of reperfused myocardial infarction with necrosis-specific and extracellular nonspecific contrast media. Circulation 2001; 103:871–876.
55. Rehwald WG, Fieno DS, Chen EL, Kim RJ, Judd RM. Myocardial magnetic resonance imaging contrast agent concentrations after reversible and irreversible ischemic injury. Circulation 2002;105:224–229.
56. Selvanayagam JB, Petersen SE, Francis JM, et al. Effects of off-pump versus on-pump coronary surgery on reversible and irreversible myocardial injury: a randomized trial using cardiovascular magnetic resonance imaging and biochemical markers. Circulation 2004; 109:345–350.
57. McCrohon JA, Moon JC, Prasad SK, et al. Differentiation of heart failure related to dilated cardiomyopathy and coronary artery disease using gadolinium-enhanced cardiovascular magnetic resonance. Circulation 2003; 108:54–59.
58. Ricciardi MJ, Wu E, Davidson CJ, et al. Visualization of discrete microinfarction after percutaneous coronary intervention associated with mild creatine kinase-MB elevation. Circulation 2001;103:2780–2783.
59. Wu KC, Lima JA. Noninvasive imaging of myocardial viability: current techniques and future developments. Circ Res 2003;93:1146–1158.
60. Shan K, Constantine G, Sivananthan M, Flamm SD. Role of cardiac magnetic resonance imaging in the assessment of myocardial viability. Circulation 2004;109: 1328–1334.
61. Kim RJ, Wu E, Rafael A, et al. The use of contrast-enhanced magnetic resonance imaging to identify reversible myocardial dysfunction. N Engl J Med 2000;343:1445–1453.
62. Mahrholdt H, Wagner A, Parker M, et al. Relationship of contractile function to transmural extent of infarction in patients with chronic coronary artery disease. J Am Coll Cardiol 2003;42:505–512.
63. Choi KM, Kim RJ, Gubernikoff G, Vargas JD, Parker M, Judd RM. Transmural extent of acute myocardial infarction predicts long-term improvement in contractile function. Circulation 2001;104:1101–1107.
64. Gerber BL, Garot J, Bluemke DA, Wu KC, Lima JA. Accuracy of contrast-enhanced magnetic resonance imaging in predicting improvement of regional myocardial function in patients after acute myocardial infarction. Circulation 2002;106:1083–1089.
65. Bello D, Shah DJ, Farah GM, et al. Gadolinium cardiovascular magnetic resonance predicts reversible myocardial dysfunction and remodeling in patients with heart failure undergoing beta-blocker therapy. Circulation 2003;108:1945–1953.
66. Knuesel PR, Nanz D, Wyss C, et al. Characterization of dysfunctional myocardium by positron emission tomography and magnetic resonance: relation to functional outcome after revascularization. Circulation 2003;108:1095–1100.
67. Wu E, Judd RM, Vargas JD, Klocke FJ, Bonow RO, Kim RJ. Visualisation of presence, location, and transmural extent of healed Q-wave and non-Q-wave myocardial infarction. Lancet 2001;357:21–28.
68. Klein C, Nekolla SG, Bengel FM, et al. Assessment of myocardial viability with contrast-enhanced magnetic resonance imaging: comparison with positron emission tomography. Circulation 2002;105:162–167.
69. Hundley WG, Morgan TM, Neagle CM, Hamilton CA, Rerkpattanapipat P, Link KM. Magnetic resonance imaging determination of cardiac prognosis. Circulation 2002;106:2328–2333.
70. Choudhury L, Mahrholdt H, Wagner A, et al. Myocardial scarring in asymptomatic or mildly symptomatic patients with hypertrophic cardiomyopathy. J Am Coll Cardiol 2002;40:2156–2164.
71. Fogel MA, Weinberg PM, Rychik J, et al. Caval contribution to flow in the branch pulmonary arteries of Fontan patients with a novel application of magnetic resonance presaturation pulse. Circulation 1999;99: 1215–1221.
72. Fratz S, Hess J, Schwaiger M, Martinoff S, Stern HC. More accurate quantification of pulmonary blood flow by magnetic resonance imaging than by lung perfusion scintigraphy in patients with Fontan circulation. Circulation 2002;106:1510–1513.
73. Bedaux WL, Hofman MB, Visser CA, van Rossum AC. Simultaneous noninvasive measurement of blood flow in the great cardiac vein and left anterior descending artery. J Cardiovasc Magn Reson 2001;3:227–235.
74. Schwitter J, DeMarco T, Kneifel S, et al. Magnetic resonance-based assessment of global coronary flow and flow reserve and its relation to left ventricular functional parameters: a comparison with positron emission tomography. Circulation 2000;101:2696–2702.
75. Taylor AM, Thorne SA, Rubens MB, et al. Coronary artery imaging in grown up congenital heart disease: complementary role of magnetic resonance and x-ray coronary angiography. Circulation 2000;101:1670–1678.
76. Brenner P, Wintersperger B, von Smekal A, et al. Detection of coronary artery bypass graft patency by contrast enhanced magnetic resonance angiography. Eur J Cardiothorac Surg 1999;15:389–393.
77. Horn M, Remkes H, Dienesch C, Hu K, Ertl G, Neubauer S. Chronic high-dose creatine feeding does not attenuate left ventricular remodeling in rat hearts post-myocardial infarction. Cardiovasc Res 1999;43:117–124.
78. Imahashi K, Kusuoka H, Hashimoto K, Yoshioka J, Yamaguchi H, Nishimura T. Intracellular sodium accumulation during ischemia as the substrate for reperfusion injury. Circ Res 1999;84:1401–1406.
79. Lamb HJ, Beyerbacht HP, van der LA, et al. Diastolic dysfunction in hypertensive heart disease is associated with altered myocardial metabolism. Circulation 1999; 99:2261–2267.
80. Neubauer S. Cardiac magnetic resonance spectroscopy. Curr Cardiol Rep 2003;5:75–82.
81. Balaban RS, Arai A. Function, metabolic, and flow heterogeneity of the heart: the view is getting better. Circ Res 2001;88:265–267.
82. Fieno DS, Kim RJ, Rehwald WG, Judd RM. Physiological basis for potassium (39K) magnetic resonance imaging of the heart. Circ Res 1999;84:913–920.

83. van der Geest RJ, Reiber JH. Quantification in cardiac MRI. J Magn Reson Imaging 1999;10:602–608.
84. Forder JR, Pohost GM. Cardiovascular nuclear magnetic resonance: basic and clinical applications. J Clin Invest 2003;111:1630–1639.
85. Kwong RY, Schussheim AE, Rekhraj S, et al. Detecting acute coronary syndrome in the emergency department with cardiac magnetic resonance imaging. Circulation 2003;107:531–537.
86. Schulz-Menger J, Gross M, Messroghli D, Uhlich F, Dietz R, Friedrich MG. Cardiovascular magnetic resonance of acute myocardial infarction at a very early stage. J Am Coll Cardiol 2003;42:513–518.
87. Winter PM, Caruthers SD, Yu X, et al. Improved molecular imaging contrast agent for detection of human thrombus. Magn Reson Med 2003;50:411–416.
88. Orlic D, Hill JM, Arai AE. Stem cells for myocardial regeneration. Circ Res 2002;91:1092–1102.
89. Kraitchman DL, Heldman AW, Atalar E, et al. In vivo magnetic resonance imaging of mesenchymal stem cells in myocardial infarction. Circulation 2003;107: 2290–2293.
90. Buecker A, Spuentrup E, Grabitz R, et al. Magnetic resonance-guided placement of atrial septal closure device in animal model of patent foramen ovale. Circulation 2002;106:511–515.
91. Rickers C, Jerosch-Herold M, Hu X, et al. Magnetic resonance image-guided transcatheter closure of atrial septal defects. Circulation 2003;107:132–138.
92. Guttman MA, Lederman RJ, Sorger JM, McVeigh ER. Real-time volume rendered MRI for interventional guidance. J Cardiovasc Magn Reson 2002;4:431–442.
93. Lederman RJ, Guttman MA, Peters DC, et al. Catheter-based endomyocardial injection with real-time magnetic resonance imaging. Circulation 2002;105: 1282–1284.
94. Dick AJ, Guttman MA, Raman VK, et al. Magnetic resonance fluoroscopy allows targeted delivery of mesenchymal stem cells to infarct borders in swine. Circulation 2003;108:2899–2904.
95. Hill JM, Dick AJ, Raman VK, et al. Serial cardiac magnetic resonance imaging of injected mesenchymal stem cells. Circulation 2003;108:1009–1014.
96. Garot J, Unterseeh T, Teiger E, et al. Magnetic resonance imaging of targeted catheter-based implantation of myogenic precursor cells into infarcted left ventricular myocardium. J Am Coll Cardiol 2003;41:1841–1846.
97. Spuentrup E, Ruebben A, Schaeffter T, Manning WJ, Gunther RW, Buecker A. Magnetic resonance-guided coronary artery stent placement in a swine model. Circulation 2002;105:874–879.
98. Duru F, Luechinger R, Scheidegger MB, Luscher TF, Boesiger P, Candinas R. Pacing in magnetic resonance imaging environment: clinical and technical considerations on compatibility. Eur Heart J 2001;22: 113–124.

4

Myocardial Perfusion Scintigraphy

Albert Flotats and Ignasi Carrió

Coronary atherosclerosis determines an altered vasoreactivity to vasodilator stimuli. As a result, impaired coronary flow reserve is one of the earliest signs of coronary artery disease (CAD), which can be assessed scintigraphically.

Myocardial perfusion scintigraphy (MPS) involves intravenous (IV) administration of a small quantity of a radioactive substance, which is avidly extracted by the myocardium in relation to myocardial blood flow (MBF) and viability. Images showing myocardial regional distribution of radioactivity are subsequently obtained, and relative MBF differences are detectable. If there is a decrease in relative regional perfusion, as seen in hemodynamically significant CAD, or loss of cell viability, as seen in myocardial infarction (MI), a reduced signal is collected scintigraphically. Usually, MPS is performed at rest and during some form of cardiovascular stress. Absence of uptake on stress images may represent areas of significantly decreased flow or areas without viable myocardium. Persistent or fixed defects on resting or baseline images depict scar. Complete defect resolution represents viable myocardium rendered ischemic during stress. Partial defect resolution is observed in areas with a mixture of scar and ischemia.

The diagnosis of CAD remains a common application of MPS, but it is increasingly being used for prognosis assessment in patients with known CAD, and for selection for revascularization and assessment of suspected acute coronary syndromes (ACS).

1. Principles of Radionuclide Imaging

Radionuclide imaging is based on the introduction into the organism of a substance with unstable atoms which emit photons, usually gamma rays and/or X-rays, when the nucleus of these atoms change from one energy level to a lower one. Thus, the body is imaged "from the inside out" by recording the distribution of radioactivity coming from internally administered radionuclides using special devices.

Radiopharmaceuticals are radionuclides that, combined or not with a chemical molecule, meet legal requirements for being administered to subjects. Radiopharmaceuticals are also known as tracers or radiotracers because they have specific organ location and no functional consequences (when given for diagnostic purposes), allowing studying or following a process without disturbing it. The radionuclide fraction of the radiopharmaceutical permits external detection, and the chemical portion is responsible for the biodistribution. For a few agents, the radionuclide itself confers the desired location properties to the radiopharmaceutical.

1.1 Gamma Scintillation Camera or Anger Camera

The scintillation camera is a device capable of detecting the radioactivity coming from organs containing radiotracers, allowing the temporal and spatial location required to generate scintigraphic images. The gamma camera consists of a radiation detector, a signal processor/event locator, and an image recording system.[1]

The detector is made from transparent sodium iodide crystal containing thallium impurities (thallium-activated sodium iodide crystal – NaI[Tl]). When gamma or X-rays enter the crystal, they impart energy to the electrons of the crystal, which give off photons of light to return to the baseline state.[1]

NaI[Tl] crystals are relatively inexpensive and afford great flexibility in size and shape. They have a good stopping power (complete energy absorption of radiation arising from the crystal) at the energy range of radiation used in clinical nuclear medicine (70–364 keV, optimally at 100–200 keV range).[2] However, they are fragile and highly hydroscopic, requiring air-tight hermetical containers, which usually consist of thin aluminum on three sides and quartz on the fourth side. This quartz window permits the light photons to reach and interact with the photocathode of a photomultiplier tube (PMT), dislodging some electrons, which are subsequently accelerated by a series of electrodes (dynodes) at gradual higher potential. As electrons are accelerated toward each dynode, they gain sufficient kinetic energy to eject several electrons at impact, with increasing the number of electrons finally collected at the anode of the PMT.[1] The multiplication factor is approximately 3–6 per dynode stage and up to several million overall. All these components are mounted on a platform made of lead or tungsten to shield them from stray radiation.

The electrical output is further amplified and the voltage pulse is processed through positioning and energy circuitries. The positioning circuitry determines the spatial location of the radiation event detected (X and Y pulses), and the energy circuitry calculates the energy deposited in the crystal (Z pulse). The location of the event in the crystal is estimated so that each tube may be thought of as having X and Y coordinates in a cartesian plane. Tubes closest to the event collect the greatest number of light photons, with lesser contributions for more remote tubes. Additionally, the output from all of the PMTs is summed and referred to as the Z pulse, which through a pulse height analyzer is used to determine whether the detected event is within the desired energy range and should be accepted in the formation of the image or whether it is of lower or higher energy and should be discriminated against and rejected.

The height of the electrical pulse recorded is proportional to the energy of the radiation initially dissipated in the crystal.[1,2] This allows discrimination between photons directly coming from the organ of interest without any previous disturbance (primary photons) and those that have undergone scatter before detection (secondary photons, less energetic than the primary photons, with lower pulse heights). Additionally, this permits distinction of radiation coming from different radionuclides, with different energies.

For image generation, only primary photons with completely perpendicular direction to the crystal detector need to be registered. Registration of secondary photons is restricted by the pulse height analyzer with an energy window setting (usually symmetrically centered at the energy peak of the radionuclide being used), and by placement of a collimator in front of the crystal detector.

The collimator is a lead foil with multiple and uniformly distributed holes, which limits the interaction of the radiation photons with the crystal to only those photons traveling parallel to the longitudinal axes of the holes, selectively absorbing the photons that strike obliquely.[1]

1.2 Creation of the Digital Image

When a radiation event is accepted for storage, it is recorded using an analog-to-digital converter on dedicated computer systems. Data recorded may be thought of as superimposed on a grid or matrix of pixels, where each X and Y pairs determine the coordinates of the event location. Each pixel of the matrix has a number corresponding to the total events accumulated during the acquisition period. The larger the matrix, the better the spatial resolution but the longer the time required to achieve adequate counting statistics in each pixel.[3] Most studies in cardiac current practice are obtained in a 64×64 or 128×128 matrix.

If time information is desired, additional time markers such as the R wave on the electrocardiogram (ECG) can be used to synchronize data collection as in gated cardiac studies. Each R-R interval is divided into a preset number of subintervals, usually 8–16. The R wave triggers data acquisition into a frame corresponding to the first subinterval. At the end of each subinterval time, data collection is switched to a frame corresponding to the next subinterval time. A new R wave will restart the cycle with data collection into the first frame of the series. The sum of data collected over several hundred cardiac cycles generates a series of images that represents a single, average cycle (representative cycle), which allows the survey of cardiac function and the assessment of wall thickening and motion when reviewed in cinematic mode. However, the presence of a fairly regular cardiac rhythm is essential.[4,5]

1.3 Data Analysis and Display

Several types of analyses can be applied to digitized images and a variety of calculations on the pixels in a "region of interest" can be performed, including the area, the total count, maximal and minimal counts, and the average counts per pixel.

With the development of computers, these devices have gained an integral role not only for image acquisition and processing but also for image management.

2. MPS Radiopharmaceuticals

Characteristics of the ideal radiopharmaceutical for MPS are summarized in Table 4.1. Currently available photon emission tracers used for MPS are divided into two groups: thallium-201 (^{201}Tl) and technetium-99m (^{99m}Tc) labeled agents.

2.1 Thallium-201

Thallium is a metallic element in group III-A of the periodic table of elements. The isotope 201 of thallium is generated in cyclotron. ^{201}Tl has a physical half-life of 73 hours and a main radioactive energy of emission of 69–83 keV (88% abundance). It is administered in the form of thallous chloride. The initial myocardial uptake of ^{201}Tl after IV administration depends on both MBF and the myocardial extraction fraction for ^{201}Tl.[6–8] Under conditions of normal flow, approximately 85% of ^{201}Tl is removed by myocardium in a single pass. Because myocardium receives 5% of the cardiac output, 4% of the total dose is taken up by myocardium (Table 4.2). ^{201}Tl myocardial uptake is proportional to regional perfusion over a wide range of flow rates. However, as flow increases, more of the tracer passes through the capillary without being extracted and will reach a plateau when flow is increased >3.5–4 times the baseline values (Figure 4.1).[9] Therefore, the uptake of ^{201}Tl at high flow rates underestimates the true

Table 4.1. Characteristics of the ideal radiopharmaceutical for MPS

Myocardial uptake in proportion to blood flow over the range of values experienced in health and disease
Efficient myocardial extraction from the blood on the first passage through the heart
Stable retention within the myocardium during image acquisition
High photon flux at an energy between 100 and 200 keV and short half-life
Rapid elimination allowing repeat studies under different conditions
Ready availability
Low cost

Table 4.2. Characteristics of major myocardial perfusion agents

	^{201}Tl	^{99m}Tc-sestamibi	^{99m}Tc-tetrofosmin
Class	Element	Isonitrile	Diphosphine
Charge	Cation	Cation	Cation
Preparation	Cyclotron	Kit boiling	Kit room temperature
Cellular uptake	Active	Passive	Passive
Average first-pass extraction fraction	0.73	0.39	0.24
Myocardial uptake at rest (%)	4	1	1.2
Flow limitation (mL/g/min)	3	2	1.5
Myocardial clearance	$t_{1/2}$ ~ 6 h	Minimal at 5 h	Minimal at 3 h
Redistribution	Significant	Minimal	None
Blood pool, initial t_ (min)	5	2.2	<5
Excretion	Renal	Hepatobiliar + renal	Hepatobiliar + renal
Liver uptake	+	+++	++
Heart-to-liver ratio at exercise (20 min p.i.)	2.6	0.65	1.2
Heart-to-liver ratio at rest (20 min p.i.)	1.4	0.5	0.78
Heart-to-lung ratio at exercise (30 min p.i.)	2.3	2.3	5.9
Start imaging time (min)	<15	>30	15
Gated SPECT	+/−	+	+
Viability assessment	Yes	Yes	Yes
Effective dose equivalent	1.6 rem/2 mCi	1.1 rem/30 mCi	0.8 rem/30 mCi

Source: Modified from Narula et al.[9]
p.i., postinjection.

myocardial flow. Additionally, at very low flow rates, the ^{201}Tl extraction fraction efficiency increases in viable cardiomyocytes because ^{201}Tl spends more time in contact with the capillary membrane, resulting in higher extraction. More than 60% of myocardial ^{201}Tl uptake occurs via the Na^+, K^+–adenosine triphosphatase active transport membrane pump, thus it cannot be removed by nonviable cardiomyocytes.[2,10]

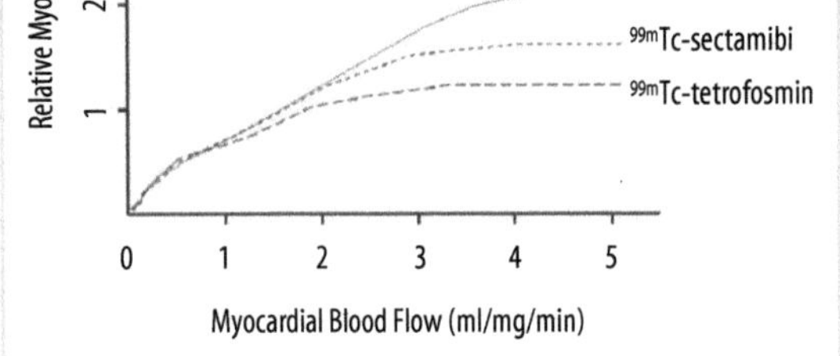

Figure 4.1. A diagrammatic representation of the relationship between myocardial uptake of different myocardial perfusion agents and MBF. [Modified from Narula et al.[9]]

Maximum myocardial ^{201}Tl uptake occurs at 10–20 minutes after IV injection, which correlates with rapid clearance of the tracer from the blood pool. The half-life of elimination from myocardium is approximately 7 hours. ^{201}Tl is principally excreted by the renal system, having a biological half-life of approximately 10 days.

There is a dynamic changing (redistribution) between the intracellular and intravascular content of ^{201}Tl along time. MPS performed early after injection reflects the MBF conditions at the time of ^{201}Tl administration. However, after the initial cellular extraction phase, ^{201}Tl continually exchanges between both compartments to meet the equilibrium. Thus, images obtained several hours after remaining at rest reflect resting MBF conditions. Redistribution results from combined effects of differential myocardial ^{201}Tl washout, which is proportional to the rate of MBF, and late ^{201}Tl uptake in hypoperfused but still viable myocardium.[2,10] Once the exercise test has been completed, image acquisition should commence within 5–10 minutes of injection, as soon as the patient's heart rate has returned to near baseline values. This prevents motion artifacts caused by the shifting position of the heart during the period of image acquisition secondary to the different amplitude of diaphragmatic excursion while recovering from the exertion ("upward creep" phenomena) and at the same time minimizes ^{201}Tl redistribution. This short delay also maximizes the ability to detect transient left ventricular dysfunction.

The major limitation of MPS with ^{201}Tl is the absence of an ideal photopeak of energy emission, which results in poor-quality images in obese patients and problems in distinguishing attenuation artifacts from defects caused by underlying CAD. Moreover, imaging must be performed very close to the stress testing because of redistribution, which also precludes repetition of image acquisition when artifacts appear.[10]

2.2 ^{99m}Technetium-labeled Agents

^{99m}Tc has become the most frequently used radionuclide for clinical imaging because of its availability, the energy characteristics (140 keV) of its principal emission, and its favorable dosimetry that is related to its short half life.

^{99m}Tc is obtained from ^{99}molybdenum (^{99}Mo)/^{99m}Tc generator systems, which consist of a longer-lived radionuclide parent (^{99}Mo, physical half-life of 66 hours), practical for the commercial shipment, and a shorter-lived radionuclide daughter (^{99m}Tc, physical half-life of 6 hours), useful for clinical applications.

^{99}Mo, produced by the fission reaction of ^{235}Uranium, is chemically purified and passed on to an anion exchange column of alumina, which binds the ^{99}Mo ions. The column is placed in a lead container with tubing attached at each end. Elution of the column with normal saline solution through a vacuum system provides ^{99m}Tc-pertechnetate. The amount of ^{99m}Tc available from a generator decreases each day as a result of decay of the ^{99}Mo parent. However, the long physical half-life of ^{99}Mo permits the same generator to be used for at least 1 week.

The short physical half-life of ^{99m}Tc allows the administration of 10-fold-larger doses of ^{99m}Tc-radiopharmaceuticals than of ^{201}Tl. Moreover, because of the energy of the gamma rays given off by ^{99m}Tc, its photons experience less scatter and attenuation than photons emitted by ^{201}Tl, which results in superior image quality.

Commercially available ^{99m}Tc agents for MPS include sestamibi (hexakis 2-methoxyisobutyl isonitrile) and tetrofosmin (1,2-bis[bis(2-ethoxyethyl) phosphino]ethane). ^{99m}Tc-sestamibi is a monovalent cation in which ^{99m}Tc is surrounded by six isonitrile ligands. ^{99m}Tc-tetrofosmin is a diphosphine. Both are prepared from a kit, but only the former requires boiling for labeling. Both agents are lipophilic cations that passively diffuse into cardiomyocytes along an electropotential gradient and are actively trapped in mitochondrias. Myocardial fixing after injection depends on both MBF and mitochondrial retention. Myocardial extraction fraction is approximately 30% in a single pass under conditions of normal MBF, lower than that of ^{201}Tl (Table 4.2).[9] As with ^{201}Tl, myocardial uptake experiences a similar roll-off phenomenon, which occurs at lower high rates of MBF, when flow increases >2.5 times the baseline values. Additionally, flow is also overestimated at low flow rates (Figure 4.1).[8,9] ^{99m}Tc agents are cleared from the blood rapidly, with hepatobiliary and renal excretion, without being secondarily released back into the blood (minimal or null redistribution). Uptake in myocardium is also rapid, but imaging requires a long delay in order to allow adequate hepatobiliary clearance of the tracer. The required imaging time after ^{99m}Tc-tetrofosmin and ^{99m}Tc-sestamibi injection is ≥10–15 minutes for exercise studies, ≥30–45 minutes for rest studies, and 45–60 minutes for pharmacologic stress studies. Because there is minimal redistribution, images can be obtained several hours after tracer injection depending on the laboratory logistics. Likewise, image acquisition can be repeated with no repercussion on image quality when artifacts are considered to be responsible for the production of a perfusion defect. The absence of redistribution, however, requires injection of tracer twice, once during stress and once at rest.[10,11]

3. Image Acquisition

Planar and tomographic imaging can be performed. Comparative studies between both methodologies showed substantially higher sensitivity with tomography for the detection of CAD. Nevertheless, the prognostic power of a normal planar scintigraphy is excellent, suggesting that the coronary lesions missed by this modality may not be prognostically significant.

3.1 Planar Imaging

Planar imaging is a two-dimensional (2D) image representation of the 3D distribution of an emitting radiation body. This compression of a 3D image into a 2D one containing the radioactivity coming from above and below the organ being imagined (background activity) results in a reduction of contrast, with decreased ability to discriminate between areas of a specific organ with normal and abnormal radioactivity count levels.

Heart anatomy is sufficiently simple to allow planar imaging to assess the location and extent of defects from several projections (or views) without need of computer reconstruction. In fact, planar imaging has good resolution and it can be the solution for patients unable to remain immobile during longer acquisition times, which is essential for single photon emission computed tomography (SPECT) studies, or for those who are very obese. An advantage of planar imaging is that a scan can be quickly repeated if the patient moves during the acquisition.

In planar MPS, it is crucial to reproduce the same position on initial and delayed images. The standard planar views are supine anterior, supine 45° left anterior oblique, and a right side decubitus 90° left lateral. The 90° left lateral view is difficult to reproduce and can be substituted by the supine 70° left anterior oblique position, which frequently is suboptimal because of occurrence of attenuation artifacts.[12,13]

In ECG gated acquisition, no beat rejection should be used in order to preserve statistical counting, because the multiple frames (usually 16) of the gated images can be summed to produce a single static planar image for conventional visual and quantitative analysis of myocardial perfusion.

Image acquisition begins by setting the energy window size. For ^{99m}Tc agents, it is symmetrically centered to 20% of 140 keV, and for ^{201}Tl to 30% of 72 keV and 167 keV. Images should contain >500 000 counts per view, which takes approximately 10 minutes for ^{201}Tl and 5 minutes for ^{99m}Tc agents. When ECG gating is used, imaging time increases by approximately 3 minutes.

3.2 SPECT Imaging

SPECT is a method that uses photon emission radionuclides for producing image sections of the body displayed as 2D images. It is considered the state-of-the-art for MPS, and it is based on a computer collection of multiple planar images obtained by the rotating scintillation detector, 180° or 360° around an underlying radiation emitting body. Transaxial, sagittal, and coronal slices are generated by computer from the 3D distribution of the tracer in the body, thus removing overlying structures that may obscure an abnormality, improving image contrast.[14] The resolution in SPECT is determined by the same mechanisms as in planar images: the collimator, the photon energy, the distance from the source to the detector, and the duration of the acquisition.

Usually, SPECT is performed with the patient lying in the supine position with elevation of the left arm above the head. Prone imaging can be added when doubts arise about possible diaphragmatic and/or breast/lateral chest-wall fat attenuation (Table 4.3).

Energy window setting is the same as that used in planar imaging. On systems with improved energy resolution, window size could be reduced, resulting in decreased scatter and improved image resolution, but increasing imaging times. ^{201}Tl SPECT uses low-energy parallel hole collimators of high sensitivity (all-purpose collimators, LEAP), whereas ^{99m}Tc agents SPECT use low-energy parallel hole collimators of high resolution (LEHR). LEHR collimators have longer bores, thinner septa, and smaller holes, as compared with LEAP collimators, which provide better resolution at the expense of reduced sensitivity.

Matrices of 64 × 64 pixels, with pixel size of 6.4 ± 0.2 mm, offer sufficient contrast and resolution for cardiac SPECT imaging. An orbit of 180° (from the 45° right anterior oblique to the 45° left posterior oblique) yields better contrast and spatial resolution and less attenuation than an orbit of 360°, because of avoiding the noise coming from the posterior projections in which the heart is fairly distant to the detector. Orbits of 360° yields better field uniformity, and for multiple detector systems, may generate similar image quality as 180° once scatter, attenuation, and variable resolution effects are corrected. Circular orbits have been widely used, although maintenance of a fixed radius of rotation results in the detector not being close to the patient, with worse spatial resolution. Recently, noncircular orbits have proliferated in conjunction with attenuation correction algorithms. Patient-contoured orbits bring the detector closer to the heart, improving spatial resolution. However, the potential of artifact production at reconstruction exists because of higher variation in spatial

Table 4.3. Image variants and artifacts of myocardial SPET with presumed explanation

Image variants and artifacts	Presumed explanation
1. Apical defect	Physiologic "apical thinning" (exaggerated by attenuation correction and elliptical orbits)
2. Basal septal defect	Physiologic membranous tissue in atrioventricular valve plane
3. Fixed/reversible anterior and/or lateral defect	Attenuation by the left breast/lateral chest wall fat
4. Fixed inferior or inferolateral defect	Attenuation by the left hemidiaphragm (mainly in men)
5. Diffusely reduced myocardial uptake	Normalization to noncardiac maximal activity
6. Fixed/reversible defects confined to the septum	LBBB causes asynchronous relaxation of the septum, resulting in shortened diastolic myocardial perfusion period in this region
7. Fixed basal inferolateral defect	Depth-dependent attenuation in obese patients
8. Anteroseptal and inferoseptal linear defects	Attenuation at the insertion points of the free wall of the RV ("11 and 7 o'clock defects"). The 11 o'clock defect is usually more marked in circular acquisition orbits of 180°
9. Opposed defects in contralateral walls	Flood field nonuniformity Errors in center of rotation Camera head tilt in multidetector systems Immediate postexercise aquisition ("upward creep") Patient motion (>2 pixels)
10. Basal defects and apical hot spot	Truncation Localized apical hypertrophy
11. Anterior defect and normal/increased inferior uptake	Scatter from subdiaphragmatic tracer accumulation artifactually increases inferior wall count density, which is erroneously taken as the reference region for image normalization (exaggerated by attenuation correction)
12. Inferior defect and increased anterior uptake	Intense subdiaphragmatic activity adjacent to the inferior wall, which is removed together with count density of the inferior wall when ramp-filtering
13. Loss of detail and contrast resolution	Increased detector-to-patient distance Decreased critical frequency of processing filter
14. Excessive noise	Decreased count density Increased critical frequency of processing filter
15. Decrease in the lateral-to-septal wall tracer activity	LV hypertrophy
16. Hot spots in the anterolateral and inferolateral walls	Hypertension with hypertrophy of papillary muscles

LV, left ventricle; LBBB, left bundle branch block; RV, right ventricle.

resolution resulting from the increased variation of source-to-detector distance.[12,14,15]

Often, the detector acquires photons throughout the orbit at preselected angles while motionless for a predetermined time, after which the detector moves to the next angular position, in a tomographic acquisition mode called "step-and-shoot." No counts are recorded as the detector moves. This process is repeated until the total number of preselected views is acquired. The optimal number of views depends on matching the number of projections to the resolution of the system. For ^{201}Tl SPECT studies, which are acquired using LEAP collimators and thus having relatively low resolution, 30 projections over an orbit of 180° are sufficient. For higher-resolution studies, such as those with ^{99m}Tc agents, acquired using LEHR collimators, ≥60 projections over an orbit of 180° are required to prevent loss of resolution.[2,12,13,16] Double number of projections is necessary when imaging throughout 360° orbits. Less widespread mode is "continuous" acquisition, for which the detector moves continuously while collecting photons, which allows increase of the number of collected counts for the same whole acquisition time. However, there is some spatial resolution loss associated with this "continuous" acquisition. A third mode is "continuous step-and-shoot" acquisition, for which the detector does not interrupt the collection of photons during its movement from one angle to the next in the step-and-shoot mode. This yields in increased counting statistics compared with the standard step-and-shoot mode while reducing most of the blurring associated with continuous acquisition.[12]

The total time for acquisition is based on the need to collect sufficient counts, but should not surpass 30 minutes, which is readily accomplished with dual-headed systems for the usual administered doses. A dual-headed system has the detectors separated by 90°, completing a 180° orbit by rotating through 90° angle, in half time compared with single-detector systems.

Images may be recorded with attenuation correction, using either an X-ray or radionuclide source for the acquisition of a transmission scan that is used to generate a reference map of the attenuation factors for the patient. Transmission images can be obtained sequentially or simultaneously to emission images.

ECG gating acquisition is frequently applied in clinical practice. Usually, data are collected in 8 or 16 time bins per cardiac cycle.[4,5]

After data acquisition, collected planar views should be reviewed in cinematic mode to identify possible source of artifacts (Table 4.3), such as breast shadow caused by attenuation, photopenic area in the fundus of the stomach caused by diaphragmatic attenuation, superimposed abdominal visceral activity, "upward creep," and patient motion, giving attention to even small variations in arm position as possible origin of shifting breast shadow artifacts. For gated studies, a full display of all time bins for each projection is required to detect gating errors, although, when the assessment is performed in the sum of all gated tomograms, most types of gating errors will become apparent as a "flashing" of image counts.

4. Image Processing

Planar MPS does not generally need any image reconstruction, but there are different quantitative programs available to quantify regional myocardial perfusion to provide a more objective means of analysis. In fact, all quantitative attempts in single photon emission imaging, either planar or SPECT, are semiquantitative, because they determine relative rather than absolute perfusion in each region of the myocardium. Hence, to determine if an individual patient's MPS is normal or abnormal, the patient's data must be compared with that of normal population.

Quantitative programs in planar MPS apply a background subtraction, which is essential in this type of image because the relative tissue distribution of the tracer at rest and after exercise may be markedly different. The software also aligns initial and delayed images, and generates a graphic displaying regional myocardial activity, generally involving a circumferential count distribution profile. This method provides a single-curve display of counts sampled around the myocardial perimeter. When compared with a normal database from "normal" subjects or normalized to each other, these profiles allow detection of the severity and extent of perfusion abnormality, and the degree of reversibility.[17]

SPECT imaging is based on the reconstruction of tomographic images from projection images. Until recently, this reconstruction has been performed by filtered backprojection. Each source of radioactivity creates spikes in the count activity profiles seen by the detector as it rotates around the patient. The counts in each profile are assumed to correspond to uniformly distributed activity perpendicular to the profile. Therefore, linear superimposition of the profiles at each projection angle back across the reconstruction matrix results in the tomographic image, but with loss of resolution and contrast as well as generation of a star artifact. Filtered backprojection solves these drawbacks of standard backprojection by filtering each profile before it is backprojected.[14,18] Currently, improvements in computer power have made possible other reconstruction approaches based on algebraic techniques that also use the projection images as input to find the mathematic solution to the problem of activity distribution in the field of view. Because the exact solution to this problem is not possible when matrix dimensions are not very small, an approximated iterative method is used instead. In iterative reconstruction, the value of all pixels is initially guessed using filtered backprojection, then successive slight transformations (iterations) of those initial values result in a tomogram consistent with the available count profiles. The iterative reconstruction makes it possible to integrate correction for many physical effects such as attenuation, scatter, variation of spatial resolution as function of depth, etc.[14,19,20]

Whether the reconstruction method is filtered backprojection or iterative, smoothing or low-pass filters are always applied to projection images before reconstruction so as to reduce statistical noise early in the processing chain. In filtered backprojection, a high-pass filter (ramp-filter) is subsequently applied to minimize the star artifact.

Tomographic reconstruction of projection images generates transaxial images, i.e., images perpendicular to the long axis of the patient. Because the orientation of the heart relative to the patient's long axis varies from patient to patient, the reconstruction process is followed by reorientation of transaxial data into the long axis of the individual patient's heart, which extends from the center of the mitral valve plane to the apex. The transaxial image data set is then resampled to generate a vertical long-axis image, on which the same operation is repeated. Then the left ventricle (LV) is successively cut through these long-axis planes, generating vertical long-axis slices (extending from the septum to the lateral wall) and horizontal long-axis slices (extending from the inferior wall to the anterior wall). Finally, sections perpendicular to both long-axis planes generate short-axis slices (extending from the apex to the base). Therefore, each plane of section is oriented at 90° angles relative to each other (Figure 4.2). Reorientation should be comparable at rest and stress studies.

Stress and rest tomographic series should be displayed normalized at peak count density within the myocardium for each set, side-by-side, appropriately aligned, and using the same color continuous scale for ready comparison of corresponding tomograms.

SPECT semiquantification of regional perfusion is achieved by commercial software programs which usually provide an average of tracer uptake throughout myocardial walls. Values obtained are normalized to the highest myocardial counts. By assuming that this maximum represents the "most normal" perfusion zone, the relative reduction of activity can be used to demarcate perfusion abnormalities. Results are displayed in a 2D circular plot referred to as a polar map or bull's eye (Figures 4.2 and 4.3; see color section). Separate databases have been used for male and female patients, but with the advent of different data sampling approaches and attenuation corrections, new normal databases are being tested.[15]

If images have been acquired by ECG gating, the individual frames of the study can be summed to create a composite data set similar to that of a nongated study, with important regional and global LV function information added, such as regional wall motion and thickening, end-diastolic (ED) and end-systolic (ES) volumes and LV ejection fraction (LVEF). Functional assessment can be both qualitative and quantitative. It is based on the changes in cavity dimensions and in count density between ED and ES frames. There are several types of well-validated and reproducible commercial software for these purposes, which have showed good agreement with other imaging techniques for the assessment of LVEF as well as for the assessment of wall motion and thickening. LV volume measurements have been less widely validated and may vary with the tracer used (^{201}Tl or ^{99m}Tc agents), and reconstruction methods (filter characteristics).[21] Potential sources of error in gated SPECT LVEF calculations are listed in Table 4.4. Global and regional LV function quantification are calculated separately using different methods based either on the detection of endocardial and epicardial edges and making geometric assumptions to estimate LV volumes, or based on peak counts measured at ED and ES to estimate thickening fractions, avoiding edge detection. Newer programs are usually a hybrid of both methods.[4,5]

5. Image Interpretation

Computer screen image assessment of the three tomographic planes is recommended to interpret correctly SPECT imaging. It permits use of cinematic displays and adjustment of the contrast, brightness, and color scales optimized to the myocardium. Initial review of the images should be performed without reference to clinical information in order to decide on major features, and then to modify the impression and decide on minor features if necessary, after review of the clinical information.

MPS may show different appearances of normally perfused myocardium on account of scatter, attenuation, and the nonuniform thickness of myocardial walls. Therefore, qualitative interpretation of MPS requires expertise for the correct evaluation of myocardial tracer distribution, including recognition of normal variants and artifacts (Table 4.3) as well as correlation of abnormalities with the known vascular territories of the three major coronary arteries. Moreover, interpretation of MPS should involve the pretest probability of CAD apart from the result of the test itself. Homogeneous LV myocardial tracer uptake indicates normally perfused and viable myocardium. The LV looks like a horseshoe on long-axis SPECT slices and on planar views (the latter may also have an ellipsoidal appearance), and it has a doughnut appearance

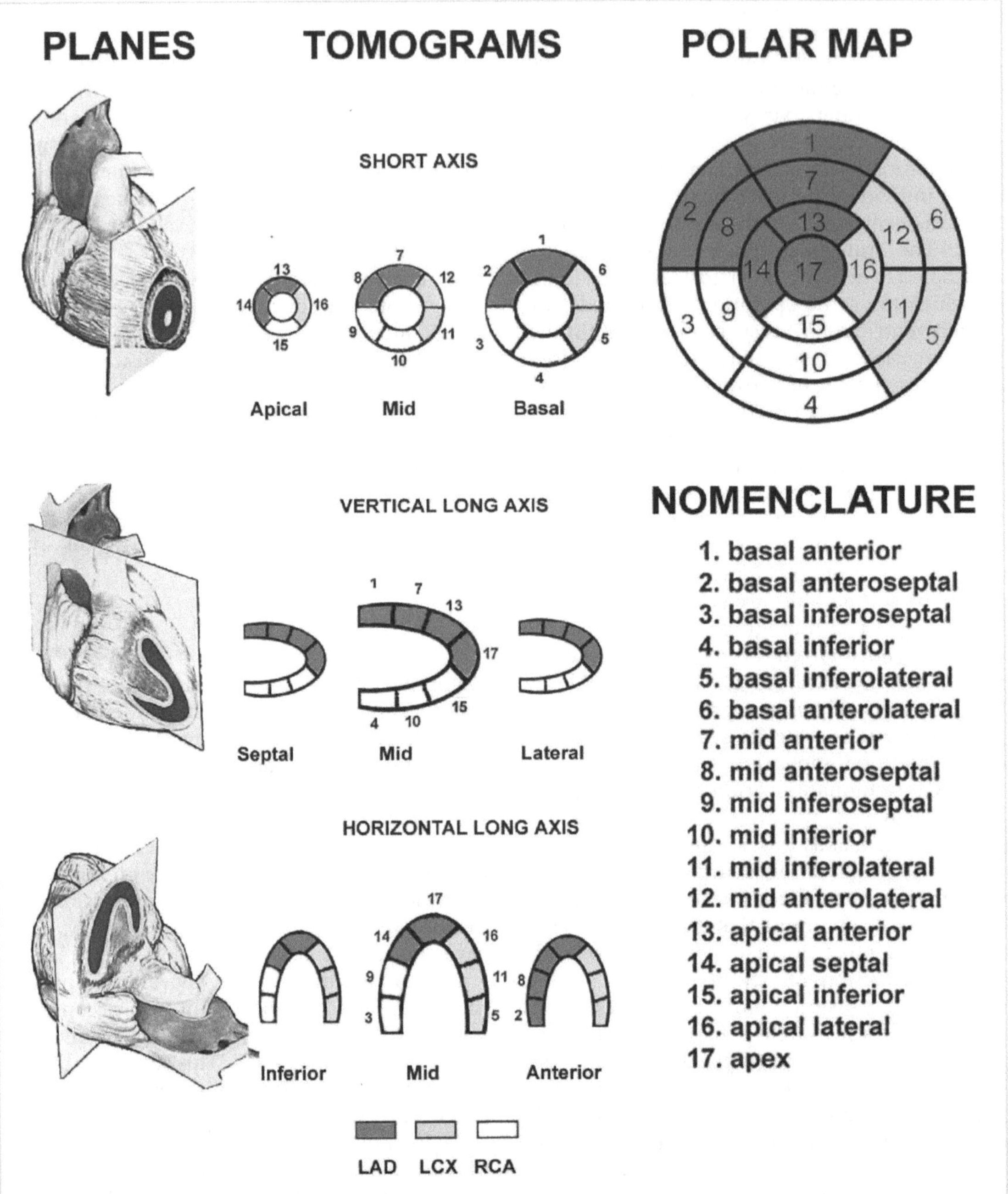

Figure 4.2. Cardiac plane definition with resultant tomograms and polar map display of the standardized 17 left ventricular myocardial segments, along with their nomenclature and correlation with coronary anatomy. LAD, left anterior descending artery; LCX, left circumflex coronary artery; RCA, right coronary artery. [Modified from Cerqueira et al.[22]]

on short-axis SPECT slices. The SPECT tomograms and polar map appearance are best explained by referring to Figure 4.2, which also shows the recommended nomenclature of the 17 LV segments with their coronary artery territory assignment.[22] In short-axis SPECT slices, the most intense activity is usually seen in the lateral wall, because it is the region closest to the detector (Figure 4.3; see color section). The right ventricle (RV) may not be seen, especially on resting

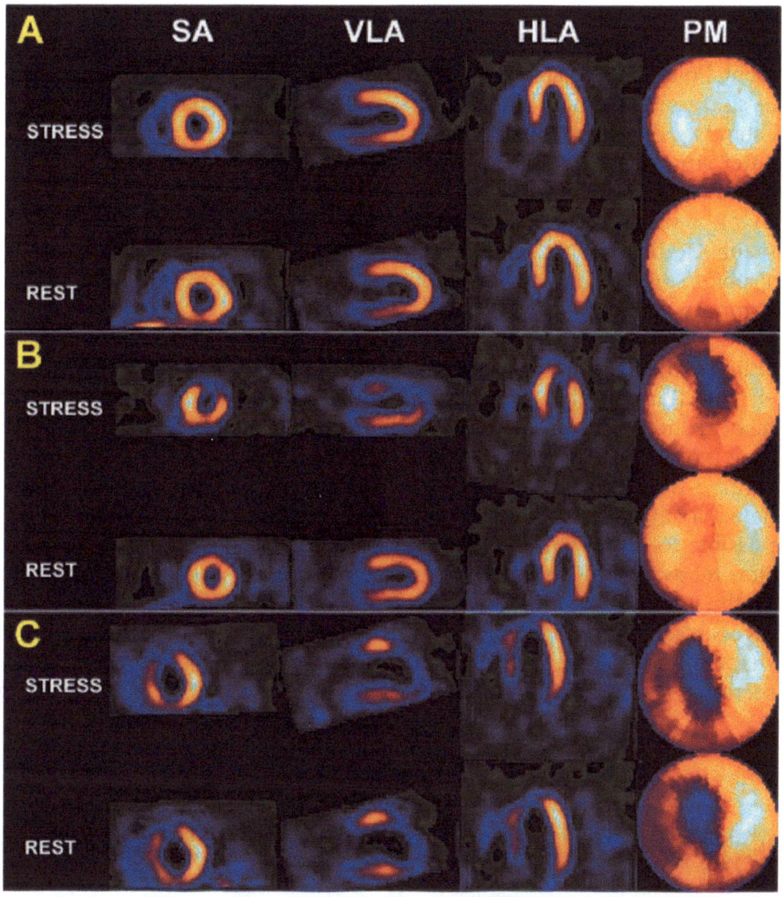

Figure 4.3. Tomograms and polar maps at stress and rest showing the three basic diagnostic patterns. **A** Normal perfusion at stress and rest. **B** Severe stress-induced perfusion abnormality in the apex and mid and apical anterior wall, with reversibility at rest, indicating ischemia in the LAD territory. **C** Extensive fixed defect in the apex extending to apical anterior and apical inferior walls, and septum representing infarction (scar). SA, short axis; VLA, vertical long axis; HLA, horizontal long axis.

^{201}Tl planar views, because of the limited thickness of its walls. It may be strikingly visible in cases of RV hypertrophy. Mild lung uptake may be seen, but when it is increased, one should consider the presence of severe CAD and/or LV dysfunction or underlying lung disease.[23,24] Liver and/or bowel tracer activity may obscure LV inferior wall.

Because blood flow is diverted from the splanchnic bed to exercising muscles during dynamic exercise, exercise stress images usually show better heart to background signal than rest images and especially than pharmacologic stress images, which increases splanchnic blood flow.

A defect of myocardial tracer uptake in the stress images that shows an improvement or normalization of the uptake in the rest images (a reversible defect) indicates inducible myocardial ischemia. A defect of myocardial tracer uptake in both stress and rest images (a fixed defect) indicates MI. On SPECT studies, defects must be present in two or more consecutive slices and two or more axes to be considered significant. The standard variables extracted from MPS are the extent (amount of segments), severity (intensity), and reversibility of defects of tracer uptake. Each of these variables has proven diagnostic and prognostic value. Different polar maps

Table 4.4. Potential sources of error in gated SPET LVEF calculations

Automatic selection of structures with intense uptake, other than LV walls, adjacent to hypoperfused myocardium:
Hepatointestinal activity in conjunction with hypoperfused inferior wall
High RV activity in conjunction with hypoperfused septa
Erroneous delineation of myocardial edges in severely hypoperfused myocardial segments
Small hearts challenge the limited reconstructed spatial resolution resulting in overestimated LVEF
Reversible stress-induced myocardial ischemia (postischemic stunning) may result in lower values of LVEF

LV, left ventricle; LVEF, LV ejection fraction; RV, right ventricle.

showing relative counts as well as defect extent, severity, and reversibility may help visual assessment. Polar maps display the LV in a circular plot of successive annular rings, where myocardium extends from apex in the center to base in the outer ring (Figure 4.2). These plots are advantageous because they display all ventricular activity on a single image. However, they generate a mapping distortion similar to that produced by a polar projection map of the earth, which hampers visual estimation of defect extent. To solve this, polar maps can be scaled accordingly either to the distance from apex to base (distance weighted) or to the different thickness of the myocardium at each level from apex to base (volume weighted). Distance-weighted and volume-weighted polar maps can yield accurate defect location and extent, respectively. It is also possible to display 3D representations of perfusion maps, which provide a visual appreciation of the magnitude and orientation of areas of myocardial scar or ischemia specific to the actual shape of each patient's LV (Figure 4.4; see color section).[12,15]

Other variables that can be derived from MPS are washout (clearance) of ^{201}Tl from the myocardium, which is related to local myocardial perfusion, and LV cavity dilatation at stress in comparison with rest, or transient ischemic dilatation, which reflects diffuse subendocardial ischemia and indicates severe and extensive CAD.[25]

Although attenuation correction algorithms are very attractive, they sometimes result in artifacts, which forces review of both uncorrected and corrected data to minimize the likelihood of misinterpretation.[26]

Functional gated planar imaging should be evaluated qualitatively because images include background activity, which impedes clear differentiation between the apparent and real endocardial edge to get precise measures of regional or global wall motion. Gated SPECT data are usually summarized with a moving five-slice display (apical, mid-ventricular, and basal short axis, along with mid-ventricular vertical and horizontal long-axis tomograms). It is important to display the computer-generated contours to

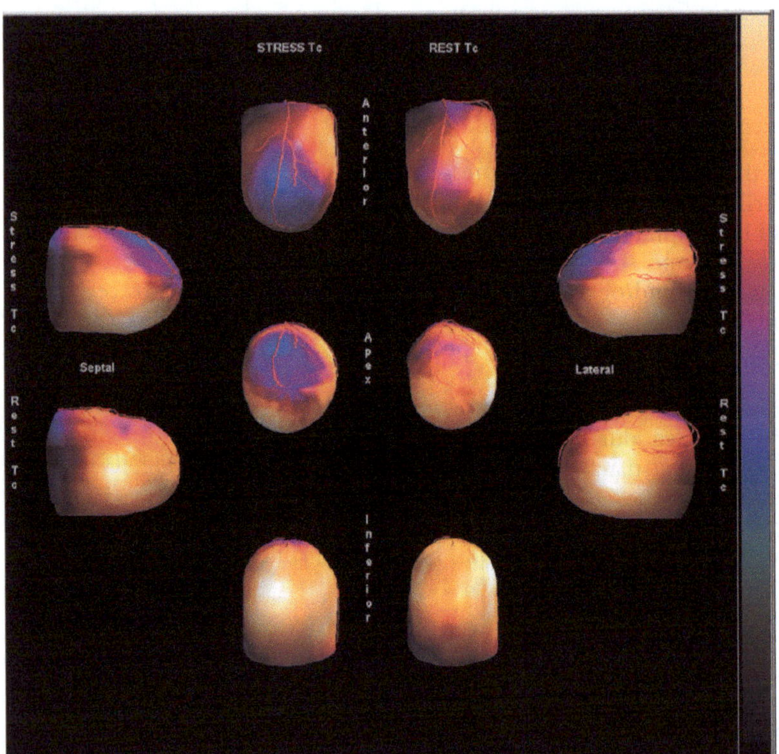

Figure 4.4. Different angle views, under stress and rest conditions, of three-dimensional left ventricle perfusion display corresponding to a woman with severe and extensive ischemia in the LAD territory. There is a reversible defect in the apex and mid and apical anterior wall.

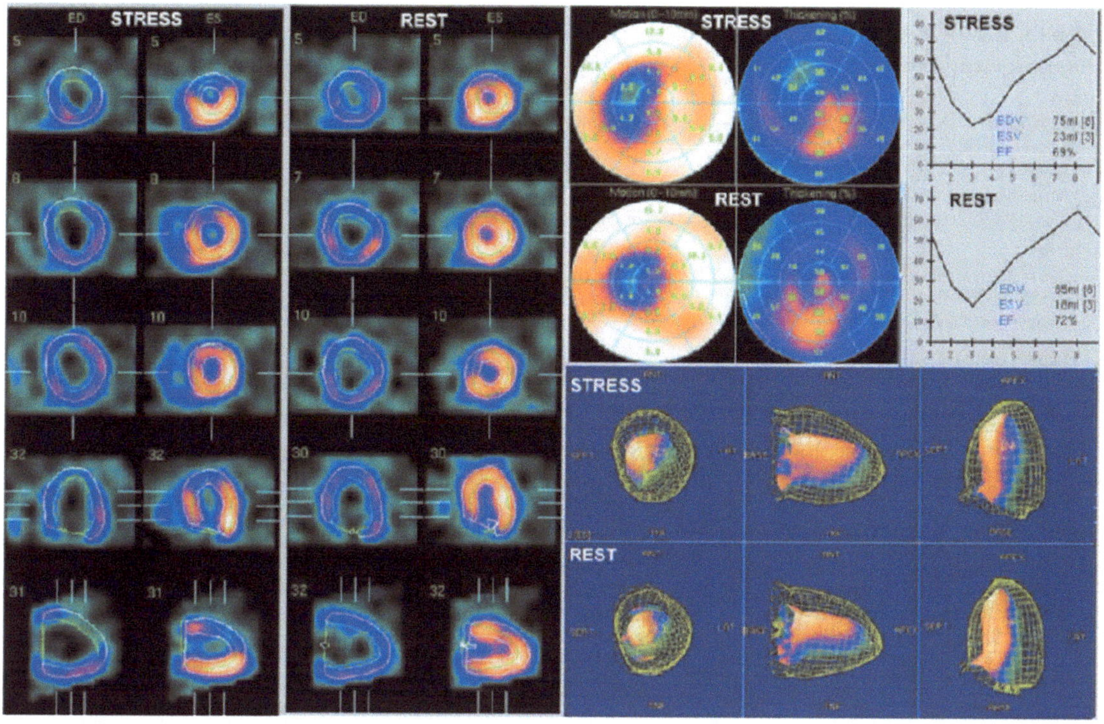

Figure 4.5. Summary of gated-SPET data of a woman with severe and extensive ischemia in the LAD territory (see Figure 4.4). Post-stress data show reduced wall thickening in the apex and mid and apical anterior wall, attributed to postischemic stunned myocardium. ED, end-diastole; ES, end-systole; EDV, ED volume; EDS, ES volume.

ensure that automatic edge detection has been correctly defined. Paper copies display an ED and ES set of images, scaled on the same intensity. Polar plots of wall motion and thickening, LV volume curve, and results of different computations are also available. Most new systems include moving 3D displays of surface-shaded representations of "beating" endocardial and epicardial surfaces, with or without a superimposed grid of the ED reference surface, which are useful for the assessment of different ventricular wall displacements during the cardiac cycle as well as for the assessment of ventricular shape (Figure 4.5; see color section). LV wall motion is best assessed in continuous gray scale, whereas wall thickening is best analyzed in continuous color scale. This latter evaluation offers better insight in the survey of functionality in areas of reduced tracer uptake, because it clearly manifests by striking increase in image brightness (Figure 4.5; see color section). Assessment of regional LV function improves the specificity of MPS for the detection of CAD by differentiating attenuation artifacts from MI, and may also be helpful for viability detection within perfusion defects.[27] Moreover, the evaluation of tracer distribution in the ED frame may also improve the sensitivity of the test, particularly in patients with LV hypertrophy by reducing the blurring effect of wall motion during heart contraction. In addition, recent reports indicate that the detection of poststress stunning by gated SPECT acquired 15–30 minutes after stress increases the sensitivity of MPS for the detection of CAD (Figure 4.5; see color section).[28]

6. Exercise and Pharmacologic Modalities Used in Stress MPS

Indications of MPS include the diagnosis of patients with an intermediate likelihood of CAD and/or risk stratification of patients with an intermediate or high likelihood of CAD, with different levels of supporting evidence (Table 4.5).

Table 4.5. Indications of myocardial perfusion scintigraphy (MPS)

Diagnosis of patients with an intermediate likelihood of CAD and/or prognostication of patients with an intermediate or high likelihood of CAD
Class I – Identification of the extent, severity, and location of ischemia in patients who have a baseline ECG abnormality that interferes with the interpretation of exercise-induced ST segment changes.* (Level of Evidence: B) – Assessment of the functional significance of intermediate (25%–75%) coronary lesions. (Level of Evidence: B) – Intermediate Duke treadmill score. (Level of Evidence: B) – After initial MPS in patients whose symptoms have changed to redefine the risk for cardiac event. (Level of Evidence: C)
Class IIa – 3–5 yr after revascularization (either PCI or CABG) in selected, high-risk asymptomatic patients. (Level of Evidence: B) – Patients who are considered to be at high risk (patients with diabetes or patients otherwise defined as having >20% 10-yr risk of a coronary heart disease event). (Level of Evidence: B)
Class IIb – 1–3 yr after initial perfusion imaging in patients with known or a high likelihood of CAD, stable symptoms, and a predicted annual mortality of >1%, to redefine the risk of a cardiac event. (Level of Evidence: C) – Assessment of the efficacy of medical therapy in patients receiving cardiac active medications after initial abnormal MPS. (Level of Evidence: C) – Symptomatic or asymptomatic patients who have severe coronary calcification (CT coronary calcium screening >75th percentile for age and sex) in the presence on the resting ECG of preexcitation (Wolff-Parkinson-White) syndrome or >1 mm ST segment depression. (Level of Evidence: B) – Asymptomatic patients who have a high-risk occupation. (Level of Evidence: B)
Patients who will undergo noncardiac surgery
Class I – Initial diagnosis of CAD in patients with intermediate pretest probability of disease and abnormal baseline ECG* or inability to exercise. (Level of Evidence: B) – Prognostic assessment of patients undergoing initial evaluation for suspected or proven CAD with abnormal baseline ECG* or inability to exercise. (Level of Evidence: B) – Evaluation of patients after a change in clinical status (e.g., ACS) with abnormal baseline ECG* or inability to exercise. (Level of Evidence: B) – Initial diagnosis and/or prognostic assessment of patients with LBBB undergoing initial evaluation for suspected (intermediate likelihood) or proven CAD, when used in conjunction with vasodilator stress. (Level of Evidence: B) – Assessment of patients with intermediate or minor clinical risk predictors† and poor functional capacity (<4 METS) who require high-risk noncardiac surgery,‡ when used in conjunction with pharmacologic stress. (Level of Evidence: C) – Assessment of patients with intermediate clinical risk predictors,† abnormal baseline ECGs,* and moderate or excellent functional capacity (>4 METS) who require high-risk noncardiac surgery. (Level of Evidence: C)
Class IIb – Routine assessment of active, asymptomatic patients who have remained stable for up to 5 yr after CABG surgery. (Level of Evidence: C) – Routine evaluation of active, asymptomatic patients who have remained stable for up to 2 yr after previous abnormal coronary angiography or noninvasive assessment of myocardial perfusion. (Level of Evidence: C) – Diagnosis of restenosis and regional ischemia in active, asymptomatic patients within weeks to months after PCI. (Level of Evidence: C) – Initial diagnosis or prognostic assessment of CAD in patients with right bundle-branch block or <1-mm ST depression on resting ECG. (Level of Evidence: C)

Source: Modified from Klocke et al.[2]

ACS, acute coronary syndromes; CT, computed tomography; CAD, coronary artery disease; ECG, electrocardiogram; LBBB, left bundle branch block; LVH, left ventricle hypertrophy; MPS, myocardial perfusion scintigraphy; PCI, percutaneous coronary intervention; CABAG, coronary artery bypass grafting.

The ACC/AHA classifications I and II as well as the levels of evidence for individual class assignments are designated as: Class I, conditions for which there is evidence and/or general agreement that a given procedure or treatment is useful and effective; Class II, conditions for which there is conflicting evidence and/or a divergence of opinion about the usefulness/efficacy of a procedure or treatment; Class IIa, weight of evidence/opinion is in favor of usefulness/efficacy; Class IIb, usefulness/efficacy is less well established by evidence/opinion.

A = data derived from multiple randomized clinical trials; B = data derived from a single randomized trial, or from nonrandomized studies; C = consensus opinion of experts.

* LBBB, ventricular pacing, ventricular preexcitation, LVH with repolarization changes, digoxin therapy, or >1 mm ST depression.

† Mild angina, prior MI, compensated or prior heart failure, diabetes, and renal insufficiency. Minor clinical risk predictors include advanced age, abnormal ECG, rhythm other than sinus, low functional capacity, history of cerebrovascular accident, and uncontrolled hypertension.

‡ Emergent operations (particularly in the elderly), aortic and other major vascular surgery, peripheral vascular surgery, and other prolonged operations during which major fluid shifts are anticipated (i.e., reported cardiac risk often >5%).

Different stress testing modalities of MPS yield comparable diagnostic value, but exercise provides additional prognostic information based on physical capacity and exercise-induced arrhythmias.

7. Exercise Stress

The preferred stress test in patients who can exercise to an adequate workload and do not have a left bundle branch block (LBBB) or electronically paced ventricular rhythm is dynamic exercise. Otherwise, pharmacologic stress should be performed. Adequate exercise is most important if the aim of the study is to detect CAD. Exercise increases myocardial oxygen demand, which, by autoregulation, increases MBF (approximately 2.5-fold above the resting condition) in normal coronary arteries, but not in arteries with fixed coronary stenoses, which can be depicted with perfusion tracers. In patients with mild and moderate CAD, MBF may become abnormal only at high heart rates [≥85% of age maximal predicted heart rate (MPHR), which is calculated as 220 – years of age] or at high double products (≥25 000). At lower heart rates, MBF may be normal and perfusion images will be correspondingly normal.[29] In patients with known CAD who are being evaluated for extent and severity of inducible myocardial ischemia, submaximal exercise can provide clinically relevant information.[2,12,13]

Gradually increasing exercise is performed with a bicycle or, more frequently, treadmill ergometer, for which different protocols are available, differing only in speed and inclination of the treadmill (Bruce protocol is the most widely used).[30] Independently of the exercise modality, a large-bore (18–20 gauge) IV cannula should be inserted for radiopharmaceutical injection during exercise.

Exercise should be symptom limited with patients achieving ≥85% of MPHR, injecting the radiopharmaceutical at peak exercise. The patients should continue the exercise for ≥1 minute after the tracer injection to maintain stable conditions over the period of extraction of tracer by the myocardium. If the patient cannot exercise to an acceptable workload, pharmacologic stress should be added.[2,31,32] Although exercise testing is relatively safe, the rate of fatal acute MI (AMI) or death is 0.01%, and the rate of nonfatal ACS is 0.02%. Contraindications of different stressing modalities and indications for early test termination are summarized in Table 4.6.

8. Pharmacological Stress

Pharmacological stress is the preferred stress modality in patients who cannot achieve an adequate heart rate and blood pressure response to exercise because of mental or physical limitations (pulmonary, peripheral vascular, or musculoskeletal abnormalities) or lack of motivation. It has the advantages of speed, reliability, and reproducibility, but the disadvantages that it is difficult to assess the adequacy of stress and it is not equivalent to the physiologic stress of everyday life.[33,34]

8.1 Adenosine

Adenosine is a natural endogenous molecule normally produced in myocardial vascular smooth muscle and endothelial cells. It is shortly present in the extracellular space, yet it has an extremely short half-life (<10 seconds) where it may bind to A_{2A} membrane cell adenosine receptors producing direct arteriolar vasodilator. In normal coronary arteries, there is an increase in MBF of approximately 4.5 fold compared to baseline, but it is of lesser magnitude through stenotic arteries, creating a flow differential and inhomogeneous distribution of perfusion tracers. However, depending on the severity of coronary stenosis and coronary flow reserve limitation, true ischemia can occur because of a coronary steal phenomenon, principally in collateral flow-dependent arteries.[2,12,33]

In addition to the common indications of pharmacologic stress testing, vasodilator stressors such as adenosine and dipyridamole are also indicated in patients with LBBB or paced ventricular rhythm[35,36] and patients with very recent AMI (<3 days) or recent (<2 weeks) angioplasty/stenting.

Adenosine should be administered through an IV line with dual-port Y-connector using an infusion pump at a rate of 140 µg/kg/min over 4–5 or 6 (standard protocol) minutes. Mild increase in heart rate and modest decrease in blood pressure result from adenosine infusion. The injection of the tracer (through the Y-connector) should be performed after 2 minutes (with 4- to 5-minute infusion protocol) or after 3 minutes (with 6-minute protocol) of the beginning of the infusion, which should be continued for another 3 minutes. The infusion may start at a lower dose (70 µg/kg/min) for patients considered to be at a higher risk for complications (recent ischemic event, borderline hypotension, inadequately controlled asthma). If this dose is well tolerated for 1 minute, the infusion rate should be increased gradually to

Table 4.6. Contraindications of stress testing and indications for early test termination

	Absolutely contraindications	Relative contraindications	Indications for early termination
Dynamic exercise	1. AMI within 2 d 2. Uncontrolled unstable angina 3. Uncontrolled cardiac arrhythmias with symptoms or hemodynamic compromise 4. Uncontrolled heart failure 5. Symptomatic severe aortic stenosis 6. Acute pulmonary embolus/infarction 7. Acute myocarditis/pericarditis 8. Acute aortic dissection 9. Severe pulmonary hypertension	1. Left main coronary stenosis 2. Moderate stenotic valvular disease 3. Hypertension ≥200/110 mm Hg) 4. Tachy/bradyarrhythmias 5. High-degree AV block 6. Outflow tract obstruction 7. Electrolyte abnormalities 8. Inability to exercise adequately	1. Severe angina 2. Ataxia, dizziness, near-syncope, marked dyspnea, or fatigue 3. Signs of poor perfusion (cyanosis or pallor) 4. ST elevation of ≥1 mm in leads without pathologic Q waves 5. Horizontal or downsloping ST depression (>2 mm) 6. Decrease in systolic blood pressure of ≥10 mm Hg from baseline 7. Sustained supra or ventricular tachycardia 8. Hypertensive response (≥250 systolic or 115 mm Hg diastolic) 9. Impossible ECG or blood pressure control
Adenosine	1. Asthma with ongoing wheezing 2. Heart block >first degree without a pacemaker 3. Sick sinus syndrome 4. Systolic blood pressure >90 mm Hg 5. Hypersensitivity to dipyridamole or adenosine 6. Use of dipyridamole >24 h 7. Use of xanthines (e.g., aminophylline, caffeine) <12 h	1. Severe sinus bradycardia (<40 bpm) 2. Recent cerebral ischemia or infarction	1. Severe hypotension (systolic blood pressure <80 mm Hg) 2. Development of symptomatic persistent second-degree or complete heart block 3. Wheezing 4. Severe chest pain associated with ≥2 mm ST depression
Dipyridamole	As for adenosine	As for adenosine	As for adenosine
Dobutamine	1. AMI <1 wk 2. Unstable angina 3. Hemodynamically significant LV outflow tract obstruction 4. Critical aortic stenosis 5. Atrial tachyarrhythmias with uncontrolled ventricular response 6. Prior history of ventricular tachycardia 7. Uncontrolled hypertension 8. Aortic dissection or large aortic aneurysm 9. β-Blockers treatment (block heart rate response)	As for dynamic exercise, Hypokalemia	As for dynamic exercise. Termination for ventricular tachycardia or ST segment elevation is more likely with dobutamine than with other pharmacologic stressors.

AMI, acute myocardial infarction; AV, atrioventricular.

140 μg/kg/min and continued for 4 minutes. The tracer should be injected 1 minute after starting the 140 μg/kg/min dose.[12]

Table 4.7 summarizes side effects attributable to different pharmacologic stressors. Those associated with adenosine usually resolve in a few seconds after discontinuation of the infusion, and only rarely is the administration of the antagonist drug (aminophylline 75–250 mg IV) required. Supplementation of adenosine infusion with low-level exercise minimizes the side effects of adenosine and improves the image quality by decreasing the artifacts caused by high hepatic tracer uptake, which is common with pharmacologic stress.[37–39] However, the low-level exercise supplementation should not be used in patients with LBBB, because, in this abnormality, it is desirable not to increase the heart rate.[2,12,13,16] First clinical trials with selective A_{2A} receptor agonists are promising, resulting in images of similar quality to those obtained with adenosine, but allowing a bolus administration and having less incidence and severity of side effects.[40,41]

8.2 Dipyridamole

Dipyridamole produces coronary arteriolar vasodilation increasing adenosine tissue levels by preventing its intracellular reuptake and deamination. The increment in coronary flow produced by dipyridamole does not differ significantly from that produced by adenosine. However, coronary hyperemia induced with dipyridamole is somewhat less predictable and lasts longer (>15 minutes) than that induced by adenosine due to the longer half-life (30 minutes) of dipyridamole.[2,12,13,16,33] Both drugs have similar indications and contraindications (Table 4.6).

Dipyridamole is administered manually as a continuous infusion at a rate of 0.56 mg/kg IV over 4 minutes. This results in a modest increase in heart rate and a modest decrease in blood pressure. The tracer is injected 3–4 minutes after the completion of dipyridamole infusion, which obviates the need for a Y-connector.

Side effects with dipyridamole (Table 4.7) are less frequent than with adenosine, but more prolonged.[33,42] They can be readily reversed with aminophylline (75–250 mg IV), although can reappear later because the half-life of dipyridamole is longer. Supplementation of dipyridamole infusion with low-level exercise for 4–6 minutes soon after the end of dipyridamole infusion, injecting the tracer during the performance of exercise, reduces the side effects of the vasodilator and improves image quality.[43] As with adenosine, low-level exercise supplementation is not recommended for patients with LBBB.

Table 4.7. Side effects (%) attributable to different pharmacologic stressors

	Adenosine	Dipyridamole	Dobutamine
Chest pain	45*	20	39
Flushing	35	3	<1
Dyspnea	33	3	6
Dizziness	9	3	4
Gastrointestinal discomfort	15	10	1
Headache	30	12	7
Hypotension	2	5	15
Arrhythmia	3	5	45
High-degree AV block	7	2	0
STΔ	6†	8	30
Bronchospasm	0.1	0.15	0
Fatal AMI/cardiac death	0	0.05	0
Nonfatal ACS	0.01	0.05	0.3
Any adverse effect	80	50	75

From References 2, 16, 33, 40.
AMI, acute myocardial infarction; AV, atrioventricular.
* Chest pain is nonspecific and not necessarily indicative of the presence of CAD.
† ST segment depression (1 mm) is indicative of significant CAD.

8.3 Dobutamine

Dobutamine is a β_1-, β_2-, and α_1-adrenergic agonist with positive inotropic and chronotropic effects, which increases myocardial oxygen demand secondarily to dose-related increase in myocardial contractility, heart rate, and blood pressure. High doses of dobutamine result in a secondary increase in MBF only within normal vascular beds (approximately three-fold increase), with the potential to provoke ischemia in vascular beds supplied by significantly stenosed arteries.[2,33]

Dobutamine stress testing is indicated in patients who cannot undergo exercise stress and have contraindications to pharmacologic vasodilator stress. It has not been studied as extensively as adenosine or dipyridamole in the evaluation and prognostication of patients with CAD.

Gradually increasing doses of dobutamine are administered through an IV line with a dual-port Y-connector using an infusion pump, starting at 5 µg/kg/min and followed by 10, 15, 20, 30, and 40 µg/kg/min, every 3–5 minutes. The tracer should be injected at ≥85% MPHR or at 1 minute into the dose of 40 µg/kg/min, continuing the infusion ≥1 minute. Atropine administration (0.25–1 mg IV) may be required to increase the heart rate response >120 beats/min with the maximum dose of dobutamine. Severe side effects (Table 4.7) may require IV administration of a short-acting β-blocker (Esmolol).

9. Currently Used Protocols

Protocols for MPS vary with regard to the radiopharmaceutical administrated, the type of stress performed (if any), and the clinical indication of the test.[44] The latter can include the diagnosis or prognosis of myocardial ischemia, the assessment of patients with suspected ACS in the emergency department, and the identification of myocardial viability.

A fast of ≥4 hours is recommended before MPS. Cardiac medications, if not contraindicated, should be suspended 24 hours before the stress MPS if imaging is performed for diagnostic purposes, especially drugs such as calcium channel blockers and β-blockers that may reduce the heart rate and blood pressure response to exercise and dobutamine stress. Additionally, caffeine and methylxanthine-containing drugs, foods or beverages, should be discontinued 24 hours before both the exercise testing and pharmacologic vasodilator testing. By preparing patients in this manner, if they are not able to achieve an acceptable exercise workload, pharmacologic vasodilator testing can be undertaken. Patients taking dipyridamole should stop the drug for ≥24 hours before pharmacologic vasodilator testing.[2,12,13,16] Sublingual nitroglycerine (0.4–0.8 μg) or isosorbide dinitrate (10–20 mg) can be administered 5 minutes before tracer injection for resting studies in order to increase regional MBF and enhance detection of ischemic but still viable myocardium.[45,46]

During the stress testing, the tracer should be injected at peak of the stress effect. Usual administered activity is 80–111 MBq for studies with ^{201}Tl and 300–925 MBq for studies with ^{99m}Tc agents. Tracer doses should be adjusted for heavier patients (0.04 mCi/kg for ^{201}Tl and by 0.31 mCi/kg for ^{99m}Tc agents). ECG should be monitored continuously and heart rate and blood pressure recorded at baseline and at the end of each stage of the stress test (or every 2 minutes). Monitoring should continue for ≥5 minutes after the termination of the stress or until patient stabilizes.

The value of giving a fatty meal between tracer injection and imaging to facilitate clearance of tracer from the liver and gall bladder is uncertain. It can result in abundant radioactivity in the upper gastrointestinal tract, which may interfere significantly with the interpretation of the inferior LV wall. Thoracic radiopaque objects should be removed before image acquisition. Registration of the patient body habitus and implanted prostheses in the thorax is also advisable.

The duration of acquisition at each stop (30–40 seconds for dual detector systems) depends on the protocol, type, and activity of radiopharmaceutical administered, patient size, gated or ungated study, and tolerance of the patient to rest without moving under the gamma camera. Total imaging time should be ≤30 minutes. Gated-SPECT acquisitions using ^{201}Tl may require increased imaging times or use of multidetector systems to collect an adequate number of counts. When using ^{99m}Tc agents, gated acquisition should be performed in both stress and rest studies, providing that there is adequate count density, particularly with regard to the lower dose acquisitions of 1-day protocols, because there is increasing evidence that post-stress global and regional LV function are not representative of basal LV function in patients with stress-induced ischemia.[28]

In the reconstruction process of SPECT data, correct filter selection is critical and depends on the specific radioisotope and protocol used. The aim of filtering is to find the optimal balance for smoothing the image while preserving its spatial resolution.[47] It is recommended that standardized filters be used for all patients undergoing the same imaging protocol.

9.1 ^{201}Tl Stress-redistribution Imaging Protocol

^{201}Tl (111 MBq) is IV administered at peak of stress. Stress imaging should begin within 5–10 minutes of injection and should be completed within 30 minutes to minimize the effects of redistribution, so that images acquired during this period reflect myocardial perfusion at peak stress despite the cessation of exercise. Redistribution imaging is usually performed 4 hours after the exercise images.

9.2 ^{201}Tl Rest-redistribution Imaging Protocol

^{201}Tl (111 MBq) is IV administered at rest, beginning image acquisition within 15 minutes. Redistribution imaging is performed ≥3 hours after the initial resting images. Additional delayed imaging at 24 hours after injection may be helpful to establish more completely redistribution in myocardial regions, which appear to have significant tracer uptake but little or no redistribution by 4 hours.

This protocol is generally considered in patients with known LV dysfunction in whom viability of a ventricular segment distal to a severe coronary artery stenosis is the clinical question to be addressed.

9.3 ^{201}Tl Stress-redistribution-reinjection Protocol

A second dose of ^{201}Tl (37 MBq) is reinjected after redistribution images are complete (the same day of the stress or the day after), and a third set of images is obtained 15 minutes later. This may enhance the amount of uptake in an initially severe defect, which shows no redistribution on delayed imaging.[48] Repeat imaging at 24 hours after reinjection may further enhance the detection of redistribution in severe defects.

9.4 ^{99m}Tc-agent Two-day Imaging Protocol (Stress–rest or Rest–stress)

^{99m}Tc agent (925 MBq) is IV administered at peak of stress. Imaging begins 15 or ≥45 minutes after tracer injection depending on the type of stress performed (exercise or pharmacologic, respectively). The day after stress imaging, the same dose of ^{99m}Tc agents is given at rest, beginning imaging ≥45 minutes later. The sequence stress–rest can be inverted to rest–stress. In patients with known CAD or with high likelihood of CAD, both imaging sequences are equally acceptable. In patients with a relatively low likelihood of CAD, it is preferable to start with stress imaging first, and if it is completely normal, rest imaging may be unnecessary.

9.5 ^{99m}Tc-agent One-day Imaging Protocol (Rest–stress or Stress–rest)

^{99m}Tc agent (250–300 MBq) is IV administered at rest, beginning imaging ≥45 minutes after tracer injection. Three hours later (to allow time for hepatobiliary and gastrointestinal clearance of the tracer from previous injection), a further injection of ^{99m}Tc agents (750–925 MBq) is administered at peak of stress. Imaging acquisition is performed 15 or ≥45 minutes after tracer injection depending on the type of stress performed (exercise or pharmacologic, respectively).

As with the previous protocol, the sequence rest–stress can be inverted. The three-times-higher dose given for the second test yields an adequate image quality without the need for subtracting the residual activity from the low dose of the first test. The rest–stress sequence allows the higher dose to be given during stress, which provides optimum imaging of stress-induced defects and may improve detection of defect reversibility compared with the alternative stress–rest sequence. However, neither the imaging sequence nor the minimum interval time between the two tracer injections is fully settled. In overweight patients (>90 kg), a low dose of ^{99m}Tc agent may result in suboptimal images; therefore, a 2-day imaging protocol is preferable. Because pharmacologic stress perfusion imaging results in higher hepatic and gastrointestinal tracer uptake with slower clearance compared with exercise studies, a rest–stress imaging sequence may offer an advantage.

9.6 One-day Dual Tracer Imaging Protocol (^{201}Tl Rest-^{99m}Tc-agent Stress)

^{201}Tl (111 MBq) is IV administered for initial rest study, imaging within 15 minutes, and ^{99m}Tc agent (925 MBq) is IV administered for stress study, imaging 15 or ≥45 minutes after tracer injection, depending on the type of stress performed (exercise or vasodilator, respectively).

This strategy allows a shorter duration of the entire imaging protocol and takes advantage of the myocardial viability properties of ^{201}Tl and the higher energy quality imaging characteristics of ^{99m}Tc agents. If fixed defects are present, additional imaging 24 hours later, centered at ^{201}Tl photopeaks, may be helpful for better detection of defect reversibility secondary to delayed redistribution. However, because of the differences between ^{201}Tl and ^{99m}Tc in terms of physical properties, this protocol requires somewhat greater experience for image interpretation. Furthermore, the approach may not be ideal for a patient population with a low likelihood of CAD, who may not require the rest study.

References

1. Ranger NT. Radiation detectors in nuclear medicine. Radiographics 1999;19:481–502.
2. Klocke FJ, Baird MG, Lorell BH, et al. ACC/AHA/ASNC guidelines for the clinical use of cardiac radionuclide imaging: a report of the American College of Cardiology/American Heart Association Task Force on Practice Guidelines (ACC/AHA/ASNC Committee to Revise the 1995 Guidelines for the Clinical Use of Cardiac Radionuclide Imaging). 2003. American College of Cardiology Web site. Available at: http: //www.acc.org/clinical/guidelines/radio/rni_fulltext.pdf.

3. Hansen CL. Digital image processing for clinicians. Part I. Basics of image formation. J Nucl Cardiol 2002;9: 343–349.
4. Cullom SJ, Case JA, Bateman TM. Electrocardiographically gated myocardial perfusion SPECT: technical principles and quality control considerations. J Nucl Cardiol 1998;5:418–425.
5. Go V, Bhatt MR, Hendel CR. The diagnostic and prognostic value of ECG-gated SPECT myocardial perfusion imaging. J Nucl Med 2004;45:912–921.
6. Strauss HW, Harrison K, Langan JK, Lebowitz E, Pitt B. Thallium-201 for myocardial imaging. Relation of thallium-201 to regional myocardial perfusion. Circulation 1975;51:641–645.
7. Weich HF, Strauss HW, Pitt B. The extraction of thallium-201 by the myocardium. Circulation 1977;56: 188–191.
8. Dahlberg ST, Leppo JA. Myocardial kinetics of radiolabeled perfusion agents: basis for perfusion imaging. J Nucl Cardiol 1994;1:189–197.
9. Narula J, Flotats A, Nunn A, Carrió I. Newer developments in radionuclide imaging of cardiovascular diseases. In: Iskandrian AE, Verani MS, eds. Nuclear Cardiac Imaging: Principles and Applications. 3rd ed. Philadelphia: FA Davis Publishing; 2003:419–456.
10. Beller GA, Bergmann SR. Myocardial perfusion imaging agents: SPECT and PET. J Nucl Cardiol 2004;11: 71–86.
11. Kailasnath P, Sinusas AJ. Comparison of Tl-201 with Tc-99m labeled myocardial perfusion agents: technical, physiologic, and clinical issues. J Nucl Cardiol 2001;8: 482–498.
12. American Society of Nuclear Cardiology. Updated imaging guidelines for nuclear cardiology procedures, Part 1. J Nucl Cardiol 2001;8: G1–58.
13. Strauss HW, Miller DD, Wittry MD, et al. Society of Nuclear Medicine procedure guideline for myocardial perfusion imaging. Version 3.0, approved June 15, 2002. Available at: http: //interactive.snm.org/index.cfm?PageID=1110&RPID=969&FileID=1302.
14. Germano G. Technical aspects of myocardial SPECT imaging. J Nucl Med 2001;42:1499–1507.
15. Garcia EV. Quantitative myocardial perfusion single-photon emission computed tomographic imaging: quo vadis? (Where do we go from here?) J Nucl Cardiol 1994; 1:83–93.
16. Anagnostopoulos C, Harbinson M, Kelion A, et al. Procedure guidelines for radionuclide myocardial perfusion imaging. Nucl Med Commun 2003;24:1105–1119.
17. Ficaro EP, Corbett JR. Advances in quantitative perfusion SPECT imaging. J Nucl Cardiol 2004;11:62–70.
18. Zubal G, Wisniewski G. Understanding space and filter selection. J Nucl Cardiol 1997;4:234–243.
19. Tsui BM, Frey EC, LaCroix KJ, et al. Quantitative myocardial perfusion SPECT. J Nucl Cardiol 1998;5: 507–522.
20. Hansen CL. Digital image processing for clinicians. Part III. SPECT reconstruction. J Nucl Cardiol 2002;9: 542–549.
21. Everaert H, Bossuyt A, Franken PR. Left ventricular ejection fraction and volumes from gated single photon emission tomographic myocardial perfusion images: comparison between two algorithms working in three-dimensional space. J Nucl Cardiol 1997;4:472–476.
22. Cerqueira MD, Weissman NJ, Dilsizian V, et al. Standardized myocardial segmentation and nomenclature for tomographic imaging of the heart: a statement for healthcare professionals from the Cardiac Imaging Committee of the Council on Clinical Cardiology of the American Heart Association. J Nucl Cardiol 2002;9: 240–245.
23. Jain D, Thompson B, Wackers FJ, Zaret BL. Relevance of increased lung thallium uptake on stress imaging in patients with unstable angina and non-Q wave myocardial infarction: results of the thrombolysis in myocardial infarction (TIMI)-IIIB study. J Am Coll Cardiol 1997;30:421–429.
24. Marcassa C, Galli M, Baroffio C, Eleuteri E, Campini R, Giannuzzi P. Independent and incremental prognostic value of (201)Tl lung uptake at rest in patients with severe postischemic left ventricular dysfunction. Circulation 2000;102:1795–1801.
25. McLaughlin MG, Danias PG. Transient ischemic dilation: a powerful diagnostic and prognostic finding of stress myocardial perfusion imaging. J Nucl Cardiol 2002;9:663–667.
26. Corbett JR, Ficaro EP. Clinical review of attenuation-corrected cardiac SPECT. J Nucl Cardiol 1999;6: 54–68.
27. Smanio PE, Watson DD, Segalla DL, et al. Value of gating of technetium-99m sestamibi single photon emission computed tomography imaging. J Am Coll Cardiol 1997;29:69.
28. Johnson LL, Verdesca SA, Aude WY, et al. Postischemic stunning can affect left ventricular ejection fraction and regional wall motion on post-stress gated sestamibi tomograms. J Am Coll Cardiol 1997;30:1641–1648.
29. Iskandrian AS, Heo J, Kong B, et al. Effects of exercise level on the ability of thallium-201 tomographic imaging in detecting coronary artery disease: analysis of 141 patients. J Am Coll Cardiol 1989;14:1477–1486.
30. Pina IL, Balady GJ, Hanson P, Labovitz AJ, Madonna DW, Myers J. Guidelines for clinical exercise testing laboratories. A statement for healthcare professionals from the Committee on Exercise and Cardiac Rehabilitation, American Heart Association. Circulation 1995;91: 912–921.
31. Candell-Riera J, Santana-Boado C, Castell-Conesa J, et al. Simultaneous dipyridamole/maximal subjective exercise with 99mTc-MIBI SPECT. Improved diagnostic yield in coronary artery disease. J Am Coll Cardiol 1997; 29:531–536.
32. Verzijlbergen JF, Vermeersch PH, Laarman GJ, Ascoop CA. Inadequate exercise leads to suboptimal imaging. Thallium-201 myocardial perfusion imaging after dipyridamole combined with low-level exercise unmasks ischemia in symptomatic patients with non-diagnostic thallium-201 scans who exercise submaximally. J Nucl Med 1991;32:2071–2078.
33. Iskandrian AS, Verani MS, Heo J. Pharmacologic stress testing: mechanism of action, hemodynamic responses, and results in detection of coronary artery disease. J Nucl Cardiol 1994;1:94–111.
34. Cerqueira MD. Pharmacologic stress versus maximal-exercise stress of perfusion imaging: which, when and why? J Nucl Cardiol 1996;3:S10–S14.
35. O'Keefe JH, Bateman TM, Barnhart CS. Adenosine thallium-201 is superior to exercise thallium-201 for detecting coronary artery disease in patients with left

bundle branch block. J Am Coll Cardiol 1993;21:1332–1338.
36. Larcos G, Brown ML, Gibbons RJ. Role of dipyridamole thallium-201 imaging in left bundle branch block. Am J Cardiol 1991;68:1097–1100.
37. Pennell DJ, Mavrogeni SI, Forbat SM, et al. Adenosine combined with dynamic exercise for myocardial perfusion imaging. J Am Coll Cardiol 1995;25:1300–1309.
38. Elliott MD, Holly TA, Leonard SM, Hendel RC. Impact of an abbreviated adenosine protocol incorporating adjunctive treadmill exercise on adverse effects and image quality in patients undergoing stress myocardial perfusion imaging. J Nucl Cardiol 2000;7:584–589.
39. Holly TA, Satran A, Bromet DS, et al. The impact of adjunctive adenosine infusion during exercise myocardial perfusion imaging: results of the Both Exercise and Adenosine Stress Test (BEAST) trial. J Nucl Cardiol 2003;10:291–296.
40. Hendel RC, Jamil T, Glover DK. Pharmacologic stress testing: new methods and new agents. J Nucl Cardiol 2003;10:197–204.
41. Udelson JE, Heller GV, Wackers FJ, et al. Randomized, controlled dose-ranging study of the selective adenosine A_{2A} receptor agonist binodenoson for pharmacological stress as an adjunct to myocardial perfusion imaging. Circulation 2004;109:457–464.
42. Taillefer R, Amyot R, Turpin S, et al. Comparison between dipyridamole and adenosine as pharmacological coronary vasodilators in detection of coronary artery disease with thallium-201 imaging. J Nucl Cardiol 1996;3:204–211.
43. Ignaszewski AP, McCormick LX, Heslip PG, McEwan AJ, Humen DP. Safety and clinical utility of combined intravenous dipyridamole/symptom-limited exercise stress test with thallium-201 imaging in patients with known or suspected coronary artery disease. J Nucl Med 1993;34:2053–2061.
44. Wackers FJ. The maze of myocardial imaging protocols in 1994. J Nucl Cardiol 1994;1:180–188.
45. Flotats A, Carrió I, Estorch M, et al. Nitrate administration to enhance detection of myocardial viability by Tc-99m-tetrofosmin SPECT. Eur J Nucl Med 1997;24:767–773.
46. He W, Acampa W, Mainolfi C, et al. Tc-99m tetrofosmin tomography after nitrate administration in patients with ischemic left ventricular dysfunction: relation to metabolic imaging by PET. J Nucl Cardiol 2003;10:599–606.
47. Hansen CL. Digital image processing for clinicians. Part II. Filtering. J Nucl Cardiol 2002;9:429–437.
48. Dilsizian V, Rocco TP, Freedman NM, Leon MB, Bonow RO. Enhanced detection of ischemic but viable myocardium by the reinjection of thallium after stress-redistribution imaging. N Engl J Med 1990;323:141–146.

5

Positron Emission Tomography

Frank M. Bengel

Positron emission tomography (PET) is a high-end imaging technique, which combines superior detection sensitivity with an almost unlimited availability of radiotracers. Short-lived positron emitters such as oxygen-15, nitrogen-13, carbon-, and fluorine-18 represent ideal isotopes for labeling of biomolecules for in vivo characterization of physiologic and biochemical processes. Dynamic data acquisition with high temporal resolution combined with attenuation correction allows for tracer kinetic modeling and calculation of truly quantitative information by noninvasive means.

After its introduction nearly 30 years ago, PET was first established in academic centers for clinical research in neurology, cardiology, and oncology. Based on promising early results, clinical applications for cardiac PET have emerged. For the assessment of myocardial viability and perfusion, PET is still widely regarded as the noninvasive gold standard. Comparison with other techniques has refined their application and allowed for improved conventional imaging approaches. Moreover, PET has substantially contributed to a better understanding of various disease processes, for example, in patients with severe coronary artery disease and ischemically compromised but viable myocardium.

A major limitation for the widespread use of PET remains the high cost, reflecting the sophisticated imaging technology and the need of a cyclotron on-site or in close proximity for production of short-lived tracers. However, simplified approaches for positron imaging have been introduced and may – together with an efficient production and distribution of radioisotopes through commercial centers – contribute to a wider clinical application of PET in the future. PET will continue to have its main role as an attractive research tool. Advances in molecular biology and progress in disease-specific therapy have prompted an increasing need for characterization of physiologic and biologic parameters in the heart. New tracer approaches aiming at molecular targets may be suited to monitor specific therapeutically induced changes in cellular function. The uniqueness of this information may contribute to define the clinical future of PET and noninvasive cardiovascular imaging in general.

This chapter highlights the potential of PET for imaging of cardiovascular disease. The methodologic background is outlined first, before major practical applications and biologic imaging targets in the heart are summarized. Finally, an outlook into the future, comprising novel molecular tracers and advanced imaging technology, is given.

1. Technical Aspects of PET Imaging

1.1 Imaging Methodology

Beta-decay of PET radiotracers results in emission of a positron, which immediately annihilates itself together with an electron. Annihilation results in emission of two 511-keV photons traveling in 180° opposite directions. Those photons are detected as coincidences in the crystal ring of the PET scanner, allowing for accurate localization of the origin of decay (Figure 5.1). The spatial resolution of currently available PET systems is in the range of 4–8 mm. Another feature of dedicated PET scanners is their high temporal resolution, allowing for dynamic imaging of radiotracer kinetics as a prerequisite for noninvasive absolute quantification of biologic processes. Correction of emission data for tissue photon attenuation is a further prerequisite for tracer quantification. This is easily and readily accomplished by performance of an additional transmission scan with external 511-keV sources, which is used for calculation of regional attenuation coefficients and subsequent correction of emission images.

Because dedicated PET scanners are expensive and not widely available, alternative strategies have been developed for imaging the cardiac distribution of PET tracers with conventional gamma cameras. One is single photon emission computed tomography (SPECT) imaging of single 511-keV photons with an ultrahigh energy collimator[1]; the other is coincidence imaging with a dual-headed gamma camera.[2] These approaches are characterized by lower spatial resolution and detection sensitivity, and do not allow for dynamic imaging and absolute quantification. But, especially for 511-keV SPECT imaging of F-18 fluorodeoxyglucose (FDG) in the assessment of myocardial viability, considerable evidence has accumulated supporting the clinical usefulness of this simplified strategy.[3]

1.2 Radioisotopes and Radiopharmaceuticals

Production of most radioisotopes for labeling of PET radiopharmaceuticals requires a cyclotron. The "medical" cyclotrons used at PET facilities accelerate either protons or deuterons onto a suitable target. Neutrons in the target nuclei are replaced by positively charged particles, resulting in short-lived isotopes that undergo β(+)-decay (Table 5.1). The most common PET radionuclide, fluorine-18, is, e.g., produced by the $^{18}O(p, n)^{18}F$ reaction. That means, a target containing oxygen-18 (in the form of ^{18}O-enriched water) is bombarded with protons, resulting in fluorine-18 by replacement of a neutron with a proton in the nucleus. Alternatively, some isotopes such as the perfusion tracer

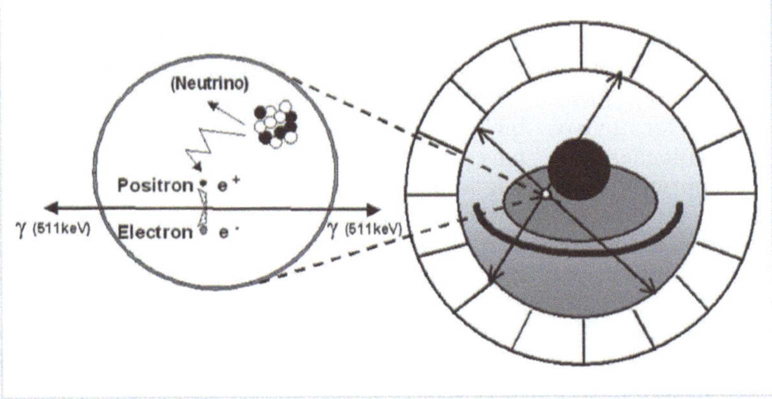

Figure 5.1. Basic principle of PET imaging. An emitted positron annihilates with an electron, causing emission of two 511-keV photons that travel in 180° opposite directions from their origin. Detection of these photons as pairs of coincidences in the PET detector ring allows for accurate localization of the radioactive decay in the target organ and the whole body.

Table 5.1. Radioisotopes used for PET imaging

Isotope	Half-life (min)	Maximum positron energy* (MeV)	Production
Carbon-11	20.4	0.96	$^{14}N(p,\alpha)^{11}C$
Nitrogen-13	9.96	1.20	$^{16}O(p,\alpha)^{13}N$
Oxygen-15	2.03	1.74	$^{15}N(p,n)^{15}O$
Fluorine-18	109.8	0.63	$^{18}O(p,n)^{18}F$
Copper-62	9.76	2.91	Generator (parent ^{62}Zn; $T_{1/2}$ 9.13 h
Rubidium-82	1.25	3.40	Generator (parent ^{82}Sr; $T_{1/2}$ 25 d
Iodine-124	6.0×10^3	2.13	$^{124}Te(d,2n)^{124}I$

* Positron energy is the major determinant of traveling range in tissue before annihilation, which is inversely related to accuracy of localization of decay.

rubidium-82 are obtained from specific generators containing longer-lived parent nuclides.

Positron-emitting isotopes of the major bioelements nitrogen, oxygen, and carbon are available, along with fluorine-18, for labeling of various biocompounds. Radiopharmaceuticals that have been applied for cardiac imaging in the clinical setting are summarized in Table 5.2. At present, these tracers target myocardial perfusion, metabolism, innervation, and receptors. Further tracers are under experimental evaluation, which aim at imaging of molecular structures such as extracellular matrix, membrane molecules, or intracellular products of gene expression. Those are expected to broaden the spectrum of biologic targets for clinical cardiac PET imaging in the future.

Table 5.2. PET radiopharmaceuticals for clinical cardiac imaging

Tracer	Biologic target
Blood flow	
N-13 ammonia	Perfusion, blood flow
O-15 water	Blood flow, perfusible tissue
Rb-82 chloride	Perfusion, Viability
Cu-62 PTSM	Perfusion
Metabolism	
F-18 fluorodeoxyglucose (FDG)	Glucose transport, hexokinase
C-11 glucose	Glucose metabolism
C-11 acetate	Oxidative metabolism (TCA cycle turnover)
C-11 palmitate	Fatty acid metabolism
F-18 FTHA	Fatty acid uptake
Innervation	
F-18 fluorodopamine	Presynaptic sympathetic function
C-11 hydroxyephedrine	Presynaptic catecholamine uptake
C-11 epinephrine	Presynaptic catecholamine uptake and storage
C-11 phenylephrine	Presynaptic catecholamine uptake and metabolism
Receptors	
C-11 CGP12177	β-Adrenergic receptor (nonselective)
C-11 MQNB	Muscarinic receptor

1.3 Noninvasive Quantification of Biologic Processes

PET is a truly quantitative imaging tool because it allows measurement of localized radiotracer concentration in the body in absolute units of radioactivity concentration with high accuracy and precision. A necessity for quantification is the routine availability of correction algorithms to eliminate sources of error in raw images. PET imaging implies corrections for random and scattered coincidences, for dead-time loss of detectors, for partial volume effects and resolution recovery, and, most importantly, for tissue attenuation of photons. The resulting images of regional radioactive tracer distribution are usefully applied to answer clinical and scientific questions. Software algorithms are available, which are similar to those applied for SPECT image display, and allow for reangulation of tomographic images along cardiac short and long axes, and for calculation of polar maps.

With the additional use of tracer kinetic modeling, however, there is the potential for substantial improvement of the type and quality of information obtained from biologic data. Kinetic modeling of tracers in the heart requires acquisition of a dynamic imaging sequence, which generates serial images at various time points after radiotracer injection. This allows for extraction of time-activity curves for myocardial segments using software algorithms. The time course of tracer concentration in arterial blood (arterial input function) is additionally obtained using a region of interest in the left ventricular cavity or left atrium. Time-activity curves are subsequently fitted to suitable compartmental models, which characterize the tissue kinetics of the respective tracers. For O-15 water as a freely diffusible perfusion tracer, e.g., this is a simple single-compartment model with one extravascular compartment.[4] For the perfusion tracer N-13 ammonia, which is taken up by tissue and subsequently used for glutamine synthesis, a two-compartment model with an extravascular

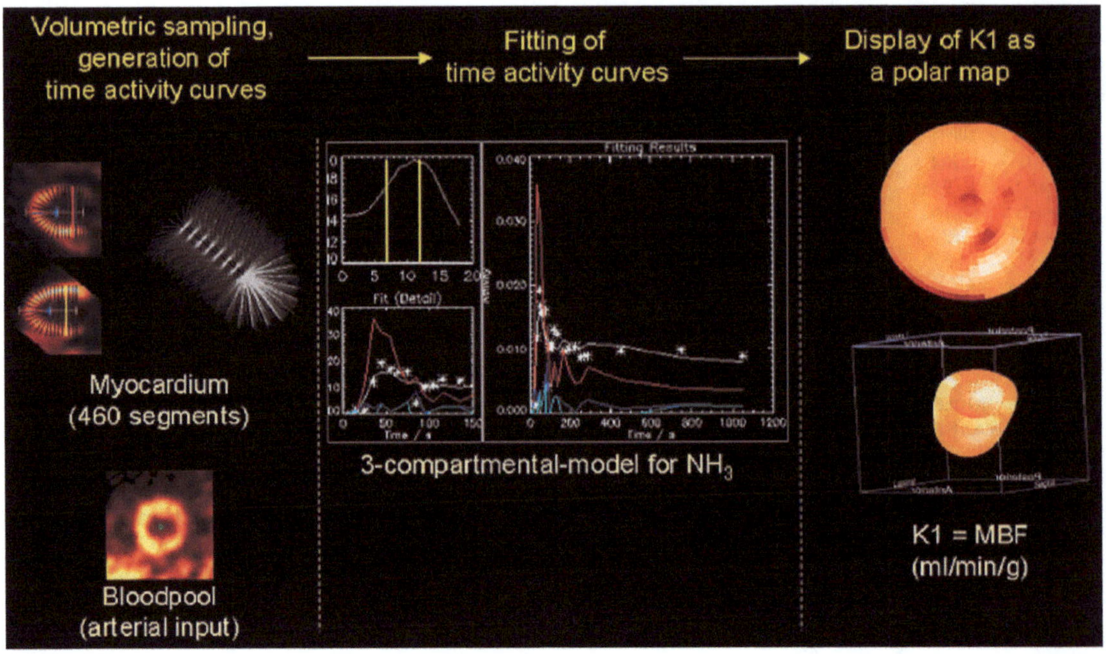

Figure 5.2. Tracer kinetic analysis for noninvasive absolute quantification. Shown are the major steps of quantification of myocardial blood flow using N-13 ammonia, as applied at the TU München. Left, Myocardial segments and blood pool are identified using software-based volumetric sampling. Time-activity curves are extracted from the dynamic imaging dataset for these segments. Middle, Individual time-activity curves are fitted to a validated three-compartment model for ammonia (white stars – measured activity over time in representative myocardial segment; white line – fitted myocardial time activity curve; red line – blood pool curve). Right, After the fitting procedure, the influx constant K1, which reflects absolute myocardial blood flow, is depicted for all myocardial segments as two- or three-dimensional polar map.

and a metabolic compartment can be applied.[5] Kinetics of the metabolic tracer F-18 FDG can be described by a three-compartment model.[6] FDG is taken up by myocardium via specific membrane glucose transporters. Intracellularly, FDG is phosphorylated by hexokinase to FDG-6-phosphate. FDG-6-phosphate is not a good substrate for further metabolism and is thus trapped intracellularly. Compartmental modeling of tracer kinetics yields rate constants that quantitatively reflect biologic processes (Figure 5.2; see color section).

2. PET Imaging of Cardiac Physiology and Biology

2.1 Myocardial Blood Flow

Myocardial perfusion PET imaging is accomplished using flow tracers at rest and during pharmacologic stress.[7,8] Dipyridamole or adenosine are applied for pharmacologic vasodilation at doses frequently used for SPECT imaging. Physical exercise is not well accepted for stress flow measurements with PET because of the high likelihood of patient motion during imaging in the ring scanner. Relative regional perfusion abnormalities are assessed from static images using N-13 ammonia and Rb-82 (Figure 5.3; see color section). The usefulness of O-15 water as a freely diffusible tracer in this regard is less well documented, because myocardial images are only obtained after application of factor analysis or blood-pool subtraction techniques.

In a clinical setting, the purpose of qualitative PET perfusion imaging is similar to that of SPECT, namely, to detect myocardial ischemia and/or infarction in patients with suspected or known coronary artery disease, to determine extent and severity of the disease, to determine individual risk for cardiac events, and to thereby guide further workup.[9–11] The diagnostic accuracy for detection of coronary artery disease is higher compared with SPECT,[12] which can be explained by higher spatial resolution, higher extraction fraction of PET flow tracers, and absence of attenuation artifacts. Incremental prognostic value of qualitative perfusion PET over clinical variables for prediction of cardiac events has been demonstrated.[13] Additionally, it has been shown that the more expensive PET perfusion imaging approach can still be cost-effective in a specific setting compared with other strategies, including exercise electrocardiogram and SPECT.[14]

The major impact of PET perfusion studies is derived from the potential for noninvasive quantification of myocardial blood flow as explained above, allowing for studies of coronary microcirculatory regulation on the resistance level. Although potentially helpful in the clinical diagnosis of coronary artery disease,[15] absolute flow measurements by PET have mainly been applied in studies to understand the effects of risk factors of coronary artery disease, such as hyperlipidemia, diabetes, and smoking, leading to an increased emphasis on preventive therapy.[16–21] With the ability to test specific components of microvascular function such as endothelial-dependent and -independent vasodilation, PET serves increasingly as an endpoint to measure effects of risk factor manipulation, new drugs, and other therapeutic approaches in the prevention of clinical coronary artery disease.

2.2 Myocardial Viability

2.2.1 Clinical Importance

PET has not only had a fundamental role in the clinical emergence of noninvasive viability imaging. Regarded as an imaging "gold standard," it has contributed to validation and refinement of other imaging approaches. The largest cumulative experience on the impact of viability imaging on patient management is derived from metabolic studies using F-18 FDG. The quantitative nature of PET has also provided significant information for a better understanding of the pathophysiologic interrelations among myocardial blood flow, metabolism, and contractile function involved in development of severely jeopardized myocardium.

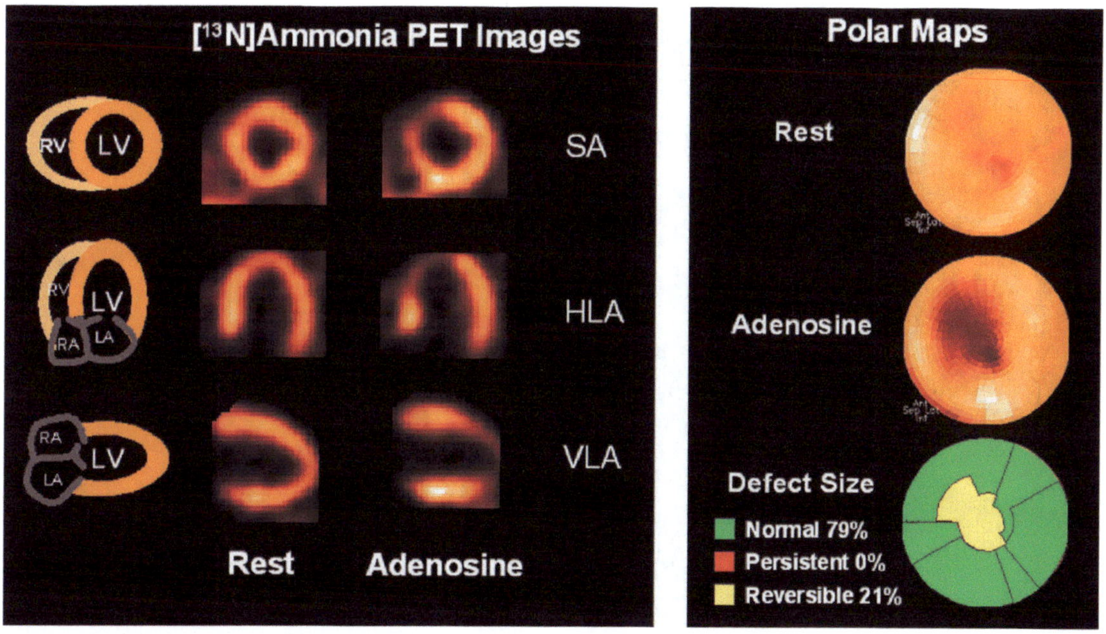

Figure 5.3. Case example of static (semiquantitative) images of myocardial perfusion at rest and during adenosine vasodilation in a patient with single-vessel coronary artery disease and stress-induced ischemia in anteroseptal myocardium.

F-18 FDG myocardial imaging is the most frequent clinical application of cardiac PET.[7,8] For assessment of myocardial viability, F-18 FDG is combined with resting perfusion measurements using either a second PET tracer in the same session, or (if performed at a place remote from a cyclotron and not equipped with a perfusion tracer generator) in combination with perfusion SPECT. PET viability imaging is obtained in patients with dysfunctional, hypoperfused myocardial regions to determine the likelihood of a benefit from revascularization. Residual metabolic activity is an indicator of myocardial viability, and thus of reversibility of contractile dysfunction. Regional reduction of FDG uptake in proportion to perfusion (perfusion/metabolism match) reflects scar and thus irreversibility of contractile dysfunction (Figure 5.4; see color section), whereas increased regional FDG uptake relative to myocardial perfusion (perfusion/metabolism mismatch) indicates ischemically compromised but viable myocardium (Figure 5.5; see color section).

Since introduction of the approach in 1986,[22] it has been shown in a variety of studies that recovery of function after revascularization can be predicted by PET with high sensitivity of 85%–90% and specificity of 75%–85%.[23]

Additionally, the importance of identification of viable myocardium has increasingly been investigated beyond the prediction of functional recovery, which is only a surrogate endpoint for clinical and prognostic importance. It has, e.g., been shown that recovery of function is coupled with improvement of heart failure symptoms.[24] Moreover, patients benefit through reduced peri- and postoperative risk when PET criteria are used for selection for bypass surgery as compared with those selected without a PET study.[25] An increased preoperative mortality and limited functional recovery were observed when revascularization was delayed after detection of viable myocardium by PET, suggesting that the hibernating state is unstable and requires immediate attention.[26] PET viability studies have a significant impact on clinical decision making in patients with coronary disease and left ventricular (LV) dysfunction.[27] Finally, randomized trials based on PET are currently underway to further establish the clinical importance of viability imaging as an evidence-based approach.

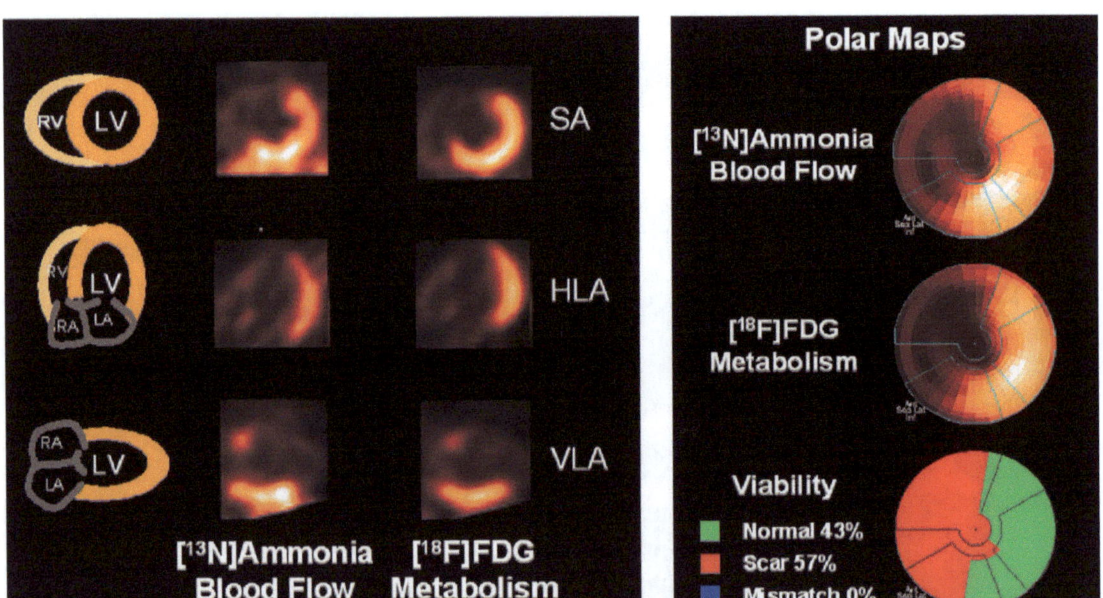

Figure 5.4. Case example of a viability scan in a patient with severe triple-vessel disease and ischemic LV dysfunction, showing a perfusion/metabolism match that indicates extensive scar.

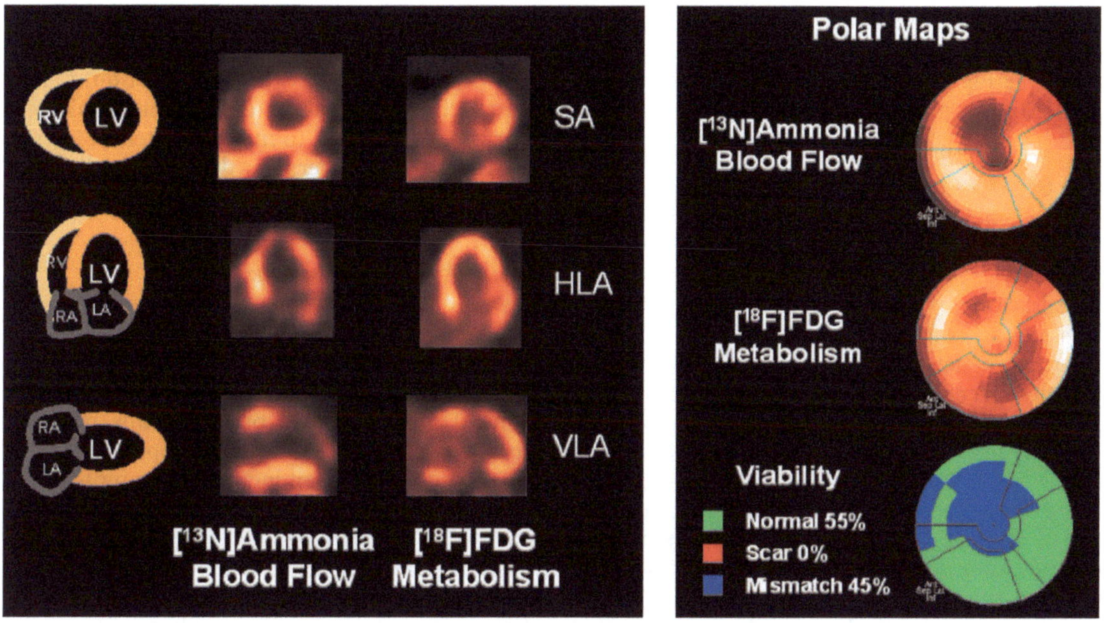

Figure 5.5. Case example of a viability scan in another patient with severe triple-vessel disease and ischemic LV dysfunction, showing a perfusion/metabolism mismatch that indicates ischemically compromised, but viable (hibernating) myocardium.

2.2.2 Metabolic Standardization

Diagnostic quality of myocardial FDG images is influenced by the concentration of tracer in myocardium and blood. Myocardial FDG uptake depends on glucose and insulin plasma concentrations as well as the rate of glucose utilization. High glucose plasma concentrations degrade the quality of the myocardial FDG uptake image.[28–30] Myocardial glucose uptake also depends on cardiac work, plasma levels of Free Fatty Acids (FFA) and other substrates, insulin, catecholamines, and oxygen supply.[31] Standardization of the metabolic environment is necessary for clinical myocardial FDG imaging.[32] There are several accepted methods for improvement of myocardial FDG PET image quality:

- Oral glucose loading is often used to stimulate insulin secretion and myocardial glucose utilization. It enhances the image quality with more homogeneously distributed FDG uptake than observed during the fasting state.[33] Despite the gain in image quality after oral glucose loading (50–75 g), diagnostically unsatisfactory images may still be obtained in 20%–25% of the patients with coronary artery disease.[29,33] Abnormal glucose handling or even type 2 diabetes that frequently have remained undetected account for the poor image quality in many of these patients.
- Euglycemic hyperinsulinemic clamping is an approach that mimics the postabsorptive steady-state,[29,34] and has become an alternative to oral glucose loading for enhancing glucose utilization.[29] Insulin clamping stimulates uptake of glucose and FDG in the myocardium and in skeletal muscle and yields images of consistently high diagnostic quality, even in patients with diabetes.
- Several studies[30,35–37] have demonstrated that oral administration of a nicotinic acid or its derivatives is another effective technique to improve FDG image quality. When combined with small amounts of short-acting insulin, good image quality can be obtained also in diabetic subjects.[35] Nicotinic acid inhibits peripheral lipolysis and thus reduces plasma FFA concentrations. Acipimox is a nicotinic acid derivative that is 20 times more potent and has more favorable kinetics than nicotinic acid.[38] Importantly, with the exception of flushing, no side effects of Acipimox have been observed.

The preparation of patients for PET studies and detailed protocols for metabolic and perfusion imaging have been described in procedural guidelines by professional societies.[7,8]

2.3 Other Imaging Targets

2.3.1 Substrate Metabolism

In addition to F-18 FDG, a variety of tracers exists to study quantitatively the complex interaction between substrate delivery, uptake, and turnover in myocardial tissue under various physiologic and pathophysiologic conditions. The myocardial metabolic rate of glucose is quantified from dynamic FDG PET,[6] or, as shown more recently, using C-11 glucose.[39] Additionally, use of fatty acids as the second major substrate can be examined using C-11 palmitate[40] or F-18 fluoro-6-thia-heptadecanoic acid (FTHA).[41]

C-11 acetate is another metabolic tracer that is extracted proportionally to myocardial blood flow, then rapidly enters the tricarboxylic acid cycle and is metabolized to carbon dioxide. Washout of C-11 from the myocardium is used to quantify turnover in the tricarboxylic acid (TCA) cycle as the final common pathway of all substrates, and thus to measure overall oxidative metabolism.[42,43] When combined with measures of cardiac contractile performance, C-11 acetate PET can be used for a noninvasive estimation of cardiac efficiency (defined as the relation between work and oxygen consumption).[44] This approach is of special interest in heart failure,[45] where it can be used to measure effects of drugs such as beta-blockers or dobutamine,[44,46] and thereby to optimize medical therapy.

2.3.2 Autonomic Innervation

The autonomic nervous system has a central role for regulation of cardiac performance under various physiologic and pathophysiologic conditions. The importance of alterations of autonomic innervation in the pathophysiology of heart disease has been increasingly emphasized. Using radiolabeled catecholamine analogs such as C-11 hydroxyephedrine (HED) or F-18 fluorodopamine, PET provides noninvasive information about global and regional myocardial sympathetic innervation. It has substantially facilitated and refined the study of the heart's nervous system in health and disease, and has significantly contributed to a continuous improvement of the understanding of cardiac pathophysiology.

In transplanted hearts, which are completely denervated early after surgery, partial sympathetic reinnervation has been identified (Figure 5.6; see color section).[47] The reinnervated heart

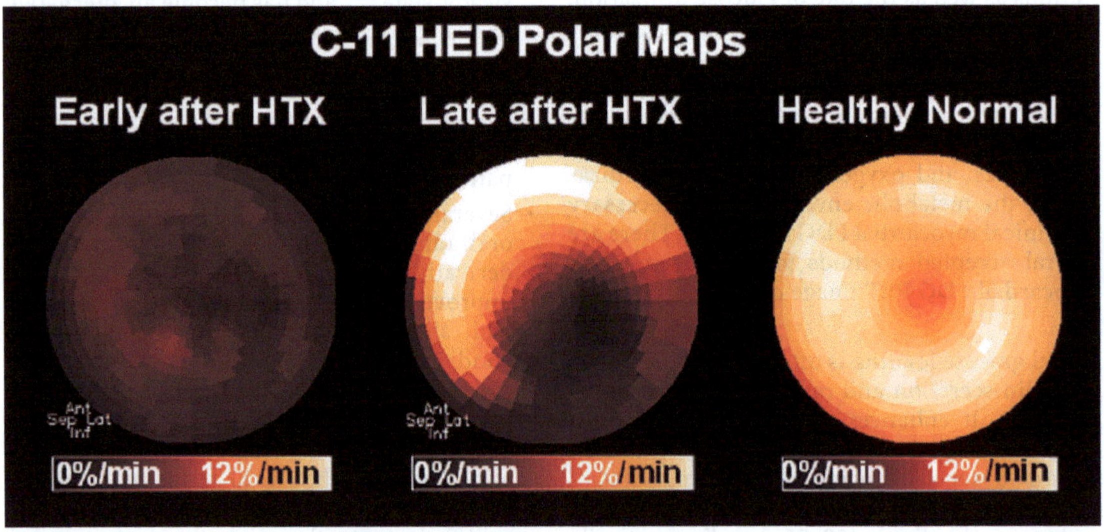

Figure 5.6. Examples of LV polar maps of myocardial retention of C-11 hydroxyephedrine (HED) in a patient early after cardiac transplantation (HTX), indicating complete sympathetic denervation (left), in a patient late after transplantation, indicating partial sympathetic reinnervation in basal anteroseptal wall (middle), and in a healthy subject (right).

was used as a model for determination of physiologic effects of innervation by intraindividual comparison of denervated and reinnervated myocardium, substantiating the role of innervation for regulation of myocardial blood flow, metabolism, and contractility.[48–50] Furthermore, alterations of cardiac innervation were identified in diabetes mellitus, ischemic syndromes,[51] arrhythmogenic diseases,[52,53] and heart failure,[54,55] and their pathophysiologic relevance[56] as well as prognostic implications[57] were identified in subsets of patients.

2.3.3 Receptors

Various myocardial receptors have been identified to have a role in cardiovascular pathophysiology, and thus represent attractive targets for imaging. The nonselective β-adrenergic receptor ligand C-11 CGP12177 has been applied to visualize down-regulation of β-receptors in heart failure,[58] and to identify pre-/postsynaptic imbalance in cardiomyopathy and arrhythmogenic diseases.[52,59] Other adrenergic receptor ligands have been introduced, but not yet applied in humans.[60,61] Furthermore, C-11 MQNB, a muscarinic receptor agonist, has been applied to describe up-regulation of myocardial muscarinic receptors in heart failure as a potential adaptive mechanism.[62] Further attractive targets for myocardial receptor imaging comprise, e.g., the opiate, endothelin, angiotensin, and adenosine receptor systems. But issues related to low selectivity and affinity, high nonspecific binding, lack of hydrophilicity (to avoid binding to internalized inactive receptors), and pharmacologic/toxicologic effects along with complicated, less reliable tracer synthesis have precluded a more widespread application of available receptor ligands for cardiac PET, and will need to be overcome in the future.

2.3.4 Further Molecular Probes

The recent advent and rapid success of molecular imaging has resulted in a series of very promising novel tracer approaches that go beyond identification of flow, metabolism, and innervation, and target further specific biomechanisms involved in disease. It has also become obvious that developments in oncologic and cardiologic research are often significantly overlapping and may benefit from each other:

- The regulation of blood vessel growth is one area of interest for both oncologists and cardiologists. $\alpha_v\beta_3$integrins are expressed on the endothelial surface during tumor angiogenesis and metastasis growth, and can be identified in the experimental setting using F-18-labeled RGD peptides.[63] These proteins are also a target for cardiac molecular imaging, when expressed during angio-/vasculogenesis, during rapid development of coronary stenosis, e.g., restenosis after interventions, or during migration of inflammatory cells.
- Apoptosis (programmed cell death) is a therapeutic target in tumor treatment, but is also known to have a pivotal role in cardiovascular disease, e.g., in transplant rejection and plaque destabilization.[64] Recently, annexin-V, a molecule that specifically binds to phosphatidylserine, which is expressed on the surface of cells entering the apoptotic cascade, has been successfully labeled with fluorine-18 and is now available for PET.[65] Previously, this tracer was available only as technetium-99m-labeled compound for conventional scintigraphy.
- Within recent years, reporter gene imaging has emerged as an innovative strategy for noninvasive visualization of genetic processes.[66] The principle of reporter gene imaging is based on vector-mediated overexpression of a transgene in host tissue which encodes for an enzyme, a receptor, or a transport protein that is normally not present in the target area. Suitable reporter probes are labeled substrates or ligands for the reporter gene product. PET can be applied to detect accumulation of the probe, which specifically identifies the reporter gene product.[67] The imaging signal thus indirectly reflects expression and transcriptional regulation of the reporter gene. An example is the use of the herpesviral thymidine kinase reporter gene and radiolabeled nucleosides as reporter probes (Figure 5.7; see color section). This technique will allow for monitoring the success of gene therapy, when reporter genes are combined and coexpressed with therapeutic genes. It may also allow for monitoring of endogenous gene expression, if reporter genes are expressed under control of specific promoters that are sensitive to endogenous gene products.[68] Or the reporter

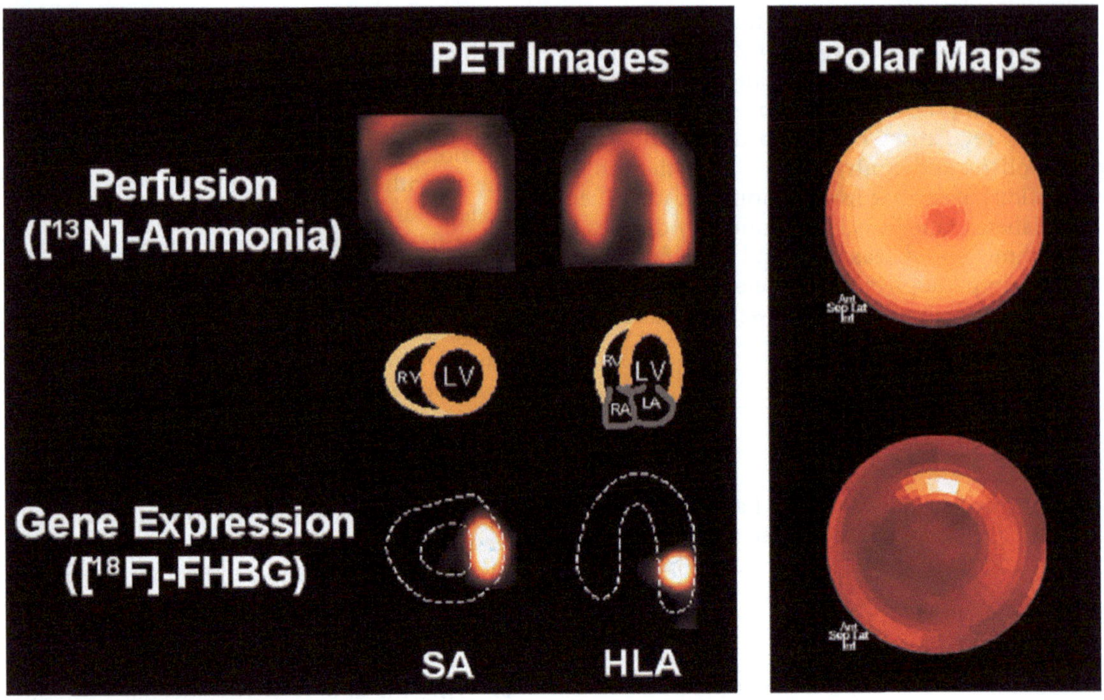

Figure 5.7. PET Imaging of myocardial reporter gene expression in a pig, 2 days after regional myocardial injection of adenovirus carrying the herpesviral thymidine kinase reporter gene (HSV1-sr39tk). High regional accumulation of the reporter probe F-18 FHBG indicates successful transfer and expression of the transgene in anterolateral myocardium.

gene can be expressed in stem cells before their transplantation for subsequent in vivo monitoring of the fate of these therapeutic cells.[69]

For all of these new molecular PET assays, the amount of signal produced, target-to-background ratios, morphologic localization, and specific probe activity are critical issues that need to be overcome for clinical application and will pose a continuous challenge for further developments in camera technology.

3. Hybrid PET/Computed Tomography Imaging

Driven by technical developments and clinical diagnostic needs in oncology, the newest generation of PET scanners is now available in combination with X-ray computed tomography (CT). These hybrid PET/CT scanners incorporate functional/biologic information from PET and morphologic information from CT into a single examination, and have been demonstrated to provide superior diagnostic accuracy for tumor staging.[70,71]

The latest generation of PET/CT scanners is equipped with ultrafast multislice CT, opening grounds for cardiac PET/CT imaging (Figure 5.8; see color section). These scanners hold great promise for a "one-stop shop" biologic/morphologic evaluation of the heart. In the future, functional PET assessment of tissue blood flow and viability will be combined with noninvasive CT assessment of coronary arteries, calcifications, and ventricular function. Furthermore, localization of highly specific molecular signals from myocardium or coronary plaques determined by PET may be facilitated through additional structural information from CT imaging.

Some technical challenges do exist for quantitative cardiac PET/CT. Because CT is acquired during breathhold, misalignment with PET data, which reflect an average over the breathing cycle, can occur. Misalignment adversely influences attenuation correction, quantification, and morphologic localization of PET tracer uptake.

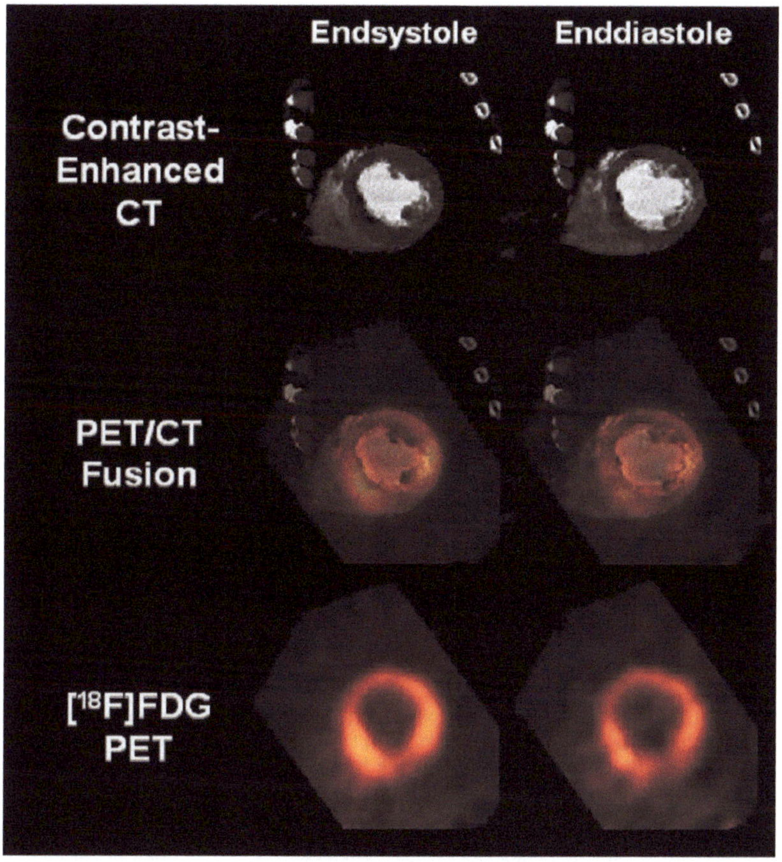

Figure 5.8. Cardiac PET/CT imaging. Coregistration and fusion of morphologic information derived from gated CT and biologic/metabolic information derived from FDG PET.

Studies addressing this issue, e.g., by respiratory gating,[72] are currently underway and will provide the methodologic background for future trials evaluating the clinical benefit of PET/CT imaging in patients with cardiac disease.

4. Summary and Future Perspectives

The application of PET as a research tool has substantially improved understanding of pathophysiologic processes in the heart. Clinical applications for assessment of myocardial viability and perfusion have emerged in the past. Knowledge derived from cardiac PET imaging has been successfully transferred to other imaging techniques, leading to refinement of their application and to increased acceptance of noninvasive cardiac imaging in general.

Clinically, PET is still regarded as the gold standard for detection of myocardial viability and for measurement of myocardial blood flow. It will continue to serve as an endpoint for evaluation of medical and interventional therapeutic approaches. High costs will remain a limitation for its use as a standard procedure, but new developments in technology may allow for a more cost-effective, widespread use of positron-emitting tracers and for integrated biologic/morphologic imaging.

The major impact of PET will continue to be derived from its application as a powerful research tool. Availability of micro PET systems for small animal imaging facilitates the evaluation of novel molecular probes and their translation to human application.[73] Combination of PET with morphologic imaging strategies will then allow for in vivo characterization and localization of molecular mechanisms in the human heart in health and disease. Thereby, PET will remain a forerunner for the future development of the entire field of cardiovascular imaging.

Acknowledgements

The author thanks Dr. Stephan Nekolla for providing material for the figures.

References

1. Bax JJ, Valkema R, Visser FC, et al. FDG SPECT in the assessment of myocardial viability. Comparison with dobutamine echo. Eur Heart J 1997;18(suppl D): D124–129.
2. Nowak B, Zimny M, Schwarz ER, et al. Diagnosis of myocardial viability by dual-head coincidence gamma camera fluorine-18 fluorodeoxyglucose positron emission tomography with and without non-uniform attenuation correction. Eur J Nucl Med 2000;27:1501–1508.
3. Bax J, Patton J, Poldermans D, Elhendy A, Sandler M. 18-Fluorodeoxyglucose imaging with positron emission tomography and single photon emission computed tomography: cardiac applications. Semin Nucl Med 2000;30:281–298.
4. Bergmann SR, Herrero P, Markham J, Weinheimer CJ, Walsh MN. Non-invasive quantitation of myocardial blood flow in human subjects with oxygen-15 labeled water and positron emission tomography. J Am Coll Cardiol 1989;14:639–652.
5. Hutchins G, Schwaiger M, Rosenspire K, Krivokapich J, Schelbert H, Kuhl D. Noninvasive quantification of regional myocardial blood flow in the human heart using N-13 ammonia and dynamic positron emission tomographic imaging. J Am Coll Cardiol 1990;15:1032.
6. Gambhir SS, Schwaiger M, Huang SC, et al. Simple noninvasive quantification method for measuring myocardial glucose utilization in humans employing positron emission tomography and fluorine-18 deoxyglucose. J Nucl Med 1989;30:359–366.
7. Bacharach SL, Bax JJ, Case J, et al. PET myocardial glucose metabolism and perfusion imaging. Part 1. Guidelines for data acquisition and patient preparation. J Nucl Cardiol 2003;10:543–556.
8. Schelbert HR, Beanlands R, Bengel F, et al. PET myocardial perfusion and glucose metabolism imaging. Part 2. Guidelines for interpretation and reporting. J Nucl Cardiol 2003;10:557–571.
9. Gould K, Goldstein R, Mullani N, et al. Clinical feasibility, sensitivity and specifically of positron cardiac imaging without a cyclotron using generator produced Rb-82 for the diagnosis of coronary artery disease. J Nucl Med 1986;27:976.
10. Schelbert HR, Wisenberg G, Phelps ME, et al. Noninvasive assessment of coronary stenoses by myocardial imaging during pharmacologic coronary vasodilation. VI. Detection of coronary artery disease in man with intravenous 13-NH3 and positron computed tomography. Am J Cardiol 1982;49:1197–1207.
11. Tamaki N, Yonekura Y, Senda M, et al. Myocardial positron computed tomography with 13N-ammonia at rest and during exercise. Eur J Nucl Med 1985;11: 246–251.
12. Schwaiger M, Melin J. Cardiological applications of nuclear medicine. Lancet 1999;354:661–666.
13. Marwick T, Shan K, Patel S, Go R, Lauer M. Incremental value of rubidium-82 positron emission tomography for prognostic assessment of known or suspected coronary artery disease. Am J Cardiol 1997;80:865–870.
14. Patterson RE, Eisner RL, Horowitz SF. Comparison of cost-effectiveness and utility of exercise ECG, single photon emission computed tomography, positron emission tomography, and coronary angiography for diagnosis of coronary artery disease. Circulation 1995; 91:54–65.
15. Muzik O, Duvernoy C, Beanlands R, et al. Assessment of diagnostic performance of quantitative flow measurements in normal subjects and patients with angiographically documented CAD by means of nitrogen-13 ammonia and using PET. J Am Coll Cardiol 1998;31: 534–540.
16. Czernin J, Barnard RJ, Sun KT, et al. Effect of short-term cardiovascular conditioning and low-fat diet on myocardial blood flow and flow reserve. Circulation 1995;92:197–204.
17. Dayanikli F, Grambow D, Muzik O, Mosca L, Rubenfire M, Schwaiger M. Early detection of abnormal coronary flow reserve in asymptomatic men at high risk for coronary artery disease using positron emission tomography. Circulation 1994;90:808–817.
18. DiCarli M, Czernin J, Hoh CK, et al. Relation among stenosis severity, myocardial blood flow, and flow reserve in patients with coronary artery disease. Circulation 1995;91:1944–1951.
19. Pitkanen O, Raitakari O, Niinikoski H, et al. Coronary flow reserve is impaired in young men with familial hypercholesterolemia. J Am Coll Cardiol 1996;28: 1705–1711.
20. Pitkanen O, Nuutila P, Raitakari O, et al. Coronary flow reserve is reduced in young men with IDDM. Diabetes 1998;47:248–254.
21. Momose M, Abletshauser C, Neverve J, et al. Dysregulation of coronary microvascular reactivity in asymptomatic patients with type 2 diabetes mellitus. Eur J Nucl Med 2002;29:1675–1679.
22. Tillisch J, Brunken R, Marshall R, et al. Reversibility of cardiac wall motion abnormalities predicted by positron tomography. N Engl J Med 1986;314:884–888.
23. Bax JJ, Wijns W, Cornel JH, Visser FC, Boersma E, Fioretti PM. Accuracy of currently available techniques for prediction of functional recovery after revascularization in patients with left ventricular dysfunction due to chronic coronary artery disease: comparison of pooled data. J Am Coll Cardiol 1997;30:1451–1460.
24. DiCarli MF, Asgarzadie F, Schelbert HR, et al. Quantitative relation between myocardial viability and improvement in heart failure symptoms after revascularization in patients with ischemic cardiomyopathy. Circulation 1995;92:3436–3444.
25. Haas F, Haehnel CJ, Picker W, et al. Preoperative positron emission tomographic viability assessment and perioperative and postoperative risk in patients with advanced ischemic heart disease. J Am Coll Cardiol 1997;30:1693–1700.
26. Beanlands R, Hendry P, Masters R, deKemp R, Woodend K, Ruddy T. Delay in revascularization is associated with increased mortality rate in patients with severe left ventricular dysfunction and viable myocardium on fluorine 18-fluorodeoxyglucose positron emission tomography imaging. Circulation 1998;98(19 suppl): II51–56.
27. Beanlands RS, deKemp RA, Smith S, Johansen H, Ruddy TD. F-18-fluorodeoxyglucose PET imaging alters clini-

cal decision making in patients with impaired ventricular function. Am J Cardiol 1997;79:1092–1095.
28. Krivokapich J, Huang SC, Selin CE, Phelps ME. Fluorodeoxyglucose rate constants, lumped constant, and glucose metabolic rate in rabbit heart. Am J Physiol 1987;252:H777–787.
29. Knuuti MJ, Nuutila P, Ruotsalainen U, et al. Euglycemic hyperinsulinemic clamp and oral glucose load in stimulating myocardial glucose utilization during positron emission tomography. J Nucl Med 1992;33:1255–1262.
30. Knuuti MJ, Yki-Jarvinen H, Voipio-Pulkki LM, et al. Enhancement of myocardial [fluorine-18]fluorodeoxyglucose uptake by a nicotinic acid derivative. J Nucl Med 1994;35:989–998.
31. Neely JR, Morgan HE. Relationship between carbohydrate and lipid metabolism and the energy balance of the heart muscle. Ann Rev Physiol 1974;36:412–459.
32. Knuuti J, Schelbert HR, Bax JJ. The need for standardisation of cardiac FDG PET imaging in the evaluation of myocardial viability in patients with chronic ischaemic left ventricular dysfunction. Eur J Nucl Med Mol Imaging 2002;29:1257–1266.
33. Berry JJ, Baker JA, Pieper KS, Hanson MW, Hoffman JM, Coleman RE. The effect of metabolic milieu on cardiac PET imaging using fluorine-18-deoxyglucose and nitrogen-13-ammonia in normal volunteers. J Nucl Med 1991;32:1518–1525.
34. DeFronzo RA, Tobin JD, Andres R. Glucose clamp technique: a method for quantifying insulin secretion and resistance. Am J Physiol 1979;237:E214–223.
35. Schinkel AF, Bax JJ, Valkema R, et al. Effect of diabetes mellitus on myocardial 18F-FDG SPECT using acipimox for the assessment of myocardial viability. J Nucl Med 2003;44:877–883.
36. Schroder O, Hor G, Hertel A, Baum RP. Combined hyperinsulinaemic glucose clamp and oral acipimox for optimizing metabolic conditions during 18F-fluorodeoxyglucose gated PET cardiac imaging: comparative results. Nucl Med Commun 1998;19:867–874.
37. Stone CK, Holden JE, Stanley W, Perlman SB. Effect of nicotinic acid on exogenous myocardial glucose utilization. J Nucl Med 1995;36:996–1002.
38. Musatti L, Maggi E, Moro E, Valzelli G, Tamassia V. Bioavailability and pharmacokinetics in man of acipimox, a new antilipolytic and hypolipemic agent. J Int Med Res 1981;9:381–386.
39. Herrero P, Weinheimer CJ, Dence C, Oellerich WF, Gropler RJ. Quantification of myocardial glucose utilization by PET and 1-carbon-11-glucose. J Nucl Cardiol 2002;9:5–14.
40. Schön HR, Schelbert HR, Robinson G, et al. C-11 labeled palmitic acid for the noninvasive evaluation of regional myocardial fatty acid metabolism with positron emission tomography. I. Kinetics of C-11 palmitic acid in normal myocardium. Am Heart J 1981;103:532–547.
41. Maki MT, Haaparanta M, Nuutila P, et al. Free fatty acid uptake in the myocardium and skeletal muscle using fluorine-18-fluoro-6-thia-heptadecanoic acid. J Nucl Med 1998;39:1320–1327.
42. Brown M, Marshall DR, Sobel BE, Bergmann SR. Delineation of myocardial oxygen utilization with carbon-11-labeled acetate. Circulation 1987;76:687–696.
43. Buxton DB, Schwaiger M, Nguyen A, Phelps ME, Schelbert HR. Radiolabelled acetate as a tracer of myocardial tricarboxylic acid cycle flux. Circ Res 1988;63:628–634.
44. Beanlands RS, Bach DS, Raylman R, et al. Acute effects of dobutamine on myocardial oxygen consumption and cardiac efficiency measured using carbon-11 acetate kinetics in patients with dilated cardiomyopathy. J Am Coll Cardiol 1993;22:1389–1398.
45. Bengel FM, Permanetter B, Ungerer M, Nekolla S, Schwaiger M. Noninvasive estimation of myocardial efficiency using positron emission tomography and C-11 acetate: comparison between the normal and failing human heart. Eur J Nucl Med 2000;27:319–326.
46. Beanlands RS, Nahmias C, Gordon E, et al. The effects of beta(1)-blockade on oxidative metabolism and the metabolic cost of ventricular work in patients with left ventricular dysfunction: a double-blind, placebo-controlled, positron-emission tomography study. Circulation 2000;102:2070–2075.
47. Bengel FM, Ueberfuhr P, Ziegler SI, Nekolla S, Reichart B, Schwaiger M. Serial assessment of sympathetic reinnervation after orthotopic heart transplantation: a longitudinal study using positron emission tomography and C-11 hydroxyephedrine. Circulation 1999;99:1866–1871.
48. Di Carli MF, Tobes MC, Mangner T, et al. Effects of cardiac sympathetic innervation on coronary blood flow. N Engl J Med 1997;336:1208–1215.
49. Bengel FM, Ueberfuhr P, Schiepel N, Nekolla SG, Reichart B, Schwaiger M. Effect of sympathetic reinnervation on cardiac performance after heart transplantation. N Engl J Med 2001;345:731–738.
50. Bengel FM, Ueberfuhr P, Ziegler SI, et al. Noninvasive assessment of the effect of cardiac sympathetic innervation on metabolism of the human heart. Eur J Nucl Med 2000;27:1650–1657.
51. Allman KC, Wieland DM, Muzik O, Degrado TR, Wolfe ER Jr, Schwaiger M. Carbon-11 hydroxyephedrine with positron emission tomography for serial assessment of cardiac adrenergic neuronal function after acute myocardial infarction in humans. J Am Coll Cardiol 1993;22:368–375.
52. Wichter T, Schafers M, Rhodes CG, et al. Abnormalities of cardiac sympathetic innervation in arrhythmogenic right ventricular cardiomyopathy: quantitative assessment of presynaptic norepinephrine reuptake and postsynaptic beta-adrenergic receptor density with positron emission tomography. Circulation 2000;101:1552–1558.
53. Calkins H, Allman K, Bolling S, et al. Correlation between scintigraphic evidence of regional sympathetic neuronal dysfunction and ventricular refractoriness in the human heart. Circulation 1993;88:172–179.
54. Ungerer M, Hartmann F, Karoglan M, et al. Regional in vivo and in vitro characterization of autonomic innervation in cardiomyopathic human heart. Circulation 1998;97:174–180.
55. Vesalainen RK, Pietila M, Tahvanainen KU, et al. Cardiac positron emission tomography imaging with [11C]hydroxyephedrine, a specific tracer for sympathetic nerve endings, and its functional correlates in congestive heart failure. Am J Cardiol 1999;84:568–574.
56. Di Carli MF, Bianco-Batlles D, Landa ME, et al. Effects of autonomic neuropathy on coronary blood flow in patients with diabetes mellitus. Circulation 1999;100:813–819.
57. Pietila M, Malminiemi K, Ukkonen H, et al. Reduced myocardial carbon-11 hydroxyephedrine retention is

associated with poor prognosis in chronic heart failure. Eur J Nucl Med 2001;28:373–376.
58. Merlet P, Delforge J, Syrota A, et al. Positron emission tomography with 11C CGP-12177 to assess beta-adrenergic receptor concentration in idiopathic dilated cardiomyopathy. Circulation 1993;87:1169–1178.
59. Schafers M, Dutka D, Rhodes CG, et al. Myocardial presynaptic and postsynaptic autonomic dysfunction in hypertrophic cardiomyopathy. Circ Res 1998;82:57–62.
60. Law MP, Osman S, Pike VW, et al. Evaluation of [11C]GB67, a novel radioligand for imaging myocardial alpha 1-adrenoceptors with positron emission tomography. Eur J Nucl Med 2000;27:7–17.
61. Momose M, Reder S, Raffel D, et al. Evaluation of cardiac β-adrenoceptors in the isolated perfused rat heart using (s)-[11C] CGP12388. J Nucl Med 2004;45:471–477.
62. Le Guludec D, Cohen-Solal A, Delforge J, Delahaye N, Syrota A, Merlet P. Increased myocardial muscarinic receptor density in idiopathic dilated cardiomyopathy: an in vivo PET study. Circulation 1997;96:3416–3422.
63. Haubner R, Wester HJ, Reuning U, et al. Radiolabeled alpha(v)beta3 integrin antagonists: a new class of tracers for tumor targeting. J Nucl Med 1999;40: 1061–1071.
64. Strauss HW, Narula J, Blankenberg FG. Radioimaging to identify myocardial cell death and probably injury. Lancet 2000;356:180–181.
65. Grierson JR, Yagle KJ, Eary JF, et al. Production of [F-18]fluoroannexin for imaging apoptosis with PET. Bioconjug Chem 2004;15:373–379.
66. Avril N, Bengel FM. Defining the success of cardiac gene therapy: how can nuclear imaging contribute? Eur J Nucl Med Mol Imaging 2003;30:757–771.
67. Bengel FM, Anton M, Richter T, et al. Noninvasive imaging of transgene expression using positron emission tomography in a pig model of myocardial gene transfer. Circulation 2003;108:2127–2133.
68. Doubrovin M, Ponomarev V, Beresten T, et al. Imaging transcriptional regulation of p53-dependent genes with positron emission tomography in vivo. Proc Natl Acad Sci USA 2001;98:9300–9305.
69. Wu JC, Chen IY, Sundaresan G, et al. Molecular imaging of cardiac cell transplantation in living animals using optical bioluminescence and positron emission tomography. Circulation 2003;108:1302–1305.
70. Bar-Shalom R, Yefremov N, Guralnik L, et al. Clinical performance of PET/CT in evaluation of cancer: additional value for diagnostic imaging and patient management. J Nucl Med 2003;44:1200–1209.
71. Lardinois D, Weder W, Hany TF, et al. Staging of non-small-cell lung cancer with integrated positron-emission tomography and computed tomography. N Engl J Med 2003;348:2500–2507.
72. Boucher L, Rodrigue S, Lecomte R, Benard F. Respiratory gating for 3-dimensional PET of the thorax: feasibility and initial results. J Nucl Med 2004;45:214–219.
73. Phelps ME. PET: the merging of biology and imaging into molecular imaging. J Nucl Med 2000;41:661–681.

6

Computed Tomography Techniques and Principles. Part a. Electron Beam Computed Tomography

Tarun K. Mittal and Michael B. Rubens

The term EBCT or electron beam computed tomography is linked to coronary artery calcification and thus diagnosis of coronary artery disease. It was in 1979 that the design of the EBCT scanner was first proposed with the aim of rapidly scanning the beating heart.[1] This gantry design did not use any moving parts and thus had much shorter scan times compared with conventional computed tomography (CT) scanners. In the early years, the EBCT scanners (also called "cine CT" or "ultrafast CT") were used to evaluate myocardial thickening, wall motion, and regional blood flow.[2] It was not, however, until 1989 that the first use of an EBCT scanner in detection of coronary artery calcification was described.[3]

Calcification in the coronary arteries as seen on fluoroscopy had been long known to predict the degree of coronary artery disease and hence the prognosis.[4,5] Because ordinary CT was highly sensitive in detecting calcium in the body, use of EBCT with its much faster temporal resolution made it ideally suited to identify coronary artery calcification.

This chapter describes the techniques and principles underlying the assessment of coronary calcium by EBCT whereas its clinical application will be discussed in Chapter 7.

1. The Scanner

The EBCT scanner, unlike conventional CT scanners, uses electromagnetically focused electrons to sweep stationary tungsten target rings to produce X-rays. There have been three iterations of EBCT scanners from the original C-100 in mid-1980s to C-150, which was introduced in 1993, and then C-300 in 2000.[6] The latest in the series is e-Speed (General Electric) introduced in 2003 and is capable of up to 33-ms true temporal resolution. In the evolution of EBCT scanners, the basic technical principle has remained unchanged, but improvements have occurred in spatial resolution, data manipulation and management, data display, and storage. Most of the literature for use of EBCT for coronary calcium scoring has been produced using C-100 and C-150 scanners with temporal resolution of 100 ms and currently no validation studies for the e-Speed scanner at high temporal resolution mode are available.

In a current-generation EBCT scanner, the electrons generated by an electron gun are accelerated up to nearly light velocity; the electron beam is then steered by an electromagnetic deflection system to sweep around the anodes (four tungsten ½ circular target rings, forming a 210-degree arc below the patient) where X-ray

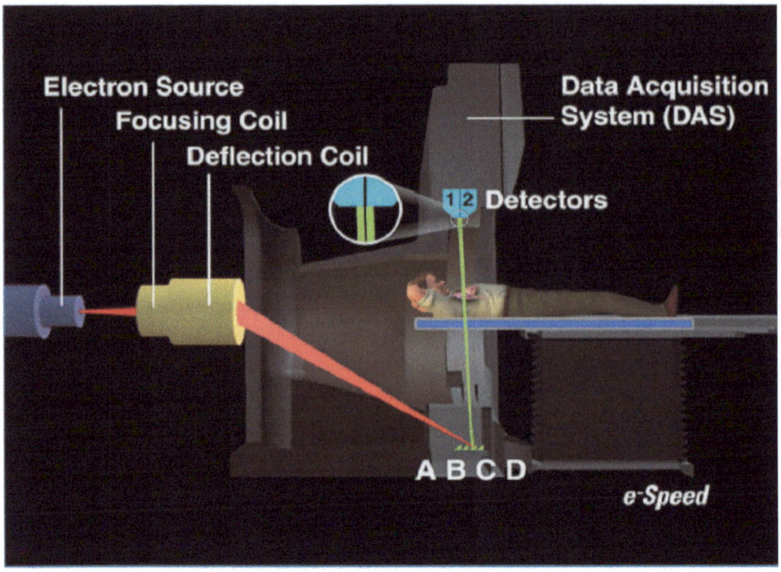

Figure 6a.1. Configuration of a typical EBCT scanner (e-Speed, General Electric).

beams are produced and directed through the patient (Figure 6a.1; see color section). The fan-shaped X-ray beams are then intercepted by stationary detector rings, forming a 216-degree arc, located above the patient, and converted into digital information by the data acquisition system. These data are then reconstructed into diagnostic images. The image acquisition is prospectively triggered with patient electrocardiogram (ECG), and temporal resolution of up to 30 frames per second can be obtained. Coronary artery calcium scoring with EBCT yields effective radiation doses of 1.0 and 1.3 mSv for male and female patients, respectively.[7]

2. Protocol for Calcium Scoring Scan

Standardized methods for imaging, identification, and quantification of coronary artery calcium using EBCT have been published.[8,9] The scanner is operated in the high-resolution, single-slice mode with continuous, non-overlapping slices of 3-mm thickness and an acquisition time of 100 ms per tomogram. Patients are positioned supine, and after localization of the main pulmonary artery, a sufficient number of tomographic slices are obtained to cover the complete heart through the left ventricular apex (usually 36–40 slices). Electrocardiographic triggering is done at end diastole at a time determined from the continuous ECG tracing recorded during scanning. Current clinical protocols of EBCT perform triggering during the cardiac cycle as varied depending on the patient's resting heart rate to minimize coronary artery motion artifacts. Coronary arteries are identified as soft tissue structures, usually surrounded by fat, in the cardiac grooves (Figure 6a.2a–d). Calcified coronary deposits are seen as bright white areas along the course of the coronary artery (Figure 6a.3a–d).

3. Scoring of Coronary Calcification

For detection and scoring of calcification in the coronary arteries, an arbitrary value of +130 Hounsfield units (HU) [HU is the attenuation value of various tissues related to water which is calibrated to zero (HU = 0)] and an area greater than 1.0 mm^2 are often used. The +130 HU level was selected because it lies well above the +30 to 50 HU of unenhanced myocardium and soft tissue. A region of interest is placed manually around the pixels thought to be in the line of the coronary arteries to separate them from the calcification in the aortic root, mitral annulus, pericardium, etc. Because individual pixels above +130 HU are frequently seen throughout the heart because of noise, a minimum area threshold of 2–4 contiguous pixels (generally 3 pixels, which represents an area of 1.03 mm^2 with a 30-cm field of view and a 512 × 512 matrix) is chosen in the evaluation of coronary calcification. Once the regions of interest have been placed, the scanner software displays the peak calcification attenuation in HU and the area in mm^2 and calculates the *Agatston score*, *volume score*, and now also the *mass measurement*.

The *Agatston score*[10] (see also Chapter 7) is the oldest and most frequently used calcium scoring system. It takes into account the peak attenuation of the calcified lesion as well its area. The area of the lesion with the peak pixel between 131 HU and 200 HU is multiplied by a factor of

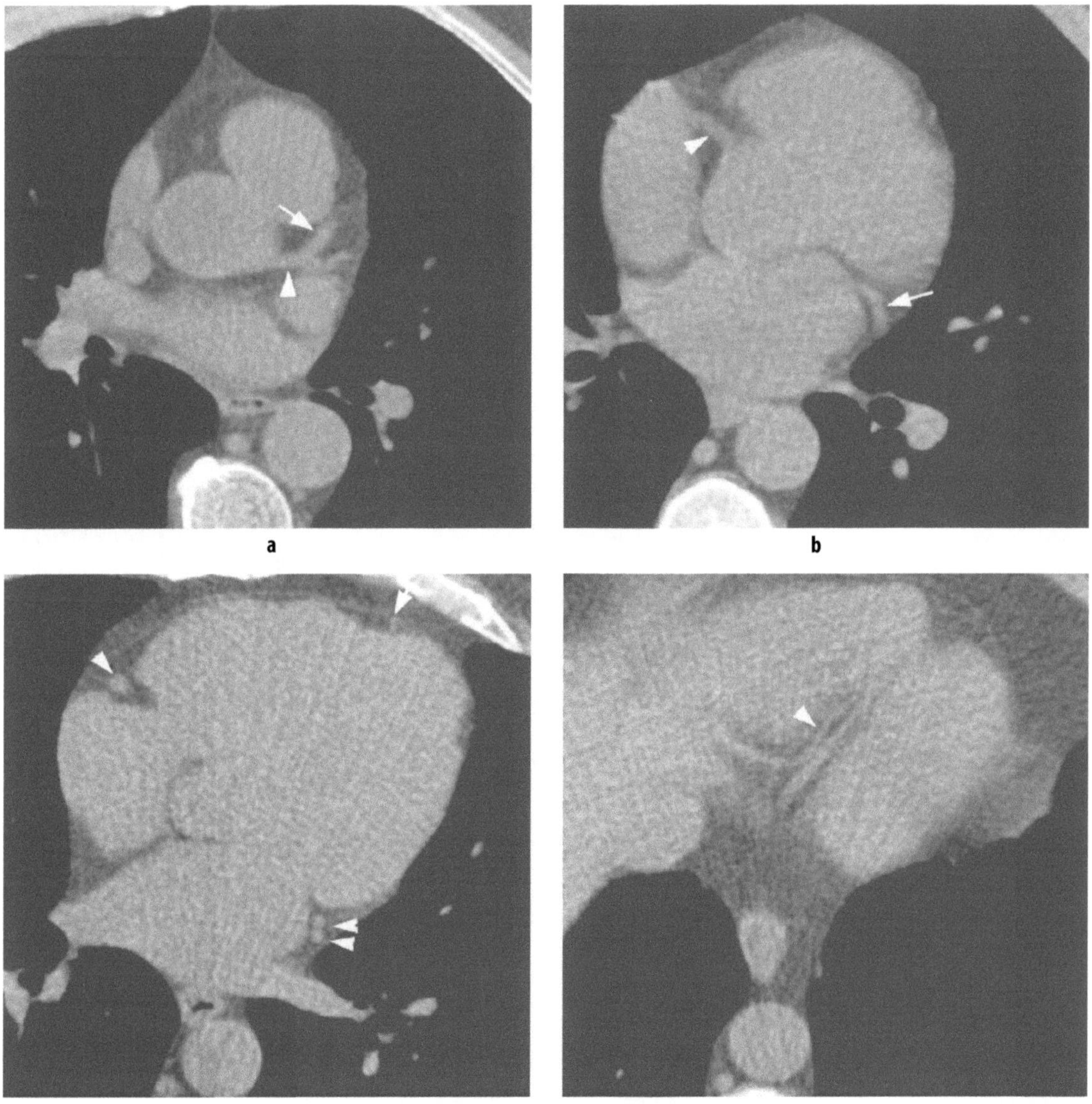

Figure 6a.2. Normal origin and course of the left main stem (arrowhead) coronary artery with continuation as left anterior descending (LAD, arrow) and diagonal branch (**a**), origin of the right coronary artery (RCA, arrowhead) anteriorly and circumflex artery (CXA, arrow) in the posterior atrioventricular groove (**b**), RCA (arrowhead), LAD (arrow), and CXA (double arrowheads) in their respective grooves along their mid course (**c**), and posterior descending branch in the inferior interventricular groove (**d**).

one, 201 HU–300 HU lesions by a factor of two, 301 HU–400 HU lesions by a factor of three, and lesions greater than 401 HU by a factor of four. The sum of the individual lesion scores is the score for that artery, and the sum of all lesion scores is the total calcification score. The *volume score* first proposed by Callister et al.[11] is the total volume of the voxels (i.e., total number of pixels × slice thickness) above the 130 HU threshold. *Calcium mass measurement* is the representation of the total mineral content of the lesion(s) as the integral (sum) of all HU in a lesion multiplied by the voxel volume in mm^3. Because a calcified lesion is a complex of different bone ash equivalent, a scaling factor specific to a scanner is used to convert the Hounsfield values to the bone ash

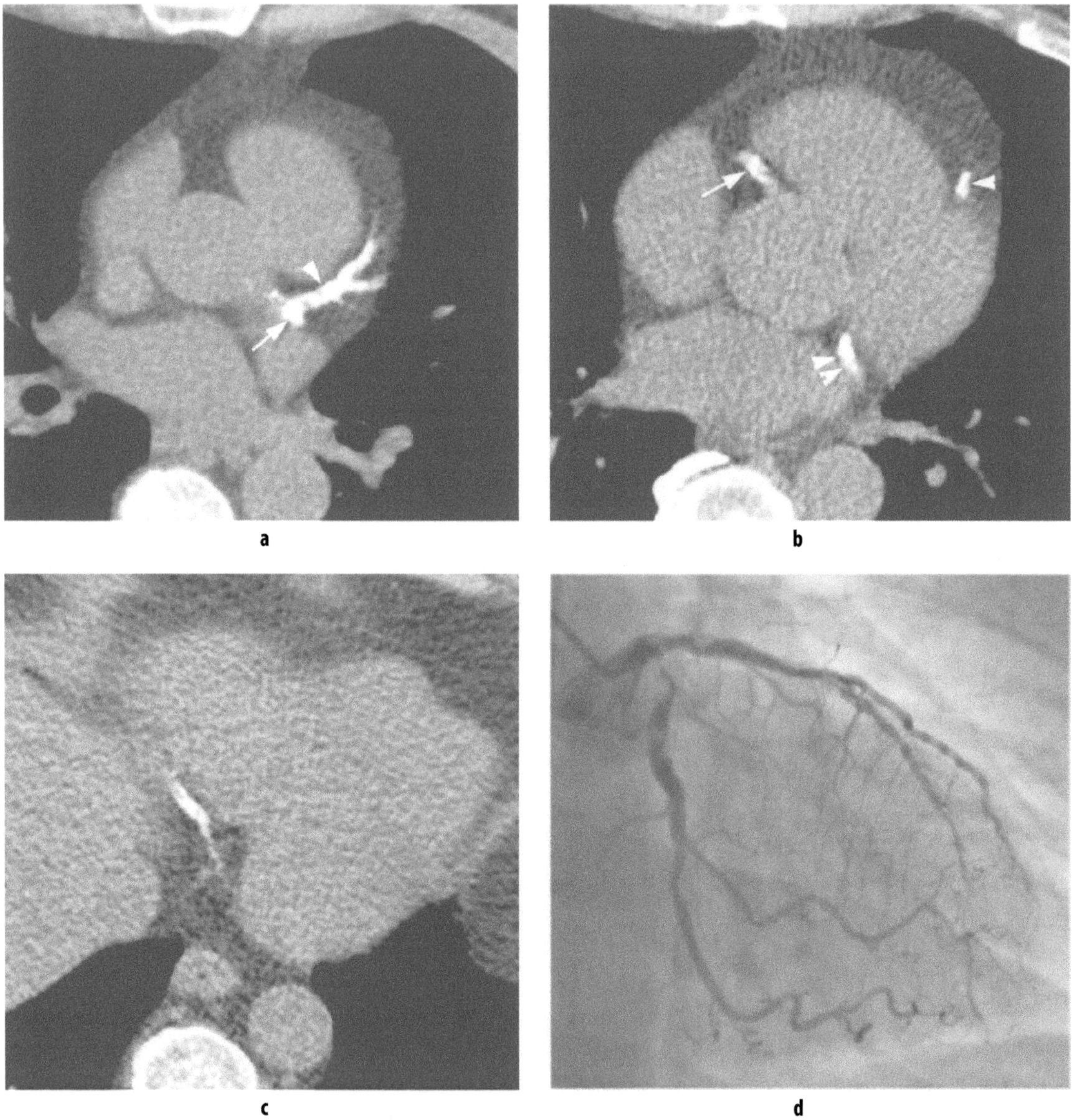

Figure 6a.3. Marked calcification along the course of proximal left anterior descending (LAD, arrowhead) and origin of the circumflex artery (CXA, arrow) (**a**), further in the right coronary artery (RCA, arrow), mid LAD (arrowhead), and CXA (double arrowheads) artery (**b**), and in the distal part of RCA (**c**). Corresponding angiogram showing significant obstructive disease in the proximal LAD and CXA artery (**d**).

Table 6a.1. Electron beam tomographic coronary artery score percentiles for men and women within each age strata

	Age (yr)								
Percentile	<40	40–44	45–49	50–54	55–59	60–64	65–69	70–74	>74
Men (25 251)	3504	4238	4940	4825	3472	2288	1209	540	235
25th	0	0	0	1	4	13	32	64	166
50th	1	1	3	15	48	113	180	310	473
75th	3	9	36	103	215	410	566	892	1071
90th	14	59	154	332	554	994	1299	1774	1982
Women (9995)	641	1024	1634	2184	1835	1334	731	438	174
25th	0	0	0	0	0	0	1	3	9
50th	0	0	0	0	1	3	24	52	75
75th	1	1	2	5	23	57	145	210	241
90th	3	4	22	55	121	193	410	631	709

Source: Reproduced with permission from Hoff et al.[13]

equivalent and thus provide the calcium mass measurement.[12] Unlike Agatston score, no arbitrary value for peak attenuation is required for such measurement, thus making it least affected by the attenuation values and also by partial volume effects caused by differences in slice thickness and slice spacing. Calcium mass estimation is thus more reproducible compared with Agatston and volume scores, and hence has more applicability between different scanner types, particularly with the increasing use of the multislice scanners.

The prevalence of coronary calcium normally increases with age, with women lagging by about 10 years with respect to men. Thus, although the total calcium score may represent the total plaque burden, the age and sex of the individual has to be taken into account to understand the significance of a particular score. Also, it has been shown by several studies that instead of absolute calcium scores, it is the percentile scores for a given age and sex that are more helpful in assessing the risk in asymptomatic individuals and in detection of obstructive disease in symptomatics, with calcium scores above the 75th percentile being more significant than scores below the 25th percentile. This has led to development of sets of nomograms for calcium scores based on age and sex and grouped by percentile ranking. The largest of these is the Kondos database (Table 6a.1), which gives the Agatston calcium scores on 35 246 asymptomatic individuals.[13] Rumberger and Kaufman[12] have provided the first normal database for volume and the mass measurements in 11 490 individuals besides the Agatston scores.

4. Reproducibility

The ability to assess progression of atherosclerotic burden over time accurately depends on the reproducibility of the technique. The median interscan variability has been shown to be 7%–12% for calcium score and 5%–11% for volume in recent studies using standard triggering technique.[14,15] Lower interscan variability has been shown with increasing calcium scores, patients with stable heart rates (heart rate changing less than 10 beats per minute during scanning), patients with no visible coronary motion, and those with an optimal ECG triggering method ($P < 0.05$ for all).[15] It has been shown that ECG trigger of 40% rather than 80% of the R-R interval significantly reduces the interscan variability.[16] Volume score diminishes the variability because it does not take into account the peak attenuation value, which is affected by image noise.[14] Similarly, measurement of mass besides reducing the interscan variability as discussed above, also has a low interobserver variability (1%–3%) in the recent studies with EBCT.[15]

5. Coronary Angiography with EBCT

Several studies have shown feasibility of performing coronary angiography with EBCT.[17–19] These studies have reported sensitivities and specificities in the range of 78%–93% and 88%–98% for the detection of significant coronary stenoses. Up to 25% of the coronary segments may, however, not be assessable using the current technology because of low contrast to noise ratio and motion artifacts caused by respiratory and cardiac movement. Also, coronary calcification can be a hindrance in evaluation of degree of stenosis, although the presence of a high calcium score by itself would indicate the presence of atheromatous disease.

6. Conclusion

EBCT is a highly sensitive technique for detection and measurement of coronary artery calcification and thus noninvasive estimation of atherosclerotic plaque burden. It offers a high spatial resolution with low acquisition time and has good reproducibility and interobserver agreement with optimized ECG triggering. EBCT is a mature technique for calcium detection with a continuously expanding literature. With growing technological advances, cardiac CT has a promising role in clinical practice as well as research.

References

1. Boyd DP, Gould RG, Quinn JR, et al. A proposed dynamic cardiac 3-D densitometer for early detection and evaluation of heart disease. IEEE Trans Nucl Sci 1979;26:2724–2727.
2. Lipton MJ, Higgins CB, Farmer D, Boyd DP. Cardiac imaging with a high-speed cine-CT scanner: preliminary results. Radiology 1984;152:579–582.
3. Tanenbaum SR, Kondos GT, Veselik KE, Prendergast MR, Brundage BH, Chomka EV. Detection of calcific deposits in coronary arteries by ultrafast computed tomography and correlation with angiography. Am J Cardiol 1989;63:870–872.
4. Lieber A, Jorgens J. Cinefluorography of coronary artery calcification: correlation with clinical arteriosclerotic heart disease and autopsy findings. Am J Roentgenol 1961;86:1063.
5. Hamby RI, Tabrah F, Wisoff BG, Hartstein ML. Coronary artery calcification: clinical implications and angiographic correlations. Am Heart J 1974;87:565–570.
6. Rumberger JA. Tomographic plaque imaging with CT: technical considerations and capabilities. Prog Cardiovasc Dis 2003;46:123–134.
7. Hunold P, Vogt FM, Schmermund A, et al. Radiation exposure during cardiac CT: effective doses at multidetector row CT and electron-beam CT. Radiology 2003;226:145–155.
8. Wexler L, Brundage B, Crouse J, et al. (AHA Writing Group). Coronary artery calcification: pathophysiology, epidemiology, imaging methods, and clinical implications – a statement for health professionals from the American Heart Association. Circulation 1996;94: 1175–1192.
9. O'Rourke RA, Brundage BH, Froelicher VF, et al. ACC/AHA expert consensus document on electron-beam computed tomography for the diagnosis and prognosis of coronary artery disease. Circulation 2000;102:126–140.
10. Agatston AS, Janowitz W, Hildner FJ, Zusmer NR, Viamonte M, Detrano R. Quantification of coronary artery calcium using ultrafast computed tomography. J Am Coll Cardiol 1990;15:827–832.
11. Callister TQ, Cooil B, Raya SP, Lippolis NJ, Russo DJ, Raggi P. Coronary artery disease: improved reproducibility of calcium scoring with an electron-beam CT volumetric method. Radiology 1998;208: 807–814.
12. Rumberger JA, Kaufman L. A rosetta stone for coronary calcium risk stratification: Agatston, volume, and mass scores in 11,490 individuals. Am J Roentgenol 2003;181:743–748.
13. Hoff JA, Chomka EV, Krainik AJ, Daviglus M, Rich S, Kondos GT. Age and gender distributions of coronary artery calcium detected by electron beam tomography in 35246 adults. Am J Cardiol 2001;87: 1335–1339.
14. Achenbach S, Ropers D, Mohlenkamp S, et al. Variability of repeated coronary artery calcium measurements by electron beam tomography. Am J Cardiol 2001; 87:210–213.
15. Lu B, Budoff MJ, Zhuang N, et al. Causes of interscan variability of coronary artery calcium measurements at electron-beam CT. Acta Radiol 2002;9:654–661.
16. Mao S, Bakhsheshi H, Lu B, Liu SCK, Oudiz RJ, Budoff MJ. Effect of electrocardiogram triggering on reproducibility of coronary artery calcium scoring. Radiology 2001;220:707–711.
17. Achenbach S, Moshage W, Ropers D, Nossen J, Daniel WG. Value of electron-beam computed tomography for the noninvasive detection of high-grade coronary-artery stenoses and occlusions. N Engl J Med 1998; 339:1964–1971.
18. Budoff MJ, Oudiz RJ, Zalace CP, et al. Intravenous three-dimensional coronary angiography using contrast enhanced electron beam computed tomography. Am J Cardiol 1999;83:840–845.
19. Schmermund A, Rensing BJ, Sheedy PF, Bell MR, Rumberger JA. Intravenous electron-beam computed tomographic coronary angiography for segmental analysis of coronary artery stenoses. J Am Coll Cardiol 1998; 31:1547–1554.

6

Computed Tomography Techniques and Principles. Part b. Multislice Computed Tomography

P.J. de Feyter, F. Cademartiri, N.R. Mollet, and K. Nieman

Invasive coronary angiography is at present the only universally accepted, widely available method for coronary artery imaging. It is highly reliable to assess the presence of coronary obstructions, but its main limitation is related to the invasive nature of the technique, requiring a short monitored hospitalization and a dedicated team consisting of a technician and cardiologist to perform the investigation, thereby making it costly. The procedure also has a small (occasionally fatal) complication rate.

A noninvasive imaging technique would be highly desirable, but to become an alternative to diagnostic invasive coronary angiography, this technique should have sufficiently high quality that it can approximate the versatility and reliability of traditional coronary angiography. This is almost impossible to achieve, but the high-quality requirements for a noninvasive coronary angiogram may be less stringent than those for invasive coronary angiography.

Noninvasive coronary angiography using electron beam tomography was initiated in 1995[1] and since then many studies using this technique have been published.[2–10] Multislice computed tomography (MS-CT) is a rapidly emerging technique, which permits noninvasive visualization of the coronary arteries.[11–17] This chapter provides the basics of MS-CT technology, gives an update on the current diagnostic performance of MS-CT coronary angiography, and discusses the potential role of MS-CT in clinical cardiology.

1. Basics of Computed Tomography

Computed tomography (CT) imaging is a cross-sectional imaging method using diagnostic X-ray radiation as the penetrating radiation source to delineate the anatomy of a slice or a section of a patient (tomogram). The cross-sectional image is reconstructed from data obtained from the specific linear X-ray attenuation of the penetrating X-ray beam. Tissues of different structures within the body have specific X-ray attenuation qualities depending on the atomic density of each tissue.

The basic design of a CT scanner is illustrated in Figure 6b.1. A rotating X-ray source produces an X-ray beam that passes through the patient.

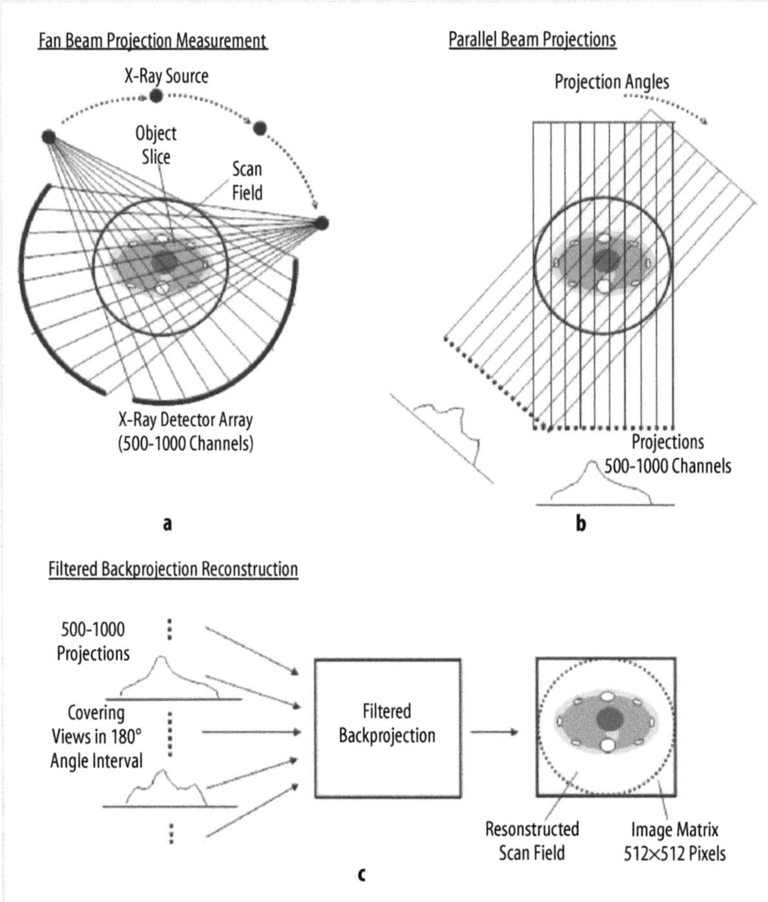

Figure 6b.1. Basic design of the CT scanner. Schematic diagram of CT data acquisition and image reconstruction. **A** A fan-shaped X-ray beam passes through the cross-section of the patient, located within the scan's field of view. The patient's morphology attenuates these X-rays after which the residual rays are registered by a detector array on the opposite side. The electrical intensity signals from the detector are converted by analog digital converters into digital intensity signals, which are transformed by computer into an attenuation projection profile. Each angular projection or attenuation profile consists of typically 500–1000 individual data points that belong to individual ray projections. A large number of attenuation profiles, from consecutive angular fan beam projections are generated and serve as basis for computation of the X-ray attenuation distribution of the patient's cross-sectional morphology that represents the image slice. **B** For most reconstruction algorithms, the measured fan beam projections are rearranged to parallel beam projections via two-dimensional interpolation algorithms. To reconstruct a slice, the minimally required amount of data is acquired during a half rotation of the X-ray source and detector array, which consists of 500–1000 parallel beam projections. **C** The final computation of the slice is performed via a so-called backprojection of the filtered parallel beam projections.

The X-ray beam is collimated as a fan beam and the width of the collimators controls the thickness of the cross-section image. The fan beam is subtended by an array of detectors at the opposite side of the X-ray source. The detectors measure the attenuation from the projection of the X-ray beam when passing through the anatomy within the slice.

An exact cross-sectional image can be constructed from the attenuation measurements obtained from a series of projections covering the full 360° round the patient. The Hounsfield unit (HU) or CT number is the attenuation value of various tissues related to water which is calibrated to zero (HU = 0). The various tissues in the body have different attenuation values (Table 6b.1). In CT imaging, tissues with a very high attenuation (such as bone) are represented on the display image as white, tissues with very low attenuation values (such as air in the lungs) are represented as dark, and tissues with moderate attenuation values are represented by various shades of gray (Figure 6b.2).

Table 6b.1. Attenuation values of various tissues in the body

A.	Structures with high density (HU range: >150)
	Metal objects
	Bones
	Iodinated contrast in blood
B.	Structures with mid-density (HU range: <150 to −50)
	Fibrotic tissue
	Water
	Soft tissues
C.	Structures with low density (HU range: −50 to −1000)
	Fat tissue
	Air

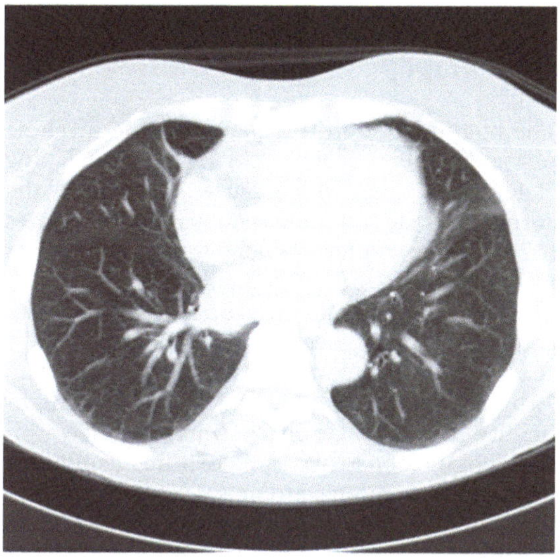

Figure 6b.2. Cross-sectional image of thorax. White = sternum and spine; dark = lung tissue; gray = myocardium.

2. Spiral CT

The basic concept of spiral CT is that the data necessary for the reconstruction of a cross-sectional image are acquired as the X-ray source rotates around the patient while the table moves continuously with a predefined speed. These two motions create a spiral volume of data. From this spiral volume of data, cross-sectional images are reconstructed using helical interpolation algorithms (Figure 6b.3).

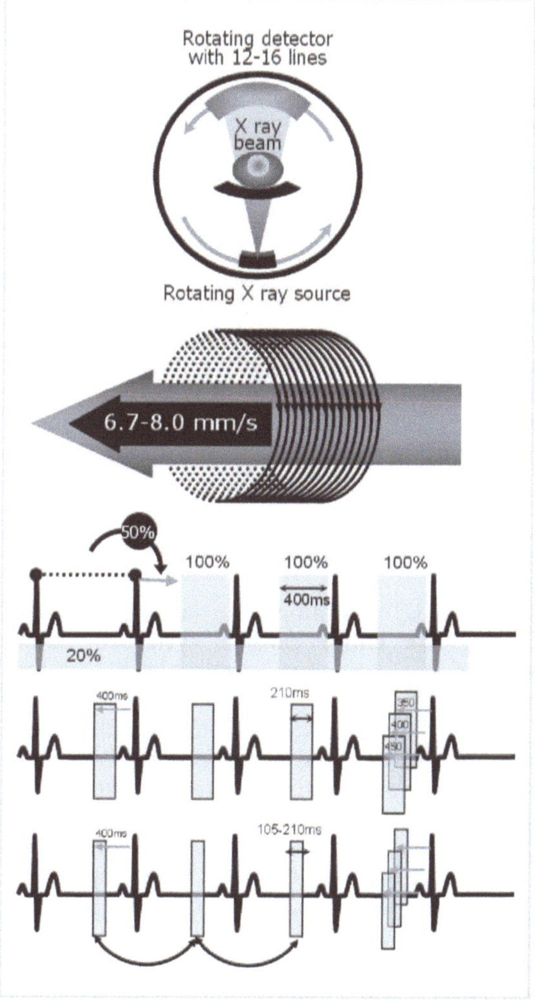

Figure 6b.3. Multislice spiral CT data acquisition and image reconstruction. Rotating around the patient are 12–16 parallel detector rows with a submillimeter slice width each. While the patient continuously moves through the scanner, the tube current is altered according to the ECG. During systole, the radiation output is lowered to 20%, whereas, during diastole, triggered at the estimated 50% RR interval time point, the nominal exposure (100%) is used during a 400-ms interval to acquire high-quality images. This way, the total dose can be reduced by 50%. From the acquired scan data, ECG synchronized cross-sectional image series are reconstructed with an overlapping increment via spiral interpolation algorithms to improve the volumetric quality of the data set. Retrospective ECG gating allows reconstruction timing related to the upcoming R wave or selective repositioning of reconstruction intervals during irregular RR intervals. By varying the position of the 210-ms reconstruction window within the 400-ms interval of nominal tube current, image data sets are retrospectively reconstructed during slightly different phases (at 350, 400, and 450 ms before the following R wave), and the most optimal result is selected for further analysis. The standard length of the reconstruction interval and temporal resolution at 0.42-s rotation time is 210 ms. Depending on the heart rate, the effective reconstruction interval can be between 105 and 210 ms by using "segmented" reconstruction algorithms, that combine data from two consecutive heart beats.

3. Multislice CT: Speed of Performance

Cardiac imaging requires fast acquisition of data, to reduce the inherent cardiac motion artifacts. The speed of MS-CT is mainly determined by the number of detector rings and the X-ray tube rotation time. The higher the number of detection rings and the faster the X-ray tube rotation, the shorter the scan time, resulting in less artifacts. MS-CT is the recent technical improvement of spiral CT. The latest generation features 64 detector arrays, which is extremely important for coronary imaging because it considerably reduces the scan time. For instance, a 1-detector ring CT would require more than 160 seconds' scan time to cover the heart, whereas this is reduced to 40 seconds with a 4-detector ring MS-CT and to 5 seconds with the 64-detector ring MS-CT. The use of the latter technique would translate into the acquisition of a MS-CT coronary angiogram within a breathhold of just a few seconds, which can be achieved in almost all patients.

The X-ray tube rotation time, which determines the speed of acquisition of a cross-section, is a significant parameter for coronary imaging. The faster the rotation, the shorter the acquisition time and thus the shorter the temporal resolution, which would result in better "motion-free" images. Technical improvements over time have significantly reduced the X-ray tube rotation time, decreasing it from 1000 ms in the early 1990s to 420 ms in 2002 to 375 ms in 2003 and 330 ms in 2004.

4. MS-CT Coronary Scan Technique

In spiral CT scanning, the data are acquired during the entire cardiac cycle. To obtain motion-free coronary images, only the data acquired in the relative motion-free diastolic phase of the cardiac cycle are used for the reconstruction of the axial cross-sections.[18–21] This is achieved by prospective or retrospective electrocardiogram (ECG) gating (Figure 6b.3), although for coronary angiography, the latter is preferable. The R wave of the ECG is used to retrospectively "gate" the scan so that only the data acquired during a predefined window in the diastolic cardiac phase are selected for reconstruction of the cross-sectional image.[18–21]

5. Heart Rate and MS-CT Coronary Angiography

The relative motion-free period in the diastolic phase of the cardiac cycle is shorter during faster heart rates, which causes blurring of the coronary image at moderately fast heart rates (±70–80 bpm) and which often precludes reconstruction of high-quality images with heart rates higher than 80 bpm.[17,22] Heart rate control by using beta-blockers before MS-CT scanning to reduce the heart rate to less than 70 bpm is a key prerequisite to produce high-quality MS-CT coronary images. New bi-segmental reconstruction algorithms using data from two or more cardiac cycles may reduce the "effective" temporal resolution to less than 100 ms.

6. Tissue Contrast and MS-CT Coronary Angiography

The attenuation values of the coronary lumen filled with blood, the coronary wall, or coronary atherosclerotic plaques have only small differences and are therefore hardly visible with MS-CT. To enhance the tissue contrast difference, an X-ray contrast intravenous injection of 80–100 mL is administered, which allows differentiating the coronary lumen from the coronary wall and atherosclerotic plaques and permits detection of coronary lumen obstructions and nonobstructive coronary plaques (Figure 6b.4).

7. Diagnostic Performance of 64-Slice MS-CT Scanner

The highest diagnostic performance is nowadays achieved with the 64-detector MS-CT scanner in combination with heart rate control using beta-blockers before scanning in case of heart rates higher than 70 bpm. The better results are obtained because of the advantages offered by the new scanner including a faster X-ray tube rotation time of 330 ms and extended number (32–64) of thinner detector rows (0.75 mm) resulting in a shorter total scan time of approximately 6–12 seconds (Figure 6b.5).

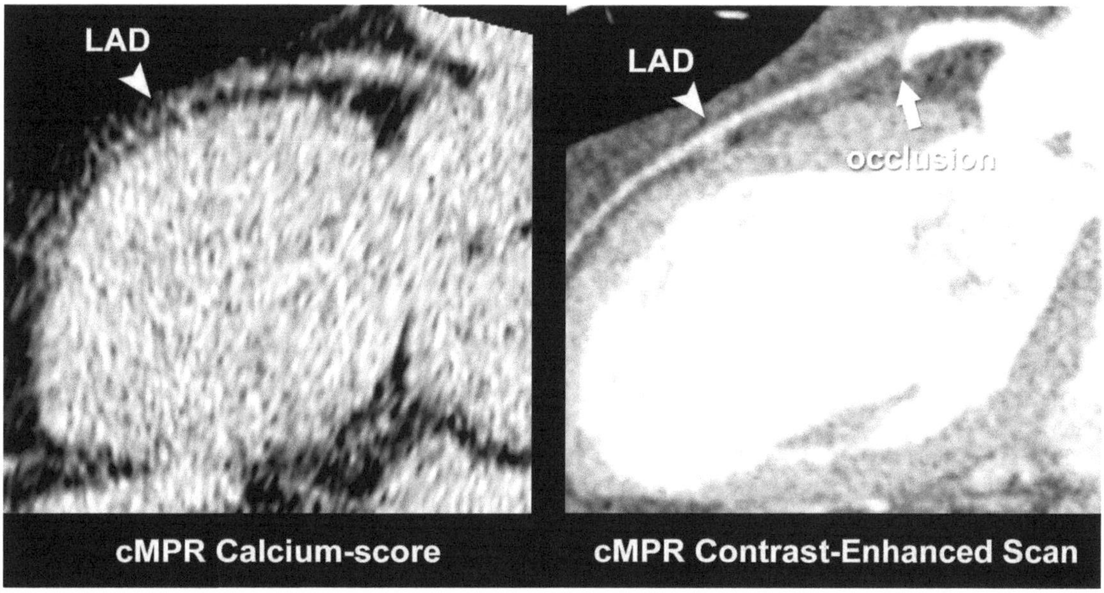

Figure 6b.4. Left anterior coronary artery (LAD) without contrast – with contrast. cMPR, curved multiplanar reconstruction.

The accuracy of MS-CT for noninvasive detection of coronary stenosis is an area of active research. Most published series have reported sensitivity values for detection of significant stenosis in proximal segments in the region of 85%–95%. Four recent studies have compared conventional coronary angiography with 64-slice MS-CT coronary angiography (Table 6b.2).[23,24] Raff et al. excluded 12% of the coronary segments from evaluation because of insufficient image quality, whereas the other investigators did not exclude coronary segments from evaluation. The sensitivity, specificity, and predictive accuracy were high in both studies. Compared with other branches of the coronary tree, the right coronary artery with its high degree of motion was still most vulnerable to image-quality degradation.

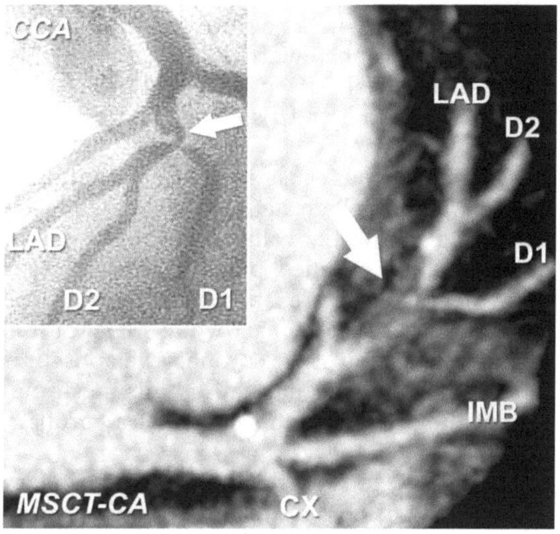

Figure 6b.5. MS-CT and invasive coronary angiography. The arrow indicates a significant obstructive coronary lesion located at the proximal LAD. CCA, conventional coronary angiography; MSCT-CA, multislice CT coronary angiography; D1, first diagonal branch; D2, second diagonal branch; LAD, left anterior descending coronary artery; arrow, left anterior descending coronary artery (LAD) with and without contrast.

Table 6b.2. Diagnostic performance of 64-slice MS-CT to detect a significant coronary stenosis (50% diameter)

	NP	Excluded vessel segments (%)	Sensitivity (%)	Specificity (%)	Positive predictive value (%)	Negative predictive value (%)
Leschka[23]	67	0	94	95	88	98
Leber[24]	55	0	76	97	75	97
Raff[25]	70	12	86	95	66	99
Mollet[26]	51	0	99	95	76	99

8. Limitations of MS-CT Coronary Angiography

As indicated in the previous section, fast heart rates adversely affect the image quality and consequently the diagnostic reliability of the images. Reduction of the heart rate with beta-blockers before the scan will resolve the problem in the majority of the cases but, unfortunately, it is not possible in all cases, particularly in patients with diabetes mellitus or with high anxiety levels, to sufficiently reduce the heart rate.

Persistent heart rhythm disturbances such as atrial fibrillation preclude MS-CT coronary angiography because of inappropriate electrocardiogram (ECG) synchronization resulting in interslice discontinuity, and differences in the volume of the ventricles caused by differences in diastolic filling times with attendant differences in three-dimensional localization within the thorax are an additional contributing factor. An occasional heart rhythm abnormality (such as an atrial or ventricular extra systole) can be corrected by retrospective editing of the ECG.

Calcium deposits cause a strong attenuation of the X-ray, causing high-density artifacts by beam hardening and partial volume effect. The consequence is that calcified plaques appear larger than they actually are, thereby increasing the apparent severity of a narrowing. In addition, severe calcification of the coronary wall obscures the coronary lumen and causes misinterpretation of the presence and severity of a coronary stenosis.

The X-ray exposure during MS-CT coronary angiography using a retrospective image reconstruction protocol is in the region of 10 mSv per investigation.[27–29] This high dose of radiation limits repeated MS-CT investigations, in particular in younger patients, and technical improvements are required to reduce the radiation exposure. One way to reduce the radiation levels is to use ECG controlled X-ray tube current modulation.[27] The radiation dose is estimated to be reduced by approximately 40% by using an R wave-triggered modulation X-ray by lowering the radiation dose during systole (data not used for reconstruction) and giving full-dose X-ray radiation only during diastole.

Table 6b.3. Diagnostic coronary angiography and MS-CT

	Diagnostic coronary angiography	MS-CT
Procedure	Cardiologist/nurse/ technician	Technician
Reading	Cardiologist	Cardiologist/radiologist
Costs	High	Low
Procedural time	30 min	10 min
Post-processing time	0	20 min
Throughput	Low	High
Radiation exposure	6–8 mSv	8–10 mSv
Resolution	High	Acceptable
Collaterals	High	Minimal
Obstruction	QCA	Visual
Nonobstructive plaque	–	+
Calcified plaque	–	++
Motion artifacts	None	Unacceptable at high HR
Availability	Worldwide	Limited

QCA, quantitative coronary angiography; HR, heart rate.

9. Clinical Implementation of MS-CT Coronary Angiography

The advantages and disadvantages of invasive and noninvasive coronary angiography are listed in Table 6b.3. It seems unlikely that MS-CT coronary angiography will be equal to the versatility and high resolution of diagnostic invasive coronary angiography, which not only is unsurpassed to detect and quantify coronary stenosis (quantitative coronary angiography) but also serves as an invaluable road map for catheter-based coronary diagnostic tools and treatment. Yet, MS-CT coronary angiography may be an acceptable alternative, now or in the foreseeable future, in a number of potential applications (Table 6b.4). The main strength of MS-CT is its noninvasive

Table 6b.4. Potential applications of MS-CT coronary angiography

1. Evaluation of chest pain in patients with a typical chest pain and an equivocal stress test
2. Evaluation of coronary anomalies
3. Alternative to invasive coronary angiography preceding percutaneous coronary intervention in hospitals without percutaneous coronary intervention (PCI) facilities
4. Early detection of atherosclerosis in high-risk individuals
5. Evaluation of obstructive coronary atherosclerosis in asymptomatic patients with known coronary artery disease
6. Coronary risk evaluation in patients undergoing major noncardiac surgery
7. Evaluation of coronary artery disease in nonischemic patients scheduled for aortic or mitral valve operations

nature, which may permit assessing early detection of nonobstructive or obstructive atherosclerotic plaques in asymptomatic individuals with multiple risk factors. (For a calcium score assessment and a comparison between multislice CT and electron beam CT, see also Chapter 7.)

10. Conclusion

The ability of CT imaging to visualize and measure disease process in the coronary arteries has increased our knowledge of atherosclerosis and coronary heart disease. Beyond feasibility studies, further well-designed, prospective single or multicenter studies are required to assess the diagnostic performance of MS-CT in various patient populations with different levels of prevalence of coronary artery disease and to establish the diagnostic role of MS-CT in cardiology before we embrace this promising technique as a clinically acceptable new diagnostic tool. Moreover, the fundamental characteristics of MS-CT such as the X-Y spatial resolution, slice thickness, and temporal resolution need to be further optimized to consider MS-CT coronary angiography as a reliable clinical diagnostic tool to detect coronary atherosclerotic obstructions. In particular, the temporal resolution needs improvement to meet the challenges of motion-free imaging also during faster heart rates.

References

1. Moshage WE, Achenbach S, Seese B, Bachmann K, Kirchgeorg M. Coronary artery stenoses: three-dimensional imaging with electrocardiographically triggered, contrast agent-enhanced, electron-beam CT. Radiology 1995;196(3):707–714.
2. Thomas PJ, McCollough CH, Ritman EL. An electron-beam CT approach for transvenous coronary arteriography. J Comput Assist Tomogr 1995;19(3):383–389.
3. Nakanishi T, Ito K, Imazu M, Yamakido M. Evaluation of coronary artery stenoses using electron-beam CT and multiplanar reformation. J Comp Assist Tomogr 1997;21:121–127.
4. Chernoff DM, Ritchie CJ, Higgins CB. Evaluation of electron beam CT coronary angiography in healthy subjects. AJR Am J Roentgenol 1997;169(1):93–99.
5. Achenbach S, Moshage W, Ropers D, Bachmann K. Curved multiplanar reconstructions for the evaluation of contrast-enhanced electron beam CT of the coronary arteries. AJR Am J Roentgenol. 1998;170(4):895–899.
6. Rensing BJ, Bongaerts A, van Geuns RJ, van Ooijen P, Oudkerk M, de Feyter PJ. Intravenous coronary angiography by electron beam computed tomography: a clinical evaluation. Circulation 1998;98(23):2509–2512.
7. Reddy GP, Chernoff DM, Adams JR, Higgins CB. Coronary artery stenoses: assessment with contrast-enhanced electron-beam CT and axial reconstructions. Radiology 1998;208(1):167–172.
8. Achenbach S, Moshage W, Ropers D, Nossen J, Daniel WG. Value of electron-beam computed tomography for the noninvasive detection of high-grade coronary-artery stenoses and occlusions. N Engl J Med 1998; 339(27):1964–1971.
9. Schmermund A, Rensing BJ, Sheedy PF, Bell MR, Rumberger JA. Intravenous electron-beam computed tomographic coronary angiography for segmental analysis of coronary artery stenoses. J Am Coll Cardiol 1998;31(7): 1547–1554.
10. Budoff MJ, Oudiz RJ, Zalace CP, et al. Intravenous three-dimensional coronary angiography using contrast enhanced electron beam computed tomography. Am J Cardiol 1999;83(6):840–845.
11. Achenbach S, Ulzheimer S, Baum U, et al. Noninvasive coronary angiography by retrospectively ECG-gated multislice spiral CT. Circulation 2000;102(23):2823–2828.
12. Nieman K, Oudkerk M, Rensing BJ, et al. Coronary angiography with multi-slice computed tomography. Lancet 2001;357(9256):599–603.
13. Achenbach S, Giesler T, Ropers D, et al. Detection of coronary artery stenoses by contrast-enhanced, retrospectively electrocardiographically-gated, multislice spiral computed tomography. Circulation 2001; 103(21):2535–2538.
14. Knez A, Becker CR, Leber A, et al. Usefulness of multislice spiral computed tomography angiography for determination of coronary artery stenoses. Am J Cardiol 2001;88(10):1191–1194.
15. Vogl TJ, Abolmaali ND, Diebold T, et al. Techniques for the detection of coronary atherosclerosis: multi-detector row CT coronary angiography. Radiology 2002;223:212–220.
16. Kopp AF, Schroeder S, Kuettner A, et al. Non-invasive coronary angiography with high resolution multidetector-row computed tomography. Results in 102 patients. Eur Heart J 2002;23(21):1714–1725.
17. Giesler T, Baum U, Ropers D, et al. Noninvasive visualization of coronary arteries using contrast-enhanced multidetector CT: influence of heart rate on image quality and stenosis detection. AJR Am J Roentgenol 2002;179(4):911–916.
18. Mao S, Lu B, Oudiz RJ, et al. Coronary artery motion in electron beam tomography. J Comput Assist Tomogr 2000;24:253–258.
19. Achenbach S, Ropers D, Holle J, Muschiol G, Daniel WG, Moshage W. In-plane coronary arterial motion velocity: measurement with electron-beam CT. Radiology 2000; 216(2):457–463.
20. Wang Y, Watts R, Mitchell I, et al. Coronary MR angiography: selection of acquisition window of minimal cardiac motion with electrocardiography-triggered navigator cardiac motion prescanning initial results. Radiology 2001;218:580–585.
21. Hong CH, Becker CR, Huber A. ECG-gated reconstructed multi-detector row CT coronary angiography: effect of varying trigger delay on image quality. Radiology 2001;220:712–717.

22. Nieman K, Rensing BJ, van Geuns RJ, et al. Non-invasive coronary angiography with multislice spiral computed tomography: impact of heart rate. Heart 2002;88:470–474.
23. Leschka S, Alkadhi H, Plass A, et al. Accuracy of MSCT coronary angiography with 64-slice technology: first experience. Eur Heart J 2005 Aug;26(15):1482–1487. Epub 2005 Apr 19.
24. Leber AW, Knez A, von Ziegler F, et al. Quantification of obstructive and nonobstructive coronary lesions by 64-slice computed tomography: a comparative study with quantitative coronary angiography and intravascular ultrasound. J Am Coll Cardiol 2005 Aug 2;46(3):552–557.
25. Raff GL, Gallagher MJ, O'Neill WW, Goldstein JA. Diagnostic accuracy of noninvasive coronary angiography using 64-slice spiral computed tomography. J Am Coll Cardiol 2005 Aug 2:46(3):552–557.
26. Mollet NRA, Cademarhri FC, Van Mieghem CAG, et al. High-resolution spiral CT coronary angiography in patients referred for diagnostic conventional coronary angiography. Circulation 2005:in press.
27. Jakobs TF, Becker CR, Ohnesorge B, et al. Multislice helical CT of the heart with retrospective ECG gating: reduction of radiation exposure by ECG-controlled tube current modulation. Eur Radiol 2002;12(5):1081–1086.
28. Hunold P, Vogt FM, Schmermund A, et al. Radiation exposure during cardiac CT: effective doses at multi-detector row CT and electron-beam CT. Radiology 2003;226(1):145–152.
29. Morin RL, Gerber TC, McCollough CH. Radiation dose in computed tomography of the heart. Circulation 2003; 107:917–922.

7

Noninvasive Assessment of Asymptomatic Individuals at Risk of Coronary Heart Disease. Part a

E.T.S. Lim, D.V. Anand, and A. Lahiri

Coronary heart disease (CHD) is a leading cause of mortality and morbidity in all the market economies,[1,2] and its incidence and prevalence is also rapidly increasing in many developing countries.[3,4] However, although clinical coronary disease is common, most patients have subclinical disease.[5,6] Studies comparing coronary angiography and intracoronary ultrasound have shown that vascular remodeling accompanies the early development of atherosclerotic plaque, and luminal narrowing does not occur until substantial amounts of plaque have accumulated.[7–9] Clinical disease therefore only manifests at a late stage.[5,6,10,11] Furthermore, because in a significant proportion of cases the initial presentation of CHD is sudden cardiac death,[12] there is no opportunity for secondary prevention. There is therefore a need to accurately identify asymptomatic individuals who have subclinical coronary artery disease[13,14] in order to institute primary preventive measures.

Cardiovascular risk can be assessed by counting the number of major coronary risk factors present (age, gender, smoking, diabetes, hyperlipidemia, hypertension, family history of premature ischemic heart disease).[15–17] Alternatively, risk functions (the prototype being the Framingham risk equation) can also be used. This is the method advocated by the National Cholesterol Education Panel Adult Treatment Panel (NCEP ATP III)[18] in the United States. Unfortunately, these approaches have limitations.[14,19] It has been estimated that approximately 20% of individuals have no cardiac risk factors before the index myocardial infarction. In 25% of cases, the index myocardial infarction will result in sudden cardiac death. Furthermore, this approach does not aid clinical decision-making for the 36 million adults in the United States classified as intermediate risk according to the NCEP ATP III standard.[16,20,21] Overall, it has been estimated that the traditional risk factors may fail to explain up to 50% of CHD morbidity and mortality.

It is likely that cardiovascular risk estimates can be improved by imaging tests. Such tests are now able to measure atherosclerotic plaque burden and character, which are key determinants of cardiovascular risk. These tests are often collectively referred to as "atherosclerosis imaging" tests. In this chapter, we will discuss the utility of such tests in the identification of asymptomatic individuals at risk of CHD.

1. Electron Beam Computed Tomography Coronary Calcium Imaging

Coronary calcification has been linked to coronary atherosclerosis,[22,23] and coronary calcium imaging is currently one of the best studied methods of noninvasive atherosclerosis imaging.[20,24,25] It is most often performed using electron beam computed tomography (EBCT) technology, although in recent years, it has also become possible to use multislice CT (MS-CT) systems. More than 300 000 EBCT coronary calcium scans are performed annually in the United States.[26] However, the use of this technique globally is variable. For example, less than 5000 such scans are performed annually in the United Kingdom.

1.2 Pathophysiologic Aspects of Coronary Calcification

1.2.1 Histologic Stages of Coronary Calcification

Histologic, sonographic and fluoroscopic studies have shown that the extent of coronary calcification is closely associated with total coronary artery atherosclerotic plaque burden[27–32] (Figure 7a.1). Coronary calcification is also

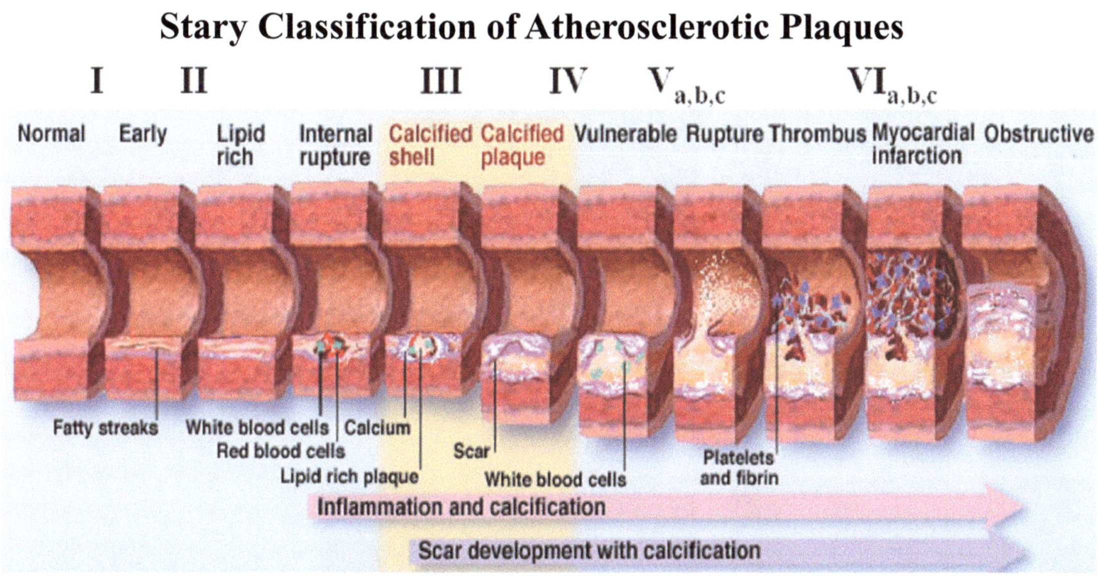

Figure 7a.1. Several histopathologic stages of atherosclerotic plaque development can be identified. Under the Stary classification,[28] early lesions are considered as types I–III, whereas advanced lesions are types IV–VI. Coronary calcification detectable using CT (stage IV lesions and beyond) usually precedes symptomatic disease by at least several (5 or more) years. (Figure courtesy of GE Healthcare.)

closely associated with coronary artery plaque on a site-by-site basis.[33–35]

Autopsy studies of persons dying in the first four decades of life from causes other than coronary artery disease show that early noncalcified atherosclerotic lesions can often be found (Figure 7a.2).[36–41] In some individuals, these lesions progress by continuing to attract lipid-droplet-laden macrophages (foam cells) and by forming an extracellular lipid core[29,42] in which microscopic calcium granules are often found. From early middle age, fibromuscular vascular changes and macroscopic calcification occur. Only at this point can coronary calcification be detected using EBCT. Nevertheless, disease at this stage is still most often clinically silent, because the plaque is usually accommodated by Glagovian vascular remodeling and does not become flow-limiting.[7,9] This process of remodeling was first demonstrated in pathologic specimens but can also be shown in vivo using intravascular ultrasound.[8,43] With further plaque growth, the likelihood of coronary artery obstruction (causing exertional angina) or plaque rupture or erosion (causing acute coronary syndromes) becomes increasingly likely. In men, this most often occurs from the fourth decade of life onward, whereas in women, it most often occurs from the fifth decade of life onward. The time between the first appearance of macroscopic coronary calcification (histologic Stary stage V disease[29]) and clinical events represents a window during which EBCT coronary calcium imaging is potentially most useful.

Because the key event in acute coronary syndromes is plaque instability,[44–46] the site of stenotic coronary artery lesions does not accurately predict the site of vessel occlusion during myocardial infarction.[10,11] It is estimated that only 30% of acute myocardial infarctions occur at the site of flow-limiting lesions. Seventy percent occur at the site of hemodynamically insignificant lesions because of disruption of plaque, distal embolization of plaque material, vessel thrombosis, and vessel closure.

The two major underlying mechanisms leading to plaque instability that have been identified are rupture and erosion.[29] Both processes coexist and can be found in coronary arteries of the same individual. Plaque rupture is more common (underlying approximately 80% of cases of acute coronary syndromes). It is associated with hyperlipidemia and male gender, whereas erosion is associated with diabetes, female gender, and young age. Ruptured plaque is frequently associated with sudden cardiac

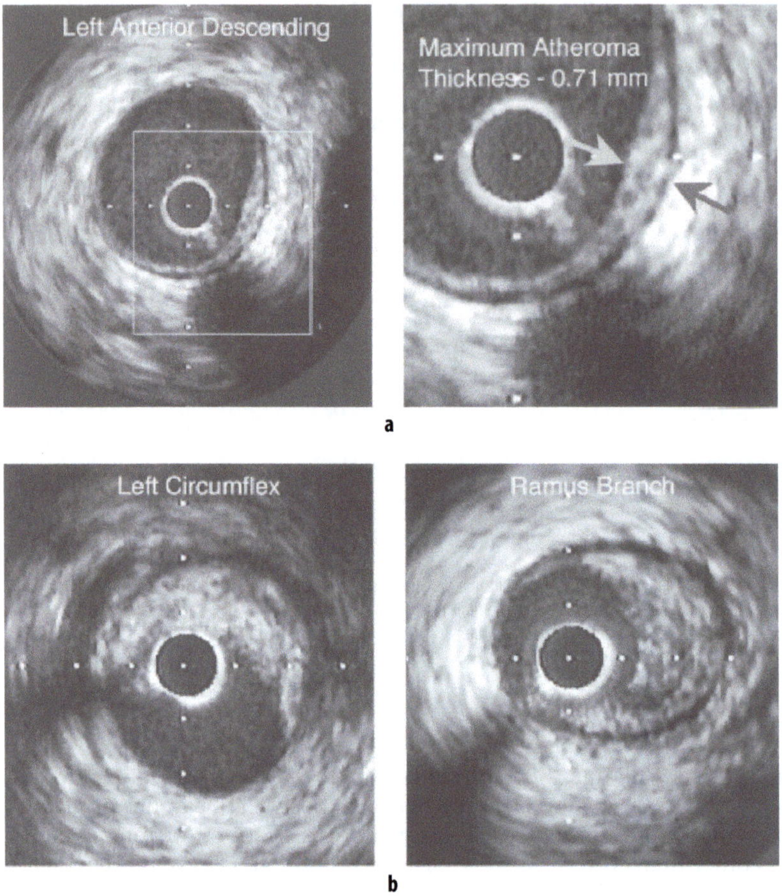

Figure 7a.2. Coronary atherosclerosis begins at a relatively young age, and becomes symptomatic only when advanced. Even the coronary arteries from transplanted hearts (in which donors are young and have no symptoms) frequently have detectable and sometimes extensive coronary atherosclerosis, using coronary intravascular ultrasound (Tuzcu et al. Circulation 2001). **a** Left anterior descending artery of 17-year-old adolescent boy. **b** Left circumflex artery of a 32-year-old woman.

death and positive vascular remodeling, and is also very likely to be calcified. In contrast, it is not clear why eroded plaque is only infrequently calcified.[28]

1.2.2 The Mechanism of Coronary Calcification

Coronary calcification is an actively regulated process, and represents the controlled deposition of calcium hydroxyapatite crystals, rather than passive precipitation.[22,47,48] It has been linked with alterations in cell differentiation at the site of atherosclerotic lesions because ectopic osseous and cartilaginous tissue is often found in atherosclerotic lesions and in animal models of vascular calcification.[22,49–51] Cells with osteoblastic characteristics have been isolated from the vascular media ("calcifying vascular cells") and it is believed that these produce matrix vesicles and osteoid in atherosclerotic lesions. The latter is an extracellular matrix that provides a permissive milieu for mineralization by calcium hydroxyapatite. All the major components of matrix vesicles and osteoid in bone that are instrumental in permitting calcification have also been found in atherosclerotic lesions; these include bone morphogenetic protein-2, osteopontin, osteoprotegerin, matrix γ-carboxylated glutamate, osteonectin, osteocalcin, and collagen type I.[48] The trigger(s) causing cell differentiation toward an osteoblast cell lineage in atherosclerotic plaque is currently under investigation.

Recently, it has been shown that matrix metalloproteinases may also be involved in vascular calcification.[52–54] This observation is of interest because matrix metalloproteinases are also expressed at the site of unstable plaque and are believed to be integral to the processes underlying plaque rupture and vascular remodeling.

1.2.3 Pathologic Consequences of Coronary Calcification

From the clinical perspective, vascular calcification serves as a marker of atherosclerotic plaque. Additionally, it is likely to have directly harmful consequences. For example, it is the single most important risk factor for coronary artery dissection during angioplasty.[47,48] Aortic calcification is also likely to reduce arterial compliance and coronary perfusion pressure (especially in combination with coronary artery stenosis).[55–57]

Whether calcification per se affects plaque stability is unclear. Recently, it was shown that monocytes purified from peripheral blood of human healthy volunteers express tumor necrosis factor-α when coincubated with calcium hydroxyapatite crystals. This observation links coronary calcification with the inflammatory process and suggests that calcium may directly destabilize plaque. However, extent of coronary calcification does not seem to be correlated with plasma high-sensitivity C-reactive protein levels (a sensitivity marker of systemic inflammation),[58,59] and furthermore, although aggressive lipid-lowering treatment lowers the risk of future cardiac events, it does not always produce a concomitant reduction in coronary calcification.[60,61]

1.3 EBCT Technology

Conventional CT is unable to image the coronary arteries accurately principally because of cardiac motion artifact.[20,62,63] EBCT was developed in the 1980s to address this shortcoming. With EBCT, this limitation is obviated because there is no mechanical gantry; instead, an electron beam is electromagnetically steered toward a tungsten target to generate X-rays. For coronary calcium scanning, images are acquired during mid-diastole to minimize coronary artery motion. Prospective electrocardiogram (ECG) gating at approximately 40% of the R-R interval is used to define the time of relative cardiac standstill (the exact timing being dependent on the heart rate). Typically, 30–40 contiguous axial slices at 3-mm intervals are taken during a single breathhold lasting approximately 25–40 seconds. No intravenous or intraarterial contrast agent is necessary, because of the great difference in CT density between coronary calcium and surrounding flowing blood, periarterial fat, and other soft tissues.

There is normally little difficulty in distinguishing coronary calcium from calcified aortic or mitral valves or calcified pericardium, which occupy characteristic positions and have a distinct configuration (Figure 7a.3 and 4; see color section). It is usually possible to distinguish the left main stem, left anterior descending, first and sometimes second diagonal branches, left circumflex, first obtuse marginal (and sometimes second obtuse marginal), right coronary artery, and posterior descending arteries.

Cardiac motion artifact is not a problem using EBCT technology. However, hardening artifact from prosthetic objects such as metallic artificial valves, pacemaker leads and stents, or in obese subjects does occur, as does misalignment of CT slices because of an inadequate breathhold. In clinical practice, these are usually not a major problem.

1.4 Radiation Exposure During EBCT Coronary Calcium Imaging

The radiation burden from EBCT coronary calcium imaging is low. Estimates of the mean effective radiation dose per scan range from 1.0 to 1.3 mSv.[64] Coronary calcium scanning can also be performed using MS-CT[65]; estimates of mean effective radiation dose range from 1.5 to 6.8 mSv, depending on the scanner and protocol used (see below).[64]

1.5 Quantification of Coronary Calcium

Unlike fluoroscopy, coronary calcium can be readily quantified using cross-sectional CT images *without the use of any intravenous contrast agent*. Four methods of quantifying coronary calcium are in widespread use, each with individual strengths and weaknesses.

The *Agatston score* was developed in 1990, and is calculated by multiplying the area of each lesion within the coronary arteries above a 130 Hounsfield unit (HU) density threshold obtained

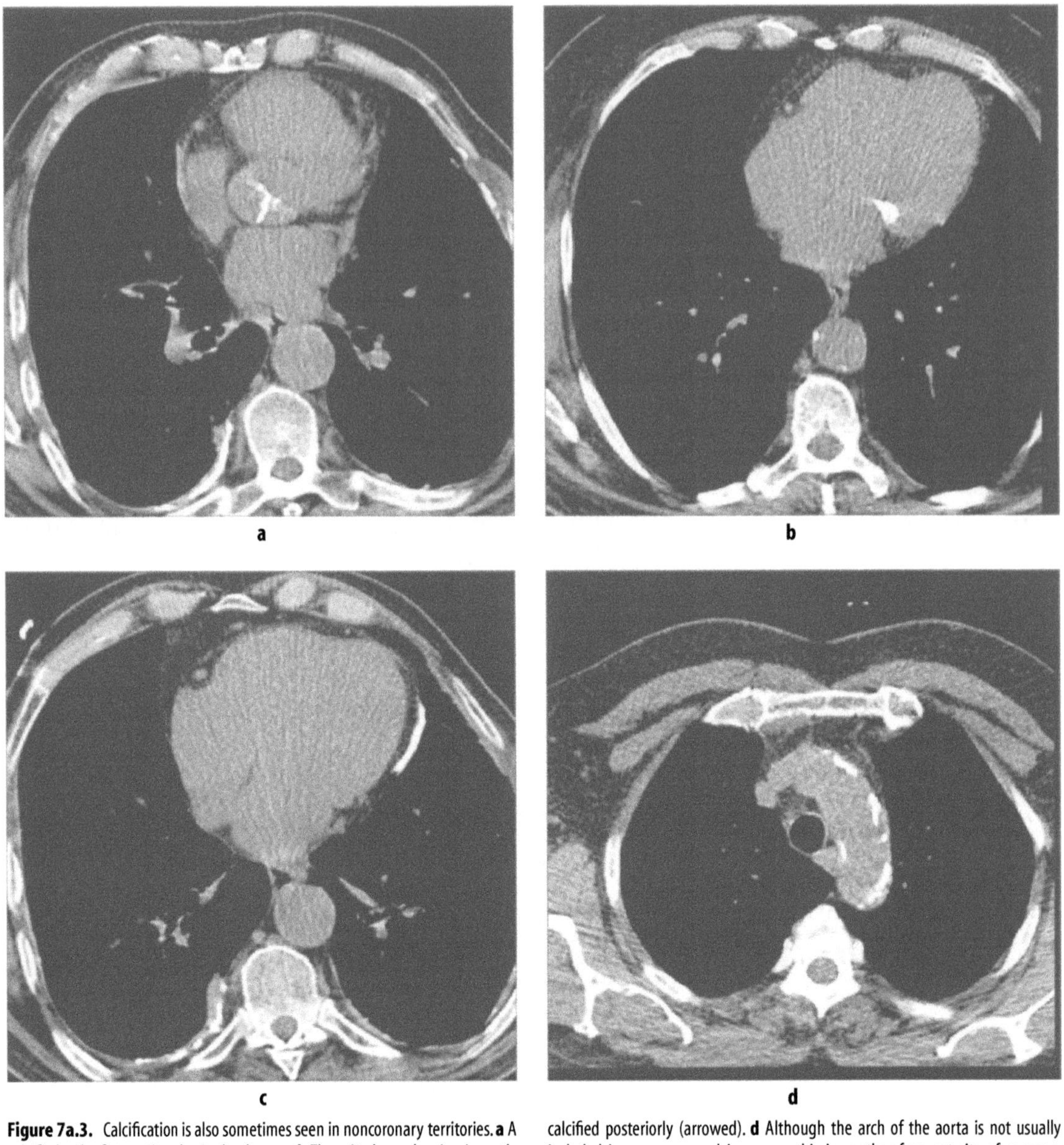

Figure 7a.3. Calcification is also sometimes seen in noncoronary territories. **a** A calcified, trileaflet aortic valve is clearly seen. **b** The mitral annular ring is partly calcified. **c** A pericardium plaque is visible. In addition, the pleura is thickened and calcified posteriorly (arrowed). **d** Although the arch of the aorta is not usually included in a coronary calcium scan, this is another frequent site of coronary calcification.

from 3-mm-thick nonoverlapping slices by a weighting factor that is dependent on the peak signal anywhere within the lesion.[66] The weighting factor is 1 for peak signal densities of 130–199 HU; 2 for densities of 200–299 HU; 3 for densities of 300–399 HU, and 4 when the density is 400 or more HU. Lesions are identified by an operator manually defining a "region of interest" by planimetry on a slice-by-slice basis. Commercial software is available for this purpose.

Because of the discrete nature of the weighting factors, one problem is that this method is highly sensitive to noise when the peak signal is near any of the threshold values, and completely insensitive away from them.[67] An alternative, more recent method of quantifying coronary calcium which is less affected by this problem is the *volume score*.[68] This linearly interpolates the data set to isotropic volumes before computing the volume above a 130-HU threshold. (An isotropic data set is one in which voxels have the same size in all three spatial dimensions.) This scoring method is vulnerable to partial volume effects, but displays reduced interscan variability in comparison to the Agatston scoring method, and is often used if serial coronary calcium scans from the same individual are being compared. *Calcium mass* measurement is another parameter that is derived by converting HU to bone ash equivalent (see also Chapter 6a).

Both the volume and Agatston scores have been validated against histologic, sonographic, and angiographic measures of coronary calcification.[66,68] Both are continuous, easily reproducible quantities. The learning curve is short, and correspondingly, the inter- and intraobserver variability is small (3% and <1%, respectively; correlation coefficients ~0.99).[63,69] Most difficulty arises when the scores are low (between 0–80 Agatston units) and any artifact is proportionally more significant.[69–71] For the majority of scans, when calcium scoring is performed for prognostication, this degree of artifact does not usually alter the overall interpretation of the scan and clinical management, because calcium scores are traditionally reported in categories (no, mild, moderate, or severe coronary calcification). However, if serial coronary calcium scoring is being performed to monitor the efficacy of lipid-lowering therapy (see later), then interscan reproducibility becomes more important. Because the median interscan variability is significant (approximately 10%–15%),[69–72] this should be taken into account during interpretation.

Because quantity of coronary calcium varies widely depending on age and sex, scores may also be expressed as age- and sex-adjusted percentiles.[25,73–75] For example, it is rare to find any coronary calcium in an asymptomatic male below the age of 35 years, whereas it is very frequent in a male above the age of 75 years. In

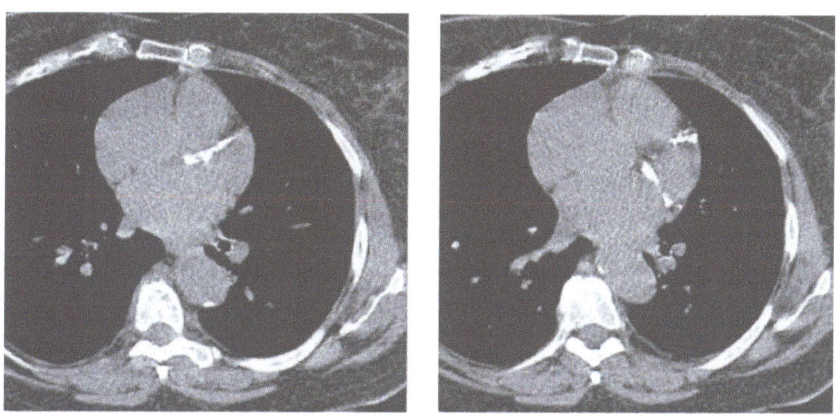

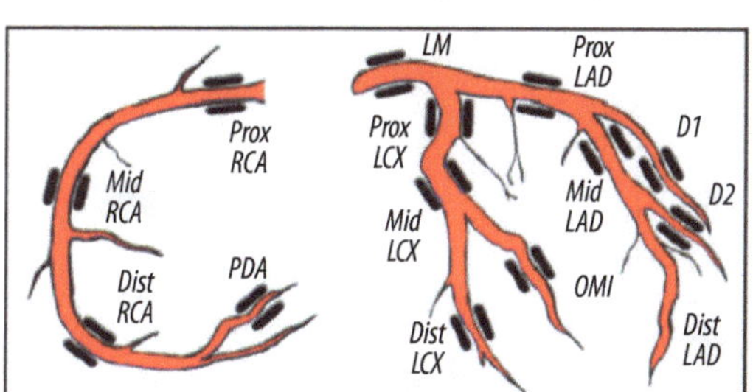

	Lesions	Volume (mm3)	AGATSTON Score
Left Main	1	168.19	195.97
Left Anterior Descending	15	1043.93	1238.51
Left Circumflex	20	1046.98	1239.54
Right Coronary Artery	39	1942.14	2399.40
Total	75	4201.24	5073.41

Figure 7a.4. Extensive calcification is evident in the left anterior descending (LAD) artery (solid arrows), left circumflex artery (LCX) (outline arrows), and right coronary artery (RCA) (not shown). With appropriate software, it is possible to quantify the extent of coronary atherosclerosis (see text). According to the frequently used Agatston scoring system, a score of ≤10 units is not significant, 10–99 units is mild, 100–399 units is moderate, 400–999 units is severe, and ≥1000 units is extensive coronary calcification. In this example, the coronary calcium score was 5073.41 units.

women, the prevalence of coronary calcium and mean calcium score is approximately half that of men until the age of 60 years, after which the difference diminishes. It has been shown that the age–sex percentile is also associated with cardiovascular risk.[74,76–78]

Age- and sex-*adjusted coronary calcium scores* can also be expressed as an equivalent "heart age."[75,79] For example, a man who has an age- and sex-adjusted percentile score of 90 could also be said to have a heart age of approximately 60 years, i.e., the age at which the individual's coronary calcium score is equivalent to the population median (50th percentile), based on age and sex. This is a useful concept because patients (as well as physicians) often find this concept more intuitive than absolute calcium scores. Additionally, it has been suggested that replacing chronological age with heart age may improve risk functions such as Framingham.[75,79]

1.6 Relationship Between Coronary Calcification and Outcomes

The most important application of coronary calcium imaging is in establishing cardiovascular prognosis. Unlike the Framingham risk function, by quantifying the atherosclerotic plaque burden, EBCT coronary calcium should potentially reflect both known and unknown (or unmeasured) risk factors, such as homocysteine, C-reactive protein, and the genetic constitution of the individual. There should therefore be a strong relationship between coronary calcium and cardiovascular mortality. Several studies provide direct support for this.

1.6.1 Retrospective Studies

Shaw et al.[76] conducted a large study of 10 377 subjects who were referred for cardiovascular risk stratification. They showed that extent of coronary calcification was closely correlated to all-cause mortality, and that risk stratification using a combination of coronary calcification and clinical variables was superior to either alone. They also showed that, for the same extent of coronary calcification, women were at significantly higher risk. However, the main outcome measure they used was all-cause mortality (and not cardiovascular mortality). Recently, this group has published a subanalysis of the diabetics referred for risk stratification,[80] and showed that diabetics with no detectable coronary calcification have similar all-cause mortality to nondiabetics with no coronary calcification, implying that coronary calcium is also a robust prognostic marker in this important patient population (Figure 7a.5).

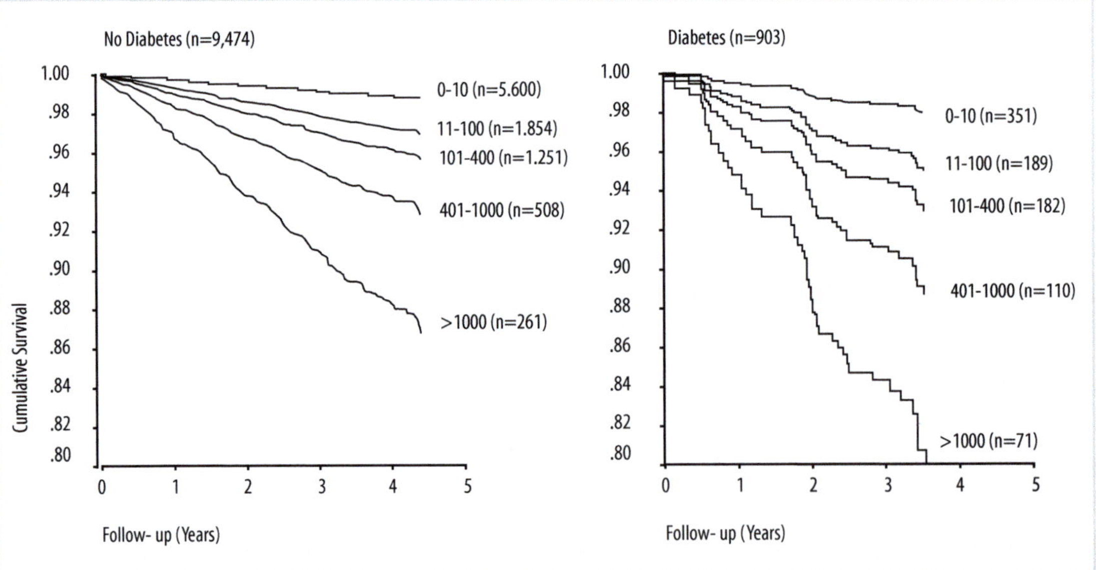

Figure 7a.5. The largest study of the prognostic power of coronary calcification included 10 377 self-referred patients. In a Cox-proportional hazards model, coronary calcium scores were powerful predictors of all-cause mortality in both nondiabetic and diabetic patients (see text; Raggi et al.[80]).

Kondos et al.[81] followed up 5635 initially asymptomatic low- to intermediate-risk adults 37 months after EBCT coronary calcium imaging. In men, coronary calcification, smoking, and diabetes were associated with a 10.5-, 1.4-, and 2-fold increase in relative risk of any cardiovascular event, respectively. In women, only coronary calcification was associated with a 2.6-fold increase in relative risk of any cardiovascular event. Coronary calcification provided incremental prognostic information in addition to age and other risk factors. However, risk factor data obtained in this study was self-reported by the patients, and although they attempted to contact all eligible subjects for follow-up, the response rate was only 64%.

1.6.2 Prospective Studies

Arad et al.[82] have conducted a prospective study of 1173 asymptomatic patients, and showed that coronary calcium was superior to traditional risk factors for the prediction of clinical cardiovascular events. The sensitivity, specificity, and negative predictive value of a coronary calcium score >160 Agatston units was 89%, 82%, and 35.4%, respectively. A coronary calcium score >100 and >160 was associated with an odds ratio of 20:1 and 35:1 for coronary events, respectively.

Raggi et al.[78] conducted a similar prospective study in 632 individuals which again associated coronary calcification with hard cardiovascular events. This study also showed that approximately two-thirds of events occurred in patients with coronary calcium scores <400 Agatston units (i.e., no more than moderate coronary atherosclerosis). They therefore adjusted for the confounding effects of age and sex, and found that a high age–sex percentile (>75th percentile) also increased cardiovascular risk, irrespective of the absolute coronary calcium score.

In contrast, Detrano et al.[83] have reported that neither EBCT coronary calcium imaging nor the Framingham risk function were strong predictors of near-term cardiovascular events in a group of 1196 high-risk adults. However, 6-mm slices were used for coronary calcium imaging, rather than the 3 mm stipulated in the original Agatston-Janowitz protocol.[84] This would have markedly reduced the sensitivity of the test. Furthermore, selection and treatment bias in this patient population is very likely to have been present[85]; >10% of the original eligible cohort were excluded because of death, angina, or acute myocardial infarction occurring within 30 months, and subjects were not blinded regarding the results of the EBCT coronary calcium scan.

In a meta-analysis of the prospective studies,[86] there was an increased risk for a combined outcome (nonfatal myocardial infarction, CHD death, or revascularization) associated with a calcium score elevated above a median value (risk ratio 8.7 [95% confidence interval (CI), 2.7–28.1]) The relative risk of hard endpoints (myocardial infarction or death) was also increased [risk ratio 4.2 (95% CI 1.6–11.3)].

Because most of these studies have compared coronary calcium scores to self-reported risk factors, and because risk factor counting was generally used in place of the Framingham risk function, a key question that remains unsettled is whether prognostication by means of coronary calcium scoring is truly superior to the Framingham risk function.[87] Three large prospective cohort studies (PACC,[88] RECALL,[89] and MESA[90]) are currently in progress to answer this question. Framingham risk and coronary calcium scores will be determined in >10 000 participants, who will be followed up for incident cardiac events and mortality; however, final results are not expected before 2010.

1.7 Relationship Between Coronary Calcification and Obstructive Coronary Artery Disease

As described earlier, the presence of coronary calcification is not synonymous with obstructive coronary artery disease.[91–95] Unsuspected intramural coronary artery plaque can frequently be demonstrated using intravascular ultrasound even in angiographically normal arteries.[7,8,43] This explains the observation that the prognostic value of EBCT coronary calcium is superior to coronary angiography, because the latter significantly underestimates the total coronary artery plaque burden. However, detecting obstructive coronary artery disease remains important because this determines those individuals most likely to benefit from coronary revascularization (percutaneous or surgical). There are, therefore, several studies on the relationship between coronary calcification and angiographic stenosis or myocardial perfusion defects.

1.7.1 Relationship with Angiographic Coronary Artery Stenosis

Nallamothu and colleagues[96,97] have conducted a meta-analysis examining the relationship of coronary calcification with angiographic coronary artery stenosis. Nine studies with a total of 1662 subjects were included.[96,97] Angiographic stenosis was defined as >50% luminal stenosis in all studies except one. The pooled sensitivity and specificity for EBCT prediction of angiographic coronary artery stenosis was 92% and 51%, respectively. Maximal joint sensitivity and specificity from a summary receiver-operating characteristic curve analysis was 75%. These figures suggest that the diagnostic accuracy of EBCT for predicting obstructive coronary artery disease is comparable to traditional exercise stress testing.

1.7.2 Relationship with Myocardial Perfusion Imaging Abnormalities

Because individuals referred for EBCT coronary calcium imaging are frequently asymptomatic, many physicians use myocardial perfusion imaging (MPI) to noninvasively detect ischemia in preference to contrast coronary angiography.[92,93,98] Three studies have established that the probability and extent of perfusion defect increase as coronary calcium score increases, even in asymptomatic individuals.[94,95,99] Two of these studies suggest that the probability and size of perfusion defect are small in individuals with a coronary calcium score <400 Agatston units, and therefore recommend that MPI be reserved for individuals with coronary calcium scores in excess of 400 Agatston units. It should be noted that because one of the studies used EBCT, and the other used multidetector CT to quantify coronary calcification, the coronary calcium scores may not be exactly comparable.

However, Anand et al.[91] showed that an even lower coronary calcium score may be associated with clinically important inducible ischemia. Using a receiver operating characteristic analysis, a coronary calcium score of 190 Agatston units maximized joint sensitivity and specificity for myocardial ischemia in their study population.[91,100] Anand et al. have also documented a significant prevalence of myocardial ischemia in asymptomatic diabetic subjects with a normal resting electrocardiogram and coronary calcium scores between 100 and 400 Agatston units.[101] These results suggest that the optimum threshold may be significantly lower than 400 Agatston units. It is possible that certain factors such as treatment with statins[60] and renal disease[57,102–104] might alter the relationship between coronary calcification and obstructive coronary artery disease, but this is so far a poorly studied area. Such factors may partially or completely account for the differences reported by the different studies.

None of these studies have been conducted in an unselected population, and except for the study by Anand et al.,[91] all have been retrospective. Prospectively conducted studies using an unselected population are underway to answer this question more fully.

1.8 Clinical Application of EBCT Coronary Calcium Imaging

At least two groups of patients *might* benefit from EBCT coronary calcium imaging.[62,63,73,75]

The first are asymptomatic patients with coronary risk factors and an intermediate pretest probability of CHD.[105–108] In the United States, this includes approximately 40% of the adult population (36 million). In this population, it has been estimated that coronary calcium imaging will reclassify patients into higher or lower risk categories 56% of the time, and therefore alter management in a substantial proportion of patients.[79] (In low-risk patients, this would occur only 2% of the time.)

Use of coronary calcium imaging in this way can be considered "screening" for cardiovascular disease. This application in particular has been highly controversial because the stringent conditions needed to conclusively show that screening is beneficial have not all been met.[109–111] These conditions include demonstrating that clinical management based on coronary calcium imaging improves patient outcome. Because the majority of contemporary studies and the ongoing prospective studies do not blind participants to the results of their coronary calcium scan,[90] and there is a natural reluctance of physicians and patients not to initiate comparatively innocuous yet highly effective therapy with HMG-CoA reductase inhibitors (statins), a substantial degree of treatment bias is likely. As noted earlier, the economic costs of screening using coronary calcium are also unclear.[21]

Because coronary calcification is not synonymous with clinically significant stenosis,[91–95,99] and because objective evidence of myocardial ischemia has been shown to predict worse outcome even in asymptomatic individuals,[112–116] it is not unreasonable to proceed to noninvasive imaging with stress myocardial perfusion scan or ECHO when significant coronary calcification is found (see earlier).

The second, perhaps less controversial category of patients who might benefit from EBCT coronary calcium imaging are those with typical or atypical cardiac symptoms,[62,73,117] but who on the basis of risk factor profile are judged to have a low to intermediate pretest probability of CHD. These patients are often referred for exercise electrocardiography despite the suboptimal positive and negative predictive value of the test in this population.[118] In contrast, the very high negative predictive value of a coronary calcium score of zero (98%) may allow coronary calcium imaging to essentially rule out atheromatous coronary artery disease.[118,119] This test is most useful in young patients (e.g., men <55 years old, women <65 years old) in whom the probability of finding minimal or no coronary calcification is very high. If significant coronary calcification is found, as is often the case in older patients, it may still be necessary to proceed to further investigation using either myocardial perfusion scan or stress ECHO.

It has also been suggested that EBCT coronary calcium imaging may be used to monitor lipid-lowering treatment.[60,120–125] An annual increase in the coronary calcium score of >20% has been associated with an annual cardiovascular event rate of 6.45%, whereas an annual increase of 1%–20% is associated with an annual cardiovascular event rate of only 1.5%. Furthermore, Achenbach et al.[60] have shown that untreated hyperlipidemia is associated with progression of coronary calcification, and that treatment with HMG-CoA inhibitors (statins) can successfully arrest this process. These are, however, preliminary observations and more data are need before the effect of statins on coronary calcification is fully understood.

At the time of this writing, the available data on its potential use for risk stratification in asymptomatic women are limited. It is possible that assessment of coronary calcium will prove to be a helpful tool in this population, but, clearly, additional high-quality data are needed that specifically address coronary artery disease outcomes in women. Until then, such assessment should be limited to clinically selected women at intermediate risk.

1.9 Economic Evaluation of EBCT Coronary Calcium Imaging as a Screening Tool for Subclinical CHD

It has been estimated that the 15% of the adult population in the United States deemed at high risk using NCEP ATP III criteria[18] represent approximately 45% of likely future coronary deaths. Coronary prevention in this population using office-based risk assessment compares favorably with other health care interventions (US $25 000 to $35 000 per quality-of-life-year saved). However, the remaining 85% of the adult population who are not deemed at high risk will account for 55% of likely future coronary deaths. Both the West of Scotland (WOSCOPS)[126] and Air Force/Texas Coronary Atherosclerosis Prevention (AFCAPS/TexCAPS) studies[127] have shown that reducing coronary mortality in this population is possible, but much less cost-effective. For example, using the WOSCOPS data, treating 1000 hypercholesterolemic middle-aged men for 5 years with a statin may be expected to prevent <50 cardiac events. In the United States, it has been estimated that approximately 50% of the adult population would meet the entry criteria for AFCAPS/TexCAPS[127]; treating this population could cost as much as US $50 billion. There is, therefore, a clear economic incentive to develop improved methods of risk prediction such as coronary calcium imaging in order to better target the "at-risk" population.

At present, it is difficult to rigorously evaluate EBCT coronary calcium imaging in economic terms because of a lack of accurate data in several areas.[21,26] A number of different forms of analysis can be used, which make varying assumptions.[26,128–130] Cost-effectiveness analysis (that is, analysis of the relative benefit purchased by adopting one strategy rather than another) can be applied, but to be most useful, benefit should preferably be expressed in units that facilitate comparison with other benchmarks (such as number of life-years saved).[26] Because a diagnostic test is being evaluated, this requires that the test results be explicitly linked to an intervention that improves patient outcome (and which preferably can be quantified as number of life-years saved). No such studies exist, and several important parameters required by such model must be extrapolated.

Alternatively, an economic model using intermediate outcome measures, such as the cost to identify coronary disease or a coronary event could be used.[94] Although such a model would not require a diagnostic test to be explicitly linked with an intervention and would involve fewer assumptions, it would not be possible to compare the calculated cost-effectiveness ratio across a broad array of alternative strategies because of the lack of a common metric.

Whatever outcome measure is used, a complete evaluation of cost should also take into account fixed ("start-up") costs in addition to the cost of each test, and "downstream" or "induced" costs. The latter includes additional testing driven by incidental findings on EBCT coronary calcium imaging and additional therapeutic interventions; these may be considerable.[131,132] For example, one study documented that 53% of patients had noncoronary abnormal findings.[132]

Two published models have compared EBCT coronary calcium imaging favorably with several alternative diagnostic pathways in symptomatic patients with a low to intermediate probability of coronary disease, based on the cost per correct diagnosis.[129,133] However, these conclusions are highly sensitive to the underlying assumptions of the model, and do not model patient outcome. A third published study modeled the costs to identify coronary events in asymptomatic subjects with one or more coronary risk factors.[21] Making the assumption that a significant proportion of coronary events could be averted by appropriate therapy (so that cost per life-year saved can be computed), this model suggested that EBCT coronary calcium imaging could be economically attractive. Sensitivity analysis showed that costs were highly dependent on the population coronary risk, with the "cost per death identified" four-fold higher in a low-risk population compared with an intermediate risk population. A fourth published model[21] has examined the incremental (marginal) cost to identify one at-risk patient, and the projected incremental cost per quality-adjusted life-year. This model studied 40 year olds, a relatively low-risk population, and used favorable assumptions of the efficacy of primary prevention and the independent prognostic value provided by EBCT coronary calcium imaging. Sensitivity analysis showed that the cost per diagnosis was most sensitive to the cost of EBCT; the projected incremental cost per quality-adjusted life-year saved was sensitive to efficacy of primary prevention, the utility placed on a year of life on medications, and the independent prognostic value of EBCT coronary calcium imaging. Overall, this model suggests that EBCT coronary calcium imaging is not economically attractive in 40 year olds; however, the results cannot be generalized to other populations. Nor can the results of any of these studies necessarily be translated into health care systems outside of the United States.

Clearly, each of these models is either simplistic in its assumptions, or is forced to make many assumptions. Before EBCT coronary calcium imaging can be widely promulgated, more data on its prognostic value in the general population and how it may be used to influence patient outcome will be necessary.

1.10 Other Emerging Issues Related to Coronary Calcium Imaging

1.10.1 Ethnic Differences in Coronary Calcification

Major, but ill-understood, differences in the incidence and prevalence of CHD exist among different ethnic groups.[90] For example, in the United Kingdom, the standardized coronary mortality rate in expatriate Indian Asians (Bangladeshis, Pakistanis, Sri Lankans, Indians) is approximately 50% higher than the national average.[134,135] In the United States, it is African Americans who have the highest overall CHD mortality of any ethnic group. The extent to which the major recognized coronary risk factors account for the excess cardiovascular mortality is uncertain, and it is possible there are important ethnic-specific differences in the mechanisms of atherogenesis, including differences in coronary calcification. In support of this, histopathologic studies suggest that aortic fibrous plaque is more likely to be calcified whereas coronary artery plaque is less likely to be calcified in American blacks compared with their Caucasian counterparts.[136] In several (although not all) EBCT studies, coronary calcification has also been observed to be significantly less frequent and less severe (despite the higher coronary mortality) in American blacks compared with Caucasians.[136–139] Only limited data are available for other ethnic groups.

Several prospective observational studies of coronary calcification in different ethnic groups are now in progress, the largest of which is the Multi-Ethnic Study of Atherosclerosis (MESA)[90] in the United States. Until such data are available, a degree of caution should be applied in the interpretation of coronary calcium scores and percentiles in non-American Caucasians.

1.10.2 MS-CT and Coronary Calcium Imaging

The emergence of MS-CT,[140,141] which is also capable of coronary calcium imaging, is an important recent development because uptake of this versatile technology has been much more widespread than EBCT.

1.10.2.1 Technological Aspects of MS-CT

The driving force motivating development of EBCT technology was the need to reduce acquisition times in order to perform cardiac imaging without motion artifact. EBCT acquisition times are very low – currently 50 milliseconds for the cine mode, and 100 milliseconds for the high-resolution mode, with the potential to improve further in the future. However, EBCT technology is expensive, has high maintenance costs, and is less versatile than "mechanical" or conventional CT.

In the last two decades, there have been significant advances in mechanical CT technology.[140–142] First, the development of slip ring gantries, high-power X-ray tubes, and improved interpolation algorithms allowed helical ("spiral") CT scanners to be developed. Using such scanners, patients are imaged during continuous X-ray tube rotation and simultaneous table translation. They allow volume acquisition while improving scanning speed as well as z-axis resolution. The second major development is MS-CT technology, which refers to the simultaneous acquisition of more than one image slice per gantry revolution. Multiple contiguous detector rows are used to achieve this; 4-, 8-, 16-, 32-slice CT is now a clinical reality, and a 64-slice CT has been recently introduced. Together with fast gantry rotation speeds, improved reconstruction algorithms, and retrospective or prospective ECG gating, acquisition times acceptable for cardiac imaging can generally be achieved.

1.10.2.2 Differences in EBCT- and MS-CT-derived Coronary Calcium Scores

There are many different MS-CT manufacturers. Each has proprietary hardware and software, including the image reconstruction algorithms used. In contrast, there is only one EBCT manufacturer (Imatron, GE, San Francisco, CA) and most centers use similar, if not identical, EBCT scanning protocols. Clearly, there are many more variables to consider when MS-CT is used to perform coronary calcium imaging compared with EBCT.[20,140,141] This includes the use of prospective or retrospective gating, slice thickness used, number of detector arrays present, variable tube current giving rise to different spatial resolution and signal-to-noise ratios, and reconstruction algorithm used. There has therefore been concern that the coronary calcium scoring packages included with all new MS-CT scanners may produce numbers that are not directly comparable with EBCT coronary calcium scores, and on which most of the current medical literature is still based.[72] Furthermore, the original Janowitz-Agatston and volumetric calcium scoring protocols developed for EBCT cannot be directly "ported" to MS-CT. Mathematical algorithms can be used to correct for these differences, but at the risk of introducing artifact.

A number of studies have attempted to address this issue by comparing EBCT- and MS-CT-derived coronary calcium scores. Generally, although the correlation coefficients are good (often <0.90), the scores themselves are not necessarily directly comparable. This seems to be particularly the case when coronary calcium scores are low.[143] Because coronary calcium scores are generally classified into one of four categories for clinical purposes, this discrepancy can impact on clinical management when the coronary calcium score is close to one of the thresholds. Stanford et al.[144] scanned 78 asymptomatic subjects who were referred for cardiovascular risk stratification using both EBCT and MS-CT, and found that management decisions might have been altered in as many as 16% of the patients. However, as MS-CT technology and standards mature, and with increasing use of 16 or more slice systems, the discrepancies between different CT systems can be expected to diminish.

A separate issue arises if MS-CT is used to track progression of disease (generally to monitor efficacy of lipid-lowering therapy) when interscan reproducibility becomes paramount. For EBCT, mean and median interscan variability is approximately 16%–19% and 4%–8%, respectively. MS-CT reproducibility seems to be less good, with mean variability as high as 36% (for volume scores) and 43% (for Agatston scores) in one study. Retrospective ECG gating and use of overlapping increments does seem to improve reproducibility significantly, however. Ohnesorge et al.[145] showed it was possible to reduce MS-CT mean and median variability to 12% and 9% for Agatston scoring, and 7.5% and 5% for volume scoring, respectively, at the cost of increased radiation burden.

1.10.2.3 MS-CT Radiation Dosimetry

The radiation dose delivered by MS-CT is highly dependent on the scanning protocol, and whether prospective or retrospective gating is used.[146] Unlike the situation with EBCT, it is possible to vary the X-ray tube current to optimize image quality, but at the expense of increased radiation burden. Most estimates of the effective dose delivered by MS-CT are higher than for EBCT (using coronary calcium protocols recommended by the CT vendor). In some cases, these differences are very substantial. Several manufacturers have therefore developed ECG- and body weight- or shape-controlled real-time dose modulation to minimize the effective delivered dose.[140] A recent study showed that ECG-controlled tube current modulation almost halved the radiation exposure when a retrospective gating protocol was used. These evolving developments contribute to the difficulty in establishing accurate dosimetry for MS-CT, but it is likely that, for similar-quality images, the effective radiation dose can be reduced to levels broadly comparable to EBCT by using the latest scanners.

1.10.2.4 Overall Comparison of MS-CT Versus EBCT

The greater versatility of MS-CT combined with its lower cost and increasing market penetration means that MS-CT coronary calcium imaging will become more widespread in the future. At the same time, the bulk of evidence supporting the use of coronary calcium imaging is currently derived from EBCT, and a number of issues will need resolution before MS-CT-derived calcium scores can be considered an adequate surrogate for EBCT-derived calcium scores. These include establishing the optimum image acquisition parameters, and ensuring MS-CT calcium scores are independent of the hardware used as well as being comparable to EBCT calcium scores. Consortia between the major industry players have recently been established to promote such developments.

A novel scoring system that estimates absolute calcium mass on the basis of calibration to a specific phantom has also recently been proposed. Calcium mass determined in this way is particularly suited for MS-CT because it is theoretically hardware independent.[67]

Until all of these issues are resolved, EBCT should be considered the imaging technology of choice for coronary calcium imaging.

1.11 CT Characterization of Soft Plaque Using CT-based Technologies

Our current understanding of vascular biology emphasizes the characteristics of the coronary vessel wall in determining cardiovascular events and outcome, rather than just the size of the vessel lumen.[5,44–46] The chief characteristics of interest are the total quantity of plaque present, as well as the physical properties of the plaque. Although CT-based technology together with coronary calcium scoring makes noninvasive assessment of total plaque burden possible for the first time, it is an incomplete picture because calcified plaque represents only a small proportion of the total plaque burden, and it remains unclear how well the calcified plaque burden reflects the quantity of vulnerable plaque (i.e., plaque prone to either rupture or erosion). The observation that lipid-lowering therapy can greatly reduce cardiovascular risk (by 10-fold or more)[60,120,121] without affecting the calcified plaque burden to any great extent suggests that the relationship between calcified plaque and vulnerable plaque can certainly be modified pharmacologically.

Recently, two CT-based approaches have been developed in an attempt to assess the "soft" plaque component of atherosclerosis in the coronary vessels. The first approach attempts to identify soft plaque by simultaneous injection of intravenous contrast agent (i.e., CT angiography).[147–149] However, the conceptual limitation of this approach is that intramural soft plaque again cannot be identified. An alternative, very different approach is to detect lipid-laden, vulnerable plaque through analysis of the full range of CT densities in the coronary arteries (rather than only those above an arbitrary chosen threshold such as 130 HU as applied by the Agatston scoring protocol). Potentially, this might identify lipid-laden plaque because the attenuation factor (in HU) for lipid is negative, whereas it is highly positive for calcium. In support of this premise, Teichholz and colleagues[150] have shown that coronary segments free of calcium in subjects with a high overall coronary calcium score have many more voxels with negative attenuation factors (i.e., suggestive of lipid-laden plaque) compared with subjects with low coronary calcium scores. This promising finding is currently under further investigation.

1.12 Summary

Coronary calcification is intimately associated with histopathologic, sonographic, and angiographic evidence of coronary atherosclerosis. EBCT and MS-CT can be used to detect and quantify the extent and severity of coronary calcification by means of coronary calcium scores. Such scores have been shown to closely reflect total coronary plaque burden and can be used to predict cardiovascular events and mortality. As a prognostic marker, the evidence suggests measures of coronary calcium could be superior to risk factor counting, and possibly, the Framingham risk function. Because coronary calcification is not synonymous with obstructive coronary artery disease, it can be usefully combined with MPI or stress ECHO as a functional test of myocardial ischemia. Coronary calcium imaging is unlikely to be cost-effective for coronary risk stratification when applied indiscriminately, but may have a role particularly when the pretest probability of coronary artery disease is intermediate.

2. MPI for Evaluation of Coronary Risk

2.1 MPI in Asymptomatic Low-risk Individuals

MPI is a well-validated technique for the detection of obstructive coronary artery disease.[151,152] It has been estimated that the overall sensitivity and specificity of MPI for obstructive coronary artery disease is approximately 85%–90%.[151] It can also be used for prognostication. A recent meta-analysis based on a pooled study population of >12 000 patients has documented a coronary event rate of only 0.6% per annum in the absence of perfusion defects.[153] Even patients with prior revascularization by coronary artery bypass and a normal MPI result have low cardiac event rates, similar to event rates seen in the general population.[154,155]

MPI is not generally used in asymptomatic individuals with a low pretest probability of coronary artery disease. In these cases, obstructive coronary artery disease is unlikely, the true positive rate is low, and the false-positive rate is high. Under these circumstances, it has not been shown to be superior to exercise ECG for either detection of obstructive coronary disease or prognostication. However, the situation may be different in diabetics.

2.2 MPI in Type II Diabetics

Type II diabetes is prevalent in the market economies, and is an emerging epidemic in many developing countries.[3,4,156,157] In 70%–80% of type II diabetics, the cause of death is cardiovascular. Frequently, however, coronary ischemia is silent in diabetics. The Framingham study suggests that one in four diabetics has ECG evidence of prior unrecognized myocardial infarction, half of whom remained asymptomatic.[158,159] Even in young asymptomatic type II diabetics with normal resting ECGs, Gokcel et al.[160] estimated that the prevalence of angiographically significant stenosis is at least 8%. Because retrospective data suggest that objective evidence of ischemia by MPI confers an adverse prognosis

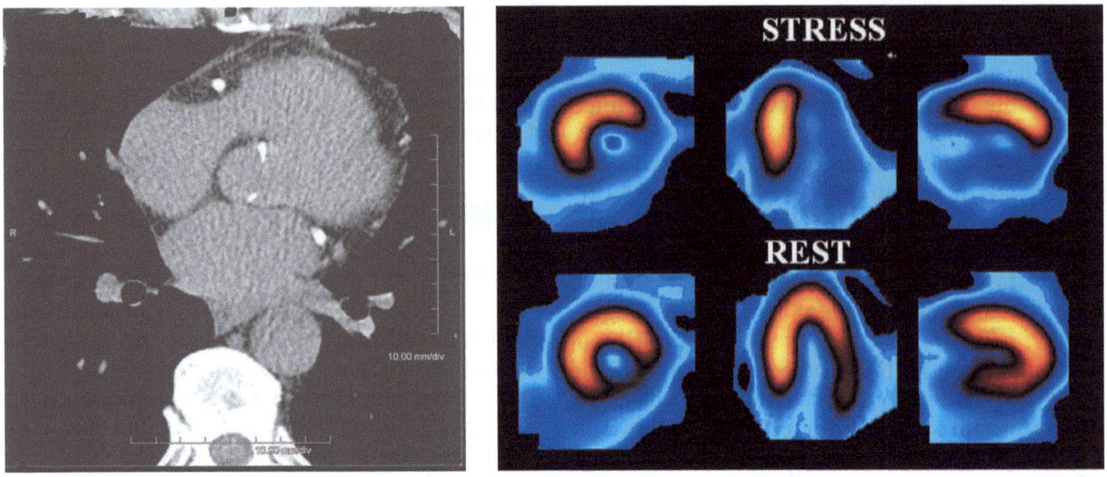

a b

Figure 7a.6. **a** EBCT scan from an asymptomatic 56-year-old diabetic with treated hyperlipidemia and hypertension. This shows significant coronary calcification in the right coronary and circumflex arteries. There is also some calcification of the aortic valve. Total Agatston score was 478 units. **b** Matching 99 m-technetium-sestamibi myocardial perfusion scan. This shows an inferolateral myocardial infarction, with extensive reversible ischemia in the same territory.

even in asymptomatic diabetics, there has been substantial interest in the use of MPI as a screening strategy for this important patient population.

Two studies have shown that the prevalence of perfusion abnormalities by stress MPI in asymptomatic diabetics is high.[161,162] In the Detection of Ischemia in Asymptomatic Patients with Diabetes (DIAD) study, the prevalence of any perfusion abnormality and severe perfusion abnormality in 522 asymptomatic type II diabetics with no history of coronary disease and a normal resting ECG was 22% and 6%, respectively.[162] In a similar patient population, De Lorenzo et al.[161] have reported a 26% and 9% prevalence of any perfusion abnormality and severe perfusion abnormality.

In contrast to these studies, Anand et al.[101] used a strategy of EBCT coronary calcium imaging to "preselect" asymptomatic type II diabetics with normal resting ECGs for subsequent MPI (Figure 7a.6; see color section). In total, 510 diabetics were enrolled. The study showed that approximately 25% of the diabetics had at least moderate coronary calcification (coronary calcium score ≥100 Agatston units). MPI restricted to this diabetic population boosted the prevalence of any perfusion abnormality and severe perfusion abnormality to 48% and 20%, respectively,[101] values that are both higher than those reported by the DIAD study (20% and 6%, respectively).

Benefit from identifying diabetics with asymptomatic perfusion abnormalities is not proven. However, clinical outcomes seem to be governed more by objective evidence of ischemia and its extent and severity than symptoms.[115,163–167] Therefore, particularly in patients with moderate-to-severe reversible perfusion defects, intensive medical therapy or even revascularization can be expected to be beneficial. Future trials will be needed to estimate the magnitude of any beneficial effect, and whether such a strategy is cost-effective. Follow-up of the 522 diabetics screened with MPI in the DIAD study[162] (see above) and comparison against a control cohort of 601 matched diabetics who were not screened by MPI will also help answer this question.

3. Carotid Artery Imaging by High-resolution Ultrasound

In 1986, through in vitro and in vivo experiments, Pignoli and colleagues[168] showed that the distance between the inner and outer echogenic lines of a high-resolution B mode ultrasound image of the common carotid artery and aorta corresponded to the distance between the adventitia-media interface and the intima-lumen interface. This measurement is of interest because of considerable experimental and clinical data showing it is involved in the atherogenesis and progression of atheroma formation and is correlated with cardiovascular and coronary risk.

3.1 Relationship with Cardiovascular Risk Factors

Carotid intima-media thickness (cIMT) has been correlated with all the major cardiovascular risk factors, including age, gender, smoking, hyperlipidemia, dyslipidemia, blood pressure, obesity, and diabetes.[169] It has also been associated with several novel cardiovascular risk factors, including homocysteine, high-sensitivity C-reactive protein (in women), and fibrinogen.[169] Furthermore, progression of cIMT thickening is predicted by many of the same risk factors, as well as several other risk factors such as factor V Leiden and platelet aggregability. Whether this is an important distinction (factors initiating atherosclerosis versus factors driving the progression of atherosclerosis) is still unclear.

3.2 Relationship with Measures of Atherosclerosis in Other Vascular Beds

As expected, cIMT has been associated with measures of atherosclerosis in other vascular beds including the coronary and peripheral circulations. For example, modest correlation has been observed between cIMT and measures of coronary atherosclerosis derived by angiography. Stronger correlations have been observed between cIMT and coronary calcification and coronary flow reserve.[170,171] An increase of 0.1 mm in common cIMT has also been linked with an age- and sex-adjusted reduction in ankle-brachial pressure index of 0.026, indicating a relationship with peripheral vascular disease also. Assessment of endothelial function of the coronary arteries rather the peripheral vessels may be a more attractive option, although still challenging when noninvasive imaging is used. Positron emission tomography, transthoracic Doppler echocardiography, which allows assessment of coronary flow velocity has been proposed and magnetic resonance (MR) methods have been applied to determine the cross-section, rather than the diameter of a vessel (see also Chapter 14).

3.3 Relationship with Clinical Outcomes

Four large prospective studies – the Atherosclerosis Risk in Communities (ARIC),[172,173] Rotterdam Study,[174] Kuopio Ischemic Heart Disease Study,[175] and Cardiovascular Health Study (CHS)[176] – have confirmed that increasing IMT is associated with clinical events, including coronary events. For example, the ARIC study[172,173] included 7289 women and 5552 men aged 45–64 years from four communities in the United States. It showed that the hazard ratio for incidents of cardiovascular events comparing mean IMT $\geq$1 mm to mean IMT <1 mm was 5.07 for women and 1.85 for men. Furthermore, although the strength of the association was attenuated by adjusting for the major cardiovascular risk factors, each one standard deviation increase in IMT still led to a 1.36 increase in relative risk of myocardial infarction or stroke ("*incremental value*"). Finally, as with coronary calcification, progression seems to be independently associated with increased cardiovascular risk. Hodis et al.[177] showed that each 0.03-mm per annum increase in cIMT was associated with a relative risk of any coronary event of 3.1.

3.4 Effect of Therapeutic Interventions on IMT

Many trials of drug intervention have substituted cIMT for hard cardiovascular end-points. This is because trials utilizing IMT and other surrogate end-points such as coronary calcium greatly improve the statistical power of a study,[90] reducing the cost and time necessary to complete the trial. However, such studies must be interpreted with caution because the assumption that IMT tracks cardiovascular mortality and morbidity accurately may not always be valid.[169] For example, although ramipril reduces stroke risk, there has been conflicting results on its effect on IMT.[178,179]

3.4.1 Lipid-lowering Trials

Six intervention studies using statins[180] (pravastatin,[178,181–184] lovastatin,[185] atorvastatin[186]) or colestipol-niacin[187,188] have also shown that aggressive lipid lowering is associated with a reduction in cIMT. In the REGRESS trial,[184] reduction of cIMT was also associated with a reduction in clinical end-points, suggesting that IMT is a valid surrogate for clinical end-points insofar as lipid-lowering therapy is concerned.

3.4.2 Intensive Insulin Therapy

Observational studies have shown that diabetics have higher cIMT than age and gender-matched nondiabetics.[189,190] In addition, the Insulin Resistance and Atherosclerosis Study (IRAS) showed that progression of common cIMT is associated with diabetes.[190] In this study, progression was most marked in undiagnosed diabetics, implying poor glycemic control may accelerate subclinical atherosclerosis. This conclusion is reinforced by the findings of the EDIC study,[191] which showed that intensive insulin therapy in type I diabetics slowed progression of cIMT, as compared with conventional therapy, implying that improved glycemic control was responsible. The thiazolidinediones[192] and more recently, metformin,[193] have also been shown to retard progression of common cIMT. These observations are interesting because it has been difficult to show that improved glycemic control has a beneficial impact on CHD.

3.4.3 Antihypertensive Therapy

Hypertension has been linked with increased IMT.[194–196] However, there is conflicting evidence of the effect of reduction of blood pressure on IMT. For example, PREVENT showed amlodipine treatment was associated with a reduction in IMT[197] but MacMahon et al.[178] did not find that ramipril treatment affected IMT.

3.4.4 Hormone Replacement Therapy

The relationship between hormone replacement therapy and cardiovascular disease has been a hotly debated topic in recent years.[198] As far as surrogate markers are concerned, there is agreement that IMT increases significantly after menopause. Furthermore, the Estrogen in the Prevention of Atherosclerosis (EPAT) trial, which enrolled healthy postmenopausal women without preexisting cardiovascular disease but low density lipoprotein (LDL) levels ≥130 mg/dL, suggests that treatment with unopposed 1-mg micronized 17β-estradiol daily can reduce progression of IMT compared with placebo (unless there was concomitant statin usage) in early atherosclerotic disease.[199]

3.5 cIMT Versus Carotid Plaque

Thickening of cIMT is not necessarily synonymous with carotid plaque formation. Pathologic studies show that increases in intimal thickness (fibromuscular hyperplasia) are associated with aging and that medial thickness (smooth muscle hypertrophy) is associated with hypertension, even in the absence of atherosclerotic plaque.[200] Using IMT as a surrogate marker for coronary artery plaque is also unsatisfactory because (1) it assumes atherosclerosis leads to a uniform increase in arterial wall thickness, whereas it is actually a focal phenomenon, and (2) it is most sensitive to changes in the media, whereas atherosclerosis is primarily confined to the intima. Furthermore, there is evidence that whereas increased common cIMT is strongly associated with risk factors for stroke, carotid plaque is better associated with prevalent coronary artery disease.[201–203] Carotid plaque area and volume are therefore now also being investigated as alternative surrogates of coronary artery disease.[201]

3.5.1 Carotid Plaque Area

Operationally, Spence[201] has defined plaque as local thickening of IMT exceeding 1 mm. Plaque area is quantified by perimetry of a cross-sectional image of the relevant magnified longitudinal view of the common, internal, and external carotid artery. This section is chosen to maximize the measured cross-sectional plaque area.

3.5.2 Carotid Plaque Volume

If three-dimensional ultrasound is available, a similar parameter can be derived from 1- to

4-mm cross-sectional slices. Plaque area in each cross-sectional slice is integrated to calculate plaque volume.

3.5.3 Assessment of Carotid Plaque Character

In addition to plaque area or volume, there is evidence that carotid plaque character as assessed by ultrasound also affects the likelihood of neurovascular symptoms.

3.5.3.1 Plaque Echodensity

Several cross-sectional studies suggest that hypoechoic plaque is more likely to be associated with symptoms.[204–206] In one study of 72 symptomatic patients and 49 asymptomatic patients,[205] type I plaque (predominantly echolucent) was found in 90% of patients with symptoms, whereas it was found in only 10% of those without symptoms. Conversely, type 4 plaque (predominantly echogenic) was found in 5% of those with symptoms, and 95% of those without symptoms. Longitudinal studies also support this conclusion.[206–208] For example, in the Cardiovascular Health Study (CHS), the age- and sex-adjusted odds ratio for incident stroke in subjects with hypoechoic carotid plaque was 2.53 (95% CI: 1.42, 4.53).[206] There is also direct evidence that hypoechoic plaque is more likely to embolize. When Tegos et al.[209] studied 59 patients with known carotid plaque using transcranial Doppler of the middle cerebral artery, they noted emboli were much more frequent when plaque was hypoechoic. Furthermore, patients with hypoechoic plaque were more likely to have discrete subcortical and cortical lesions on brain CT, consistent with embolic stroke. Clinicopathologic studies show that hypoechoic plaque contain lipid or blood (intraplaque hemorrhage), whereas hyperechoic plaque have a large collagen content and are fibrous.[210] These studies therefore also support the idea that hypoechoic lesions are unstable and prone to embolization.

3.5.3.2 Plaque Surface Characteristics

A number of pathologic,[211–213] angiographic,[214–217] and sonographic[218,219] studies suggest that ulcerated carotid plaque is more likely to embolize, particularly when it is deep or complicated. Other (generally older) studies have failed to document such a relationship.[204,220–222]

3.5.3.3 Classifying Plaque Morphology

Plaque character is currently classified according to whether it is homogenous or heterogenous, plaque echodensity, and plaque surface characteristics.[210] However, several classification systems are in current use.[223]

3.5.3.3.1 Echodensity. Three-,[208] four-,[224] and five-category[205] classifications are in use. For example, in the Gray-Weale classification, four plaque types are recognized:

- Type 1: Predominantly echolucent with a thin echo genic cap
- Type 2: Intermediate echolucent lesions with small areas of echogenicity
- Type 3: Intermediate echogenic lesions with small areas of echolucency (<25%)
- Type 4: Uniformly echogenic lesions (equivalent to homogenous)

A fifth type has been added in one modification of this classification to include plaque that cannot be classified because of acoustic shadowing artifact.[205] This kind of plaque is frequently calcified.

Plaque echodensity is usually assessed visually. However, this is affected by machine settings, and is observer-dependent, and objective, quantitative methods of classification using digital image processing have also been proposed.[204,210,223]

3.5.3.3.2 Surface Characteristics. Again, there are no consistent standards for classifying plaque surface characteristics. At the simplest level, plaque can be classified as regular (when blood lesion interface is smooth and unbroken), or irregular (when there is a break in the echoreflective surface of the lesion).[225] Color flow Doppler can be used to refine this assessment. Sitzer and colleagues[226] have defined carotid plaque as ulcerated if there is a plaque niche filled with reversed flow on color Doppler on longitudinal views, found at the same location on transverse views, without evidence of aliasing phenomena.

3.6 Measuring IMT – Technical Considerations

Currently, there are no standardized protocols for measuring IMT. Important technical considerations include[227]:

1. Number and location of arterial segments that are imaged. IMT can be determined in the proximal internal carotid artery, carotid bulb, mid-common carotid artery, or even the femoral artery.
2. Whether the near or far arterial wall will be used for measurements. (The far wall of the mid-common carotid artery is most often used, because it can be easily and consistently imaged.)
3. Number of imaging angles used.
4. How images are captured (videotape or digitally; loops or R wave-gated still frames).
5. Whether mean or maximal thickness will be measured.
6. What measurement techniques will be used (manual or semiautomated; if semiautomated techniques are used, what software will be used).
7. If plaque character will also be recorded; if so, what classification will be used.
8. Hardware that will be used (including the ultrasound probes).

The usual reasons for inaccurate IMT measurements have been reviewed by Mitchell et al.[227] These include (1) poor image quality, (2) drifting, (3) suboptimal machine settings, and (4) difficult patient anatomy. Nevertheless, with careful attention to detail, cIMT measurements have been shown to be reproducible and reliable.[227,228] For example, in the Tromso study[228] (which used highly trained sonographers and a semiautomated software package to measure IMT), the mean between-observer difference in IMT of the far wall of the mid-common carotid artery was 0.08 mm. The corresponding within-observer difference was 0.06 mm.

It is important to note that published studies are unlikely to reflect "real-world" practice. In the Tromso study, three highly trained sonographers conducted all the studies (including a neurologist with >10 years' experience in carotid imaging). Because the difference between a normal and abnormal study is only hundredths of a millimeter, issues pertaining to training and quality control must be addressed before widespread measurement of IMT can be advocated.

3.7 Contrast-enhanced Carotid Imaging

The near wall of the carotid artery is often difficult to discern clearly. Consequently, ultrasound underestimates near-wall cIMT by as much as 20% compared with histologic sections.[229] Although not used routinely, it has recently been shown that intravenous microbubble echocontrast agents can be used to improve definition of both the near and far wall IMT.[230,231] Any atherosclerotic plaque present can also be defined more precisely. This includes plaque size, anatomic location, and morphology.

It was also shown recently that echocontrast allows real-time visualization of the vasa vasorum of the carotid artery, and associated neovascularization of any carotid plaque. This finding may eventually have clinical ramifications because occlusive atherosclerotic plaque has been correlated with the presence and degree of neovascularization within the vasa vasorum and plaque,[232–234] and may be an important determinant of plaque stability. This is an area of ongoing research.

3.8 Utilizing Carotid Ultrasonography for Cardiovascular Risk Stratification in Clinical Practice

In 2000, the American Heart Association (AHA) Prevention Conference V writing group concluded that, "in asymptomatic persons >45 years old, carefully performed carotid ultrasound examination with IMT measurement can add incremental information to traditional risk factor assessment," based on the evidence outlined above.[235] The patients most likely to benefit from carotid ultrasonography are those at intermediate risk of cardiovascular disease, when it might aid clinical decision-making. For example, Bard et al.[236] showed that carotid plaque area and cIMT measurements reclassified at least 63% of patients with intermediate Framingham risk scores into either a higher or lower risk category. As with coronary calcium imaging, however, there is as yet no proof that this will lead to improved clinical outcomes.

Currently, there are no established treatment guidelines based on cIMT measurements. In the absence of guidance, we use the following for clinical decision-making:

1. Asymptomatic patients with extreme IMT (≥1 mm) or evidence of plaque should be considered high risk, and any risk factors need to be identified and treated aggressively. The incremental value provided by assessment of plaque type (echogenic, echolucent, mixed, calcified) is not clear, and should probably not affect clinical decision-making.

2. It may be helpful to transform IMT into an age- and sex-adjusted percentile, to obtain a "vascular age"[237,238] – analogous to coronary calcium imaging-derived "heart age"[75,79] described earlier. Patients with a high vascular age should probably also be considered to be at increased risk.

3. The role of any adjunctive testing or imaging (such as exercise stress testing or MPI) is unclear, but should be considered if any suggestive symptoms develop.

It has also been suggested that cIMT may be useful in assessing efficacy of therapeutic interventions. There are several difficulties with this approach. First, as outlined earlier, there are limited and sometimes conflicting data on whether IMT is an accurate reflection of therapeutic efficacy. Second, the difference in change of IMT between adequately and inadequately treated patients may be very small. For example, in the EDIC study,[191] the change in IMT in diabetics receiving intensive insulin therapy versus those receiving conventional therapy was 0.032 and 0.046 mm over the 6.5-year period of the study. For lipid-lowering trials, cIMT changes are typically of the order of 0.01 mm/year, which is substantially lower than cIMT measurement error. Serial cIMT measures are therefore unlikely to be helpful over the time period during which clinicians typically titrate therapy.

4. Other Imaging Technologies and the Future

Accumulating evidence suggests that atherogenesis can be viewed as the vascular response to chronic inflammation.[239–242] Factors initiating atherogenesis have been shown to lead to endothelial dysfunction and subsequent expression of inflammatory cytokines, chemokines, and adhesion molecules.[240] This leads to recruitment of monocyte-derived macrophage T cells and enhanced endothelial permeability, lipid insudation of the vessel wall, and formation of the characteristic atherosclerotic lesion. However, plaque character and propensity for either rupture or erosion varies both between individuals and even within the same individual, as described previously. Imaging technologies that can explore various aspects of the processes underlying plaque growth and identify vulnerable plaque have been developed in animal models and, more recently, in humans. These include MR imaging (MRI), LDL imaging, apoptosis imaging, and metabolic plaque imaging,[243] together with CT-based methods of soft plaque characterization (see earlier). However, such imaging is challenging because of the small size of coronary plaque relative to the spatial and temporal resolution that can be achieved using most techniques.[243] Plaque dimensions are typically 1–2 cm, but are very thin so that plaque volume is often less than 0.1 mL.

4.1 Cardiovascular MRI

Cardiovascular MRI is a rapidly evolving technology that is able to noninvasively evaluate the location and volume of atherosclerotic plaque.[244–248] Currently, the limited spatial and temporal resolution of MR limits its clinical application to large vessels such as the carotid and femoral arteries. In these vessels, using MR, it has been shown that statin therapy is able to induce regression of plaque in asymptomatic hypercholesterolemic patients.[249]

However, the ultimate goal is to use MR in clinical settings to define coronary artery lumen size *and* coronary artery wall characteristics. Because different components of plaque have different biophysical and biochemical properties, plaque can be characterized by means of the signal intensity in T1-weighted, T2-weighted, and proton-density weighted sequences. The morphologic appearance of plaque can also be assessed. Fayad and Fuster[250] showed that coronary plaque characterization is possible in humans, using high-resolution black-blood MRI (this nulls the signal from blood in order to visualize the coronary wall). Novel MR contrast agents are also in development to further aid plaque characterization. These include fibrin-targeted paramagnetic lipid-encapsulated perfluorocarbon nanoparticles, which might be able to detect microthrombus formation on vulnerable plaque,[251] and superparamagnetic iron oxides particles. Ruehm et al.[252] have shown that the latter are phagocytosed by macrophages in hypercholesterolemic rabbits and localize to aortic atherosclerotic plaque; plaque may then be detected because superparamagnetic iron oxides induce a susceptibility effect that leads to low signal intensity on T2- and gradient echo T2-weighted images.

Studies to identify the MR features of plaque linked to adverse outcome ("*vulnerable* plaque") are now needed, together with improvements in MR technology in order to bring this technique into the clinical arena.

4.2 Molecular Nuclear Techniques

Nuclear techniques are versatile because they use different radiolabeled molecules to localize and characterize plaque.[243] For example, radiolabeled LDL,[141,253] oxidized LDL,[254] or high density lipoprotein[254] can be used to define the lipid component of plaque, 18-fluorodeoxyglucose can be used to image metabolic activity within plaque,[255] and annexin V imaging[256] can be used to image apoptosis within plaque.

However, significant technical difficulties must be overcome before these techniques can be applied in the clinical setting.[243] Single photon imaging cameras have a spatial resolution of approximately 4mm at the surface of the collimator, but this decreases to 8–10mm at the center of the object with planar imaging and only 10–12mm with single photon emission computer tomography. Although detection of lesions remains achievable, because the lesion size is less than the imaging spatial resolution, very high lesion-to-background ratios are required. In the future, development of highly specific labeling agents, and, possibly, gamma camera technology, may bring such techniques closer to the clinical arena.

5. Summary

Cardiovascular risk estimates can be improved by several noninvasive imaging techniques, collectively called atherosclerosis imaging. Clinically useful techniques currently include coronary calcium imaging and carotid ultrasound. Both these tests are most valuable in intermediate-risk patients, in whom a significant proportion will be reassigned into either a higher- or lower-risk category. However, before widespread adoption of any of these techniques takes place, studies to establish treatment protocols based on atherosclerosis imaging tests and to determine the cost-effectiveness of atherosclerosis imaging tests are needed.

References

1. Braunwald E. Shattuck lecture – cardiovascular medicine at the turn of the millennium: triumphs, concerns, and opportunities. N Engl J Med 1997;337(19): 1360–1369.
2. Arias E, Anderson RN, Kung HC, Murphy SL, Kochanek KD. Deaths: final data for 2001. Natl Vital Stat Rep 2003;52(3):1–115.
3. Reddy KS, Yusuf S. Emerging epidemic of cardiovascular disease in developing countries. Circulation 1998;97(6):596–601.
4. Yusuf S, Reddy S, Ounpuu S, Anand S. Global burden of cardiovascular diseases. Part I. General considerations, the epidemiologic transition, risk factors, and impact of urbanization. Circulation 2001;104(22): 2746–2753.
5. Corti R, Fuster V. New understanding, diagnosis, and prognosis of atherothrombosis and the role of imaging. Am J Cardiol 2003;91(3A):17A–26A.
6. Worthley SG, Helft G, Zaman AG, Fuster V, Badimon JJ. Atherosclerosis and the vulnerable plaque – pathogenesis. Part I. Aust N Z J Med 2000;30(5):600–607.
7. Topol EJ, Nissen SE. Our preoccupation with coronary luminology. The dissociation between clinical and angiographic findings in ischemic heart disease. Circulation 1995;92(8):2333–2342.
8. Nissen S. Coronary angiography and intravascular ultrasound. Am J Cardiol 2001;87(4A):15A–20A.
9. Glagov S, Weisenberg E, Zarins CK, Stankunavicius R, Kolettis GJ. Compensatory enlargement of human atherosclerotic coronary arteries. N Engl J Med 1987; 316(22):1371–1375.
10. Giroud D, Li JM, Urban P, Meier B, Rutishauer W. Relation of the site of acute myocardial infarction to the most severe coronary arterial stenosis at prior angiography. Am J Cardiol 1992;69(8):729–732.
11. Moise A, Lesperance J, Theroux P, Taeymans Y, Goulet C, Bourassa MG. Clinical and angiographic predictors of new total coronary occlusion in coronary artery disease: analysis of 313 nonoperated patients. Am J Cardiol 1984;54(10):1176–1181.
12. Thaulow E, Erikssen J, Sandvik L, Erikssen G, Jorgensen L, Cohn PF. Initial clinical presentation of cardiac disease in asymptomatic men with silent myocardial ischemia and angiographically documented coronary artery disease (the Oslo Ischemia Study). Am J Cardiol 1993;72(9):629–633.
13. Hecht HS, Superko HR. Electron beam tomography and National Cholesterol Education Program guidelines in asymptomatic women. J Am Coll Cardiol 2001; 37(6):1506–1511.

14. Grover SA, Coupal L, Hu XP. Identifying adults at increased risk of coronary disease. How well do the current cholesterol guidelines work? JAMA 1995; 274(10):801–806.
15. Neaton JD, Wentworth D. Serum cholesterol, blood pressure, cigarette smoking, and death from CHD. Overall findings and differences by age for 316,099 white men. Multiple Risk Factor Intervention Trial Research Group. Arch Intern Med 1992;152(1):56–64.
16. Wilson PW, D'Agostino RB, Levy D, Belanger AM, Silbershatz H, Kannel WB. Prediction of coronary heart disease using risk factor categories. Circulation 1998;97(18):1837–1847.
17. Kannel WB, Neaton JD, Wentworth D, et al. Overall and coronary heart disease mortality rates in relation to major risk factors in 325,348 men screened for the MRFIT. Multiple Risk Factor Intervention Trial. Am Heart J 1986;112(4):825–836.
18. Executive Summary of The Third Report of The National Cholesterol Education Program (NCEP) Expert Panel on Detection, Evaluation, And Treatment of High Blood Cholesterol in Adults (Adult Treatment Panel III). JAMA 2001;285(19):2486–2497.
19. Heller RF, Chinn S, Pedoe HD, Rose G. How well can we predict coronary heart disease? Findings in the United Kingdom Heart Disease Prevention Project. Br Med J (Clin Res Ed) 1984;288(6428):1409–1411.
20. Budoff MJ. Atherosclerosis imaging and calcified plaque: coronary artery disease risk assessment. Prog Cardiovasc Dis 2003;46(2):135–148.
21. Shaw LJ, Raggi P, Berman DS, Callister TQ. Cost effectiveness of screening for cardiovascular disease with measures of coronary calcium. Prog Cardiovasc Dis 2003;46(2):171–184.
22. Speer MY, Giachelli CM. Regulation of cardiovascular calcification. Cardiovasc Pathol 2004;13(2):63–70.
23. Parry C. Inquiry into the symptoms and causes of syncopa anginosa, commonly called angina pectoris. 1799.
24. Redberg RF, Vogel RA, Criqui MH, Herrington DM, Lima JA, Roman MJ. 34th Bethesda Conference: task force #3 – what is the spectrum of current and emerging techniques for the noninvasive measurement of atherosclerosis? J Am Coll Cardiol 2003;41(11):1886–1898.
25. Anand DV, Lahiri A, Lipkin D. EBCT coronary calcium imaging for the early detection of coronary artery disease in asymptomatic individuals. Br J Cardiol 2003;10:273–280.
26. Mark DB, Shaw LJ, Lauer MS, O'Malley PG, Heidenreich P. 34th Bethesda Conference: task force #5 – is atherosclerosis imaging cost effective? J Am Coll Cardiol 2003;41(11):1906–1917.
27. Wexler L, Brundage B, Crouse J, et al. Coronary artery calcification: pathophysiology, epidemiology, imaging methods, and clinical implications. A statement for health professionals from the American Heart Association Writing Group. Circulation 1996;94(5):1175–1192.
28. Stary HC. The development of calcium deposits in atherosclerotic lesions and their persistence after lipid regression. Am J Cardiol 2001;88(2A):16E–19E.
29. Stary HC, Chandler AB, Dinsmore RE, et al. A definition of advanced types of atherosclerotic lesions and a histological classification of atherosclerosis. A report from the Committee on Vascular Lesions of the Council on Arteriosclerosis, American Heart Association. Circulation 1995;92(5):1355–1374.
30. Mautner GC, Mautner SL, Froehlich J, et al. Coronary artery calcification: assessment with electron beam CT and histomorphometric correlation. Radiology 1994; 192(3):619–623.
31. Baumgart D, Schmermund A, Goerge G, et al. Comparison of electron beam computed tomography with intracoronary ultrasound and coronary angiography for detection of coronary atherosclerosis. J Am Coll Cardiol 1997;30(1):57–64.
32. Schmermund A, Baumgart D, Gorge G, et al. Coronary artery calcium in acute coronary syndromes: a comparative study of electron-beam computed tomography, coronary angiography, and intracoronary ultrasound in survivors of acute myocardial infarction and unstable angina. Circulation 1997;96(5): 1461–1469.
33. Simons DB, Schwartz RS, Edwards WD, Sheedy PF, Breen JF, Rumberger JA. Noninvasive definition of anatomic coronary artery disease by ultrafast computed tomographic scanning: a quantitative pathologic comparison study. J Am Coll Cardiol 1992;20(5):1118–1126.
34. Rumberger JA, Schwartz RS, Simons DB, Sheedy PF 3rd, Edwards WD, Fitzpatrick LA. Relation of coronary calcium determined by electron beam computed tomography and lumen narrowing determined by autopsy. Am J Cardiol 1994;73(16):1169–1173.
35. Kajinami K, Seki H, Takekoshi N, Mabuchi H. Coronary calcification and coronary atherosclerosis: site by site comparative morphologic study of electron beam computed tomography and coronary angiography. J Am Coll Cardiol 1997;29(7):1549–1556.
36. Mann GV, McNamara JJ, Macomber PB, Wroblewski R. Coronary artery disease in Vietnam casualties. JAMA 1971;217(4):478–479.
37. Strong JP, Malcom GT, Oalmann MC, Wissler RW. The PDAY Study: natural history, risk factors, and pathobiology. Pathobiological Determinants of Atherosclerosis in Youth. Ann NY Acad Sci 1997;811:226–235; discussion 235–237.
38. Wissler RW. New insights into the pathogenesis of atherosclerosis as revealed by PDAY. Pathobiological Determinants of Atherosclerosis in Youth. Atherosclerosis 1994;108(suppl):S3–20.
39. Stary HC. The sequence of cell and matrix changes in atherosclerotic lesions of coronary arteries in the first forty years of life. Eur Heart J 1990;11(suppl E): 3–19.
40. Stary HC. Atlas of Atherosclerosis Progression and Regression. London: Parthenon Publishing; 1999.
41. Strong JP. Landmark perspective: coronary atherosclerosis in soldiers. A clue to the natural history of atherosclerosis in the young. JAMA 1986;256(20):2863–2866.
42. Detrano RC, Doherty TM, Davies MJ, Stary HC. Predicting coronary events with coronary calcium: pathophysiologic and clinical problems. Curr Probl Cardiol 2000;25(6):374–402.
43. Tobis JM, Mallery J, Mahon D, et al. Intravascular ultrasound imaging of human coronary arteries in vivo. Analysis of tissue characterizations with comparison to in vitro histological specimens. Circulation 1991; 83(3):913–926.

44. Falk E, Shah PK, Fuster V. Coronary plaque disruption. Circulation 1995;92(3):657–671.
45. Maseri A, Fuster V. Is there a vulnerable plaque? Circulation 2003;107(16):2068–2071.
46. Schaar JA, Muller JE, Falk E, et al. Terminology for high-risk and vulnerable coronary artery plaques. Report of a meeting on the vulnerable plaque, June 17 and 18, 2003, Santorini, Greece. Eur Heart J 2004; 25(12):1077–1082.
47. Bostrom K. Insights into the mechanism of vascular calcification. Am J Cardiol 2001;88(2A):20E–22E.
48. Bostrom K, Demer LL. Regulatory mechanisms in vascular calcification. Crit Rev Eukaryot Gene Expr 2000;10(2):151–158.
49. Galvin KM, Donovan MJ, Lynch CA, et al. A role for smad6 in development and homeostasis of the cardiovascular system. Nat Genet 2000;24(2):171–174.
50. Luo G, Ducy P, McKee MD, et al. Spontaneous calcification of arteries and cartilage in mice lacking matrix GLA protein. Nature 1997;386(6620):78–81.
51. Bucay N, Sarosi I, Dunstan CR, et al. Osteoprotegerin-deficient mice develop early onset osteoporosis and arterial calcification. Genes Dev 1998;12(9):1260–1268.
52. Chase AJ, Bond M, Crook MF, Newby AC. Role of nuclear factor-kappa B activation in metalloproteinase-1, -3, and -9 secretion by human macrophages in vitro and rabbit foam cells produced in vivo. Arterioscler Thromb Vasc Biol 2002;22(5):765–771.
53. Molloy KJ, Thompson MM, Jones JL, et al. Unstable carotid plaques exhibit raised matrix metalloproteinase-8 activity. Circulation 2004;110(3):337–343.
54. Shah PK. Mechanisms of plaque vulnerability and rupture. J Am Coll Cardiol 2003;41(4 suppl S):15S–22S.
55. Glasser SP. On arterial physiology, pathophysiology of vascular compliance, and cardiovascular disease. Heart Dis 2000;2(5):375–379.
56. Atkinson J. Arterial calcification. Mechanisms, consequences and animal models. Pathol Biol (Paris) 1999;47(7):677–684.
57. Haydar AA, Covic A, Colhoun H, Rubens M, Goldsmith DJ. Coronary artery calcification and aortic pulse wave velocity in chronic kidney disease patients. Kidney Int 2004;65(5):1790–1794.
58. Hunt ME, O'Malley PG, Vernalis MN, Feuerstein IM, Taylor AJ. C-reactive protein is not associated with the presence or extent of calcified subclinical atherosclerosis. Am Heart J 2001;141(2):206–210.
59. Redberg RF, Rifai N, Gee L, Ridker PM. Lack of association of C-reactive protein and coronary calcium by electron beam computed tomography in postmenopausal women: implications for coronary artery disease screening. J Am Coll Cardiol 2000;36(1):39–43.
60. Achenbach S, Ropers D, Pohle K, et al. Influence of lipid-lowering therapy on the progression of coronary artery calcification: a prospective evaluation. Circulation 2002;106(9):1077–1082.
61. Callister TQ, Raggi P, Cooil B, Lippolis NJ, Russo DJ. Effect of HMG-CoA reductase inhibitors on coronary artery disease as assessed by electron-beam computed tomography. N Engl J Med 1998;339(27):1972–1978.
62. Callister TQ, Raggi P. Electron beam tomography for early detection of coronary heart disease. In: Braunwald E, ed. Harrison's Advances in Cardiology. Boston: McGraw-Hill; 2003:226–233.
63. Agatston A. electron beam tomography in the prevention of coronary artery disease. In: Foody JM, ed. Preventive Cardiology: Strategies for the Prevention and Treatment of Coronary Artery Disease. Totowa, NJ: Humana Press; 2001:303–324.
64. Hunold P, Vogt FM, Schmermund A, et al. Radiation exposure during cardiac CT: effective doses at multi-detector row CT and electron-beam CT. Radiology 2003;226(1):145–152.
65. Jakobs TF, Wintersperger BJ, Herzog P, et al. Ultra-low-dose coronary artery calcium screening using multi-slice CT with retrospective ECG gating. Eur Radiol 2003;13(8):1923–1930.
66. Agatston AS, Janowitz WR, Hildner FJ, Zusmer NR, Viamonte M Jr, Detrano R. Quantification of coronary artery calcium using ultrafast computed tomography. J Am Coll Cardiol 1990;15(4):827–832.
67. Rumberger JA, Kaufman L. A rosetta stone for coronary calcium risk stratification: Agatston, volume, and mass scores in 11,490 individuals. AJR Am J Roentgenol 2003;181(3):743–748.
68. Callister TQ, Cooil B, Raya SP, Lippolis NJ, Russo DJ, Raggi P. Coronary artery disease: improved reproducibility of calcium scoring with an electron-beam CT volumetric method. Radiology 1998;208(3): 807–814.
69. Kaufmann RB, Sheedy PF 2nd, Breen JF, et al. Detection of heart calcification with electron beam CT: interobserver and intraobserver reliability for scoring quantification. Radiology 1994;190(2):347–352.
70. Bielak LF, Kaufmann RB, Moll PP, McCollough CH, Schwartz RS, Sheedy PF 2nd. Small lesions in the heart identified at electron beam CT: calcification or noise? Radiology 1994;192(3):631–636.
71. McCollough CH, Kaufmann RB, Cameron BM, Katz DJ, Sheedy PF 2nd, Peyser PA. Electron-beam CT: use of a calibration phantom to reduce variability in calcium quantitation. Radiology 1995;196(1):159–165.
72. Nasir K, Budoff MJ, Post WS, et al. Electron beam CT versus helical CT scans for assessing coronary calcification: current utility and future directions. Am Heart J 2003;146(6):969–977.
73. Callister T, Raggi P. Electron-beam computed tomography: a Bayesian approach to risk assessment. Am J Cardiol 2001;88(2A):39E–41E.
74. Raggi P, Callister TQ, Cooil B. Calcium scoring of the coronary artery by electron beam CT: how to apply an individual attenuation threshold. AJR Am J Roentgenol 2002;178(2):497–502.
75. Anand DV, Lipkin D, Lahiri A. Finding the age of the patient's heart. BMJ 2003;326(7398):1045–1046.
76. Shaw LJ, Raggi P, Schisterman E, Berman DS, Callister TQ. Prognostic value of cardiac risk factors and coronary artery calcium screening for all-cause mortality. Radiology 2003;228(3):826–833.
77. Wong ND, Budoff MJ, Pio J, Detrano RC. Coronary calcium and cardiovascular event risk: evaluation by age- and sex-specific quartiles. Am Heart J 2002; 143(3):456–459.
78. Raggi P, Callister TQ, Cooil B, et al. Identification of patients at increased risk of first unheralded acute myocardial infarction by electron-beam computed tomography. Circulation 2000;101(8):850–855.
79. Callister T. Heart age. EBT Symposium. New Orleans; 2002.

80. Raggi P, Shaw LJ, Berman DS, Callister TQ. Prognostic value of coronary artery calcium screening in subjects with and without diabetes. J Am Coll Cardiol 2004; 43(9):1663–1669.
81. Kondos GT, Hoff JA, Sevrukov A, et al. Electron-beam tomography coronary artery calcium and cardiac events: a 37-month follow-up of 5635 initially asymptomatic low- to intermediate-risk adults. Circulation 2003;107(20):2571–2576.
82. Arad Y, Spadaro LA, Goodman K, et al. Predictive value of electron beam computed tomography of the coronary arteries: 19-month follow-up of 1173 asymptomatic subjects. Circulation 1996;93(11):1951–1953.
83. Detrano RC, Wong ND, Doherty TM, et al. Coronary calcium does not accurately predict near-term future coronary events in high-risk adults. Circulation 1999; 99(20):2633–2638.
84. Janowitz WR. Coronary calcium does not accurately predict near-term future coronary events in high-risk adults. Circulation 2000;102(2):E20–21.
85. Pitt B, Rubenfire M. Risk stratification for the detection of preclinical coronary artery disease. Circulation 1999;99(20):2610–2612.
86. O'Malley PG, Taylor AJ, Jackson JL, Doherty TM, Detrano RC. Prognostic value of coronary electron-beam computed tomography for coronary heart disease events in asymptomatic populations. Am J Cardiol 2000;85(8):945–948.
87. Grundy SM. Coronary calcium as a risk factor: role in global risk assessment. J Am Coll Cardiol 2001; 37(6):1512–1515.
88. O'Malley PG, Taylor AJ, Gibbons RV, et al. Rationale and design of the Prospective Army Coronary Calcium (PACC) Study: utility of electron beam computed tomography as a screening test for coronary artery disease and as an intervention for risk factor modification among young, asymptomatic, active-duty United States army personnel. Am Heart J 1999; 137(5):932–941.
89. Schmermund A, Mohlenkamp S, Stang A, et al. Assessment of clinically silent atherosclerotic disease and established and novel risk factors for predicting myocardial infarction and cardiac death in healthy middle-aged subjects: rationale and design of the Heinz Nixdorf RECALL Study. Risk factors, evaluation of coronary calcium and lifestyle. Am Heart J 2002;144(2):212–218.
90. Bild DE, Bluemke DA, Burke GL, et al. Multi-ethnic study of atherosclerosis: objectives and design. Am J Epidemiol 2002;156(9):871–881.
91. Anand DV, Lim E, Raval U, Lipkin D, Lahiri A. Prevalence of silent myocardial ischemia in asymptomatic individuals with subclinical atherosclerosis detected by electron beam tomography. J Nucl Cardiol 2004; 11(4):450–457.
92. Berman DS. Complementary roles of coronary calcium scanning and myocardial perfusion SPECT. J Nucl Cardiol 2004;11(4):379–381.
93. Berman DS, Schisterman EF, Miranda R, et al. Nuclear cardiology and electron-beam computed tomography: competitive or complementary? Am J Cardiol 2001; 88(2A):51E–55E.
94. Berman DS, Wong ND, Gransar H, et al. Relationship between stress-induced myocardial ischemia and atherosclerosis measured by coronary calcium tomography. J Am Coll Cardiol 2004;44(4):923–930.
95. He ZX, Hedrick TD, Pratt CM, et al. Severity of coronary artery calcification by electron beam computed tomography predicts silent myocardial ischemia. Circulation 2000;101(3):244–251.
96. Nallamothu BK, Saint S, Bielak LF, et al. Electron-beam computed tomography in the diagnosis of coronary artery disease: a meta-analysis. Arch Intern Med 2001; 161(6):833–838.
97. Budoff MJ, Georgiou D, Brody A, et al. Ultrafast computed tomography as a diagnostic modality in the detection of coronary artery disease: a multicenter study. Circulation 1996;93(5):898–904.
98. Thompson R, McGhie IA, Moser K, O'Keefe JH Jr, Bateman TM. Coronary calcium scoring in selected patients after normal or equivocal myocardial perfusion imaging studies, clinical usefulness. J Nucl Cardiol 2004;11(4):S35.
99. Moser KW, O'Keefe JH Jr., Bateman TM, McGhie IA. Coronary calcium screening in asymptomatic patients as a guide to risk factor modification and stress myocardial perfusion imaging. J Nucl Cardiol 2003;10(6): 590–598.
100. Lim E, Anand DV, Raval U, Lipkin D, Lahiri A. Relationship between coronary calcium and 99 m-Tc sestamibi SPECT myocardial perfusion abnormalities. Heart 2004;(suppl 2):A56.
101. Anand DV, Hopkins D, Sharp P, et al. Prevalence of silent myocardial ischemia in asymptomatic type 2 diabetic patients with subclinical atherosclerosis. JACC 2004;43(5 suppl A):816–6-349A.
102. Ketteler M, Bongartz P, Westenfeld R, et al. Association of low fetuin-A (AHSG) concentrations in serum with cardiovascular mortality in patients on dialysis: a cross-sectional study. Lancet 2003;361(9360):827–833.
103. Ketteler M, Vermeer C, Wanner C, Westenfeld R, Jahnen-Dechent W, Floege J. Novel insights into uremic vascular calcification: role of matrix Gla protein and alpha-2-Heremans Schmid glycoprotein/ fetuin. Blood Purif 2002;20(5):473–476.
104. Ketteler M, Wanner C, Metzger T, et al. Deficiencies of calcium-regulatory proteins in dialysis patients: a novel concept of cardiovascular calcification in uremia. Kidney Int Suppl 2003(84):S84–87.
105. Greenland P. Improving risk of coronary heart disease: can a picture make the difference? JAMA 2003;289(17): 2270–2272.
106. Greenland P, Gaziano JM. Clinical practice. Selecting asymptomatic patients for coronary computed tomography or electrocardiographic exercise testing. N Engl J Med 2003;349(5):465–473.
107. Greenland P, Knoll MD, Stamler J, et al. Major risk factors as antecedents of fatal and nonfatal coronary heart disease events. JAMA 2003;290(7):891–897.
108. Greenland P, LaBree L, Azen SP, Doherty TM, Detrano RC. Coronary artery calcium score combined with Framingham score for risk prediction in asymptomatic individuals. JAMA 2004;291(2):210–215.
109. Wilson JM, Jungner YG. Principles and practice of mass screening for disease. Bol Oficina Sanit Panam 1968;65(4):281–393.
110. Thompson GR, Partridge J. Coronary calcification score: the coronary-risk impact factor. Lancet 2004; 363(9408):557–559.
111. Hamilton M. Rapid responses: coronary artery calcification scoring. BMJ.com 2003.

112. Almeda FQ, Kason TT, Nathan S, Kavinsky CJ. Silent myocardial ischemia: concepts and controversies. Am J Med 2004;116(2):112–118.
113. Deedwania PC. Silent ischemia predicts poor outcome in high-risk healthy men. J Am Coll Cardiol 2001; 38(1):80–83.
114. Bonou M, Benroubis A, Kranidis A, et al. Functional and prognostic significance of silent ischemia during dobutamine stress echocardiography in the elderly. Coron Artery Dis 2001;12(6):499–506.
115. Solomon H, DeBusk RF. Contemporary management of silent ischemia: the role of ambulatory monitoring. Int J Cardiol 2004;96(3):311–319.
116. Cosson E, Guimfack M, Paries J, Paycha F, Attali JR, Valensi P. Are silent coronary stenoses predictable in diabetic patients and predictive of cardiovascular events? Diabetes Metab 2003;29(5):470–476.
117. Georgiou D, Budoff MJ, Kaufer E, Kennedy JM, Lu B, Brundage BH. Screening patients with chest pain in the emergency department using electron beam tomography: a follow-up study. J Am Coll Cardiol 2001;38(1):105–110.
118. Lamont DH, Budoff MJ, Shavelle DM, Shavelle R, Brundage BH, Hagar JM. Coronary calcium scanning adds incremental value to patients with positive stress tests. Am Heart J 2002;143(5):861–867.
119. Schmermund A, Baumgart D, Sack S, et al. Assessment of coronary calcification by electron-beam computed tomography in symptomatic patients with normal, abnormal or equivocal exercise stress test. Eur Heart J 2000;21(20):1674–1682.
120. Budoff MJ. Tracking progression of heart disease with cardiac computed tomography. J Cardiovasc Pharmacol Ther 2004;9(2):75–82.
121. de Feyter PJ, Vos J, Deckers JW. Progression and regression of the atherosclerotic plaque. Eur Heart J 1995;16(suppl I):26–30.
122. Hecht HS, Harman SM. Comparison of the effects of atorvastatin versus simvastatin on subclinical atherosclerosis in primary prevention as determined by electron beam tomography. Am J Cardiol 2003; 91(1):42–45.
123. Shemesh J, Koren-Morag N, Apter S, et al. Accelerated progression of coronary calcification: four-year follow-up in patients with stable coronary artery disease. Radiology 2004;233(1):201–209.
124. Wong ND, Teng W, Abrahamson D, et al. Noninvasive tracking of coronary atherosclerosis by electron beam computed tomography: rationale and design of the Felodipine Atherosclerosis Prevention Study (FAPS). Am J Cardiol 1995;76(17):1239–1242.
125. Budoff MJ, Lane KL, Bakhsheshi H, et al. Rates of progression of coronary calcium by electron beam tomography. Am J Cardiol 2000;86(1):8–11.
126. Shepherd J, Cobbe SM, Ford I, et al. Prevention of coronary heart disease with pravastatin in men with hypercholesterolemia. West of Scotland Coronary Prevention Study Group. N Engl J Med 1995; 333(20):1301–1307.
127. Downs JR, Clearfield M, Weis S, et al. Primary prevention of acute coronary events with lovastatin in men and women with average cholesterol levels: results of AFCAPS/TexCAPS. Air Force/Texas Coronary Atherosclerosis Prevention Study. JAMA 1998;279(20): 1615–1622.
128. O'Malley PG, Greenberg B, Taylor AJ. What is the marginal cost-effectiveness of EBCT in an asymptomatic screening population? [abstract] Circulation 2001(104).
129. Rumberger JA, Behrenbeck T, Breen JF, Sheedy PF 2nd. Coronary calcification by electron beam computed tomography and obstructive coronary artery disease: a model for costs and effectiveness of diagnosis as compared with conventional cardiac testing methods. J Am Coll Cardiol 1999;33(2):453–462.
130. Shaw L, Callister T, Raggi P. Establishing cost effective thresholds for coronary disease screening: a predictive model with risk factors and coronary calcium [abstract]. Circulation 2002(104):478–479.
131. Elgin EE, O'Malley PG, Feuerstein I, Taylor AJ. Frequency and severity of "incidentalomas" encountered during electron beam computed tomography for coronary calcium in middle-aged army personnel. Am J Cardiol 2002;90(5):543–545.
132. Hunold P, Schmermund A, Seibel RM, Gronemeyer DH, Erbel R. Prevalence and clinical significance of accidental findings in electron-beam tomographic scans for coronary artery calcification. Eur Heart J 2001;22(18):1748–1758.
133. Raggi P, Callister TQ, Cooil B, Russo DJ, Lippolis NJ, Patterson RE. Evaluation of chest pain in patients with low to intermediate pretest probability of coronary artery disease by electron beam computed tomography. Am J Cardiol 2000;85(3):283–288.
134. Petersen S, Peto V, Rayner M. Coronary Heart Disease Statistics. London: British Heart Foundation; 2004.
135. Heartstats. Coronary heart disease statistics. www.heartstats.org. 2004.
136. Doherty TM, Tang W, Detrano RC. Racial differences in the significance of coronary calcium in asymptomatic black and white subjects with coronary risk factors. J Am Coll Cardiol 1999;34(3):787–794.
137. Hatwalkar A, Agrawal N, Reiss DS, Budoff MJ. Comparison of prevalence and severity of coronary calcium determined by electron beam tomography among various ethnic groups. Am J Cardiol 2003;91(10):1225–1227.
138. Khurana C, Rosenbaum CG, Howard BV, et al. Coronary artery calcification in black women and white women. Am Heart J 2003;145(4):724–729.
139. Lee TC, O'Malley PG, Feuerstein I, Taylor AJ. The prevalence and severity of coronary artery calcification on coronary artery computed tomography in black and white subjects. J Am Coll Cardiol 2003;41(1):39–44.
140. Ohnesorge BM. Multislice CT Cardiac Imaging. 1st ed. New York: Springer-Verlag; 2002.
141. Dawson P, Lees WR. Multi-slice technology in computed tomography. Clin Radiol 2001;56(4):302–309.
142. Fuchs T, Kachelriess M, Kalender WA. Technical advances in multi-slice spiral CT. Eur J Radiol 2000;36(2):69–73.
143. Knez A, Becker C, Becker A, et al. Determination of coronary calcium with multi-slice spiral computed tomography: a comparative study with electron-beam CT. Int J Cardiovasc Imaging 2002;18(4):295–303.
144. Stanford W, Thompson BH, Burns TL, Heery SD, Burr MC. Coronary artery calcium quantification at multidetector row helical CT versus electron-beam CT. Radiology 2004;230(2):397–402.

145. Ohnesorge B, Flohr T, Fischbach R, et al. Reproducibility of coronary calcium quantification in repeat examinations with retrospectively ECG-gated multisection spiral CT. Eur Radiol 2002;12(6):1532–1540.
146. Goldin JG, Yoon HC, Greaser LE 3rd, et al. Spiral versus electron-beam CT for coronary artery calcium scoring. Radiology 2001;221(1):213–221.
147. Achenbach S, Moselewski F, Ropers D, et al. Detection of calcified and noncalcified coronary atherosclerotic plaque by contrast-enhanced, submillimeter multidetector spiral computed tomography: a segment-based comparison with intravascular ultrasound. Circulation 2004;109(1):14–17.
148. Schroeder S, Kuettner A, Leitritz M, et al. Reliability of differentiating human coronary plaque morphology using contrast-enhanced multislice spiral computed tomography: a comparison with histology. J Comput Assist Tomogr 2004;28(4):449–454.
149. Schroeder S, Kuettner A, Kopp AF, et al. Noninvasive evaluation of the prevalence of noncalcified atherosclerotic plaques by multi-slice detector computed tomography: results of a pilot study. Int J Cardiol 2003;92(2–3):151–155.
150. Teichholz LE, Petrillo S, Larson AJ, Klig V. Quantitative assessment of atherosclerosis by electron beam tomography. Am J Cardiol 2002;90(12):1416–1419.
151. Underwood SR, Anagnostopoulos C, Cerqueira M, et al. Myocardial perfusion scintigraphy: the evidence. Eur J Nucl Med Mol Imaging 2004;31(2):261–291.
152. New insights into myocardial perfusion imaging: adding value in diagnosis and management decision-making in coronary artery disease. Eur Heart J 2001;3(suppl F):F1–F20.
153. Iskander S, Iskandrian AE. Risk assessment using single-photon emission computed tomographic technetium-99 m sestamibi imaging. J Am Coll Cardiol 1998;32(1):57–62.
154. Brown KA. Prognostic value of myocardial perfusion imaging: state of the art and new developments. J Nucl Cardiol 1996;3(6 pt 1):516–537.
155. Allman KC, Thomson LE. Prognostic value of myocardial perfusion imaging in patients with known or suspected coronary artery disease. Eur Heart J 2001;3(suppl F):F5–F7.
156. Beller GA. The epidemics of obesity and type 2 diabetes: implications for noninvasive cardiovascular imaging. J Nucl Cardiol 2004;11(2):105–106.
157. Beller GA. President's page: the epidemic of type 2 diabetes and obesity in the U.S.: cause for alarm. J Am Coll Cardiol 2000;36(7):2348–2350.
158. Kannel WB, Abbott RD. Incidence and prognosis of unrecognized myocardial infarction. An update on the Framingham study. N Engl J Med 1984;311(18):1144–1147.
159. Niakan E, Harati Y, Rolak LA, Comstock JP, Rokey R. Silent myocardial infarction and diabetic cardiovascular autonomic neuropathy. Arch Intern Med 1986;146(11):2229–2230.
160. Gokcel A, Aydin M, Yalcin F, et al. Silent coronary artery disease in patients with type 2 diabetes mellitus. Acta Diabetol 2003;40(4):176–180.
161. De Lorenzo A, Lima RS, Siqueira-Filho AG, Pantoja MR. Prevalence and prognostic value of perfusion defects detected by stress technetium-99 m sestamibi myocardial perfusion single-photon emission computed tomography in asymptomatic patients with diabetes mellitus and no known coronary artery disease. Am J Cardiol 2002;90(8):827–832.
162. Wackers FJ, Young LH, Inzucchi SE, et al. Detection of silent myocardial ischemia in asymptomatic diabetic subjects: the DIAD study. Diabetes Care 2004;27(8):1954–1961.
163. Zellweger MJ, Hachamovitch R, Kang X, et al. Prognostic relevance of symptoms versus objective evidence of coronary artery disease in diabetic patients. Eur Heart J 2004;25(7):543–550.
164. Bergmann SR, Giedd KN. Silent ischemia: unsafe at any time. J Am Coll Cardiol 2003;42(1):41–44.
165. Davies RF. The need for a prognosis trial of revascularization and aggressive medical therapy in patients with asymptomatic cardiac ischemia. ACIP Investigators. Asymptomatic Cardiac Ischemia Pilot. Clin Cardiol 1998;21(3):154–156.
166. Davies RF, Goldberg AD, Forman S, et al. Asymptomatic Cardiac Ischemia Pilot (ACIP) study two-year follow-up: outcomes of patients randomized to initial strategies of medical therapy versus revascularization. Circulation 1997;95(8):2037–2043.
167. Stone PH, Chaitman BR, Forman S, et al. Prognostic significance of myocardial ischemia detected by ambulatory electrocardiography, exercise treadmill testing, and electrocardiogram at rest to predict cardiac events by one year (the Asymptomatic Cardiac Ischemia Pilot [ACIP] Study). Am J Cardiol 1997;80(11):1395–1401.
168. Pignoli P, Tremoli E, Poli A, Oreste P, Paoletti R. Intimal plus medial thickness of the arterial wall: a direct measurement with ultrasound imaging. Circulation 1986;74(6):1399–1406.
169. Mancini GB, Dahlof B, Diez J. Surrogate markers for cardiovascular disease: structural markers. Circulation 2004;109(25 suppl 1):IV22–30.
170. Sonoda M, Yonekura K, Yokoyama I, Takenaka K, Nagai R, Aoyagi T. Common carotid intima-media thickness is correlated with myocardial flow reserve in patients with coronary artery disease: a useful non-invasive indicator of coronary atherosclerosis. Int J Cardiol 2004;93(2–3):131–136.
171. Takiuchi S, Rakugi H, Fujii H, et al. Carotid intima-media thickness is correlated with impairment of coronary flow reserve in hypertensive patients without coronary artery disease. Hypertens Res 2003;26(12):945–951.
172. Chambless LE, Heiss G, Folsom AR, et al. Association of coronary heart disease incidence with carotid arterial wall thickness and major risk factors: the Atherosclerosis Risk in Communities (ARIC) Study, 1987–1993. Am J Epidemiol 1997;146(6):483–494.
173. Chambless LE, Folsom AR, Clegg LX, et al. Carotid wall thickness is predictive of incident clinical stroke: the Atherosclerosis Risk in Communities (ARIC) Study. Am J Epidemiol 2000;151(5):478–487.
174. Bots ML, Hoes AW, Koudstaal PJ, Hofman A, Grobbee DE. Common carotid intima-media thickness and risk of stroke and myocardial infarction: the Rotterdam Study. Circulation 1997;96(5):1432–1437.
175. Salonen JT, Salonen R. Ultrasound B-mode imaging in observational studies of atherosclerotic progression. Circulation 1993;87(3 suppl):II56–65.

176. O'Leary DH, Polak JF, Kronmal RA, Manolio TA, Burke GL, Wolfson SK Jr. Carotid-artery intima and media thickness as a risk factor for myocardial infarction and stroke in older adults. Cardiovascular Health Study Collaborative Research Group. N Engl J Med 1999; 340(1):14–22.
177. Hodis HN, Mack WJ, LaBree L, et al. The role of carotid arterial intima-media thickness in predicting clinical coronary events. Ann Intern Med 1998;128(4): 262–269.
178. MacMahon S, Sharpe N, Gamble G, et al. Randomized, placebo-controlled trial of the angiotensin-converting enzyme inhibitor, ramipril, in patients with coronary or other occlusive arterial disease. PART-2 Collaborative Research Group. Prevention of Atherosclerosis with Ramipril. J Am Coll Cardiol 2000;36(2):438–443.
179. Lonn E, Yusuf S, Dzavik V, et al. Effects of ramipril and vitamin E on atherosclerosis: the study to evaluate carotid ultrasound changes in patients treated with ramipril and vitamin E (SECURE). Circulation 2001; 103(7):919–925.
180. Kastelein JJ, Wiegman A, de Groot E. Surrogate markers of atherosclerosis: impact of statins. Atheroscler Suppl 2003;4(1):31–36.
181. Byington RP, Furberg CD, Crouse JR 3rd, Espeland MA, Bond MG. Pravastatin, lipids, and atherosclerosis in the carotid arteries (PLAC-II). Am J Cardiol 1995; 76(9):54C–59C.
182. Salonen R, Nyssonen K, Porkkala-Sarataho E, Salonen JT. The Kuopio Atherosclerosis Prevention Study (KAPS): effect of pravastatin treatment on lipids, oxidation resistance of lipoproteins, and atherosclerotic progression. Am J Cardiol 1995;76(9):34C–39C.
183. Salonen R, Nyyssonen K, Porkkala E, et al. Kuopio Atherosclerosis Prevention Study (KAPS). A population-based primary preventive trial of the effect of LDL lowering on atherosclerotic progression in carotid and femoral arteries. Circulation 1995;92(7):1758–1764.
184. de Groot E, Jukema JW, van Boven AJ, et al. Effect of pravastatin on progression and regression of coronary atherosclerosis and vessel wall changes in carotid and femoral arteries: a report from the Regression Growth Evaluation Statin Study. Am J Cardiol 1995;76(9): 40C–46C.
185. Furberg CD, Adams HP Jr, Applegate WB, et al. Effect of lovastatin on early carotid atherosclerosis and cardiovascular events. Asymptomatic Carotid Artery Progression Study (ACAPS) Research Group. Circulation 1994;90(4):1679–1687.
186. Taylor AJ, Kent SM, Flaherty PJ, Coyle LC, Markwood TT, Vernalis MN. ARBITER: Arterial Biology for the Investigation of the Treatment Effects of Reducing Cholesterol: a randomized trial comparing the effects of atorvastatin and pravastatin on carotid intima medial thickness. Circulation 2002;106(16):2055–2060.
187. Blankenhorn DH, Selzer RH, Crawford DW, et al. Beneficial effects of colestipol-niacin therapy on the common carotid artery. Two- and four-year reduction of intima-media thickness measured by ultrasound. Circulation 1993;88(1):20–28.
188. Mack WJ, Selzer RH, Hodis HN, et al. One-year reduction and longitudinal analysis of carotid intima-media thickness associated with colestipol/niacin therapy. Stroke 1993;24(12):1779–1783.
189. Howard G, O'Leary DH, Zaccaro D, et al. Insulin sensitivity and atherosclerosis. The Insulin Resistance Atherosclerosis Study (IRAS) Investigators. Circulation 1996;93(10):1809–1817.
190. Wagenknecht LE, D'Agostino R Jr, Savage PJ, O'Leary DH, Saad MF, Haffner SM. Duration of diabetes and carotid wall thickness. The Insulin Resistance Atherosclerosis Study (IRAS). Stroke 1997;28(5):999–1005.
191. Nathan DM, Lachin J, Cleary P, et al. Intensive diabetes therapy and carotid intima-media thickness in type 1 diabetes mellitus. N Engl J Med 2003;348(23): 2294–2303.
192. Minamikawa J, Tanaka S, Yamauchi M, Inoue D, Koshiyama H. Potent inhibitory effect of troglitazone on carotid arterial wall thickness in type 2 diabetes. J Clin Endocrinol Metab 1998;83(5):1818–1820.
193. Matsumoto K, Sera Y, Abe Y, Tominaga T, Yeki Y, Miyake S. Metformin attenuates progression of carotid arterial wall thickness in patients with type 2 diabetes. Diabetes Res Clin Pract 2004;64(3):225–228.
194. Tartiere JM, Kesri L, Safar H, et al. Association between pulse pressure, carotid intima-media thickness and carotid and/or iliofemoral plaque in hypertensive patients. J Hum Hypertens 2004;18(5):325–331.
195. Bots ML, Hofman A, de Bruyn AM, de Jong PT, Grobbee DE. Isolated systolic hypertension and vessel wall thickness of the carotid artery. The Rotterdam Elderly Study. Arterioscler Thromb 1993;13(1):64–69.
196. Lemne C, Jogestrand T, de Faire U. Carotid intima-media thickness and plaque in borderline hypertension. Stroke 1995;26(1):34–39.
197. Pitt B, Byington RP, Furberg CD, et al. Effect of amlodipine on the progression of atherosclerosis and the occurrence of clinical events. PREVENT Investigators. Circulation 2000;102(13):1503–1510.
198. Hodis HN, Mack WJ. Atherosclerosis imaging methods: assessing cardiovascular disease and evaluating the role of estrogen in the prevention of atherosclerosis. Am J Cardiol 2002;89(12A):19E–27E; discussion 27E.
199. Hodis HN, Mack WJ, Lobo RA, et al. Estrogen in the prevention of atherosclerosis. A randomized, double-blind, placebo-controlled trial. Ann Intern Med 2001;135(11):939–953.
200. Mayet J, Stanton AV, Chapman N, Foale RA, Hughes AD, Thom SA. Is carotid artery intima-media thickening a reliable marker of early atherosclerosis? J Cardiovasc Risk 2002;9(2):77–81.
201. Spence JD. Ultrasound measurement of carotid plaque as a surrogate outcome for coronary artery disease. Am J Cardiol 2002;89(4A):10B–15B; discussion 15B–16B.
202. Ebrahim S, Papacosta O, Whincup P, et al. Carotid plaque, intima media thickness, cardiovascular risk factors, and prevalent cardiovascular disease in men and women: the British Regional Heart Study. Stroke 1999;30(4):841–850.
203. Griffin M, Nicolaides AN, Belcaro G, Shah E. Cardiovascular risk assessment using ultrasound: the value of arterial wall changes including the presence, severity and character of plaques. Pathophysiol Haemost Thromb 2002;32(5–6):367–370.
204. Tegos TJ, Kalomiris KJ, Sabetai MM, Kalodiki E, Nicolaides AN. Significance of sonographic tissue and

surface characteristics of carotid plaques. AJNR Am J Neuroradiol 2001;22(8):1605–1612.
205. Geroulakos G, Ramaswami G, Nicolaides A, et al. Characterization of symptomatic and asymptomatic carotid plaques using high-resolution real-time ultrasonography. Br J Surg 1993;80(10):1274–1277.
206. Polak JF, Shemanski L, O'Leary DH, et al. Hypoechoic plaque at US of the carotid artery: an independent risk factor for incident stroke in adults aged 65 years or older. Cardiovascular Health Study. Radiology 1998; 208(3):649–654.
207. Langsfeld M, Gray-Weale AC, Lusby RJ. The role of plaque morphology and diameter reduction in the development of new symptoms in asymptomatic carotid arteries. J Vasc Surg 1989;9(4):548–557.
208. Johnson JM, Kennelly MM, Decesare D, Morgan S, Sparrow A. Natural history of asymptomatic carotid plaque. Arch Surg 1985;120(9):1010–1012.
209. Tegos TJ, Sabetai MM, Nicolaides AN, et al. Correlates of embolic events detected by means of transcranial Doppler in patients with carotid atheroma. J Vasc Surg 2001;33(1):131–138.
210. Geroulakos G, Sabetai MM. Ultrasonic carotid plaque morphology. Arch Hellen Med 2000;17(2):141–145.
211. Park AE, McCarthy WJ, Pearce WH, Matsumura JS, Yao JS. Carotid plaque morphology correlates with presenting symptomatology. J Vasc Surg 1998;27(5): 872–878; discussion 878–879.
212. Bassiouny HS, Sakaguchi Y, Mikucki SA, et al. Juxtalumenal location of plaque necrosis and neoformation in symptomatic carotid stenosis. J Vasc Surg 1997; 26(4):585–594.
213. Sterpetti AV, Hunter WJ, Schultz RD. Importance of ulceration of carotid plaque in determining symptoms of cerebral ischemia. J Cardiovasc Surg (Torino) 1991;32(2):154–158.
214. Dixon S, Pais SO, Raviola C, et al. Natural history of nonstenotic, asymptomatic ulcerative lesions of the carotid artery. A further analysis. Arch Surg 1982;117(11):1493–1498.
215. Eliasziw M, Streifler JY, Fox AJ, Hachinski VC, Ferguson GG, Barnett HJ. Significance of plaque ulceration in symptomatic patients with high-grade carotid stenosis. North American Symptomatic Carotid Endarterectomy Trial. Stroke 1994;25(2):304–308.
216. Ricotta JJ, Schenk EA, Ekholm SE, DeWeese JA. Angiographic and pathologic correlates in carotid artery disease. Surgery 1986;99(3):284–292.
217. Moore WS, Boren C, Malone JM, et al. Natural history of nonstenotic, asymptomatic ulcerative lesions of the carotid artery. Arch Surg 1978;113(11):1352–1359.
218. Steinke W, Hennerici M, Rautenberg W, Mohr JP. Symptomatic and asymptomatic high-grade carotid stenoses in Doppler color-flow imaging. Neurology 1992;42(1):131–138.
219. Iannuzzi A, Wilcosky T, Mercuri M, Rubba P, Bryan FA, Bond MG. Ultrasonographic correlates of carotid atherosclerosis in transient ischemic attack and stroke. Stroke 1995;26(4):614–619.
220. Kroener JM, Dorn PL, Shoor PM, Wickbom IG, Bernstein EF. Prognosis of asymptomatic ulcerating carotid lesions. Arch Surg 1980;115(11):1387–1392.
221. Imparato AM, Riles TS, Gorstein F. The carotid bifurcation plaque: pathologic findings associated with cerebral ischemia. Stroke 1979;10(3):238–245.
222. Harward TR, Kroener JM, Wickbom IG, Bernstein EF. Natural history of asymptomatic ulcerative plaques of the carotid bifurcation. Am J Surg 1983;146(2): 208–212.
223. Debray JM, Baud JM, Dauzat M. Consensus concerning the morphology and the risk of carotid plaques. Cerebrovasc Dis 1997;7:289–296.
224. Gray-Weale AC, Graham JC, Burnett JR, Byrne K, Lusby RJ. Carotid artery atheroma: comparison of preoperative B-mode ultrasound appearance with carotid endarterectomy specimen pathology. J Cardiovasc Surg (Torino) 1988;29(6):676–681.
225. Fitzgerald DE, O'Farrell CM. Prognostic value of ultrasound morphology in carotid atherosclerosis. Int Angiol 1993;12(4):337–341.
226. Sitzer M, Muller W, Rademacher J, et al. Color-flow Doppler-assisted duplex imaging fails to detect ulceration in high-grade internal carotid artery stenosis. J Vasc Surg 1996;23(3):461–465.
227. Mitchell CK, Aeschlimann SE, Korcarz CE. Carotid intima-media thickness testing: technical considerations. J Am Soc Echocardiogr 2004;17(6):690–692.
228. Stensland-Bugge E, Bonaa KH, Joakimsen O. Reproducibility of ultrasonographically determined intima-media thickness is dependent on arterial wall thickness. The Tromso Study. Stroke 1997;28(10): 1972–1980.
229. Wong M, Edelstein J, Wollman J, Bond MG. Ultrasonic-pathological comparison of the human arterial wall. Verification of intima-media thickness. Arterioscler Thromb 1993;13(4):482–486.
230. Macioch JE, Robin J, Liebson PR, et al. Effect of contrast enhancement on measurement of carotid artery intima medial thickness. Am J Vasc Med 2004;9(1):7–12.
231. Rajaram V, Pandhya S, Patel S, et al. Role of surrogate markers in assessing patients with diabetes mellitus and the metabolic syndrome and in evaluating lipid-lowering therapy. Am J Cardiol 2004;93(11A):32C–48C.
232. Moulton KS. Plaque angiogenesis and atherosclerosis. Curr Atheroscler Rep 2001;3(3):225–233.
233. Barger AC, Beeuwkes R 3rd, Lainey LL, Silverman KJ. Hypothesis: vasa vasorum and neovascularization of human coronary arteries. A possible role in the pathophysiology of atherosclerosis. N Engl J Med 1984;310(3):175–177.
234. Mofidi R, Crotty TB, McCarthy P, Sheehan SJ, Mehigan D, Keaveny TV. Association between plaque instability, angiogenesis and symptomatic carotid occlusive disease. Br J Surg 2001;88(7):945–950.
235. Greenland P, Abrams J, Aurigemma GP, et al. AHA Scientific Statement, Prevention Conference V, Beyond Secondary Prevention: Identifying the High-Risk Patient for Primary Prevention: Noninvasive Tests of Atherosclerotic Burden: Writing Group III. Circulation 2000;101:e16–22.
236. Bard RL, Kalsi H, Rubenfire M, et al. Effect of carotid atherosclerosis screening on risk stratification during primary cardiovascular disease prevention. Am J Cardiol 2004;93(8):1030–1032.
237. Stein JH. Carotid intima-media thickness and vascular age: you are only as old as your arteries look. J Am Soc Echocardiogr 2004;17(6):686–689.
238. Stein JH, Fraizer MC, Aeschlimann SE, Nelson-Worel J, McBride PE, Douglas PS. Vascular age: integrating carotid intima-media thickness measurements with

global coronary risk assessment. Clin Cardiol 2004; 27(7):388–392.
239. Libby P. Atherosclerosis: the new view. Sci Am 2002; 286(5):46–55.
240. Libby P. Inflammation in atherosclerosis. Nature 2002; 420(6917):868–874.
241. Libby P, Ridker PM, Maseri A. Inflammation and atherosclerosis. Circulation 2002;105(9):1135–1143.
242. Lusis AJ. Atherosclerosis. Nature 2000;407(6801): 233–241.
243. Strauss HW, Grewal RK, Pandit-Taskar N. Molecular imaging in nuclear cardiology. Semin Nucl Med 2004; 34(1):47–55.
244. Fayad ZA, Fuster V. Detection of vulnerable plaque using magnetic resonance imaging. In: Braunwald E, ed. Harrison's Advances in Cardiology. Boston: McGraw-Hill; 2003:220–225.
245. Choi CJ, Kramer CM. MR imaging of atherosclerotic plaque. Radiol Clin North Am 2002;40(4):887–898.
246. Kramer CM. Magnetic resonance imaging to identify the high-risk plaque. Am J Cardiol 2002;90(10C): 15L–17L.
247. Kramer CM. Current and future applications of cardiovascular magnetic resonance imaging. Cardiol Rev 2000;8(4):216–222.
248. Corti R, Fuster V, Badimon JJ, Hutter R, Fayad ZA. New understanding of atherosclerosis (clinically and experimentally) with evolving MRI technology in vivo. Ann NY Acad Sci 2001;947:181–195; discussion 195–198.
249. Corti R, Fayad ZA, Fuster V, et al. Effects of lipid-lowering by simvastatin on human atherosclerotic lesions: a longitudinal study by high-resolution, noninvasive magnetic resonance imaging. Circulation 2001;104(3):249–252.
250. Fayad ZA, Fuster V. The human high-risk plaque and its detection by magnetic resonance imaging. Am J Cardiol 2001;88(2A):42E–45E.
251. Flacke S, Fischer S, Scott MJ, et al. Novel MRI contrast agent for molecular imaging of fibrin: implications for detecting vulnerable plaques. Circulation 2001; 104(11):1280–1285.
252. Ruehm SG, Corot C, Vogt P, Kolb S, Debatin JF. Magnetic resonance imaging of atherosclerotic plaque with ultrasmall superparamagnetic particles of iron oxide in hyperlipidemic rabbits. Circulation 2001; 103(3):415–422.
253. Leitha T, Staudenherz A, Gmeiner B, Hermann M, Huttinger M, Dudczak R. Technetium-99 m labelled LDL as a tracer for quantitative LDL scintigraphy. II. In vivo validation, LDL receptor-dependent and unspecific hepatic uptake and scintigraphic results. Eur J Nucl Med 1993;20(8):674–679.
254. Shaish A, Keren G, Chouraqui P, Levkovitz H, Harats D. Imaging of aortic atherosclerotic lesions by (125)I-LDL, (125)I-oxidized-LDL, (125)I-HDL and (125)I-BSA. Pathobiology 2001;69(4):225–229.
255. Rudd JH, Warburton EA, Fryer TD, et al. Imaging atherosclerotic plaque inflammation with [18F]-fluorodeoxyglucose positron emission tomography. Circulation 2002;105(23):2708–2711.
256. Blankenberg FG. Recent advances in the imaging of programmed cell death. Curr Pharm Des 2004;10(13): 1457–1467.

7

Noninvasive Assessment of Asymptomatic Individuals at Risk of Coronary Heart Disease. Part b

Dhrubo Rakhit and Thomas H. Marwick

1. Background

Silent myocardial ischemia may occur at rest and on exertion[1,2] and the prevalence of undiagnosed coronary artery disease (CAD) in asymptomatic 50 year olds has been estimated at 15%–20% in men and 5% in women.[3] Although coronary angiography is the current gold standard in detection of CAD, American Heart Association (AHA)/American College of Cardiology guidelines recommend "that coronary angiography is indicated for patients found to have high-risk abnormalities on noninvasive testing and that noninvasive procedures for identifying patients with stress-induced ischemia, should remain the primary means of risk stratification."[4]

This second part of Chapter 7 deals with the role of noninvasive imaging in assessing asymptomatic individuals and particularly specific higher-risk groups such as patients with diabetes mellitus, end-stage renal failure (ESRF), cardiac transplant, and those awaiting surgery for peripheral vascular disease. It complements the first part not only by the shift of the emphasis on specific groups but also by its focus on echocardiography. The latter is a versatile modality with very good diagnostic and prognostic value[5–7] that does not use ionizing radiation and is therefore a very attractive option for assessing the patients discussed in this chapter.

2. Screening

The value of screening is to reduce morbidity and mortality from a disease. For screening to be effective, the disease should have an early asymptomatic stage and have important health consequences. A screening test should be cost effective, have a low false-positive and false-negative rate, be able to detect disease earlier than it would otherwise present and there must be an appropriate therapy to prevent the outcome that would have ensued.[8] Specifically, screening in high-risk patients can only be justified if a) a suitable cost-effective approach to identify CAD is available, and b) a treatment strategy for positive cases identified by the screening procedure is feasible.

There are several social reasons why asymptomatic individuals request screening for CAD. These include family history, presence of risk factors, anxiety, dangerous or important occupation (e.g., airline pilots or executives). From a medical standpoint, the main rationale is the detection of asymptomatic CAD, which is thought to account for 20%–25% of cases of sudden death.[9] It has been proposed that the most effective primary prevention of sudden death may be prevention of coronary events.[10]

3. Statistical Considerations and the Clinical Detection of Risk

Bayes' theory states that the probability of a disease being present after a positive or negative test depends on the pretest probability of the disease.[11] Therefore, if the pretest probability of a disease is low, then even with a highly sensitive or specific test, the posttest probability will be low (see Figure 7b.1).

To maximize the chances of obtaining a positive test, a low-risk ("screening") group should undergo some process whereby the patients at lowest risk are removed from the screening program. This process effectively enriches the testing group with individuals at higher risk. Indeed, the use of stress echocardiography (SE) in a group of low-risk patients is not cost effective,[12] whereas in patients at higher risk it has been shown to provide incremental benefit in risk evaluation.[13]

Various clinical approaches to allocating risk are available and include coronary prediction models, such as those based on Framingham data[14] for long-term outcome or Eagle's criteria[15] for perioperative outcome. Because stress-induced wall motion abnormalities may be manifested even before symptoms occur (Figure 7b.3) sE has been used to identify CAD in the high-

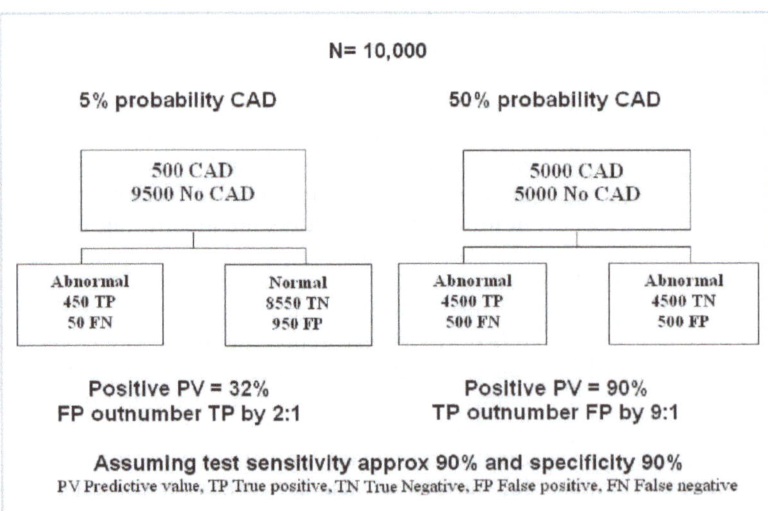

Figure 7b.1. Importance of pretest probability. Even with the most sensitive possible test, testing of low-probability patients is associated with high numbers of false-positive results.

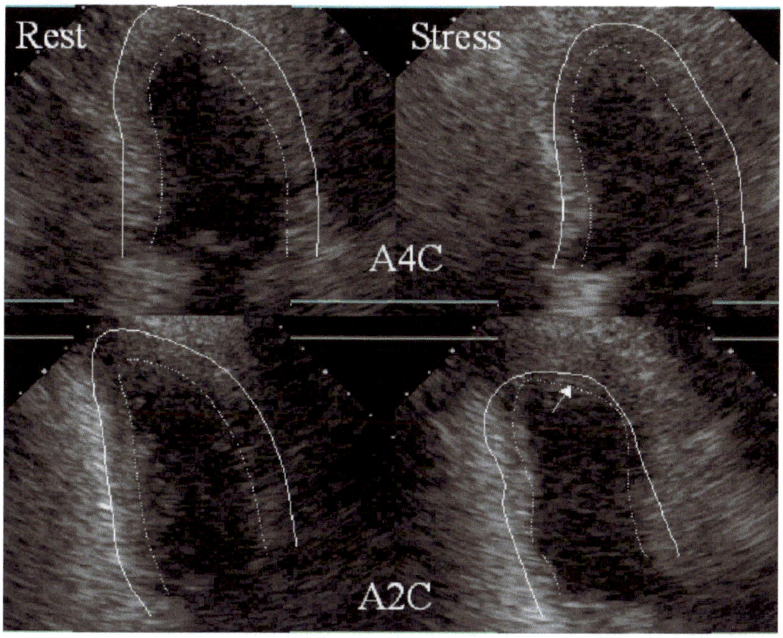

Figure 7b.2. Wall motion abnormalities during exercise echocardiography. End-systolic freeze-frame images (endocardial contour marked by dotted line, contrast with end-diastolic marked by continuous line) shows normal thickening in all walls at rest. Postexercise images show an inducible wall motion abnormality in the anterior wall. A4C, apical 4-chamber; A2C, apical 2-chamber.

risk groups that include asymptomatic patients with diabetes mellitus,[16] renal[17] or cardiac transplants,[18] ESRF[19] or metabolic syndrome,[20] those with established peripheral vascular disease,[21] and those with multiple risk factors.[22] Recently, the practice of SE in screening certain high-risk groups for noncardiac surgery has become more common.[15]

4. Echocardiography as a Screening Tool

4.1 Prognostic Value of Resting Echocardiography

The prevalence of asymptomatic left ventricular dysfunction has been estimated at 0.9%–12.9%.[23] Resting left ventricular systolic dysfunction is a predictor of outcome when applied to asymptomatic individuals from a randomly selected population.[24] The likely cause of resting left ventricular systolic dysfunction is CAD and early intervention in these individuals with medical treatment such as angiotensin-converting enzyme inhibitors, β-blockers, or antiplatelet agents may prevent progression to more severe degrees of heart failure, although current evidence in support of a screening program using resting echo alone is inadequate.[23]

4.2 Stress Echo as Screening Tool

SE is considered a useful, feasible, and safe technique for detecting the presence, localization, and extent of CAD.[25] In comparison with myocardial perfusion imaging (MPI), SE is more specific but has a lower sensitivity for the detection of CAD[26,27] – this may actually be of some benefit in its application to a screening population. SE has been shown to be of prognostic and/or diagnostic value in patients with right bundle branch block (RBBB) and left anterior hemiblock,[28] hypertension and RBBB,[29] and in patients with chest pain of unknown origin[30] (Figure 7b.2).

5. Management Implications of Positive Stress Echocardiograms

The finding of a positive SE carries implications for both medical management and revascularization. Because a positive test signifies the presence of underlying CAD, an aggressive risk factor management approach should be adopted. In addition, the physician responsible for the patient's care may elect to proceed to coronary angiography with a view to revascularization. Data supporting the latter option are limited. One positive study, the Asymptomatic Cardiac Ischemia Pilot Study[31] enrolled 558 patients who had coronary anatomy suitable for revascularization, ischemia during exercise or pharmacologic stress testing, and at least one episode of asymptomatic ischemia during 48-hour ambulatory electrocardiogram (ECG) monitoring. Patients were angina-free or had few symptoms on therapy and were randomized to one of three treatment options: angina-guided medical treatment, ischemia-guided medical treatment, or revascularization. Results at 2-year follow-up showed that mortality was 6.6% in the angina-guided strategy, 4.4% in the ischemia-guided strategy, and 1.1% in the revascularization strategy. In a recent review, reduction of ischemia, either by medical therapy or revascularization in patients with silent myocardial ischemia was thought to be of benefit.[2] These data justify the referral at least, of selected patients for revascularization.

6. Use of Stress Echo in High-risk Patient Groups

6.1 Multiple Risk Factors (Including Metabolic Syndrome/Obesity)

6.1.1 Clinical

As discussed in the introduction, the standard approach to the noninvasive evaluation of CAD precludes investigation of all asymptomatic patients because the probability of disease is considered low in the absence of chest pain, irrespective of age and gender.[32] However, prognostic studies of stress testing have shown that the identification of CAD increases the relative risk of these patients significantly,[33,34] even though their absolute risk remains low. Consequently, standard guidelines classify functional testing in patients with multiple risk factors to be a class IIb indication for testing. However, it must be recognized that this recommendation is restricted to definite risk factor criteria, and even favorable studies do not reflect application of standard risk scores such as the Framingham score.[35]

6.1.2 Echocardiography

Almost all of the screening studies reported in patients with multiple risk factors have been performed with the exercise ECG. The use of exercise echocardiography has been compared with the Duke treadmill score in a recent study of 1832 patients without evidence of CAD, who were followed up over 10 years.[36] Although exercise provoked significant (>0.1 mV) ST segment depression more often than wall motion abnormalities (12% versus 8%), which might suggest more false-positive results, Duke treadmill score (RR 0.9, $P < .0001$) and resting left ventricular (LV) dysfunction (RR 1.9, $P <$

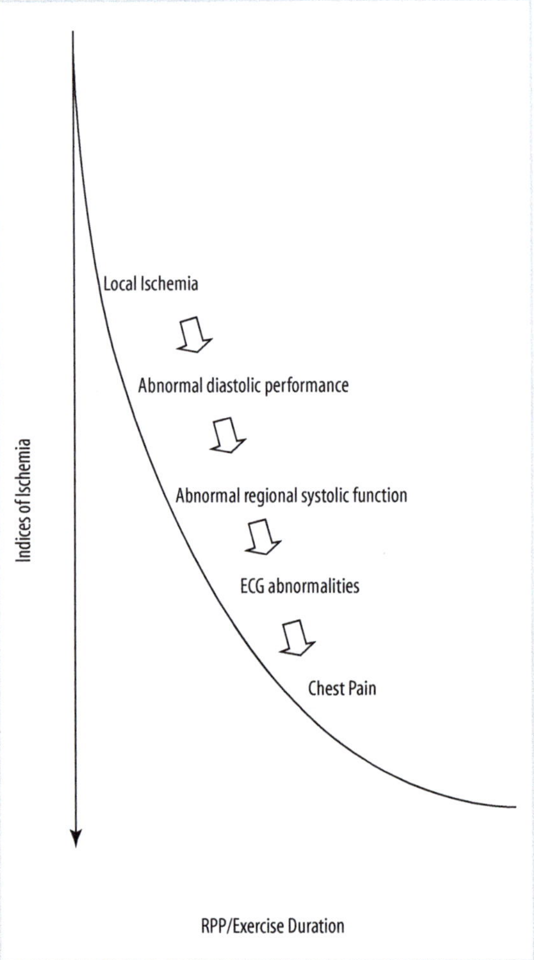

Figure 7b.3. The ischemic cascade. The development of chest pain and electrocardiographic (ECG) changes of ischemia occur at a greater level of cardiovascular stress than wall motion or perfusion abnormalities.

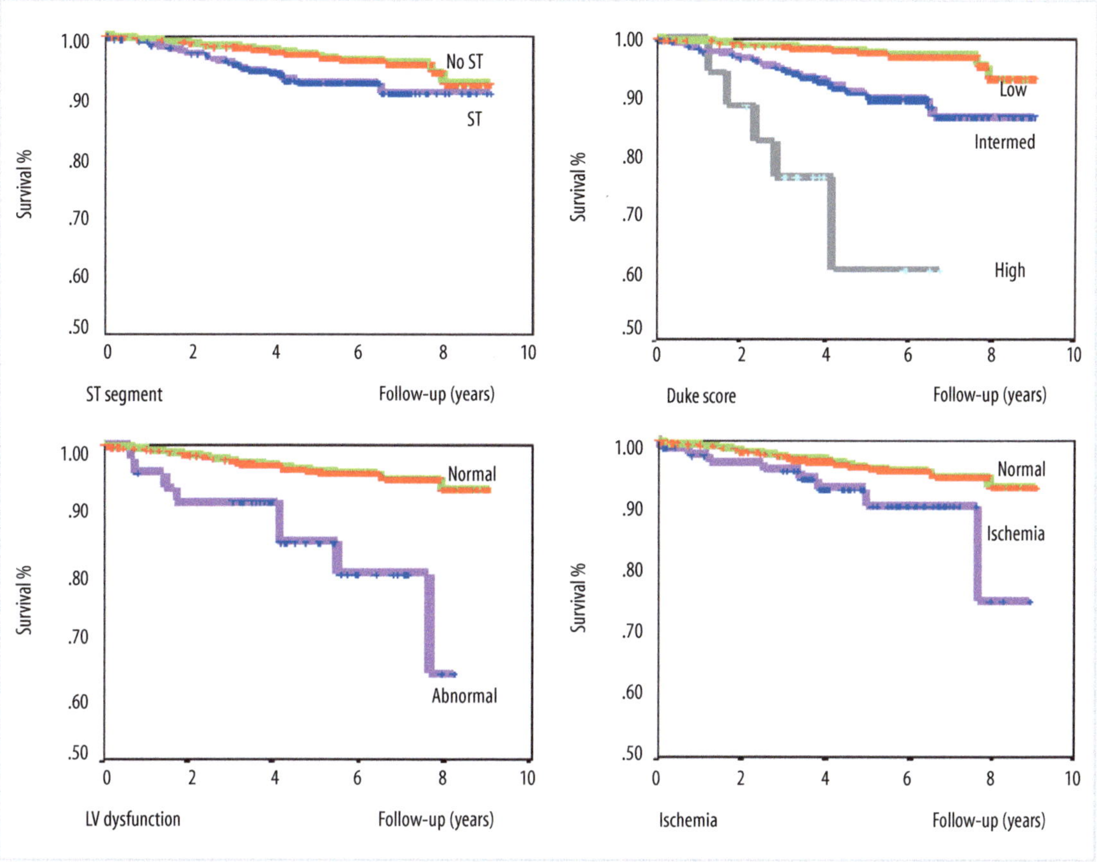

Figure 7b.4. Kaplan-Meier survival curves of patients with and without ST depression, LV dysfunction, and ischemia and in each risk level of the Duke treadmill score. (Reproduced from Marwick et al.[36]).

.04), but not ischemia at exercise echocardiography, were predictors of events, even in patients with multiple risk factors (Figure 7b.4; see color section).

6.1.3 Alternate Strategies for Screening

Myocardial perfusion scintigraphy (MPS) has been shown to be useful in this setting and particularly for the identification of disease in relatives of patients with premature CAD. Its value is stronger when it is performed after a positive exercise ECG.[37,38] Electron beam computed tomography (EBCT) or multislice computed tomography, followed, depending on the results, by MPS is another possibility. For a more detailed discussion on the role of these techniques and also for the assessment of endothelial function, see Chapters 7a and 14, respectively.

6.1.4 Appropriate Responses

A summary report from an AHA prevention conference outlined a strategy to identify high-risk asymptomatic individuals, who would be appropriate for aggressive risk-factor modification.[39] In accordance with ATP III[40] and JNC-VII[41] guidelines, high-risk asymptomatic individuals should have all cardiovascular risk factors treated and modified in an attempt at primary prevention. There are limited data to support revascularization of some patients in this category.

6.2 Diabetes Mellitus

6.2.1 Clinical

The problem with testing patients with multiple risk factors is that these carry varying levels of risk. In contrast, by restricting the screened group to patients with type II diabetes (>90% of all diabetic patients), the risk of CAD is increased two- to six-fold.[50–52] There is no uniform policy regarding screening diabetic patients for CAD. Some authors suggest that "screening would make no useful contribution to management."[53] Others suggest that approximately 20% of asymptomatic type II male diabetics have significant CAD and do recommend screening in male diabetics in whom the duration of the disease is longer than 10 years or if one additional risk factor is present.[54] Methods of enriching the group screened include applying Framingham model to the selected population as a whole and screening only those who are high risk (i.e., those who have a >1% risk of events per year).

6.2.2 Echocardiography

It has been suggested that diabetic cardiomyopathy should be screened for using cardiac ultrasound,[47] and tissue Doppler techniques may be able to identify subclinical disease.[48] However, these patients show a normal stress response and therefore CAD is not an etiologic factor.[49] For identification of CAD, a number of studies, shown in Tables 7b.1a and 7b.1b, have used SE in diabetic patients. Some of these have been in symptomatic rather than asymptomatic patients, but overall, it seems that SE is a valid and informative technique for screening diabetic patients.

6.2.3 Alternate Strategies for Screening

Other screening tests for CAD have been evaluated in asymptomatic diabetic patients. These include exercise tolerance testing (ETT), MPS, and EBCT. In a cohort of 206 patients who underwent ETT, 29% were unable to exercise sufficiently[61] and this has implications for the sensitivity and specificity of the test in this patient group. Other studies have screened using the combination of ETT and MPI[46] or EBCT alone.[65] The use of ETT, MPI, and SE in asymptomatic diabetics[57] has been compared. In this study, predictive positive value was 69% for dobutamine stress echocardiography (DSE), 75% for MPS using 201Tl single photon emission computed tomography (SPECT) and 60% for ETT. For a further discussion on the role of these techniques in this group of patients, see also Chapter 7a.

6.2.4 Appropriate Responses

All patients with diabetes should have aggressive risk-factor modification according to American Diabetes Association guidelines.[66] For those who are revascularized, even after revascularization, there is a high frequency of silent myocardial ischemia – in one study this was reported as 43%.[64] Diabetic patients tend to have more

Table 7b.1a. Diagnostic use of SE in patients with diabetes mellitus

Author	Group	Test used	Asymptomatic	Results
Bacci et al.[50]	35 DM unable to exercise	DSE and CA	Yes	Sensitivity 21%, specificity 94%
Coisne et al.[51]	49 DM and 63 nondiabetics	DSE and CA	Yes	Positive DSE in 3 of 49 DM (confirmed by angio)
Elhendy et al.[52]	1446 patients, 184 DM	DSE and CA	?	Sensitivity 81%, specificity 85%
Gaddi et al.[53]	24 DM with positive thallium	DiSE and CA	Yes	Sensitivity 92%, specificity 100%
Griffin et al.[54]	18 DM and nephropathy	DSE and CA	Yes	7 positive DSE with 2 positive angios
Hennessy et al.[55]	52 DM for cardiac opinion	DSE and CA	?	Sensitivity 82%, specificity 54%
Hung et al.[56]	338 patients post-AMI, 116 DM	DSE and CA	?	Sensitivity 71.8%, specificity 50%
Penfornis et al.[57]	56 DM	SPECT, ExECG, DSE, and CA	Yes	Sensitivity 69%, specificity 89%

CA, coronary angiography; DSE, dobutamine stress echo; DiSE, dipyridamole stress echo; ExECG, exercise ECG; SPECT, single photon emission computed tomography; DM, diabetes mellitus; AMI, acute myocardial infarction.

Table 7b.1b. Prognostic use of SE in patients with diabetes mellitus

Author	Group	Test used	Asymptomatic	Result
Bates et al.[58]	53 IDDM for kidney/pancreas Tx	DSE	Yes	Event rates 45% in those with abnormal DSE (38%) vs 6% with normal DSE
Bigi et al.[59]	259 DM, 108 DSE, 151 DiSE, 120 ExSE	DSE, DiSE ExECG	No	SE positive in 65% with FU events and 39% without. SE negative in 35% with FU events and 61% without.
D'Andrea et al.[60]	325 DM (128 diagnosis, 197 risk stratify)	195 DSE, 130 DiSE	No	45.8% positive SE hazard ratio 2.9 for death
Elhendy et al.[61]	563 DM	ExSE	?No	41% ExSE positive. Event rate lower in normal ExSE vs abnormal ExSE at 1 yr (0% vs 1.9%), 3 yr (1.8% vs 11.9%), and 5 yr (7.6% vs 23.3%)
Hung et al.[56]	338 patients post-AMI, 116 DM	DSE and CA	?	38.9% events in DM with positive DSE; 20% in DM with negative DSE
Kamalesh et al.[62]	239 patients, 89 DM negative ExSE/DSE	DSE	?	FU 25 ± 7 mo DM had higher incidence of cardiac events (19% vs 9.7%)
Marwick et al.[16]	937 DM for symptoms (42%) and FU CAD	DSE	No	165/370 with rest or stress WMA died during FU (M 3.9 yr)
Sozzi et al.[63]	396 DM unable to exercise	DSE	?No	DSE abnormal in 82% abnormal vs normal DSE death rate: 1 yr 9 vs 3% 3 yr 29 vs 11% 5 yr 31 vs 24%

CA, coronary angiography; DSE, dobutamine stress echo; DiSE, dipyridamole stress echo; ExECG, exercise ECG; ExSE, exercise stress echo; DM, diabetes mellitus; Tx, transplant; FU, follow-up; WMA, wall motion abnormalities; IDDM, insulin dependent diabetes mellitus; AMI, acute myocardial infarction; SE, stress echo.

diffuse CAD than their nondiabetic counterparts and often have poor target vessels, which may contribute to worse outcomes after revascularization. Nonetheless, the data in Table 7b.1b indicate that diabetes and ischemia are a potent combination in terms of provoking subsequent events, and although no strong evidence base is yet available, it seems reasonable to consider revascularization, at least for selected patients. In randomized studies comparing revascularization by either coronary bypass surgery (CABG) or percutaneous intervention (PCI), diabetic patients who undergo CABG have a survival benefit over diabetics who have PCI.[76,77] In addition, patients with diabetes have higher restenosis rates after PCI.[78,79]

6.3 End-stage Renal Failure

6.3.1 Clinical

Patients with end-stage renal disease are prone to coronary events, partly because of the high prevalence of risk factors (hypertension, diabetes, dyslipidemia), and partly because uremia itself provides an atherogenic milieu.[72] Moreover, the number of patients requiring dialysis is increasing with both the aging of the population and the epidemic of diabetes mellitus (Figure 7b.5; http://www.usrds.org).

Disturbingly, the cardiovascular mortality in young patients on dialysis is similar to that of older patients, and several orders of magnitude greater than the general population, matched for age.[73]

There is no consensus about how best to go about the process of detecting CAD in patients with end-stage renal disease. In many centers, some form of testing is routinely performed at the time of transplant evaluation, with the hope of decreasing the risk of surgery and also reduce the prospect of "wasting" a donated kidney if the patient were to succumb to a coronary event post-transplantation. However, the restriction of testing to this time frame does not account for the risks associated with the predialysis population, as well as those dialysis patients who are not candidates for transplant.

The only clinical tool developed to facilitate risk prediction in this population was reported by Le et al.,[74] who identified three groups. Those with low risk (<0.5% per year over 4 years) were aged <50 years, nondiabetic, asymptomatic for either coronary disease or heart failure, and with a normal ECG. Intermediate risk patients (0.5%–4% annualized event rate) were also asymptomatic, but >50 years old or diabetic, and

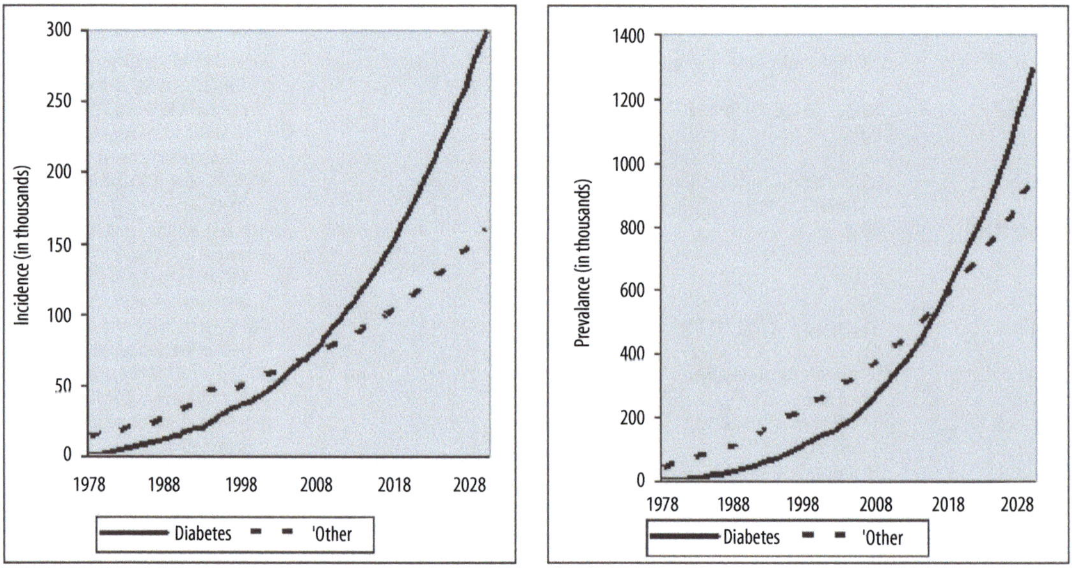

Figure 7b.5. Projected growth of the incident and prevalent ESRD populations, by primary cause of renal failure.

high risk (>4% annualized risk) were symptomatic for either coronary disease or heart failure.

6.3.2 Echocardiography

Resting echocardiography is very often abnormal in this patient group, showing either LV hypertrophy, LV enlargement, or systolic dysfunction.[75] These abnormalities are associated with adverse outcome, and many renal units perform routine resting echos on a regular basis to identify these abnormalities.

SE has also been used in ESRF patients, usually at the time of transplant evaluation. Table 7b.2a illustrates the reported sensitivity and specificity of dobutamine echo in ESRF; it seems that its sensitivity is somewhat less than in the normal population, reflecting the difficulties posed by attaining peak stress in these patients – many of whom are taking β-blockers or hypertensive.

Data have also been obtained regarding the prognostic implications of stress testing in patients with ESRF (Table 7b.2b). Generally,

Table 7b.2b. Prognostic implications of DSE in ESRF

Study	Stress	Group	Outcomes
Reis et al.[80]	DSE	97 Tx and HD patients	PV negative test 97% over 12 mo
Brennan et al.[82]	DSE	47 ESRF patients	PV negative test 95% over 20 mo
Marwick et al.[19]	DSE	193 ESRF patients	Predicted early but not late events

DSE, dobutamine stress echo; Tx, transplant; HD, haemodialysis; PV, predictive value; ESRF, end stage renal failure; MO, months.

Table 7b.2a. Diagnostic use of DSE or thallium scans in ESRF

Study	Stress	Group	Sensitivity (%)	Specificity (%)
Boudreau et al.[76]	Dip-Tl	40 patients with DM and ESRF	86	72
Marwick et al.[77]	Dip-Tl	45 Tx candidates	37	73
Vandenberg et al.[78]	Dip-Tl	41 Tx patients	53	73
Dahan et al.[79]	Dip-Tl	60 asymptomatic HD patients	92	89
Reis et al.[80]	DSE	97 ESRF patients	95	86
Herzog et al.[81]	DSE	50 Tx candidates	75	76

DM, diabetes mellitus; ESRF, end stage renal failure; Tx, transplant; Dip T1, dipyridamole thallium; HD, haemodialysis; DSE, dobutamine stress echo.

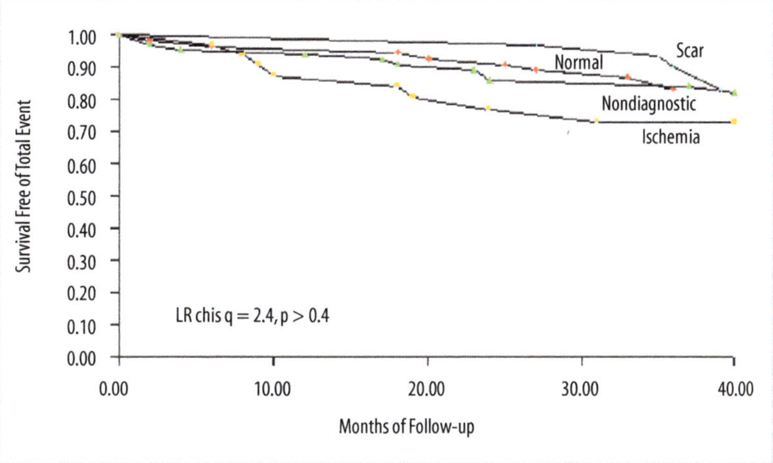

Figure 7b.6. Event-free survival of patients with end-stage renal disease. Curves reflect outcomes with ischemia, scar, nondiagnostic, and normal dobutamine echocardiography. (Reproduced from Marwick et al.[19]).

these patients are debilitated and pharmacologic stress testing is necessary. The presence of a normal scan does imply a favorable prognosis in this patient group, although the warranty of a normal test result (2 years) is somewhat shorter than in other circumstances (Figure 7b.6; see color section). Ischemia is associated with an adverse outcome in ESRF, as in other diseases.

6.3.3 Alternate Strategies for Screening

Other screening tests for CAD have also been evaluated in ESRF. From a diagnostic standpoint, dipyridamole thallium scanning has a somewhat lower specificity (probably reflecting false positives because of LV hypertrophy) (Table 7b.2a). Various explanations for its lower sensitivity have been proposed – abnormalities or myocardial perfusion and disturbances of adenosine metabolism being the most plausible. The prognostic findings have also been somewhat variable (Table 7b.2c).

A number of other markers of risk have been reported in ESRF. These include biomarkers of both subclinical cardiac damage (e.g., troponin) and vascular inflammation (e.g., C-reactive protein), genetic markers, and vascular function parameters (e.g., pulse wave velocity). Coronary calcium is often observed in ESRF – being primarily associated with age, duration on dialysis, and disturbances of calcium metabolism,[91] and does not seem to be a good surrogate for CAD in this group.

Table 7b.2c. Prognostic findings of thallium scanning in renal patients

Study	Stress agent	Group	Outcomes
Morrow et al.[83]	Ex-T1	85 Tx and HD patients	T1 predictive but not more than Hx CAD/ECG
Brown et al.[84]	Dip-T1	65 DM and non-DM Tx patients	Ischemia and EF predicted outcome
Marwick et al.[77]	Dip-T1	45 Tx candidates	T1 did not predict outcome
Camp et al.[85]	Dip-T1	40 DM Tx candidates	Only patients with T1 defects had events
Holley et al.[86]	Ex-T1	141 DM Tx candidates	T1 did not predict perioperative risk
Derfler et al.[87]	Dip-T1	59 asymptomatic/symptomatic ESRF	T1 predicted events, not death
Brown et al.[88]	Ex-T1	103 asymptomatic ESRF	Sensitivity 88%, specificity 70% for events
Le et al.[74]	Ex-T1	95 high-risk Tx patients	T1-ischemia/scar predicted outcomes
Lewis[89]	Ex-T1	112 high risk pts	T1-ischemia/scar predicted outcomes
Vandenberg et al.[78]	Dip-T1	41 Tx patients	Outcome same with + or – scan
Heston et al.[90]	Dip-T1	95 Tx patients; T1 and neural net	Sensitivity 82%, specificity 77% for events
Dahan et al.[879]	Dip-T1	60 asymptomatic HD patients	Sensitivity 92%, specificity 89% for CAD; 3 yr FU: NPV 91%, PPV 47%

T1, thallium scintigraphy; HD, hemodialysis; CAD, coronary artery disease; DM, diabetes mellitus; EF, ejection fraction; Tx, transplant; NPV, negative predictive value; PPV, positive predictive value; Ex, exercise; Dip, dipyridamole; HX, history; FU, follow up; ESRF, end stage renal failure.

Table 7b.3a. Accuracy of DSE for diagnosis of CAD in cardiac transplant patients

Author	Group	Test used	Sensitivity (%)	Specificity (%)
Akosah et al.[98]	41	DSE and CA	95	55
Akosah et al.[99]	82 (45 had CA)	DSE induced angina and CA	33	95
Bacal et al.[100]	39	24-h Holter, thallium scintigraphy, ETT, DSE	64	91
Ciliberto et al.[101]	68	DSE and CA	100	87
Derumeaux et al.[102]	37	DSE and CA at 37 and 56 mo post-OCT	(37 mo) 65, (56 mo) 92	95, 73
Derumeaux et al.[103]	55	DSE and CA	85	93
Derumeaux et al.[104]	37	DSE and CA	86	91
Gunther et al.[105]	20	DSE and CA	50	100
Herregods et al.[106]	28	DSE and CA	0	100
Spes et al.[107]	46	DSE, IVUS, and CA	(CA) 83, (IVUS) 79	56, 83
Spes et al.[108]	80	DSE, IVUS, and CA	85	71
Spes et al.[109]	109	DSE, IVUS, and CA	85	82

CA, coronary angiography; DSE, dobutamine stress echo; IVUS, intracoronary ultrasound; OCT, orthotopic cardiac transplant; ETT, exercise treadmill testing; MO, months.

6.3.4 Appropriate Responses

Patients with renal disease should have cardiovascular risk-factor modification[99] whether or not they have established cardiac disease. For patients with positive stress echoes who undergo coronary angiography, there is a risk of further impairment of renal reserve by contrast mediated nephropathy, particularly in those patients who are not dialysis dependent.[100] A recent review has suggested that patients with ESRF benefit from coronary revascularization either by CABG or PCI.[101] However, large randomized controlled trial data are required to support this and the value of this in a screening group needs to be defined.

6.4 Cardiac Transplants

6.4.1 Clinical

In patients with cardiac transplants, the risk of CAD is increased and the prevalence 5 years posttransplantation has been estimated at 42%.[96] Denervation of the transplanted heart removes warning symptoms of CAD such as angina and so screening for CAD is usually performed by coronary angiography. An alternative approach may be to use noninvasive methods to predict cardiac events, and some centers, however, have abandoned routine angiography.[97]

6.4.2 Echocardiography

A number of studies shown in Tables 7b.3a and 7b.3b have used SE in cardiac transplant patients. Recently recorded levels of sensitivity have been acceptable. The disease is often a diffuse process, so that angiography alone is suboptimal as the gold standard.

6.4.3 Alternate Strategies for Screening

MPS could be a useful alternative but other noninvasive tests, such as exercise testing or radionuclide ventriculography, have not been shown to be useful as screening tests.[112,113] EBCT is emerging as a promising technique[114,115] for assessment of CAD after transplantation.

Table 7b.3b. Prediction of events using DSE in cardiac transplant patients

Author	Group	Test used	Result	Outcome
Akosah et al.[98]	77	DSE	DSE positive in 57	33% had cardiac events in 2 yr FU
Akosah et al.[99]	22	DSE and CA	11 had persistent WMA	8/11 had events over mean FU 32 mo; no events in 11 patients with negative DSE
Ciliberto et al.[101]	68	DSE and CA	21 positive DSE	11/21 had cardiac events
Lewis et al.[111]	63	DSE	21 positive DSE, 42 negative DSE	5 events in 21, 1 event in 42

DSE, dobutamine stress echocardiography; CA, coronary angiography; WMA, wall motion abnormalities; MO, months.

6.4.4 Appropriate Responses

Revascularization in patients with cardiac transplants is complicated by the nature of the diffuse disease in graft coronary disease. For this reason, the use of CABG is limited.[116] PCI is more successful[117] and should be considered for severe lesions.

6.5 Noncardiac (Vascular) Surgery

6.5.1 Clinical

Patients undergoing surgery for peripheral vascular disease represent a high-risk group for silent coronary disease, even if they are asymptomatic.[118] From the standpoint of perioperative risk evaluation, the clinical risk factors as designated by Eagle et al.[119] usually determine the use of other testing to designate risk, because they are predictive of perioperative events.[120] Although patients without these predictors may very well have coronary disease and occasionally have positive studies (Figure 7b.7[121]), they rarely have events.[122]

The paucity of data regarding the screening of patients without these risk predictors reflects the age and comorbidity of this patient group, which tend to focus the process of screening on perioperative rather than long-term risk.

6.5.2 Echocardiography

Resting echocardiography is often requested in this patient group but has limited value as a routine test. In patients with a history of unexplained dyspnoea or previous heart failure diagnosis without an estimation of ejection fraction, the test may indeed guide perioperative therapy, especially regarding fluid management. Unfortunately, the value of routine echocardiography seems restricted to the prediction of perioperative heart failure, with a slightly higher frequency of sudden death in those with LV dysfunction.[123] Moreover, although the test is sometimes performed to identify silent ischemic heart disease, it is ischemia that determines risk – much more than infarction – so that patients with clinical risk variables warrant a stress test, not a resting echocardiogram.

SE is widely performed in at-risk patients undergoing major surgery. Because many such patients are unable to exercise, either because of peripheral vascular disease or other comorbidity, pharmacologic stress echo is usually performed – the most widely used stressor being dobutamine. Cardiac complications occur very rarely in those patients with normal studies, usually expressed as a very high negative predictive value (Table 7b.4).

The frequency of events in those with positive tests is about 20% overall (Table 7b.4) and may be substratified based on the number of clinical risk predictors (Figure 7b.8[139]).

An asymptomatic patient may score up to three Eagle factors for age, diabetes mellitus, and ECG evidence of silent infarction.

The other determinant of outcome in patients with a positive stress echocardiogram is the ischemic threshold,[121] which is the heart rate at which ischemia is first identified. Its importance

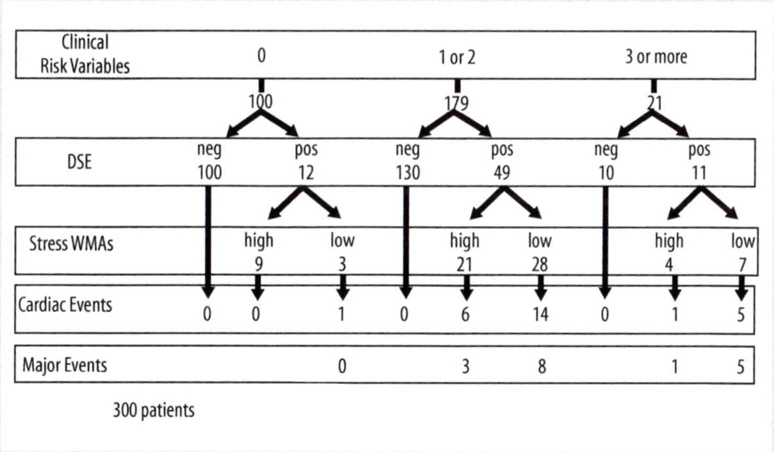

Figure 7b.7. Clinical variables and DSE results for perioperative outcome. WMAs, wall motion abnormalities; DSE, dobutamine stress echocardiography.

Table 7b.4. Predictive value of SE in perioperative outcomes

	n	PPV (%)	NPV (%)	Events
Lane et al.[124]	57	21	100	CD, MI, UA
Poldermans et al.[121]	300	38	100	CD, MI, UA, HF
Lalka et al.[125]	60	29	95	CD, MI, UA
Davila-Roman et al.[126]	93	83	100	CD, MI, UA, HF
Eichelberger et al.[127]	70	19	100	MI, UA
Langan et al.[128]	74	17	100	MI
Tischler et al.[129]	109	78	99	CD, MI, UA
Rossi et al.[130]	110	23	94	CD, MI, UA, HF
Pasquet et al.[131]	129	23	95	CD, MI, UA
Sicari et al.[132]	509	28	99	CD, MI, UA

PPV, positive predictive value; NPV, negative predictive value; CD, cardiovascular death; MI, myocardial infarction; UA, unstable angina; HF, heart failure.

mandates sequential videotape or digital recording of wall motion during the study; development of ischemia at a heart rate <70% of predicted maximum identifies the patient as being at particularly high risk of perioperative events – as high as 30%–50% in the presence of three or more risk factors. Whereas the use of dobutamine stress facilitates the acquisition of data at intermediate stages, gauging the time of onset of abnormal wall motion remains subjective. Interestingly, the extent of ischemia, although not a predictor of perioperative outcome, is a determinant of long-term outcome.[133]

6.5.3 Alternate Strategies for Screening

As mentioned above, exercise testing is rarely used in this patient population because the ability to exercise maximally is compromised by their underlying disease.

MPS has also been used extensively in risk evaluation of patients undergoing noncardiac surgery (see also Chapter 9b). The results of these studies have been closely analogous to those obtained with stress echo, with a very high negative predictive value and a positive predictive value usually in the 20% range. With this test, the extent of ischemia has been identified as an important determinant of risk.[134] Stress echo and nuclear approaches have been compared in head-to-head studies[135] and meta-analyses.[136] The results of these studies have shown equivalence between the two tests.

6.5.4 Appropriate Responses

In the diagnostic setting, the usual response to a positive stress echo is the performance of coronary angiography. This needs careful consideration in the vascular surgery group for several reasons. First, the risk of the procedure is greater than usual, with respect to both complicated atheroma and concomitant disease, which may, for example, increase the risk of renal sequelae. Second, the evidence to support percutaneous revascularization as a means of reducing perioperative risk is scant, and although there are some data in favor of selective surgical revascularization,[137] many such patients are not good candidates for cardiac surgery on the basis of age or comorbidity. However, β-adrenoceptor blockers have been shown to be effective,[138] although

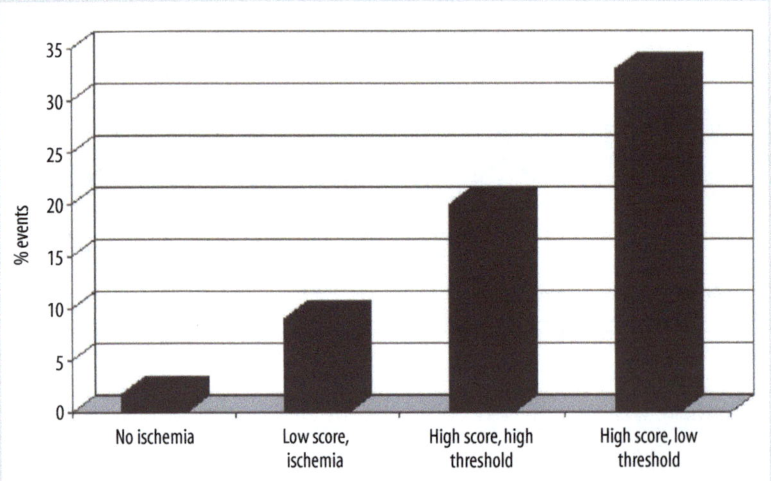

Figure 7b.8. Risk of perioperative events in patients with and without ischemia at high and low threshold and clinical risk variables.

not in the highest-risk patients. Therefore, the allocation of risk on the basis of clinical status and stress testing results may facilitate selection of individualized therapy.

7. Conclusion

Echocardiography provides useful information for high-risk asymptomatic patients. When combined with stress, a powerful prognostic tool is available that can unmask previously undiagnosed CAD. The application of this to screening is constrained by overall low disease probability in unselected asymptomatic patients, but the use of clinical tools, such as the Framingham risk score, can define a subgroup, which will be enriched with high-risk individuals.

We have examined the role of SE and other imaging modalities in various high-risk subgroups. Overall, SE seems to have a good predictive value comparable to that of MPS and in certain cases may avoid the need for coronary angiography. For those who have abnormalities on a noninvasive imaging test and are asymptomatic, a management plan needs to be defined. This includes a choice of addressing cardiac risk factors, or invasive assessment of coronary anatomy by angiography with a view to possible revascularization if necessary. In many of the high-risk subgroups we have discussed, the decision to proceed to revascularization is hampered by the lack of large randomized trials to support this approach. Although SE and MPS can provide prognostic data in high-risk subgroups, further clarification with multicenter studies is required to assess under what circumstances revascularization can alter prognosis in high-risk patients who are truly asymptomatic.

References

1. Lindsey HE Jr, Cohn PF. "Silent" myocardial ischemia during and after exercise testing in patients with coronary artery disease. Am Heart J 1978;95:441–447.
2. Almeda FQ, Kason TT, Nathan S, Kavinsky CJ. Silent myocardial ischemia: concepts and controversies. Am J Med 2004;116:112–118.
3. Gandelman G, Bodenheimer MM. Screening coronary arteriography in the primary prevention of coronary artery disease. Heart Dis 2003;5:335–344.
4. Scanlon PJ, Faxon DP, Audet AM, et al. ACC/AHA guidelines for coronary angiography: executive summary and recommendations. A report of the American College of Cardiology/American Heart Association Task Force on Practice Guidelines (Committee on Coronary Angiography) developed in collaboration with the Society for Cardiac Angiography and Interventions. Circulation 1999;99:2345–2357.
5. Sicari R, Pasanisi E, Venneri L, Landi P, Cortigiani L, Picano E. Stress echo results predict mortality: a large-scale multicenter prospective international study. J Am Coll Cardiol 2003;41:589–595.
6. Marwick TH, Case C, Sawada S, et al. Prediction of mortality using dobutamine echocardiography. J Am Coll Cardiol 2001;37:754–760.
7. Pizzuto F, Voci P, Romeo F. Value of echocardiography in predicting future cardiac events after acute myocardial infarction. Curr Opin Cardiol 2003;18:378–384.
8. Butler JR. Economic evaluations of screening programs: a review of methods and results. Clin Chim Acta 2002;315:31–40.
9. Myerburg RJ, Kessler KM, Castellanos A. Sudden cardiac death – epidemiology, transient risk, and intervention assessment. Ann Intern Med 1993;119: 1187–1197.
10. Kannel WB, Doyle JT, McNamara PM, Quickenton P, Gordon T. Precursors of sudden coronary death. Factors related to the incidence of sudden death. Circulation 1975;51:606–613.
11. Diamond GA, Forrester JS. Analysis of probability as an aid in the clinical diagnosis of coronary-artery disease. N Engl J Med 1979;300:1350–1358.
12. Elhendy A, Shub C, McCully RB, Mahoney DW, Burger KN, Pellikka PA. Exercise echocardiography for the prognostic stratification of patients with low pretest probability of coronary artery disease. Am J Med 2001; 111:18–23.
13. Hennessy TG, Codd MB, Kane G, McCarthy C, McCann HA, Sugrue DD. Dobutamine stress echocardiography in the detection of coronary artery disease: importance of the pretest likelihood of disease. Am Heart J 1997;134:685–692.
14. Wilson PW, D'Agostino RB, Levy D, Belanger AM, Silbershatz H, Kannel WB. Prediction of coronary heart disease using risk factor categories. Circulation 1998;97:1837–1847.
15. Eagle KA, Brundage BH, Chaitman BR, et al. Guidelines for perioperative cardiovascular evaluation for noncardiac surgery. Report of the American College of Cardiology/American Heart Association Task Force on Practice Guidelines (Committee on Perioperative Cardiovascular Evaluation for Noncardiac Surgery). J Am Coll Cardiol 1996;27:910–948.
16. Marwick TH, Case C, Sawada S, Vasey C, Short L, Lauer M. Use of stress echocardiography to predict mortality in patients with diabetes and known or suspected coronary artery disease. Diabetes Care 2002;25: 1042–1048.
17. Herzog CA, Marwick TH, Pheley AM, White CW, Rao VK, Dick CD. Dobutamine stress echocardiography for the detection of significant coronary artery disease in renal transplant candidates. Am J Kidney Dis 1999;33:1080–1090. With Dussol B, Bonnet JL, Sampol J, Savin B, De La FC, Mundler D, et al. Prognostic value of inducible myocardial ischemia in predicting cardiovascular events after renal transplantation. Kidney Int 2004;66:1633–1639.
18. Akosah KO, McDaniel S, Hanrahan JS, Mohanty PK. Dobutamine stress echocardiography early after heart transplantation predicts development of allograft

coronary artery disease and outcome. J Am Coll Cardiol 1998;31:1607–1614.
19. Marwick TH, Lauer MS, Lobo A, Nally J, Braun W. Use of dobutamine echocardiography for cardiac risk stratification of patients with chronic renal failure. J Intern Med 1998;244:155–161.
20. Madu EC. Transesophageal dobutamine stress echocardiography in the evaluation of myocardial ischemia in morbidly obese subjects. Chest 2000; 117:657–661.
21. Mocini D, Uguccioni M, Galli C, et al. Dipyridamole echocardiography and 99mTc-MIBI SPECT dipyridamole scintigraphy for cardiac evaluation prior to peripheral vascular surgery. Minerva Cardioangiol 1995;43:185–190.
22. Davar JI, Roberts EB, Coghlan JG, Evans TR, Lipkin DP. Prognostic value of stress echocardiography in women with high (≥80%) probability of coronary artery disease. Postgrad Med J 2001;77:573–577.
23. Wang TJ, Levy D, Benjamin EJ, Vasan RS. The epidemiology of "asymptomatic" left ventricular systolic dysfunction: implications for screening. Ann Intern Med 2003;138:907–916.
24. McDonagh TA, Cunningham AD, Morrison CE, et al. Left ventricular dysfunction, natriuretic peptides, and mortality in an urban population. Heart 2001;86: 21–26.
25. Geleijnse ML, Fioretti PM, Roelandt JR. Methodology, feasibility, safety and diagnostic accuracy of dobutamine stress echocardiography. J Am Coll Cardiol 1997; 30:595–606.
26. Geleijnse ML, Elhendy A. Can stress echocardiography compete with perfusion scintigraphy in the detection of coronary artery disease and cardiac risk assessment? Eur J Echocardiogr 2000;1:12–21.
27. Schinkel AF, Bax JJ, Geleijnse ML, et al. Noninvasive evaluation of ischemic heart disease: myocardial perfusion imaging or stress echocardiography? Eur Heart J 2003;24:789–800.
28. Cortigiani L, Bigi R, Gigli G, et al. Prognostic implications of intraventricular conduction defects in patients undergoing stress echocardiography for suspected coronary artery disease. Am J Med 2003;115: 12–18.
29. Cortigiani L, Bigi R, Rigo F, et al. Diagnostic value of exercise electrocardiography and dipyridamole stress echocardiography in hypertensive and normotensive chest pain patients with right bundle branch block. J Hypertens 2003;21:2189–2194.
30. Amici E, Cortigiani L, Coletta C, et al. Usefulness of pharmacologic stress echocardiography for the long-term prognostic assessment of patients with typical versus atypical chest pain. Am J Cardiol 2003; 91:440–442.
31. Davies RF, Goldberg AD, Forman S, et al. Asymptomatic Cardiac Ischemia Pilot (ACIP) study two-year follow-up: outcomes of patients randomized to initial strategies of medical therapy versus revascularization. Circulation 1997;95:2037–2043.
32. Gibbons RJ, Balady GJ, Bricker JT, et al. ACC/AHA 2002 guideline update for exercise testing: summary article: a report of the American College of Cardiology/American Heart Association Task Force on Practice Guidelines (Committee to Update the 1997 Exercise Testing Guidelines). Circulation 2002;106: 1883–1892.
33. Ekelund LG, Suchindran CM, McMahon RP, et al. Coronary heart disease morbidity and mortality in hypercholesterolemic men predicted from an exercise test: the Lipid Research Clinics Coronary Primary Prevention Trial. J Am Coll Cardiol 1989;14:556–563.
34. Rautaharju PM, Prineas RJ, Eifler WJ, et al. Prognostic value of exercise electrocardiogram in men at high risk of future coronary heart disease: Multiple Risk Factor Intervention Trial experience. J Am Coll Cardiol 1986;8:1–10.
35. Gibbons LW, Mitchell TL, Wei M, Blair SN, Cooper KH. Maximal exercise test as a predictor of risk for mortality from coronary heart disease in asymptomatic men. Am J Cardiol 2000;86:53–58.
36. Marwick TH, Case C, Short L, Thomas JD. Prediction of mortality in patients without angina: use of an exercise score and exercise echocardiography. Eur Heart J 2003;24:1223–1230.
37. Blumenthal RS, Becker DM, Moy TF, Coresh J, Wilder LB, Becker LC. Exercise thallium tomography predicts future clinically manifest coronary heart disease in a high-risk asymptomatic population. Circulation 1996; 93:915–923.
38. Fleg JL, Gerstenblith G, Zonderman AB, et al. Prevalence and prognostic significance of exercise-induced silent myocardial ischemia detected by thallium scintigraphy and electrocardiography in asymptomatic volunteers. Circulation 1990;81:428–436.
39. Smith SC Jr, Greenland P, Grundy SM. AHA Conference Proceedings. Prevention conference V: beyond secondary prevention: identifying the high-risk patient for primary prevention: executive summary. American Heart Association. Circulation 2000;101: 111–116.
40. Third Report of the National Cholesterol Education Program (NCEP) Expert Panel on Detection, Evaluation, and Treatment of High Blood Cholesterol in Adults (Adult Treatment Panel III) Final Report. Circulation 2002;106:3143.
41. Chobanian AV, Bakris GL, Black HR, et al. Seventh report of the Joint National Committee on prevention, detection, evaluation, and treatment of high blood pressure. Hypertension 2003;42:1206–1252.
42. Pan WH, Cedres LB, Liu K, et al. Relationship of clinical diabetes and asymptomatic hyperglycemia to risk of coronary heart disease mortality in men and women. Am J Epidemiol 1986;123:504–516.
43. Stamler J, Vaccaro O, Neaton JD, Wentworth D. Diabetes, other risk factors, and 12-yr cardiovascular mortality for men screened in the Multiple Risk Factor Intervention Trial. Diabetes Care 1993;16:434–444.
44. Wilson PW, Cupples LA, Kannel WB. Is hyperglycemia associated with cardiovascular disease? The Framingham Study. Am Heart J 1991;121:586–590.
45. Sayer JW, Timmis AD. Investigation of coronary artery disease in diabetes: is screening of asymptomatic patients necessary? Heart 1997;78:525–526.
46. Janand-Delenne B, Savin B, Habib G, Bory M, Vague P, Lassmann-Vague V. Silent myocardial ischemia in patients with diabetes: who to screen. Diabetes Care 1999;22:1396–1400.
47. Picano E. Diabetic cardiomyopathy: the importance of being earliest. J Am Coll Cardiol 2003;42:454–457.

48. Fang ZY, Yuda S, Anderson V, Short L, Case C, Marwick TH. Echocardiographic detection of early diabetic myocardial disease. J Am Coll Cardiol 2003;41:611–617.
49. Fang ZY, Najos-Valencia O, Leano R, Marwick TH. Patients with early diabetic heart disease demonstrate a normal myocardial response to dobutamine. J Am Coll Cardiol 2003;42:446–453.
50. Bacci S, Russo A, Rauseo A, Fanelli R, Trischitta V. The role of dobutamine stress echocardiography in detecting severe coronary artery disease in asymptomatic at high risk type 2 diabetic patients. Diabetes Care 2002;25:1659.
51. Coisne D, Donal E, Torremocha F, Christiaens L, Allal J. Dobutamine stress echocardiography response of asymptomatic patients with diabetes. Echocardiography 2001;18:373–379.
52. Elhendy A, van Domburg RT, Poldermans D, et al. Safety and feasibility of dobutamine-atropine stress echocardiography for the diagnosis of coronary artery disease in diabetic patients unable to perform an exercise stress test. Diabetes Care 1998;21:1797–1802.
53. Gaddi O, Tortorella G, Picano E, et al. Diagnostic and prognostic value of vasodilator stress echocardiography in asymptomatic type 2 diabetic patients with positive exercise thallium scintigraphy: a pilot study. Diabet Med 1999;16:762–766.
54. Griffin ME, Nikookam K, Teh MM, McCann H, O'Meara NM, Firth RG. Dobutamine stress echocardiography: false positive scans in proteinuric patients with type 1 diabetes mellitus at high risk of ischemic heart disease. Diabet Med 1998;15:427–430.
55. Hennessy TG, Codd MB, Kane G, McCarthy C, McCann HA, Sugrue DD. Evaluation of patients with diabetes mellitus for coronary artery disease using dobutamine stress echocardiography. Coron Artery Dis 1997;8:171–174.
56. Hung MJ, Wang CH, Cherng WJ. Can dobutamine stress echocardiography predict cardiac events in nonrevascularized diabetic patients following acute myocardial infarction? Chest 1999;116:1224–1232.
57. Penfornis A, Zimmermann C, Boumal D, et al. Use of dobutamine stress echocardiography in detecting silent myocardial ischemia in asymptomatic diabetic patients: a comparison with thallium scintigraphy and exercise testing. Diabet Med 2001;18:900–905.
58. Bates JR, Sawada SG, Segar DS, et al. Evaluation using dobutamine stress echocardiography in patients with insulin-dependent diabetes mellitus before kidney and/or pancreas transplantation. Am J Cardiol 1996;77:175–179.
59. Bigi R, Desideri A, Cortigiani L, Bax JJ, Celegon L, Fiorentini C. Stress echocardiography for risk stratification of diabetic patients with known or suspected coronary artery disease. Diabetes Care 2001;24:1596–1601.
60. D'Andrea A, Severino S, Caso P, et al. Prognostic value of pharmacological stress echocardiography in diabetic patients. Eur J Echocardiogr 2003;4:202–208.
61. Elhendy A, Arruda AM, Mahoney DW, Pellikka PA. Prognostic stratification of diabetic patients by exercise echocardiography. J Am Coll Cardiol 2001;37:1551–1557.
62. Kamalesh M, Matorin R, Sawada S. Prognostic value of a negative stress echocardiographic study in diabetic patients. Am Heart J 2002;143:163–168.
63. Sozzi FB, Elhendy A, Roelandt JR, et al. Prognostic value of dobutamine stress echocardiography in patients with diabetes. Diabetes Care 2003;26:1074–1078.
64. Bacci S, Villella M, Villella A, et al. Screening for silent myocardial ischemia in type 2 diabetic patients with additional atherogenic risk factors: applicability and accuracy of the exercise stress test. Eur J Endocrinol 2002;147:649–654.
65. Wolfe ML, Iqbal N, Gefter W, Mohler ER III, Rader DJ, Reilly MP. Coronary artery calcification at electron beam computed tomography is increased in asymptomatic type 2 diabetics independent of traditional risk factors. J Cardiovasc Risk 2002;9:369–376.
66. Standards of medical care for patients with diabetes mellitus. Diabetes Care 2002;25:33S–49.
67. L'huillier I, Cottin Y, Touzery C, et al. Predictive value of myocardial tomoscintigraphy in asymptomatic diabetic patients after percutaneous coronary intervention. Int J Cardiol 2003;90:165–173.
68. Seven-year outcome in the Bypass Angioplasty Revascularization Investigation (BARI) by treatment and diabetic status. J Am Coll Cardiol 2000;35:1122–1129.
69. King SB III, Kosinski AS, Guyton RA, Lembo NJ, Weintraub WS. Eight-year mortality in the Emory Angioplasty versus Surgery Trial (EAST). J Am Coll Cardiol 2000;35:1116–1121.
70. Schofer J, Schluter M, Rau T, Hammer F, Haag N, Mathey DG. Influence of treatment modality on angiographic outcome after coronary stenting in diabetic patients: a controlled study. J Am Coll Cardiol 2000;35:1554–1559.
71. Abizaid A, Kornowski R, Mintz GS, et al. The influence of diabetes mellitus on acute and late clinical outcomes following coronary stent implantation. J Am Coll Cardiol 1998;32:584–589.
72. Kennedy R, Case C, Fathi R, Johnson D, Isbel N, Marwick TH. Does renal failure cause an atherosclerotic milieu in patients with end-stage renal disease? Am J Med 2001;110:198–204.
73. Sarnak MJ, Levey AS. Epidemiology of cardiac disease in dialysis patients. Semin Dial 1999;12:69–76.
74. Le A, Wilson R, Douek K, et al. Prospective risk stratification in renal transplant candidates for cardiac death. Am J Kidney Dis 1994;24:65–71.
75. Foley RN, Parfrey PS, Harnett JD, et al. Clinical and echocardiographic disease in patients starting end-stage renal disease therapy. Kidney Int 1995;47:186–192.
76. Boudreau RJ, Strony JT, duCret RP, et al. Perfusion thallium imaging of type I diabetes patients with end stage renal disease: comparison of oral and intravenous dipyridamole administration. Radiology 1990;175:103–105.
77. Marwick TH, Steinmuller DR, Underwood DA, et al. Ineffectiveness of dipyridamole SPECT thallium imaging as a screening technique for coronary artery disease in patients with end-stage renal failure. Transplantation 1990;49:100–103.
78. Vandenberg BF, Rossen JD, Grover-McKay M, Shammas NW, Burns TL, Rezai K. Evaluation of diabetic patients for renal and pancreas transplantation: noninvasive screening for coronary artery disease using radionuclide methods. Transplantation 1996;62:1230–1235.

79. Dahan M, Viron BM, Faraggi M, et al. Diagnostic accuracy and prognostic value of combined dipyridamole-exercise thallium imaging in hemodialysis patients. Kidney Int 1998;54:255–262.
80. Reis G, Marcovitz PA, Leichtman AB, et al. Usefulness of dobutamine stress echocardiography in detecting coronary artery disease in end-stage renal disease. Am J Cardiol 1995;75:707–710.
81. Herzog CA, Marwick TH, Pheley AM, White CW, Rao VK, Dick CD. Dobutamine stress echocardiography for the detection of significant coronary artery disease in renal transplant candidates. Am J Kidney Dis 1999;33:1080–1090.
82. Brennan DC, Vedala G, Miller SB, et al. Pretransplant dobutamine stress echocardiography is useful and cost-effective in renal transplant candidates. Transplant Proc 1997;29:233–234.
83. Morrow CE, Schwartz JS, Sutherland DE, et al. Predictive value of thallium stress testing for coronary and cardiovascular events in uremic diabetic patients before renal transplantation. Am J Surg 1983; 146:331–335.
84. Brown KA, Rimmer J, Haisch C. Noninvasive cardiac risk stratification of diabetic and nondiabetic uremic renal allograft candidates using dipyridamole-thallium-201 imaging and radionuclide ventriculography. Am J Cardiol 1989;64:1017–1021.
85. Camp AD, Garvin PJ, Hoff J, Marsh J, Byers SL, Chaitman BR. Prognostic value of intravenous dipyridamole thallium imaging in patients with diabetes mellitus considered for renal transplantation. Am J Cardiol 1990;65:1459–1463.
86. Holley JL, Fenton RA, Arthur RS. Thallium stress testing does not predict cardiovascular risk in diabetic patients with end-stage renal disease undergoing cadaveric renal transplantation. Am J Med 1991; 90:563–570.
87. Derfler K, Kletter K, Balcke P, Heinz G, Dudczak R. Predictive value of thallium-201-dipyridamole myocardial stress scintigraphy in chronic hemodialysis patients and transplant recipients. Clin Nephrol 1991; 36:192–202.
88. Brown JH, Vites NP, Testa HJ, et al. Value of thallium myocardial imaging in the prediction of future cardiovascular events in patients with end-stage renal failure. Nephrol Dial Transplant 1993;8:433–437.
89. Lewis MS, Wilson RA, Walker KW, Wilson DJ, Norman DJ, Barry JM, et al. Validation of an algorithm for predicting cardiac events in renal transplant candidates. Am J Cardiol 2002;89:847–850.
90. Heston TF, Norman DJ, Barry JM, Bennett WM, Wilson RA. Cardiac risk stratification in renal transplantation using a form of artificial intelligence. Am J Cardiol 1997;79:415–417.
91. Goodman WG, Goldin J, Kuizon BD, et al. Coronary-artery calcification in young adults with end-stage renal disease who are undergoing dialysis. N Engl J Med 2000;342:1478–1483.
92. Hatada K, Sugiura T, Nakamura S, et al. Coronary artery diameter and left ventricular function in patients on maintenance hemodialysis treatment: comparison between diabetic and nondiabetic patients. Nephron 1998;80:269–273.
93. Jaradat MI, Molitoris BA. Cardiovascular disease in patients with chronic kidney disease. Semin Nephrol 2002;22:459–473.
94. Gruberg L, Mintz GS, Mehran R, et al. The prognostic implications of further renal function deterioration within 48 h of interventional coronary procedures in patients with pre-existent chronic renal insufficiency. J Am Coll Cardiol 2000;36:1542–1548.
95. Keeley EC, McCullough PA. Coronary revascularization in patients with end-stage renal disease: risks, benefits, and optimal strategies. Rev Cardiovasc Med 2003;4:125–130.
96. Costanzo MR, Naftel DC, Pritzker MR, et al. Heart transplant coronary artery disease detected by coronary angiography: a multiinstitutional study of preoperative donor and recipient risk factors. Cardiac Transplant Research Database. J Heart Lung Transplant 1998;17:744–753.
97. Grant SC, Brooks NH, Levy RD. Routine coronary angiography after heart transplantation. Heart 1997; 78:101–102.
98. Akosah KO, Mohanty PK, Funai JT, et al. Noninvasive detection of transplant coronary artery disease by dobutamine stress echocardiography. J Heart Lung Transplant 1994;13:1024–1038.
99. Akosah K, Olsovsky M, Mohanty PK. Dobutamine stress-induced angina in patients with denervated cardiac transplants. Clinical and angiographic correlates. Chest 1995;108:695–700.
100. Bacal F, Stolf NA, Veiga VC, et al. Noninvasive diagnosis of allograft vascular disease after heart transplantation. Arq BrasCardiol 2001;76:29–42.
101. Ciliberto GR, Parodi O, Cataldo G, et al. Prognostic value of contractile response during high-dose dipyridamole echocardiography test in heart transplant recipients. J Heart Lung Transplant 2003;22:526–532.
102. Derumeaux G, Redonnet M, Soyer R, Cribier A, Letac B. Assessment of the progression of cardiac allograft vasculopathy by dobutamine stress echocardiography. J Heart Lung Transplant 1998;17:259–267.
103. Derumeaux G, Redonnet M, Mouton-Schleifer D, Cribier A, Soyer R, Letac B. [Value of dobutamine echocardiography in the detection of coronary disease in heart transplant patient. Groupe de Recherche VACOMED.] Arch Mal Coeur Vaiss 1996;89:687–694.
104. Derumeaux G, Redonnet M, Mouton-Schleifer D, et al. Dobutamine stress echocardiography in orthotopic heart transplant recipients. VACOMED Research Group. J Am Coll Cardiol 1995;25:1665–1672.
105. Gunther F, Schwammenthal E, Rahmel A, et al. [Initial experiences with dobutamine stress echocardiography in heart transplant patients.] Z Kardiol 1995;84: 411–418.
106. Herregods MC, Anastassiou I, Van Cleemput J, et al. Dobutamine stress echocardiography after heart transplantation. J Heart Lung Transplant 1994;13: 1039–1044.
107. Spes CH, Mudra H, Schnaack SD, et al. Dobutamine stress echocardiography for noninvasive diagnosis of cardiac allograft vasculopathy: a comparison with angiography and intravascular ultrasound. Am J Cardiol 1996;78:168–174.
108. Spes CH, Klauss V, Mudra H, et al. [Quantitative dobutamine stress echocardiography in follow-up of heart transplantation: normal values and findings in patients with transplant vasculopathy.] Z Kardiol 1997;86:868–876.

109. Spes CH, Klauss V, Mudra H, et al. Diagnostic and prognostic value of serial dobutamine stress echocardiography for noninvasive assessment of cardiac allograft vasculopathy: a comparison with coronary angiography and intravascular ultrasound. Circulation 1999;100:509–515.
110. Akosah KO, Olsovsky M, Kirchberg D, Salter D, Mohanty PK. Dobutamine stress echocardiography predicts cardiac events in heart transplant patients. Circulation 1996;94:II283–II288.
111. Lewis JF, Selman SB, Murphy JD, Mills RM Jr, Geiser EA, Conti CR. Dobutamine echocardiography for prediction of ischemic events in heart transplant recipients. J Heart Lung Transplant 1997; 16:390–393.
112. Fang JC, Rocco T, Jarcho J, Ganz P, Mudge GH. Noninvasive assessment of transplant-associated arteriosclerosis. Am Heart J 1998;135:980–987.
113. Smart FW, Ballantyne CM, Cocanougher B, et al. Insensitivity of noninvasive tests to detect coronary artery vasculopathy after heart transplant. Am J Cardiol 1991;67:243–247.
114. Ludman PF, Lazem F, Barbir M, Yacoub M. Incidence and clinical relevance of coronary calcification detected by electron beam computed tomography in heart transplant recipients. Eur Heart J 1999;20: 303–308.
115. Knollmann FD, Bocksch W, Spiegelsberger S, Hetzer R, Felix R, Hummel M. Electron-beam computed tomography in the assessment of coronary artery disease after heart transplantation. Circulation 2000;101: 2078–2082.
116. Musci M, Pasic M, Meyer R, et al. Coronary artery bypass grafting after orthotopic heart transplantation. Eur J Cardiothorac Surg 1999;16:163–168.
117. Parry A, Roberts M, Parameshwar J, Wallwork J, Schofield P, Large S. The management of post-cardiac transplantation coronary artery disease. Eur J Cardiothorac Surg 1996;10:528–532.
118. Hertzer NR. Basic data concerning associated coronary disease in peripheral vascular patients. Ann Vasc Surg 1987;1:616–620.
119. Eagle KA, Coley CM, Newell JB, et al. Combining clinical and thallium data optimizes preoperative assessment of cardiac risk before major vascular surgery. Ann Intern Med 1989;110:859–866.
120. Eagle KA, Berger PB, Calkins H, et al. ACC/AHA guideline update for perioperative cardiovascular evaluation for noncardiac surgery – executive summary: a report of the American College of Cardiology/ American Heart Association Task Force on Practice Guidelines (Committee to Update the 1996 Guidelines on Perioperative Cardiovascular Evaluation for Noncardiac Surgery). J Am Coll Cardiol 2002;39:542–553.
121. Poldermans D, Arnese M, Fioretti PM, et al. Improved cardiac risk stratification in major vascular surgery with dobutamine-atropine stress echocardiography. J Am Coll Cardiol 1995;26:648–653.
122. Kertai MD, Klein J, van Urk H, Bax JJ, Poldermans D. Cardiac complications after elective major vascular surgery. Acta Anaesthesiol Scand 2003;47:643–654.
123. Halm EA, Browner WS, Tubau JF, Tateo IM, Mangano DT. Echocardiography for assessing cardiac risk in patients having noncardiac surgery. Study of Perioperative Ischemia Research Group. Ann Intern Med 1996;125:433–441.
124. Lane RT, Sawada SG, Segar DS, et al. Dobutamine stress echocardiography for assessment of cardiac risk before noncardiac surgery. Am J Cardiol 1991;68: 976–977.
125. Lalka SG, Sawada SG, Dalsing MC, et al. Dobutamine stress echocardiography as a predictor of cardiac events associated with aortic surgery. J Vasc Surg 1992;15:831–840.
126. Davila-Roman VG, Waggoner AD, Sicard GA, Geltman EM, Schechtman KB, Perez JE. Dobutamine stress echocardiography predicts surgical outcome in patients with an aortic aneurysm and peripheral vascular disease. J Am Coll Cardiol 1993;21:957–963.
127. Eichelberger JP, Schwarz KQ, Black ER, Green RM, Ouriel K. Predictive value of dobutamine echocardiography just before noncardiac vascular surgery. Am J Cardiol 1993;72:602–607.
128. Langan EM III, Youkey JR, Franklin DP, Elmore JR, Costello JM, Nassef LA. Dobutamine stress echocardiography for cardiac risk assessment before aortic surgery. J Vasc Surg 1993;18:905–911.
129. Tischler MD, Lee TH, Hirsch AT, et al. Prediction of major cardiac events after peripheral vascular surgery using dipyridamole echocardiography. Am J Cardiol 1991;68:593–597.
130. Rossi E, Citterio F, Vescio MF, et al. Risk stratification of patients undergoing peripheral vascular revascularization by combined resting and dipyridamole echocardiography. Am J Cardiol 1998;82:306–310.
131. Pasquet A, D'Hondt AM, Verhelst R, Vanoverschelde JL, Melin J, Marwick TH. Comparison of dipyridamole stress echocardiography and perfusion scintigraphy for cardiac risk stratification in vascular surgery patients. Am J Cardiol 1998;82:1468–1474.
132. Sicari R, Ripoli A, Picano E, et al. Perioperative prognostic value of dipyridamole echocardiography in vascular surgery: a large-scale multicenter study in 509 patients. EPIC (Echo Persantine International Cooperative) Study Group. Circulation 1999;100: II269–II274.
133. Poldermans D, Arnese M, Fioretti PM, et al. Sustained prognostic value of dobutamine stress echocardiography for late cardiac events after major noncardiac vascular surgery. Circulation 1997;95:53–58.
134. Lette J, Waters D, Lassonde J, et al. Multivariate clinical models and quantitative dipyridamole-thallium imaging to predict cardiac morbidity and death after vascular reconstruction. J Vasc Surg 1991;14:160–169.
135. van Daele ME, McNeill AJ, Fioretti PM, et al. Prognostic value of dipyridamole sestamibi single-photon emission computed tomography and dipyridamole stress echocardiography for new cardiac events after an uncomplicated myocardial infarction. J Am Soc Echocardiogr 1994;7:370–380.
136. Shaw LJ, Eagle KA, Gersh BJ, Miller DD. Meta-analysis of intravenous dipyridamole-thallium-201 imaging (1985 to 1994) and dobutamine echocardiography (1991 to 1994) for risk stratification before vascular surgery. J Am Coll Cardiol 1996;27:787–798.
137. Landesberg G, Mosseri M, Wolf YG, et al. Preoperative thallium scanning, selective coronary revasculariza-

tion, and long-term survival after major vascular surgery. Circulation 2003;108:177–183.
138. Kertai MD, Boersma E, Bax JJ, et al. Optimizing long-term cardiac management after major vascular surgery: role of beta-blocker therapy, clinical characteristics, and dobutamine stress echocardiography to optimize long-term cardiac management after major vascular surgery. Arch Intern Med 2003;163: 2230–2235.
139. Torres MR, Short L, Baglin T, Case C, Gibbs H, Marwick TH. Usefulness of clinical risk markers and ischemic threshold to stratify risk in patients undergoing major noncardiac surgery. Am J Cardiol 2002; 90:238–242.

8

Diagnosis of Coronary Artery Disease

Eliana Reyes, Nicholas Bunce, Roxy Senior,
and Constantinos D. Anagnostopoulos

An estimated 16.7 million people die of cardiovascular diseases every year with 43% of these deaths being attributed to atheromatous coronary artery disease (CAD).[1] CAD represents the leading cause of death worldwide, with most cases occurring in developing nations. In recent years, there has been a decline in mortality rate associated with CAD in developed countries that has been attributed to a better identification of high-risk subjects, availability and rapid access to accurate diagnostic procedures, and also development of highly effective therapeutic interventions, all of which have contributed to a substantial increase of costs in health care. At times of economic constraints, it has become of paramount importance to ensure that medical care is delivered in the most cost-effective way around the world. A clear understanding of the disease and methods used for its identification would provide the basis for a judicious management and a more efficient use of resources. In this regard, noninvasive diagnostic procedures have demonstrated to have a major role in the assessment of patients investigated for CAD.

Exercise electrocardiogram (ECG), myocardial perfusion scintigraphy (MPS), and stress echocardiography are the most frequently used techniques for this purpose. Exercise radionuclide ventriculography has been used in the past for the diagnosis of CAD but, currently, stress MPS is the preferred radionuclide technique for this purpose. Although still an evolving modality, cardiovascular magnetic resonance (CMR) has demonstrated to be highly effective in the detection of myocardial ischemia and, more recently, multislice computed tomography (MS-CT) has been introduced as a promising modality for assessment of coronary artery anomalies and also for identification of lesions and assessment of calcium in the coronaries. The clinical potential of the latter and also of electron beam computed tomography (EBCT) has been discussed in the previous chapter. Herein, after a short discussion on the initial approach to patients presenting with symptoms of CAD, we focus on the characteristics and role of the mainstream noninvasive imaging modalities and their relative strengths and limitations for diagnosing CAD.

1. Clinical Diagnosis of CAD

1.1 Medical History and Physical Examination

The medical history remains the first and most important diagnostic tool available to the physician, because a decision to investigate further relies on the initial clinical impression. Angina, the most specific symptom for myocardial ischemia secondary to obstructive CAD, is classically defined as a retrosternal, pressure-like discomfort or central chest tightness precipitated by exertion or emotional stress, accompanied by a sense of uneasiness, and relieved within minutes by rest or sublingual glyceryl trinitrate. However, not all patients with CAD present with typical angina, and thus it is a relatively insensitive marker of disease. In many patients, myocardial ischemia is associated with less typical features, including discomfort in one or both arms, shoulders, jaw, or epigastrium, as well as nonexertional symptoms. Moreover, comorbidities such as diabetes mellitus and ischemia-induced left ventricular dysfunction may affect the quality of anginal symptoms resulting in a wide constellation of manifestations, which are often referred to as angina equivalents. In the presence of typical symptoms of angina, the clinical diagnosis is straightforward and additional noninvasive testing might be indicated to assess the extent and severity of underlying myocardial ischemia. A complete medical history may therefore provide the correct diagnosis in some cases, and may also help identify cardiovascular risk factors, such as smoking and family history, which increase the probability of coronary disease and have important prognostic implications.[2,3]

Along with the clinical history, a complete physical examination may contribute to the diagnosis of CAD, although in the great majority of patients it will be normal. However, a careful examination may reveal signs associated with an increased risk of coronary disease, such as xanthelasma, corneal arcus, elevated blood pressure, and abnormal pulses suggestive of peripheral vascular disease. Moreover, it may help identify conditions that precipitate myocardial ischemia, such as thyroid disease, anemia, valvular heart disease, and hypertrophic cardiomyopathy, whereas signs of ventricular failure would suggest the presence of severe underlying CAD. Finally, it is important to consider conditions other than coronary disease that may compromise myocardial blood flow (MBF) and provoke ischemia, such as anomalous coronary arteries, vasculitis, Kawasaki's disease, and coronary embolization secondary to atrial tumor or thrombus (see also Chapter 14).

1.2 Resting Electrocardiography

The easy access to portable electrocardiographic equipment has made the ECG a readily available tool that alongside the clinical history and the physical examination aids in the diagnosis of CAD. When present, dynamic ST-segment and T-wave changes strongly suggest the presence of obstructive coronary disease. However, most patients with stable angina and angiographically proven coronary stenosis will have a normal ECG.[4] In the remainder, abnormal Q waves or repolarization changes suggestive of myocardial injury, and atrioventricular or intraventricular conduction abnormalities [i.e., left bundle branch block (LBBB) and left anterior fascicular block] secondary to underlying ischemia can be observed. All these changes are nonspecific with an increased prevalence in the elderly as well as in hypertensive subjects and in those taking antiarrhythmic medication. Therefore, both the sensitivity and specificity of electrocardiographic findings are relatively low, adding little to the diagnosis of CAD.[5]

1.3 Chest X-ray

Normal in the majority of patients with chronic stable chest pain, a well-performed posteroanterior or frontal projection can provide additional information to the diagnosis of CAD. More importantly, it can be helpful in the differential diagnosis of chest pain (Table 8.1). An enlarged cardiac silhouette, opacification of lung fields with prominent upper lobe vessels, or interlobular septal lines or Kelley B lines, and pleural effusion can be observed in patients with significantly impaired left ventricular function secondary to severe ischemia. All these radiographic signs are, however, nonspecific because they can also be seen in patients with ventricular dysfunction of nonischemic cause.

Table 8.1. Common causes of chest pain

Cardiovascular		
	Ischemic	
		Coronary artery disease
		Anomalous coronary artery
		Muscle bridging
		Aortic valve stenosis
		Hypertrophic cardiomyopathy
		Severe hypertension and LVH
		Vasculitis
		Coronary emboli
	Nonischemic	
		Aortic dissection
		Pericarditis
		Mitral valve prolapse
Noncardiac		
	Respiratory	
		Pneumonia
		Pulmonary embolism/infarction
		Pleurisy
		Pneumothorax
	Gastrointestinal	
		Gastroesophageal reflux
		Esophageal spasm/rupture
		Esophagitis, gastritis
		Peptic ulcer
		Cholecystitis, pancreatitis
	Neuromusculoskeletal	
		Costochondritis (Tietze's syndrome)
		Cervical/thoracic spine disease
		Thoracic outlet syndrome
		Herpes zoster
	Others	
		Severe anemia, hypoxemia
		Psychosomatic disorders

LVH, left ventricular hypertrophy.

1.4 Assessment of Likelihood of CAD

To determine the need for further investigation, it is essential to estimate the pretest probability of angiographically significant coronary disease. In this regard, the American College of Cardiology (ACC) and the American Heart Association (AHA) guidelines on the management of chronic stable angina recommend the use of validated predictive nomograms.[5] The Diamond and Forrester predictive table integrates three clinical variables – quality of chest pain, gender, and age – to provide an estimate of the risk of significant coronary stenosis as defined by coronary angiography (Table 8.2).[6] This approach can be refined by incorporating other powerful predictors, such as serum cholesterol levels, systolic blood pressure, and diabetes.[7] Most predictive tables and nomograms clearly separate low- from high-risk subjects. However, most patients will have an intermediate pretest probability of CAD,[6] and thus will need further stratification.

1.5 Application of Bayes' Theorem

The Bayes' theorem is a basic principle to bear in mind when requesting, performing, and interpreting diagnostic tests. The application of the Bayesian analysis to the currently available techniques for the diagnosis of CAD indicates that the diagnostic power of any test that is not 100% accurate is highly dependent on the prevalence of disease in the population studied. According to this, a positive test in a population with a low prevalence of coronary disease (<10%) is likely to be false positive, and thus investigations will only increase costs while exposing subjects to unnecessary procedures and risk. Conversely, most patients with a high pretest likelihood of disease (>90%) can confidently be referred for coronary angiography with a view to intervening. Although noninvasive tests can be performed

Table 8.2. Pretest likelihood of angiographically significant coronary artery disease according to age, gender, and chest pain quality[9]

Age (yr)	Gender	Typical angina	Atypical angina	Nonanginal chest pain	Asymptomatic
30–39	Men	Intermediate	Intermediate	Low	Very low
	Women	Intermediate	Very low	Very low	Very low
40–49	Men	High	Intermediate	Intermediate	Low
	Women	Intermediate	Low	Very low	Very low
50–59	Men	High	Intermediate	Intermediate	Low
	Women	Intermediate	Intermediate	Low	Very low
60–69	Men	High	Intermediate	Intermediate	Low
	Women	High	Intermediate	Intermediate	Low

for other reasons (i.e., risk stratification and prognosis), it is important to bear in mind that a negative result in this group is likely to be false negative and thus disease cannot be ruled out. Additional diagnostic testing is therefore most valuable in patients with an intermediate probability of CAD, as further stratification is needed.

2. Exercise Electrocardiography

Since the introduction of the first standardized protocol in the late 1920s,[8] exercise ECG has remained the most frequently performed stress procedure for the assessment of patients with stable chest pain. Furthermore, current practice guidelines recommend exercise ECG as the initial diagnostic test in patients with an intermediate pretest likelihood of coronary disease and a normal resting ECG.[5,9] Its major advantages are its wide availability, relatively low cost, and ability to provide a dynamic assessment of the significance of coronary stenosis by reproducing the patient's symptoms and unveiling ischemia-induced electrocardiographic and hemodynamic changes.

2.1 Procedure

All currently available exercise protocols involve continuous exercise with incremental workloads between multiple stages, producing a progressive increase in myocardial oxygen demand up to the patient's maximal level. The choice of one protocol over the others depends on physical conditioning and familiarity to exercise (i.e., walking versus cycling). The treadmill Bruce protocol is the most popular test, with modified versions available for patients with limited exercise tolerance. Regardless of the protocol used, an optimal exercise test should last at least 6 minutes, ideally between 8–12 minutes, with patients achieving at least 85% of the age- and gender-adjusted maximum predicted heart rate (MPHR), unless limiting symptoms develop. The classical criterion of an electrocardiographically positive exercise ECG is the occurrence of ≥1 mm horizontal or down-sloping ST-segment depression calculated at 60–80 milliseconds after the J point in three or more consecutive beats on any ECG lead. Exercise-induced ST-segment depression is the result of diffuse subendocardial ischemia, and thus does not localize the site of coronary stenosis, nor does its magnitude correlate with the severity or extent of CAD.[10] In contrast, exercise-induced ST-segment elevation, which results from transmural involvement, does localize the vascular bed, but occurs rarely during diagnostic exercise testing.[11,12] Dynamic electrocardiographic changes therefore aid in the detection of myocardial ischemia but are limited in their ability to provide information on the magnitude of underlying disease. Because of the reduced value of electrocardiographic changes alone, other exercise variables including cardiac symptoms, exercise capacity, and hemodynamic response must be considered before reaching a conclusion.[9] An exercise ECG test is terminated when the patient achieves his/her MPHR, develops limiting symptoms, or produces an abnormal test. Exercise testing not only allows an objective assessment of patients' symptoms and their relation with electrocardiographic and hemodynamic changes, but also provides information on exercise capacity, an important independent prognostic marker of future cardiac events.[13]

Overall, exercise ECG performs relatively well for the detection of flow-limiting epicardial coronary stenosis, although its diagnostic accuracy is not as high as that observed with imaging techniques. In the largest meta-analysis of 147 studies of 24 074 patients, 58 studies were considered free of bias, and they showed that the mean sensitivity of exercise ECG for diagnosis of CAD was 67%, with a specificity of 72%.[9] This varied according to the severity of underlying disease, with the highest sensitivity in patients with severe multivessel disease, and the lowest accuracy for single-vessel coronary stenosis. One approach to improving the diagnostic accuracy of the test is through the use of score systems that integrate several exercise parameters. The Duke treadmill score, a composite index that combines physical capacity measured in minutes of exercise, severity of angina, and magnitude of ST-segment changes to provide an estimate of risk of future cardiac events,[14] can also be used to stratify patients further according to their probability of having angiographically significant coronary stenosis.[15] This predictive tool provides both diagnostic and prognostic information that guide recommendations for optimal management according to risk categories (Figure 8.1).[16]

2.2 Limitations of Exercise ECG

From an electrocardiographic viewpoint, baseline abnormalities [e.g., LBBB, left ventricular hypertrophy (LVH) with repolarization changes, preexcitation syndromes, ST-segment depression of >1 mm] as well as digitalis therapy may complicate the interpretation of dynamic changes. Because the diagnostic performance of exercise testing is highly dependent on the patient's motivation and physical capacity to achieve an adequate workload, the value of the test is limited in populations with orthopedic, respiratory, or neurologic disorders (Table 8.3). Even after an optimal test is performed, conflicting findings such as borderline ST-segment or T-wave changes in the absence of symptoms are not uncommon and may lead to inconclusive results. Moreover, an inadequate hemodynamic response to exercise or the development of arrhythmias during the test, albeit nonspecific, warrants further evaluation, because these responses may be the result of significant CAD. In all these circumstances, the correct diagnosis of significant coronary disease

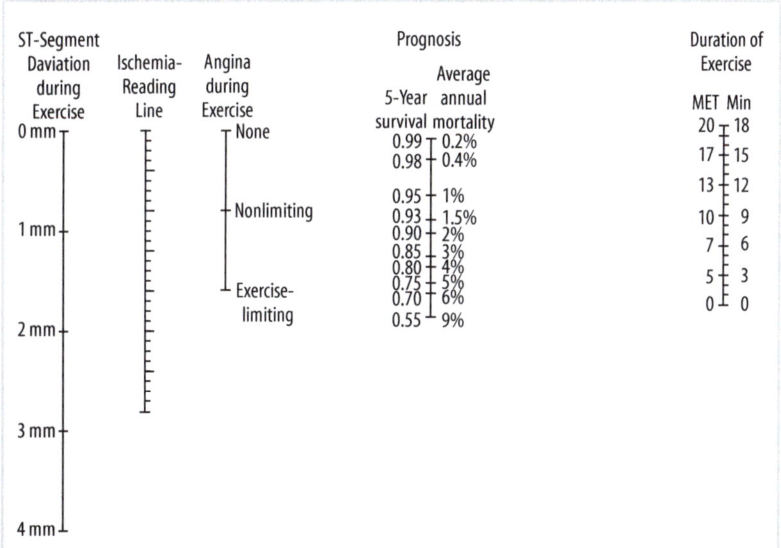

Figure 8.1. Nomogram of the Duke University prognostic treadmill score. Survival estimation is based on 1) the magnitude of exercise-induced ST-segment deviation from the isoelectric line expressed in millimeters; 2) development of chest pain, and 3) cardiac workload achieved measured in multiples of basal resting requirements (METS) or duration of exercise in minutes. The ST-segment deviation and the angina score points are connected with a straight line to determine the point on the ischemia reading line. A line is then drawn between this point and the maximal METS achieved or minutes of exercise performed to determine the point of intersection on the prognosis line. Information on prognosis is expressed as 5-year cardiovascular survival rate and average annual cardiovascular mortality. A patient who exercises for 6 minutes on the treadmill and develops 2-mm ST-segment depression associated with exercise-limiting angina has a 5-year survival rate in the region of 75% (average annual mortality rate, 5%) according to the nomogram.[16] (Reproduced with permission.)

Table 8.3. Contraindications to exercise testing

Absolute	
	Recent/unstable acute coronary syndrome
	Known significant left main stem stenosis
	Heart failure with resting symptoms
	Acute inflammatory process of the heart
	Myocarditis
	Pericarditis
	Endocarditis
	Life-threatening arrhythmias
	Severe fixed or dynamic left ventricular outflow tract obstruction
	Aortic stenosis
	Obstructive hypertrophic cardiomyopathy
	Uncontrolled hypertension
	Pulmonary embolism or infarction
	Thrombophlebitis or deep vein thrombosis
Relative	
	Orthopedic, neurologic, or respiratory disorders that limit exercise capacity
	Poor motivation to perform the test

could be jeopardized, and thus before embarking upon treatment strategies, an alternative diagnostic modality should be considered.

Exercise ECG has demonstrated to be less accurate in women than in men. In a meta-analysis of 19 studies in women undergoing exercise ECG for the diagnosis of coronary disease, the test had a weighted mean sensitivity of 61% and specificity of 70%.[17] This reduced diagnostic accuracy of exercise ECG in women has been attributed to the lower prevalence of disease, particularly among premenopausal patients,[18,19] the digitalis-like effect of estrogen responsible for repolarization changes, and the lower exercise tolerance of women compared with men.[20] Hormonal variations, higher prevalence of mitral valve prolapse, and abnormalities of microvascular function have also accounted for the suboptimal performance of exercise ECG in women.[20,21] However, higher accuracy can be achieved with the inclusion of additional parameters (e.g., functional capacity, treadmill scores) to the interpretation of the ST-segment response to exercise. Indeed, obstructive disease is more prevalent in women with high Duke treadmill score (see above) and they could benefit from referral to coronary angiography.

3. Stress Radionuclide MPS

Since its introduction 30 years ago, MPS has become an established technique for the detection of CAD, with important advantages over other diagnostic modalities. MPS is a robust technique that has demonstrated to be highly sensitive for the diagnosis of angiographically significant coronary stenosis by means of the detection of regional abnormalities of myocardial perfusion. Furthermore, myocardial perfusion imaging (MPI) overcomes the various diagnostic limitations of exercise ECG previously described. Myocardial perfusion can also be assessed accurately by positron emission tomography (PET) but, at present, its role in clinical practice is constrained by high cost and poor availability.

3.1 Procedure

In the ischemic cascade, impaired myocardial blood flow (MBF) reserve is one of the earliest events in the progression of disease from atherosclerotic changes to obstructive coronary lesions (Figure 8.2). MPS enables detection of such abnormality and provides accurate information on the state of myocardial perfusion that has both diagnostic and prognostic implications. MPS also assists in the identification of viable myocardium, which is facilitated by the simultaneous assessment of perfusion and function using ECG-gated imaging.

MPS relies on a camera that detects photons (usually gamma rays and/or X-rays), and the administration of a "perfusion tracer" (i.e., thallium-201, technetium-99m sestamibi, technetium-99m tetrofosmin) that is taken up by the myocytes in proportion to regional blood flow during stress as well as resting conditions (see also Chapter 4). In routine clinical practice,

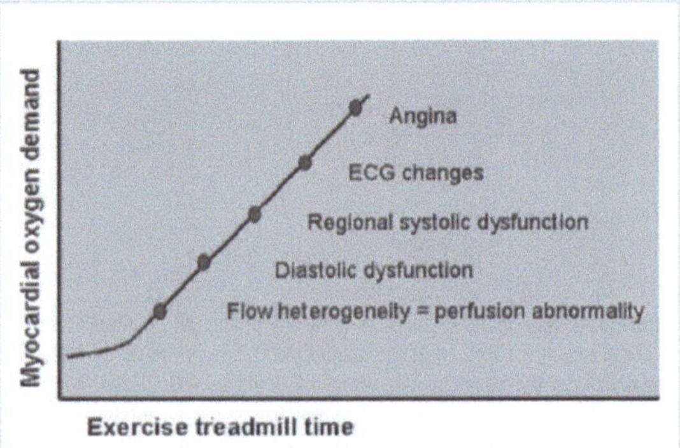

Figure 8.2. Ischemic cascade.

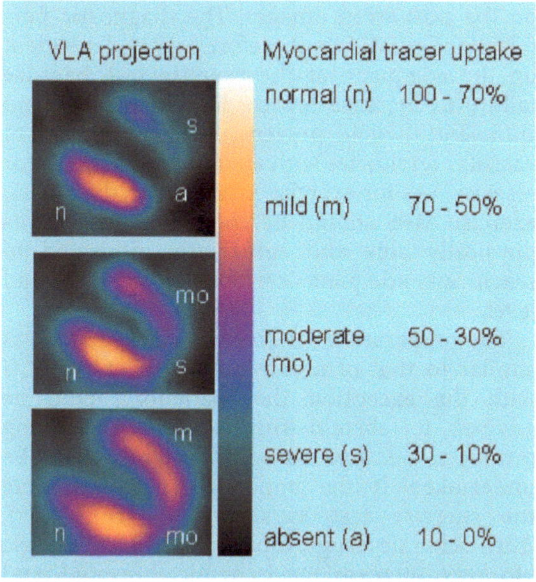

Figure 8.3. Tracer uptake within each myocardial wall or segment can be defined as normal, reduced, or absent. A segment of reduced tracer uptake can be further described as mildly, moderately, or severely reduced. These categories reflect the counts as a percentage of maximum in the whole set of tomographic projections. For instance, anything between 70%–100% of maximal myocardial tracer uptake is considered normal – this corresponds to the colors orange, yellow, and white on the Cool color scale. VLA: vertical long axis.

image interpretation relies on visual assessment of tracer uptake and its distribution into the myocardium (Figure 8.3; see color section). However, with advances in automated software algorithms and the availability of validated normal databases, quantitative analysis is becoming increasingly popular, and could be used to support visual interpretation (see Chapter 4).

3.1.1 Thallium MPS

Thallium-201 was the first perfusion tracer identified to image myocardial perfusion. Thallium-201 is a potassium analog that is rapidly transported into the myocytes through the Na-K adenosine triphosphatase pump, an active, energy-dependent mechanism. A small proportion enters the myocardial cell passively through an electropotential gradient and accumulates into the cytoplasm. After an injection of thallium-201 at peak stress, the tracer is rapidly extracted by the myocardium with a first-pass extraction fraction of 88%.[22] Thallium-201 uptake is proportional to blood flow until it reaches values >3 mL/min/g; at this point uptake levels off (roll-off phenomenon) despite further increments in blood flow.[23] Thallium-201 starts redistributing shortly after injection, and thus imaging 3–4 hours later allows assessment of resting perfusion and myocardial viability.[24] Comparison between the stress and redistribution images distinguishes between the reversible defect of inducible hypoperfusion and the fixed defect of myocardial necrosis, although, in some cases, redistribution may be incomplete at 4 hours. A second injection of thallium can then be given and reinjection images acquired for a more accurate assessment of myocardial viability.[25] In addition, administration of nitrates before a resting injection of thallium-201 (nitrate-enhanced thallium reinjection imaging) has been shown to improve the detection of viability.[26] Therefore, a resting injection of thallium increases the pool of circulating tracer whereas nitrates augment its delivery by increasing blood flow through collateral circulation.

Thallium-201 MPS is highly accurate for the diagnosis of CAD. Typical values of sensitivity and specificity are in the region of 85%–90% and 75%, respectively.[27] Thallium-201 imaging is used in many centers worldwide, although it is being largely superseded by the technetium tracers because of their superior imaging characteristics.

3.1.2 Technetium-99m MPS

Technetium-99m sestamibi and technetium-99m tetrofosmin are both well-validated perfusion tracers that can be used alone or in combination with thallium-201 imaging for the assessment of patients with suspected CAD. These agents are less vulnerable to attenuation and scatter, and therefore produce better-quality images, particularly in overweight and female patients with dense breast tissue. Because they exhibit minimal redistribution over time, imaging can be delayed for some time after the stress injection, and there is no need to inject close to the gamma camera. Injections can be given during treadmill exercise testing, in the catheter laboratory, or in the coronary care unit immediately before thrombolysis. In addition, because of the higher doses that can be used with technetium-99m, ventricular function can be assessed either by first-pass imaging of the tracer as it passes through the central circulation or by ECG-gated acquisition of the myocardial perfusion images. In comparison with thallium-201, they are extracted less avidly from the circulation, with a first-pass extraction fraction in the region of 50%–55%,[28,29] and an early roll-off at blood flow velocities exceeding 2 mL/min/g myocardium.[23] In theory, these tracers will be less capable of tracking MBF at high flow velocities. Indeed, experimental models have demonstrated the nonlinear relation between myocardial tracer uptake and blood flow at high flow velocities for all available tracers, with the best uptake/flow relation for thallium-201, and the least favorable relation for technetium-99m sestamibi and technetium-99m tetrofosmin.[23] It has also been shown that technetium-99m MPS is less sensitive for the detection of mild coronary stenosis (≤70% luminal diameter reduction) than thallium-201 imaging.[28,30] However, such differences may not be important in clinical practice and indeed a large body of evidence indicates that the average diagnostic accuracy of technetium-99m MPS is similar to that observed with thallium-201 imaging.[27]

3.1.3 Exercise MPS

The addition of radionuclide imaging to conventional exercise stress testing not only enhances its diagnostic performance significantly but at the same time offers incremental prognostic information above that obtained by the exercise ECG data, thus allowing accurate stratification of patients into low- and high-risk groups of future coronary events.[31] Such classification is highly important for patients' management, because low-risk individuals are unlikely to benefit from further investigation and are best managed medically, whereas those with significant ischemia will usually be referred for coronary angiography.[32]

The diagnosis of flow-limiting coronary disease is based on the ability of exercise testing to decrease coronary arteriolar resistance as myocardial oxygen consumption increases. In the presence of a flow-limiting stenosis, a reduced vasodilator reserve will produce a heterogeneous distribution of tracer identifiable on the post-stress images. The diagnostic performance of MPS is therefore highly dependent on the adequacy of the exercise test, because failure to increase myocardial oxygen demand sufficiently would prevent the identification of vascular territories with an impaired vasodilator reserve.[33] As for exercise ECG testing, diagnostic exercise MPS should be conducted in patients physically able and sufficiently motivated to reach an adequate cardiovascular workload level.

The preparation for an exercise MPS study is similar to that of a conventional exercise ECG with the exception that patients should be advised to abstain from caffeine-containing products, because vasodilator stress may be undertaken if the patient fails to complete the exercise test satisfactorily (see below). Anti-ischemic drugs, especially beta-adrenergic blockers, increase the ischemic threshold, and should therefore be discontinued for a minimum of four half-lives before the test. Ideally, the exercise test should be symptom-limited, with patients achieving their maximal workload level or at least 85% MPHR unless cardiac symptoms and ECG changes suggestive of significant myocardial ischemia develop (>1 mm ST-segment elevation in non-Q waves leads or ≥2 mm horizontal or down-sloping ST-segment depression). The perfusion tracer is administered at peak stress, and the patient should continue exercising for 1–2 minutes to allow for adequate myocardial extraction of tracer.[34]

There is some variation in published data on the diagnostic accuracy of exercise MPS, partly because of differences in imaging protocols and standards of interpretation; however, well-designed studies have found high values of sensitivity and specificity (approximately 85% and 75%, respectively).[26] After exclusion of patients with documented previous myocardial infarction (MI), exercise MPS maintains its high sensitivity (87%) for the detection of disease.[26] Likewise, specificity for the identification of normal coronary arteries is good,[35–37] although most of the studies are influenced by referral bias, which leads to overestimation of sensitivity and underestimation of specificity, because most patients with a normal scan are spared from coronary angiography. To reduce the effect of referral bias on specificity, the performance of MPS in patients without disease is best assessed as normalcy. Based on estimation of the proportion of normal MPS studies in populations with a low pretest likelihood of CAD (<10%), the normalcy rate of exercise MPS is in the region of 81%–95%.[33,38,39]

In addition to the traditional contraindications to exercise testing (see also Chapter 4), exercise should be avoided in patients with LBBB and electronically paced ventricular rhythm. Near half of patients with LBBB may develop perfusion defects in the interventricular septum and adjacent myocardial segments during exercise MPS in the absence of obstructive coronary disease (Figure 8.4; see color section).[40] The exact underlying mechanism remains unknown; however, there is evidence suggesting that, in LBBB, the temporal delay between left and right ventricular activation results in a prolonged systole and a reduced diastolic filling time for the septum. Because most coronary flow occurs in diastole, this has the effect of reducing septal myocardial perfusion, which would be exacerbated by increments in heart rate. Thus, any maneuver that increases heart rate (e.g., exercise, inotropic agents) should be avoided, because this increases the likelihood of perfusion defects arising from the conduction abnormality. Vasodilator stress has been found to increase the specificity of the technique by 40%, indicating that vasodilator MPS is the modality of choice in these patients (Figure 8.5; see color section).[40,41]

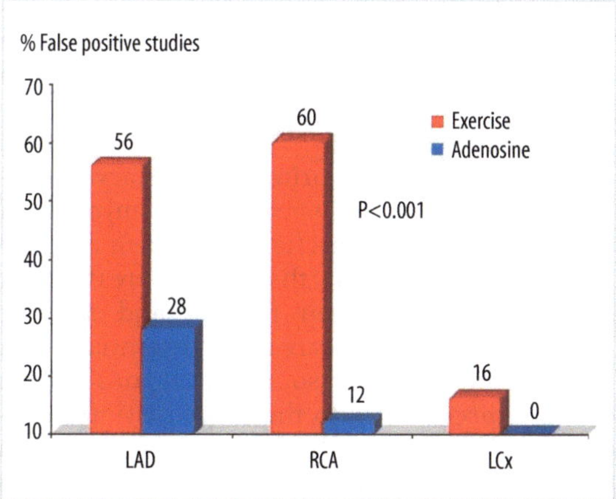

Figure 8.5. False-positive studies (%) in patients with LBBB undergoing exercise versus adenosine myocardial perfusion scintigraphy. LAD, left anterior descending coronary artery; RCA, right coronary artery; LCx, left circumflex coronary artery.

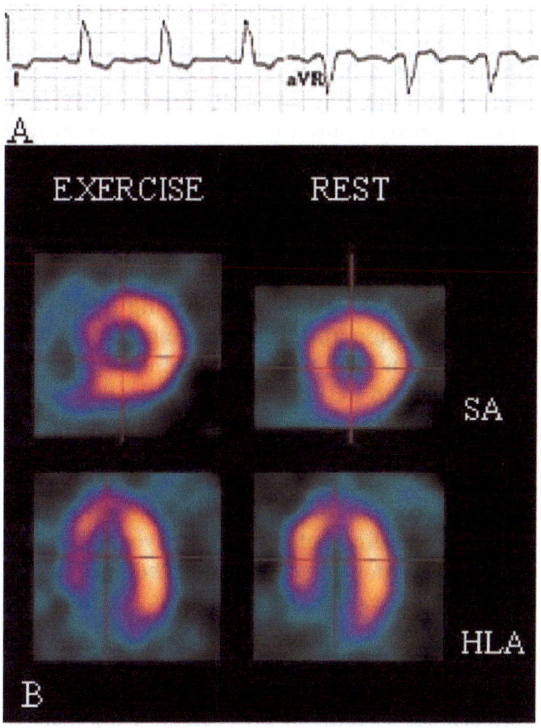

Figure 8.4. A 54-year-old man with atypical chest pain and no history of coronary artery disease underwent exercise thallium-201 myocardial perfusion scintigraphy. **A** ECG showing complete LBBB. **B** Short-axis and horizontal long-axis views showing exercise-induced septal hypoperfusion that normalizes at rest. Subsequent X-ray coronary angiography revealed normal coronary arteries.

3.1.4 Pharmacologic MPS

One of the major advantages of radionuclide imaging is its versatility among the different stress modalities currently available. MPS can be combined with a pharmacologic stress agent that mediates either direct (e.g., adenosine, dipyridamole, and selective $A2_A$ receptor agonists) or indirect (e.g., dobutamine) coronary vasodilation if exercise is contraindicated or discontinued.

3.1.4.1 Vasodilator MPS. Dipyridamole and adenosine are the two currently available vasodilators for the assessment of myocardial perfusion. Both drugs act via the activation of adenosine $A2_A$ receptors located on the membrane of the smooth muscle cells of the small resistance vessels, producing direct coronary arteriolar dilation and increasing MBF to a level comparable to that achieved with intracoronary papaverine.[42] Dipyridamole and adenosine increase MBF up to 4 times its resting level, with absolute values in the region of 3.5–4 and 4–5 mL/min/g, respectively.[42,43] Contrary to exercise, vasodilators produce primary coronary arteriolar dilation and only rarely true myocardial ischemia through a mechanism known as coronary steal. During this, the driving pressure for collateral flow between normal and stenotic coronary territories decreases substantially as a result of the greater vasodilator response of the normal vascular bed to these agents (intercoronary steal).[44] This may lead to profound ischemia with the potential for myocyte injury.[45] Although this phenomenon seems to be uncommon, it is more prevalent in the elderly as well as in patients with long-standing CAD who have developed collateral circulation between obstructed and nonstenotic coronary vascular territories. Blood flow diversion from the subendocardial to subepicardial layer can also occur as the former is subjected to the highest wall stress (intracoronary steal).

Preparation for vasodilator stress testing requires the abstention from caffeine-containing beverages and food for a minimum of 12 hours, as well as discontinuation of aminophylline and theophylline for at least 48 hours. Methylxanthines, such as caffeine and theophylline, are nonselective competitive antagonists of adenosine receptors that have been found to reduce the sensitivity of vasodilator stress for the detection of coronary stenosis.[46] Dipyridamole should also be discontinued 24–48 hours before the test. The role of antianginal medications in vasodilator stress is not clear, although recent observations mainly from studies performed with dipyridamole indicate that they may reduce sensitivity and should be discontinued if the scan is performed for diagnostic purposes.[47] Data with adenosine are still sparse and further research is essential before final recommendations.

Adenosine is administered as an intravenous infusion at 140 µg/kg/min for 6 minutes with tracer injection after 3–4 minutes of infusion. Because of the rapid onset of action of adenosine on the coronary vasculature (84 ± 46 seconds),[42] several studies have evaluated the effectiveness of shorter protocols, observing a similar overall predictive accuracy for the detection of angiographic coronary stenosis with a 4–5- versus 6-minute infusion.[48] Shorter protocols (≤3-minute infusion) may adversely affect the diagnostic and prognostic value of the test by reducing the extent of perfusion abnormality and should therefore be avoided.[49,50] The potential for increasing patient throughput and reducing costs has encouraged the implementation of 4- and 5-minute adenosine protocols in nuclear cardiology laboratories worldwide. Despite this, the 6-minute adenosine infusion remains the standard clinical protocol. Dipyridamole is given intravenously at 140 µg/kg/min for 4 min (0.56 mg/kg), and the perfusion tracer administered 3–4 minutes after termination of the infusion.

Summarized data demonstrate that the diagnostic accuracy of vasodilator MPS is similar to that of exercise imaging. This has been confirmed in studies performed with either thallium-201 or technetium-99m sestamibi; however, data from studies with tetrofosmin are less consistent, with some studies reporting good accuracy with vasodilators and others showing it to be less sensitive than Tl-201 or sestamibi for detection of mild-to-moderate angiographic disease.[51,52]

Vasodilator stress is well tolerated and has an excellent safety profile (≤0.05% risk of nonfatal MI or major cardiac complications),[53,54] and a high success rate because little cooperation is needed to complete the test satisfactorily. The addition of dynamic exercise has demonstrated to reduce significantly the intensity and frequency of side effects resulting from peripheral vasodilation (e.g., headache, flushing, hypotension) as well as the incidence of atrioventricular conduction abnormalities.[55,56] Exercise also enhances image quality by provoking splanchnic vasoconstriction and thus reducing extracardiac accumulation of tracer and increasing heart-to-background activity ratio.[57] The addition of submaximal exercise to vasodilator stress has also been found to increase the sensitivity of the test,[55,58] and this seems to be independent of the effect of exercise on quality and image interpretation. A combined effect on the myocardial perfusion system has been postulated,[59] although the exact mechanism is not known. Adding exercise reduces but does not abolish vasodilator-induced side effects, and thus their impact on test compliance continues to be a matter of concern. As a result of this, selective agonists to the adenosine $A2_A$ receptors have been developed,[60] and preliminary data suggest that these new agents are associated with fewer side effects.[61] The effectiveness of $A2_A$ receptor agonists seems to be similar to that of adenosine.[62]

3.1.4.2 Dobutamine MPS. Dobutamine can also be used in combination with MPS to determine the presence of significant coronary artery stenosis in patients with clinically suspected CAD. Dobutamine has not been studied as extensively as the vasodilators, and published estimates of its diagnostic accuracy vary markedly.[27] This has been largely attributed to inadequate stress protocols, lack of standardized test endpoints, and other factors independent of the test such as the concomitant use of beta-adrenergic blockers. Dobutamine stress is therefore a less well-established protocol and should be limited to patients unable to exercise who have a contraindication to vasodilator stress. As for exercise testing, the sensitivity of dobutamine for the detection of CAD is highly dependent on the level of cardiac work achieved. Beta-blockers increase the threshold at which abnormalities of myocardial perfusion would become apparent; hence, these agents should be discontinued before the test. Overall, dobutamine MPS has a sensitivity for the detection of significant coronary stenosis in the region of 80%–90% and a specificity ranging between 64%–100%[27] with the higher values recorded more often with thallium-201 than with technetium-99m labeled tracers. This is probably because dobutamine produces an increase in calcium flux into the myocytes that may affect the ability of monovalent cations such as sestamibi to bind to the mitochondrial membrane, reducing its intracellular uptake.

Dobutamine is given as an intravenous infusion, starting at 5 µg/kg/min and increasing to 10, 20, 30, and 40 µg/kg/min at 3- to 5-minute intervals. The tracer is injected after 3–5 minutes on the maximal dose of 40 µg/kg/min unless the patient develops limiting symptoms or the age- and gender-adjusted MPHR is reached. Tracer injection at low dobutamine rates (<20 µg/kg/min) should be avoided whenever possible. Atropine is often given during dobutamine echocardiography if 85% of MPHR is not reached at peak dobutamine infusion. This practice may not be necessary for perfusion imaging as long as the patient is not taking beta-blockers because of the primary vasodilator effect of dobutamine.[63] Other protocols combining exercise with dobutamine or atropine have been investigated; however, their use in clinical practice is limited.

3.1.5 ECG-gated MPS

The diagnostic accuracy of MPS improves further by incorporating information on global and regional left ventricular function to myocardial perfusion with the use of ECG-gated MPS imaging. For this purpose, image acquisition is synchronized with the QRS complex of the ECG signal, and sets of 8–16 frames are acquired, each frame corresponding to a specific part of the cardiac cycle. Automated algorithms are applied to the acquired data to obtain an accurate estimation of ventricular volumes, left ventricular ejection fraction, mass and regional wall motion and thickening. Over the last decade, ECG-gated MPS has been validated in many studies, comparing favorably with other well-established imaging modalities, including radionuclide ventriculography, echocardiography, and magnetic resonance imaging.[64–67]

The addition of functional information derived from ECG-gated MPS to perfusion data not only improves substantially the specificity of MPS by differentiating myocardial scar from artifact but it may also increase the sensitivity of the technique for detecting CAD. Moreover, it provides incremental prognostic information above that obtained from perfusion assessment alone in patients with suspected or known CAD (see next chapter). Because of the minimal added cost, ECG-gated MPS has become a routine procedure in most nuclear cardiology departments (Figure 8.6; see color section).

3.1.6 Advantages of MPS

The increasing use of MPS for the diagnosis of clinically important CAD is the direct result of its strengths; MPS is a robust and highly validated technique, widely available, with a clear role in the assessment of patients investigated for CAD as stated by national and internationally published guidelines.[5,68,69] With very few exceptions, MPS can be performed to virtually all patients presenting with stable chest pain. Its versatility allows the technique to be adjusted to patients' needs and medical status, whether exercise or pharmacologic stress is being performed.

The diagnostic superiority of MPS over conventional exercise testing relies on the ability of

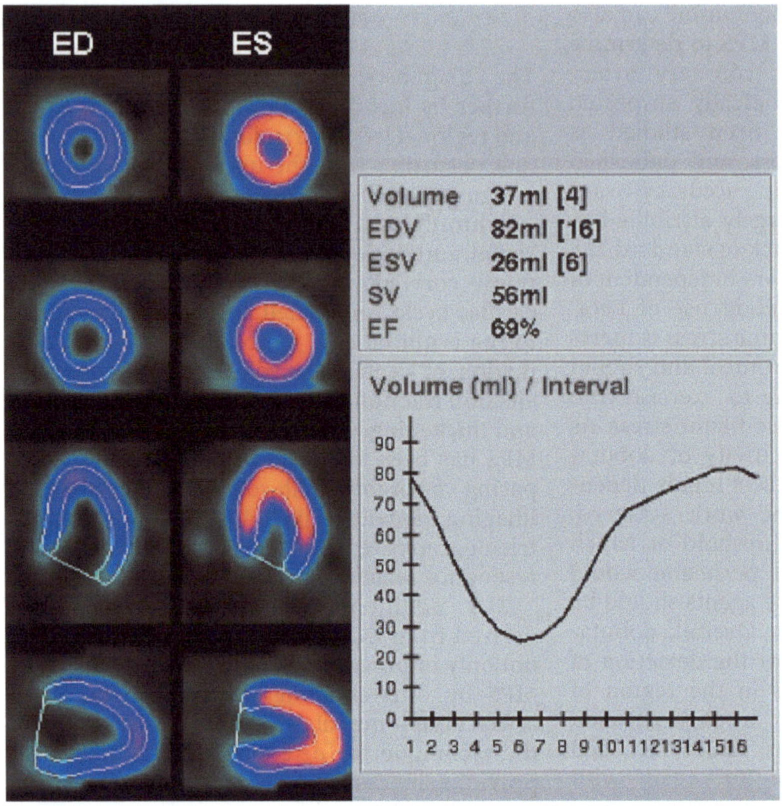

Figure 8.6. Quantitative gated SPECT (QGS) analysis of a 62-year-old woman with atypical chest pain of recent onset. The resting left ventricular ejection fraction (EF) is normal at 69% with normal left ventricular end-diastolic volume (EDV) and end-systolic volume (ESV).

the technique to identify one of the earliest manifestations of CAD. MPS not only allows the detection of early abnormalities of myocardial perfusion but also defines the extent and magnitude of involvement of the vascular bed distal to the coronary stenosis and is the more sensitive test for detection of single-vessel coronary disease.

Radionuclide imaging has recently demonstrated to be more accurate than conventional exercise ECG for diagnosing CAD in women. In the past, MPS was highly vulnerable to soft tissue attenuation artifacts, producing a large proportion of false-positive tests in women. Modern camera technology and increasing use of high-energy tracers have both contributed to enhance the accuracy of MPS in women by reducing significantly the incidence of false-positive scans and increasing confidence in reporting.[70]

One of the most important advantages of MPS over other techniques is its high prognostic value. A normal MPS study not only suggests the absence of flow-limiting coronary disease, but it is also associated with a low likelihood of nonfatal MI or cardiac death (<1%/year). Conversely, an abnormal scan indicates the presence of significant CAD, and provides valuable incremental prognostic information that is based on the extent and severity of a perfusion abnormality, as well as the presence of other adverse prognostic signs, such as increased lung tracer uptake, transient left ventricular dilation, and global and regional left ventricular dysfunction (see next chapter). Reliable prognostication guides the selection of patients for further interventions, such as revascularization. This in turn allows more appropriate utilization of resources, with the potential for improved clinical outcomes and greater cost-effectiveness. Evidence from modeling and observational studies supports the enhanced cost-effectiveness associated with MPS use. In patients presenting with stable chest pain, strategies of investigation involving MPS are more cost-effective than those not using the technique (Figure 8.7; see color section).[71,72] MPS also has particular advantages over exercise ECG in the management of a number of patient

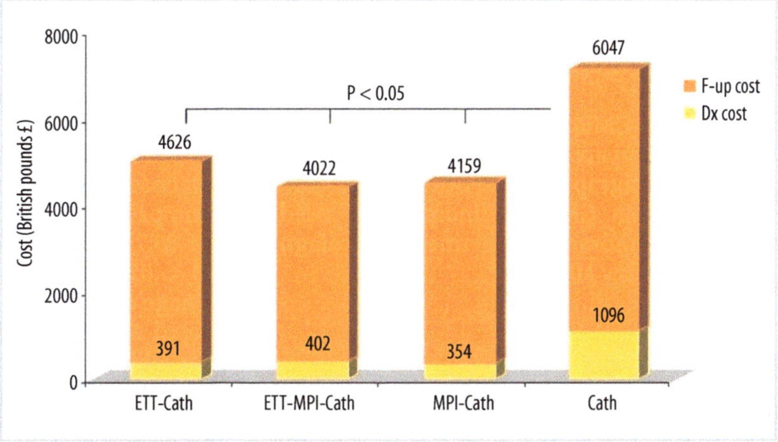

Figure 8.7. The Economics of Myocardial Perfusion Imaging (MPI) in Europe (EMPIRE) study explored the economic impact of four diagnostic strategies that combined exercise testing, MPI, and coronary angiography for the assessment of patients with chronic chest pain. The study, comprising 396 patients from eight hospitals in the United Kingdom, France, Italy, and Germany, showed significantly lower diagnostic and 2-year management costs when MPI was used as the gatekeeper to coronary angiography compared with direct referral to catheterization, with no effect on outcome. Dx, diagnostic; and F-up, follow-up costs of care estimated in British pounds (£).[71] (By permission of Oxford University Press on behalf of The European Society of Cardiology.)

subgroups, including the elderly[73] and those with diabetes,[74,75] and its use will have a favorable impact on cost-effectiveness in these groups. The high diagnostic and prognostic value of MPS in the setting of stable chest pain syndromes and chronic stable angina is widely recognized and MPS has become an integral part of the investigative strategies recommended by both European and American guidelines.

3.1.7 Disadvantages of MPS

Its vulnerability to artifacts has been largely recognized as the major limitation of radionuclide imaging. However, continuous improvement in imaging technology has had a tremendous impact on the diagnostic performance of the MPS, producing a significant reduction in the incidence of artifacts and thus improving the specificity of the technique. The increasing availability of automated software that allows quantitative analysis using normal databases has also contributed substantially to enhance the diagnostic profile of the technique over the last few years. ECG-gated MPS, motion, attenuation, and scatter-correction algorithms are available in most modern equipment. The correct use and application of these new tools may lead to a more accurate diagnosis of myocardial ischemia. Furthermore, dynamic cardiac single photon emission computed tomography (SPECT) based on the principle of tracer kinetics is another direction of current research that opens new horizons for the development of a potentially more sensitive tool for detecting myocardial ischemia.

The agreement between the magnitude of a perfusion abnormality and the severity of angiographically defined coronary stenosis is frequently referred to as moderate (60%–80%).[76] Initially considered as a potential disadvantage of MPS, it is now accepted that this is the result of the inability of conventional coronary angiography to fully assess the hemodynamic significance of coronary lesions.[77,78] Moreover, coronary angiography can underestimate the effect of diffusely distributed coronary atherosclerosis on distal perfusion, an observation that has been largely supported by numerous experimental studies showing the close relation between stress perfusion defects and coronary blood flow reserve.[76,79] Other potential causes of the discordance between MPI and coronary angiography are the presence of collateral blood flow, coronary vasospasm, and abnormalities of endothelial function and regulation of microcirculation.[80,81]

4. Cardiovascular Magnetic Resonance

In CMR, two main techniques are used in the assessment of CAD:

- Dobutamine stress CMR (DSCMR) – using the infusion of incremental doses of dobutamine to induce wall motion abnormalities as determined with high-resolution cine-CMR
- Adenosine perfusion CMR – using an infusion of adenosine as a coronary vasodilator to induce regional perfusion abnormalities, detected with the administration of a gadolinium contrast agent

CMR angiography is also feasible but, at present, is of limited value in the patients discussed here (see more in Chapters 3, 14, and 15).

Although CMR is a relatively new imaging modality compared with echocardiography and nuclear scintigraphy, both DSCMR and adenosine perfusion CMR are increasingly used in large cardiothoracic departments to diagnose coronary artery stenoses.

4.1 Dobutamine Stress CMR

Dobutamine has been extensively combined with echocardiography as a noninvasive diagnostic test for coronary artery stenoses, although diagnostic images may not be possible in obese patients or patients with bronchial asthma. Dobutamine increases myocardial contractility, heart rate, and systemic blood pressure, which increase myocardial oxygen consumption. In the presence of a significant coronary artery stenosis, this will produce myocardial ischemia leading to regional wall motion abnormalities, surface ECG changes, and the development of angina. "High-dose" dobutamine (30–40 μg/kg/min) is a safe agent to produce myocardial ischemia, but does have a small rate of serious complications in approximately 0.25% of patients, including MI (0.07%), ventricular fibrillation (0.07%), and sustained ventricular tachycardia (0.1%).[82,83]

DSCMR was used by Pennell et al.[84] in 1992 in the investigation of 25 patients with angina and an abnormal exercise tolerance test. Using a dobutamine infusion to a maximum of 20 μg/kg/min and non-breathhold gradient-echo cine imaging in two short-axis and two long-axis planes, they demonstrated inducible wall motion abnormalities in 20 of 21 patients with reversible ischemia on thallium tomography. Baer et al.,[85] using a similar technique in 28 patients with coronary artery stenoses, obtained sensitivity and specificity values for the detection of significant coronary artery stenoses of 87% and 100% for the left anterior descending, 62% and 93% for the left circumflex, and 78% and 88% for the right coronary artery, respectively. In a study of 45 patients, van Rugge[86] obtained an overall sensitivity for the detection of CAD of 81%, with a specificity of 100%. "High-dose" dobutamine (up to 40 μg/kg/min) with atropine (0.25 mg repeated up to 1.0 mg) to reach a target heart rate (>85% maximal predicted), was used by Nagel et al.,[87] in a large study (208 patients) that compared DSCMR with dobutamine stress echocardiography (DSE). The protocol was well tolerated with no significant adverse events. For the detection of significant coronary artery stenoses, the sensitivity of DSCMR was 86.2% compared with 74.3% for DSE, with a specificity of 85.7% for DSCMR and 69.8% for DSE (both $P < .05$). Of particular note was the improved image quality with DSCMR, with 69% of images rated as very good, compared with only 19.6% for DSE. In fact, 8.8% of DSE images were nondiagnostic, as compared with 1.6% for DSCMR. With the addition of myocardial tagging, Kuijpers et al.[88] were able to demonstrate an improved detection of CAD, and of 68 patients identified as having abnormal wall motion, 65 had significant ischemic heart disease with 62 needing revascularization. In the 112 patients with normal DSCMR, there was an event-free rate of 98.2% at a mean follow-up of 17.3 months.

4.1.1 Procedure

The patient is prepared for the scanner following standard procedures, including the checklist of contraindications to CMR. In addition, patients with specific contraindications to high-dose dobutamine (e.g., recent acute coronary syndrome, ventricular tachyarrhythmia) are excluded. Patients are asked to discontinue beta-blockers 48–72 hours before the examination. A 12-lead ECG and baseline observations (heart rate and blood pressure) are obtained. An intravenous cannula is inserted into a large peripheral vein and connected to a saline-flushed long-line. Continuous ECG monitoring and automated blood pressure recording are connected. The patient is then positioned in the magnet bore. Using rapid pilot scans for accurate positioning, multiple breathhold cardiac-gated cine images are acquired of the vertical long-axis, horizontal long-axis, and a stack of short-axis planes from the base to the apex of the left ventricle (Figure 8.8). The dobutamine infusion is then commenced at a rate of 5 μg/kg/min for 5–10 minutes. The dobutamine infusion rate is increased at 5 or 10 μg/kg/min doses until the heart rate increases by 10% over baseline. At this "low-dose" level, cine imaging is repeated in all planes to detect inotropic reserve in myocardial

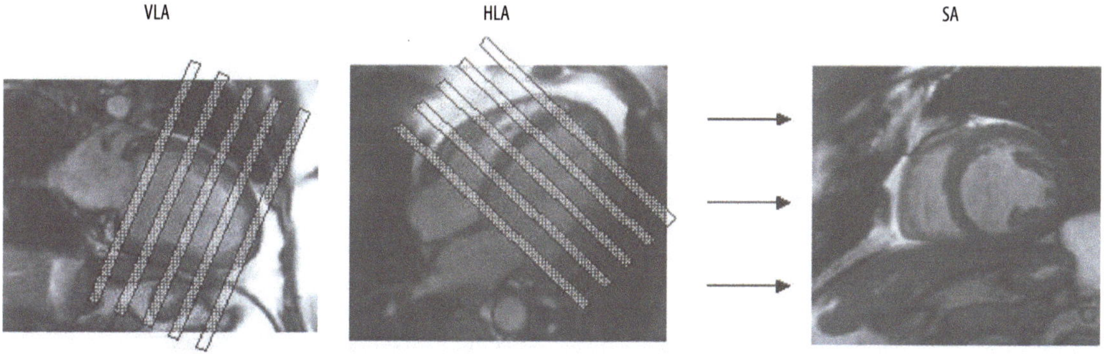

Figure 8.8. Rest and stress images are acquired in the vertical long axis (VLA) and horizontal long axis (HLA) of the left ventricle. These axes are used to pilot the short axis (SA) slices from the base to the apex of the left ventricle.

segments with resting abnormal wall motion. The dobutamine infusion rate is then increased at regular intervals until the target heart rate is obtained. After each incremental dose increase, it is important to perform a rapid visual analysis of the myocardial wall motion to avoid prolonging the study once wall motion abnormalities are induced. Blood pressure measurements and continuous ECG monitoring are performed. At this "high-dose" level, cine imaging is repeated in all planes. In some patients, atropine 0.5–3.0 mg may be necessary to allow the patient to reach the target heart rate. Once the study is complete, the patient can be removed from the magnet bore and allowed to recover. Analysis of the DSCMR is performed using a 17-segment model (6 basal-, 6 mid-, and 4-apical short-axis segments as well as the apical cap; Figure 8.9; see color section). At rest, each segment is scored as normal, hypokinetic, akinetic, dyskinetic. The scores are repeated for the "low-dose" – viability, and the "high-dose" – ischemia levels. A viable but ischemic segment (attributed to a critical coronary artery stenosis) may be scored hypokinetic at rest, normal at "low-dose," and hypokinetic at "high dose." In addition to the wall motion score, baseline and peak left ventricular ejection fraction can be calculated by summating the volume of each short-axis slice. Further quantitative information can be obtained including radial thickening, cardiac output, left ventricular volume-loops, and with the use of

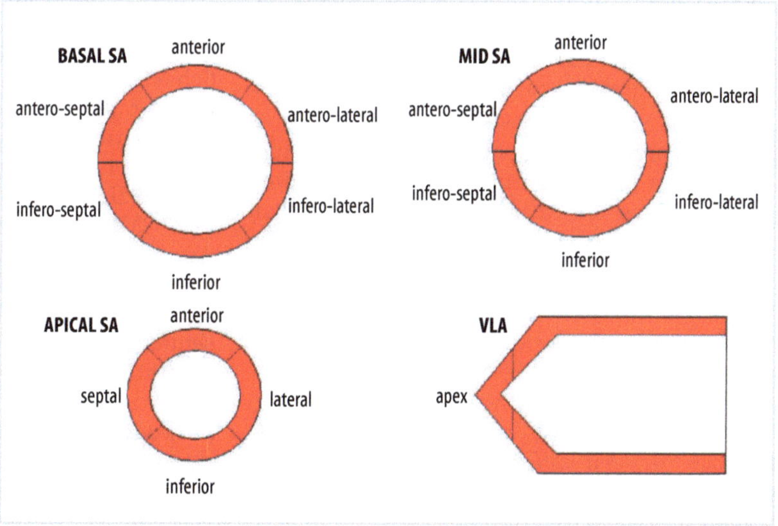

Figure 8.9. Analysis of dobutamine CMR is performed using a 17-segment model.

"tagging lines" complex three-dimensional data can be processed.

4.1.2 Advantages of DSCMR

DSCMR has certain advantages compared with DSE:

- DSCMR can produce high-quality images in almost all subjects. DSE can be limited by patients with poor echo windows because of obesity or chronic lung disease. In particular, the lateral wall can be problematic for DSE.
- Unlike DSE, which requires considerable operator skill in acquisition and interpretation, DSCMR is less operator dependent because the standard imaging planes can be acquired by most CMR technicians.

4.1.3 Disadvantages of DSCMR

The main disadvantages of performing dobutamine stress in a CMR environment result from the static and gradient magnetic fields:

- Monitoring equipment must be compatible with the static magnetic field and be remotely operated. In addition, the magnetic field distorts the surface ECG making ST-segment analysis difficult, although cardiac arrhythmias can be safely detected.
- Although dobutamine stress is a safe technique, there is a small risk of inducing a significant cardiac arrhythmia, e.g., ventricular tachycardia or ventricular fibrillation. Resuscitation must be performed outside the static magnetic field and so the patient needs to be rapidly extracted from the magnet bore. Regular simulated cardiac arrest training sessions are therefore essential.
- A small percentage of people experience claustrophobia inside the magnet bore. Performing a stress test on these patients (which can produce unpleasant symptoms) may not be possible.

4.2 Adenosine Perfusion CMR

MPI has been extensively performed with SPECT using exercise or vasodilator stress to produce regional differences in the uptake of radioactive tracers. Both adenosine and dipyridamole agents have more recently been used with CMR. The CMR sequences use a presaturation or inversion prepulse to null signal from the myocardium. An intravenous gadolinium-based contrast agent is then rapidly administered via a large peripheral vein. The gadolinium shortens the T1 of the blood pool and then the myocardium, which results in more signal being obtained and the images appear bright. In a normal subject, there will be homogenous myocardial enhancement with the gadolinium. A segment of myocardium supplied by a stenosed coronary artery will enhance slower than the surrounding myocardium and may reach a lower peak signal intensity. Infarcted myocardium with an occluded vessel and microvascular obstruction may remain black because no gadolinium can reach the tissue. These relative changes in signal intensity after gadolinium may be assessed qualitatively with a visual assessment by a trained observer, or semiquantitatively with the use of signal-intensity-time curves.

CMR-perfusion techniques were investigated in the early 1990s using single-slice inversion recovery (IR) gradient-echo sequences. The IR techniques were sensitive to heart rate variability and had limited spatial coverage. In 1990, Atkinson et al.[89] demonstrated the feasibility of CMR-perfusion in animal and human studies, using 0.1 mmol/kg gadolinium-DTPA, acquiring 32 ultrafast images in a transverse plane. In 1991, Manning et al.[90] studied 17 patients with chest pain, 12 of whom had significant coronary artery stenoses. They used 0.04 mmol/kg gadolinium-DTPA and were able to demonstrate that in myocardium supplied by a coronary stenosis, there was a lower peak signal intensity after gadolinium, and a lower up-slope. In 1992, Schaefer et al.[91] compared the results of thallium scintigraphy with dipyridamole CMR-perfusion in six patients with coronary artery stenoses and four normal volunteers. There were nine myocardial regions supplied by stenosed vessels, and CMR-perfusion matched the scintigraphy results in eight of them. In 1993 and 1995, Wilke et al.[92,93] performed quantitative studies in animal models. They used an IR Turbo-FLASH sequence combined with dipyridamole and a central injection of 0.05 mmol/kg gadolinium-DTPA in dogs. They found a linear relationship between the gadolinium concentration and the myocardial signal intensity at administered doses of between 0.2 and 1.2 mmol/L. Using an intravascular contrast agent (polylysine gadolinium-

DTPA), they produced good correlation with microspheres to accurately determine MBF and volume. In 1994, Eichenberger et al.[94] used gadolinium DOTA at 0.05 mmol/kg in 10 patients with >75% coronary artery stenosis, at rest and after dipyridamole administration. They were able to acquire three short-axis slices (one every heart beat), and obtained a sensitivity of 65%, specificity of 76%, and an accuracy of 74%, using thallium scintigraphy and coronary angiography as the gold standard. In 1995, Saeed et al.[95] performed rest-stress perfusion CMR in dogs with a critical circumflex artery stenosis. Measuring the peak signal intensity, they determined that at rest there was no difference between the myocardium with a normal blood supply compared with the myocardium subtended by the stenosed vessel. However, after dipyridamole, the normal territory increased signal intensity by a factor of three, compared with the stenosed region that increased signal intensity by a factor of two. In 1995, Walsh et al.[96] used a "key-hole" acquisition (only reacquiring the center of K-space every two heart beats and interpolating the data), with a small field-of-view, in 46 patients undergoing thallium scintigraphy. In 28 of 46 patients, there was 100% agreement (4 of 28 both normal, 24 of 28 both defects). In 8 of 46 patients, there were defects in both scans but not matched; in 5 of 46, the CMR was abnormal but SPECT was normal. In 5 of 46 patients, the CMR acquisition was not sufficient (one no gating, four not enough slices). A similar study was performed by Matheijssen et al.[97] in 1996, in which CMR-perfusion visually matched SPECT imaging in 90% of cases. Further analysis of the signal-intensity-time curves and a linear-fit approach, identified that the slope and the peak signal intensity increase were useful parameters. In 1997, Wilke et al.[98] used a central injection of gadolinium-DTPA to obtain a myocardial perfusion reserve index (MPRI) to differentiate between myocardium supplied by a normal coronary artery and that with a stenosed vessel. They produced a linear correlation between microspheres and MPRI in pigs, and between intracoronary Doppler flow and MPRI in humans. In 1999, Cullen et al.[99] studied the MPRI in 20 patients with ischemic heart disease and five normal volunteers. The MPRI in control patients was 4.21 ± 1.16 compared with 2.02 ± 0.7 for patients with ischemic heart disease. There also seemed to be a negative correlation between the MPRI and the diameter stenosis – >40% stenosis MPRI 2.8, >40% stenosis MPRI 1.93. In 2000, Al-Saadi et al.[100] performed a prospective study using single-slice CMP-perfusion and obtained sensitivity of 90% and specificity of 83% for detection of coronary stenoses >75%. In 2001, Schwitter et al.[101] studied 48 patients using a multislice hybrid echo planar imaging (EPI) sequence with 0.1 mmol/kg Omniscan (gadodiamide). Using parametric maps of the signal intensity up-slope, they obtained sensitivity of 91% and a specificity of 94% compared with PET. In 2003, Nagel et al.[102] performed rest-stress CMR-perfusion in 84 patients awaiting coronary angiography. Using Turbo-GRE/hybrid EPI sequence, they were able to obtain five slices per heart beat. The prevalence of CAD was 51%. They used an MPRI of 1.1 as a cut-off between normal and abnormal myocardium, and obtained sensitivity of 88%, specificity of 90%, and an accuracy of 89% for the detection of CAD. In patients with cardiac syndrome X, Panting et al.[103] identified subendocardial perfusion defects after adenosine vasodilatation, which could explain the angina symptoms and ECG abnormalities in these patients with normal epicardial coronary arteries.

4.2.1 Procedure

The patient is prepared for the scanner following standard procedures, including the checklist of contraindications to CMR. In addition, patients with specific contraindications to adenosine (e.g., bronchial asthma, patients taking dipyridamole) are excluded. Patients are asked to stop caffeine ingestion 24 hours before the examination, because caffeine reduces the vasodilator effects of adenosine. A 12-lead ECG is performed to exclude patients with second- and third-degree heart block. Baseline observations (heart rate and blood pressure) are obtained. Two intravenous cannulae are inserted into large peripheral veins, one connected to a saline-flushed long-line for the adenosine infusion, and the second to the gadolinium pump. Continuous ECG monitoring and automated blood pressure recording are connected. The patient is then positioned in the magnet bore. Using rapid pilot scans for accurate positioning, the perfusion slices are defined – this may include 2–5 short-axis slices, or a combination of short-axis and long-axis slices. A resting perfusion scan is then acquired using a saturation-recovery or inversion-recovery sequence with ultrafast gradient-echo or EPI. The acquisition is obtained with the patient performing a breath-hold or very shallow breathing, to minimize respiratory artifacts. During the acquisition, gadolinium is injected at a dose of 0.01–0.05 mmol/kg and between 50–60 images are obtained for each slice. The sequential effects of gadolinium on the signal intensity of the blood pool and myocardium are demonstrated in Figure 8.10. After the rest acquisition, it is necessary to wait for 20–30 minutes to allow the gadolinium to disperse from the myocardium, before proceeding to the stress study. The adenosine infusion is then commenced at a rate of 140 μg/kg/min for 4–6 minutes, when the perfusion acquisition is repeated. Blood pressure measurements and continuous ECG monitoring is performed. Once the study is complete, the patient can be removed from the magnet bore and allowed to recover. Analysis of the adenosine perfusion CMR may be performed using a 17-segment model [six basal-, six mid-, and four-apical short-axis segments as well as the apical cap; Figure 8.9 (see color section)]. However, it is important that the images are analyzed with reference to coronary artery territory. The analysis can be performed qualitatively (by visually reviewing the images as a cine-movie; Figure 8.11) or semiquantitatively with the use of signal-intensity-time curves (Figure 8.12). For visual analysis, delayed signal intensity increase in a myocardial segment is consistent with a significant coronary artery stenosis or previous MI. A fixed defect (present on the rest and the stress images) may represent a previous full-thickness or subendocardial MI. This can be demonstrated with "delayed-enhancement" gadolinium imaging, and will exclude artifacts. An inducible perfusion defect (present only on the stress images) represents an area subtended by a critically stenosed coronary artery. Semi-quantitative assessment with signal-intensity-time curves and myocardial perfusion reserve indices can also be used for the detection of coronary artery stenoses.

4.2.2 Advantages of Adenosine Perfusion CMR

Adenosine stress CMR has certain advantages compared with MPS:

- There is no radiation exposure with CMR. This enables the safe study of women of child-bearing age, pregnant women, children, and for many follow-up and research studies that would otherwise represent a significant cumulative radiation dose.
- CMR has superior resolution that results in the ability to detect subendocardial perfusion defects.

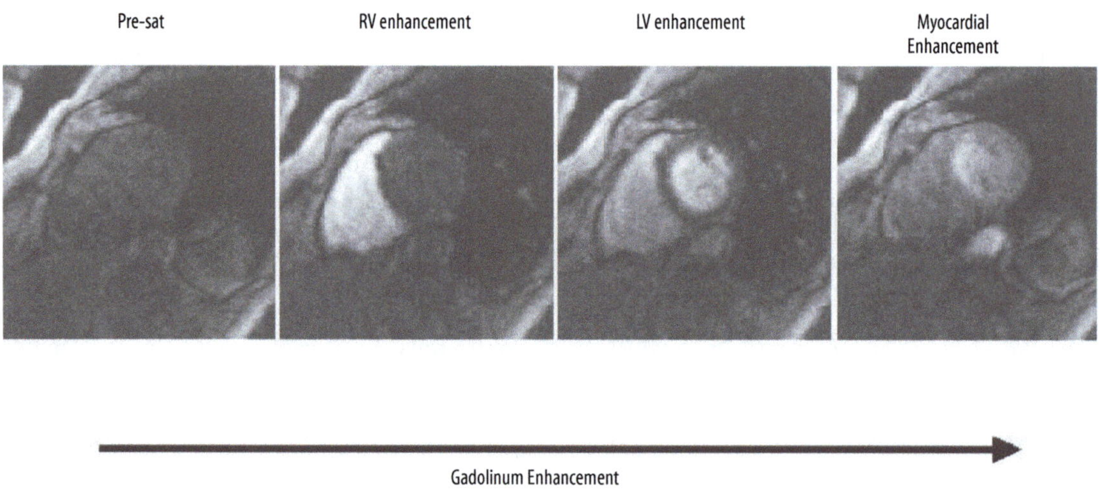

Figure 8.10. Before contrast administration, the saturation pulse nulls signal from the myocardium and blood pool. The gadolinium contrast enters the right ventricular (RV) blood pool producing "white-blood" images. The contrast rapidly transits the lungs and enters the left ventricle. The contrast then produces signal enhancement of the left ventricular (LV) myocardium. In a normal subject, there is uniform enhancement.

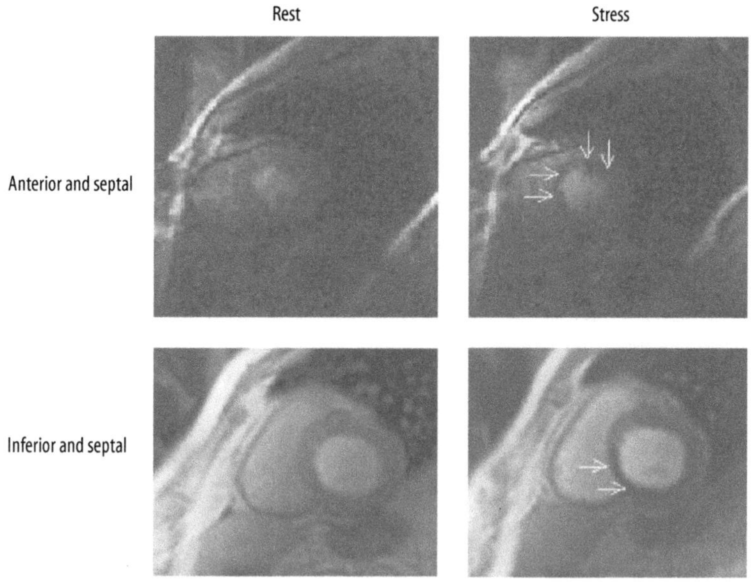

Figure 8.11. CMR perfusion images. The top panel demonstrates an inducible per-fusion defect in the anterior wall and anteroseptum consistent with significant disease in the left coronary artery. The lower panel demonstrates an inducible perfusion defect in the inferior wall and inferoseptum consistent with significant disease in the right coronary artery.

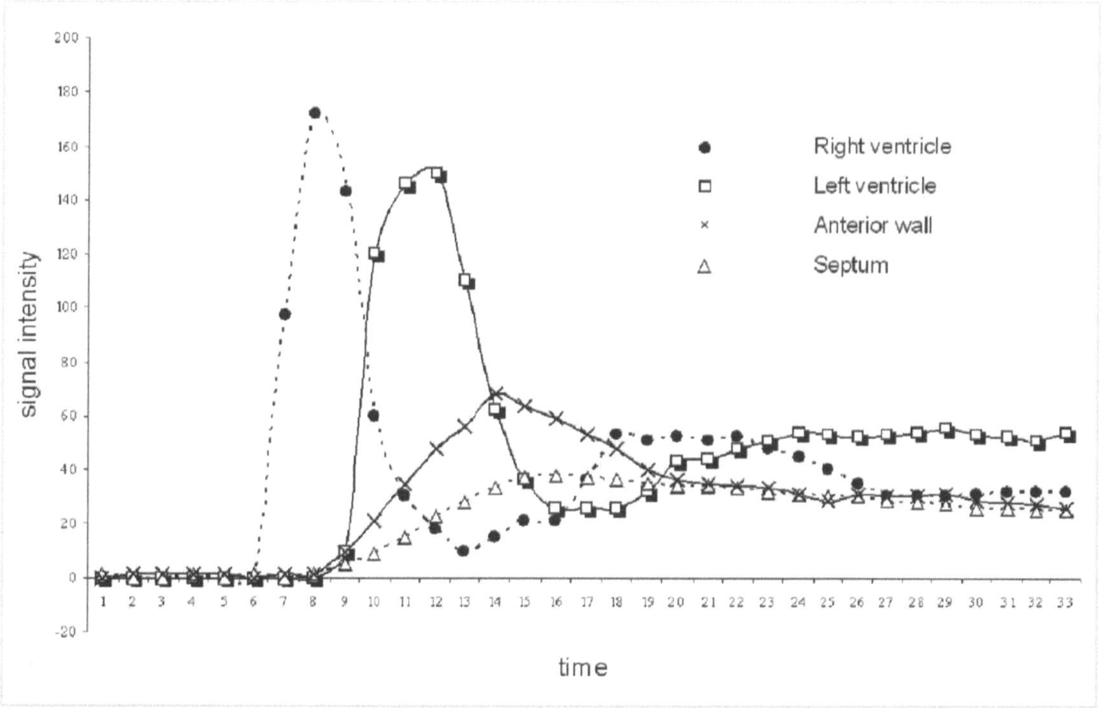

Figure 8.12. Signal-intensity-time curves. The left and right ventricular blood pools show a rapid up-slope and high peak signal intensity. The curve for the anterior wall is much steeper and reaches a higher peak compared with the septum (data plotted for the patient images in Figure 8.11 with an inferior and inferoseptal defect).

- CMR does not suffer from attenuation artifacts caused by breast or diaphragm that can reduce the accuracy of MPS.
- An adenosine perfusion CMR study can be performed in <60 minutes, which makes it more convenient for the patient than either the 1-day or 2-day MPS protocol.

4.2.3 Disadvantages of Adenosine Perfusion CMR

The main disadvantage of adenosine perfusion CMR compared with MPS or DSE is the novelty of the technique and its limited availability.

- SPECT and DSE are established techniques for the detection of CAD for male and female patients. In addition, both have prognostic data that can predict a future high or low likelihood of cardiovascular events.
- At present, there are limited data on detection of CAD in women and on cost-effectiveness.
- Because the administration of adenosine to a patient can produce unpleasant systemic side effects (flushing, abdominal pain, chest pain), patients with significant claustrophobia may not tolerate the scan.

5. Echocardiography

CAD can also be diagnosed with echocardiography by the presence of a regional wall motion abnormality that is seen at rest or during stress. Echocardiography, with its high spatial and temporal resolution, is an ideally suited noninvasive method of assessing such changes in wall motion. In the acute setting, the ability to detect these abnormalities can be very useful in the early detection of myocardial ischemia, even preceding changes on ECG. Equally, in patients presenting acutely with chest pain but inconclusive ECGs, normal regional wall motion may help exclude underlying ischemia. In nonacute situations, the presence of regional wall motion abnormalities and extent of left ventricular wall thinning can provide valuable information regarding the site and severity of damage together with the extent of remodeling. In patients with suspected CAD but no wall motion abnormality at rest, this may be induced by stress testing and detected by echocardiography. The improved image quality, particularly with harmonic imaging has allowed regional wall motion assessment to be much more reliable. Newer techniques that further improve endocardial definition, such as the use of contrast agents, now allow accurate assessment of wall motion in all vascular territories with improved reproducibility.

5.1 Regional Wall Motion Abnormality – How Does It Occur?

There is a well-established relationship between regional coronary blood flow and contractile function in the corresponding territory. In patients with normal coronary arteries, myocardial perfusion is maintained even when the oxygen demands of the tissue are increased. In patients with CAD, resting regional blood flow remains normal, despite severe stenosis of the supplying artery. This is achieved by compensatory vasodilation of the arterioles, which maintains resting MBF until the stenosis severity exceeds 80%–90% (although collaterals may maintain normal MBF even in this situation). As a result, resting wall motion may be entirely normal in patients with significant coronary disease. However, if the oxygen demand of the tissue is increased (e.g., during stress), because the vasodilator response is nearly exhausted, there is an inability to increase myocardial perfusion appropriately to that area. This leads to a reduction in the contractile function of that segment and, hence, to a regional wall motion abnormality. When the oxygen demands of that tissue are reduced and return to normal, there is resolution of the ischemia and wall motion returns to normal. However, severe CAD can give rise to prolonged persistence of wall motion abnormalities.

Acute coronary artery occlusion as seen in acute MI (AMI) leads to a rapid reduction in resting MBF and hence cessation of muscular contraction in the area supplied, leading to a reduction in ventricular function. Relief of the occlusion, either spontaneously or by treatment (such as thrombolysis) can lead to recovery of regional wall motion, but this depends on the duration of the occlusion and the extent of myocardial necrosis that has occurred as a result. The duration and severity of myocardial ischemia determines the degree of wall motion abnormality and indeed wall motion may not return to normal for several hours after the acute episode ("stunned myocardium").

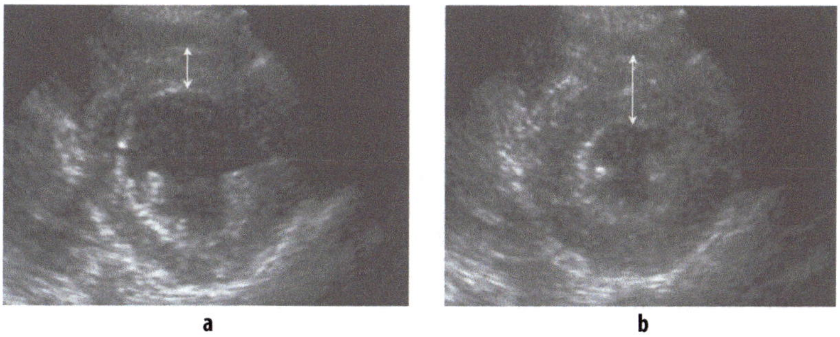

Figure 8.13. Parasternal short-axis views of the left ventricle during (**a**) diastole and (**b**) systole demonstrating normal systolic wall thickening.

In chronic CAD, progressive reduction in MBF caused by the progression of CAD may result in down-regulation of myocardial contractile function with preserved metabolic activity ("hibernating myocardium"). Diminished contractile function in chronic CAD may also occur as a result of myocardial stunning caused by repetitive episodes of ischemia followed by reperfusion. These episodes may either occur at rest (vasospasm) or during increased myocardial oxygen demand such as exercise. The detection of wall motion abnormalities during stress is the basis for diagnosis of CAD in patients without resting abnormalities. The wall motion abnormalities occur early in the "ischemic cascade," preceding ECG changes and symptoms (Figure 8.2).

5.2 Wall Motion Versus Systolic Wall Thickening for the Assessment of CAD

There are some limitations to using wall motion as the sole criterion for ischemia. The movement of any given segment of the ventricle is influenced by the adjacent muscle to which it is attached. For example, in a chamber with a dyskinetic ischemic segment, some of the adjacent normal tissue may appear hypokinetic because its motion is influenced by the attached dyskinetic muscle. The reverse phenomenon can also occur. If vigorously contracting normal muscle is next to an ischemic area, the hyperdynamic segment may pull the ischemic muscle toward the cavity, which may mask the abnormally perfused area. In general, wall motion abnormalities alone overestimate the degree of ischemia seen in the myocardium.

A more specific finding of ischemia is a deterioration of systolic wall thickening. Normal myocardial muscle increases in thickness during systole (Figure 8.13). During ischemia, there is a reduction or absence of systolic wall thickening. Indeed, there may also be systolic thinning during acute ischemia; i.e., wall thickening is greater in diastole compared with systole (Figure 8.14). It has been shown that the extent and severity of wall thickening abnormality

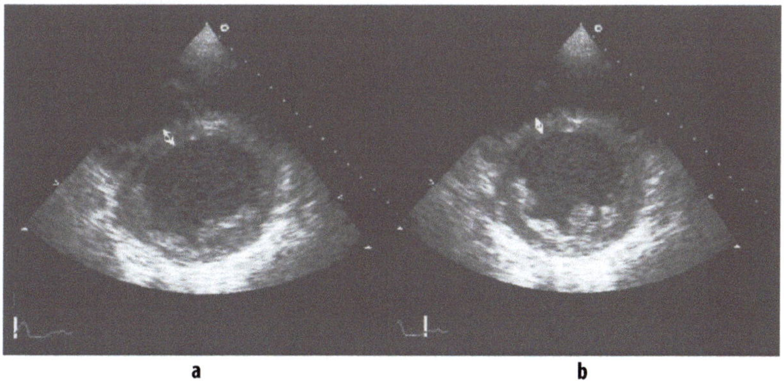

Figure 8.14. Parasternal short-axis views of (**a**) diastole and (**b**) systole of wall thickening in AMI.

is superior to that of wall motion abnormality evaluation for predicting outcome after AMI.[104]

Situations in which wall motion may be abnormal with preserved wall thickening include LBBB, Wolf-Parkinson-White syndrome, and when the patient has a paced rhythm. The presence of preserved systolic wall thickening in these conditions confirms that the wall motion abnormalities are not caused by underlying CAD.

5.3 Basic Anatomy and Echocardiographic Findings

The changes seen in regional wall motion correlate closely with the blood supply to that area of myocardium. Several methods have been used to portray the left ventricle in order that regional wall motion can be accurately described, although the basic principles remain the same. The ventricle is divided into three sections: base, mid-ventricular cavity, and the apex. Each section is then divided into segments that correspond to areas in the left ventricle wall. The most recent recommendations from the ACC and AHA[105] is to use a 17-segment model (Figure 8.15). This divides the base and mid-ventricular cavity into six segments each, with the apical section having four segments. A final segment is a very distal apical "cap" which is best assessed in the apical two- and four-chamber views. Often, a "bull's-eye" plot of all of these segments is used to note the individual segment scores,

Left Ventricular Segmentation

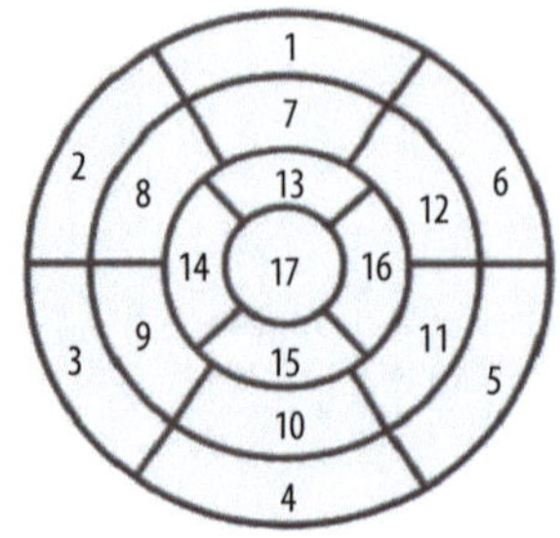

1. base anterior
2. basal anteroseptal
3. basal ingeroseptal
4. basal inferior
5. basal inferolateral
6. basal anterolateral
7. mid anterior
8. mid anteroseptal
9. mid inferoseptal
10. mid inferior
11. mid inferolateral
12. mid anterolateral
13. apical anterior
14. apical septal
15. apical inferior
16. apical lateral
17. apex

Figure 8.15. Diagram of the "bull's-eye" plot representing the 17 left ventricular segments in the recommended model.[105]

with the basal segments on the outside, followed by the mid-cavity and then the apex. This allows clear localization of any defect on a single form with an indication of vascular supply (Figure 8.16).

Once these changes have been established, wall motion can be scored according to a four-point semiquantitative scale:

1. Normal
2. Hypokinetic – normally directed motion, but reduced endocardial excursion and wall thickening

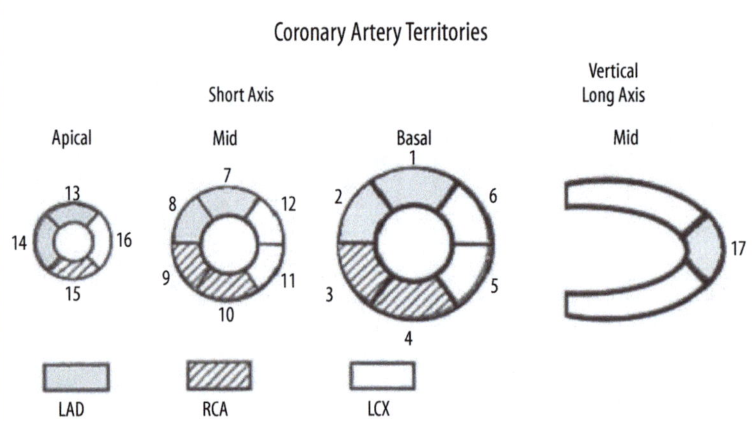

Figure 8.16. Assignment of the 17 myocardial segments to the territories of the left anterior descending (LAD), right coronary artery (RCA), and left circumflex artery (LCx).[105]

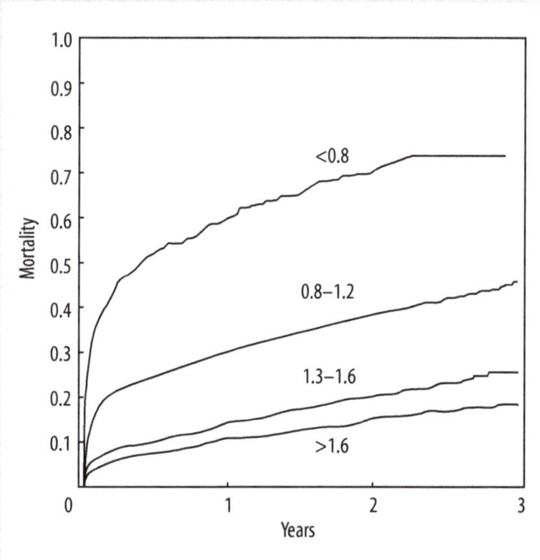

Figure 8.17. Graph demonstrating relationship between mortality and wall motion score index (WMSI).[106] (By permission of Oxford University Press on behalf of The European Society of Cardiology.)

3. Akinetic – absent wall motion/thickening
4. Dyskinetic – systolic bulging of the wall with no thickening

The sum of the individual segment scores gives a wall motion score (WMS), which can be used to give an indication of the severity of ischemia found; a WMS index (WMSI) can also be used (WMS divided by the number of segments assessed) and has been shown to be an important prognostic indicator in patients with CAD (Figure 8.17).[106,107]

5.4 Stress Echocardiography

5.4.1 Procedure and Interpretation

Stress echocardiography, which was first introduced in the early 1980s, has matured over the years as a reliable and cost-effective method for both the diagnosis and risk stratification of patients with suspected or known CAD (see also Chapters 2 and 9). It can be performed in conjunction with dynamic exercise (treadmill or bicycle). In patients who are unable to exercise, pharmacologic agents may be used, i.e., dobutamine or dipyridamole. With any form of stress testing, echocardiographic images are first acquired digitally during rest in parasternal and apical views. These views of the heart visualize all three vascular territories. Subsequently, stress images are acquired during low, intermediate, and peak stress, except for treadmill exercise in which images may be acquired immediately (60–90 seconds) after peak stress for optimal imaging. Stress and rest images are arranged digitally side by side in each view for analysis and archiving.

Rest and stress images are interpreted for global and regional left ventricular size, shape, and function. A normal response is when, during stress, the left ventricular size becomes smaller compared with rest while the shape is maintained and there is increased endocardial excursion and systolic wall thickening (Figure 8.18). Figure 8.19 is an example of a patient who had undergone exercise echocardiography, demonstrating a dilated left ventricular cavity with change in shape with marked reduction of systolic wall thickening of the septum, anterior and inferior wall suggestive of multivessel disease. Prolonged persistence of a systolic wall thickening abnormality may also identify severe CAD.[108]

Dobutamine echocardiography is particularly useful in patients with an existing resting wall thickening abnormality. Low-dose dobutamine increases myocardial perfusion, recruits potentially contractile myocardium, and hence increases myocardial contractility in dysfunctional myocardium if there is sufficient contractile reserve. At high dose, however, dobutamine increases myocardial O_2 demand and, in the presence of a flow-limiting stenosis, will result in demand/supply mismatch leading to myocardial ischemia and hence deterioration of regional function.[109] Thus, dobutamine at low doses depicts the presence of myocardial viability whereas at high dose, myocardial ischemia (biphasic response; Figure 8.20).

Dobutamine is also widely used as an alternative test in patients who are unable to exercise. Figure 8.21 describes the various myocardial responses to dobutamine in patients with and without resting wall thickening abnormality. Dipyridamole is used in some centers as a form of stress test but the study may be negative even in the presence of a significant flow-limiting coronary stenosis.[110]

5.4.2 Accuracy of Stress Echocardiography

The accuracy of stress echo, and other noninvasive imaging tests, for the detection of CAD is

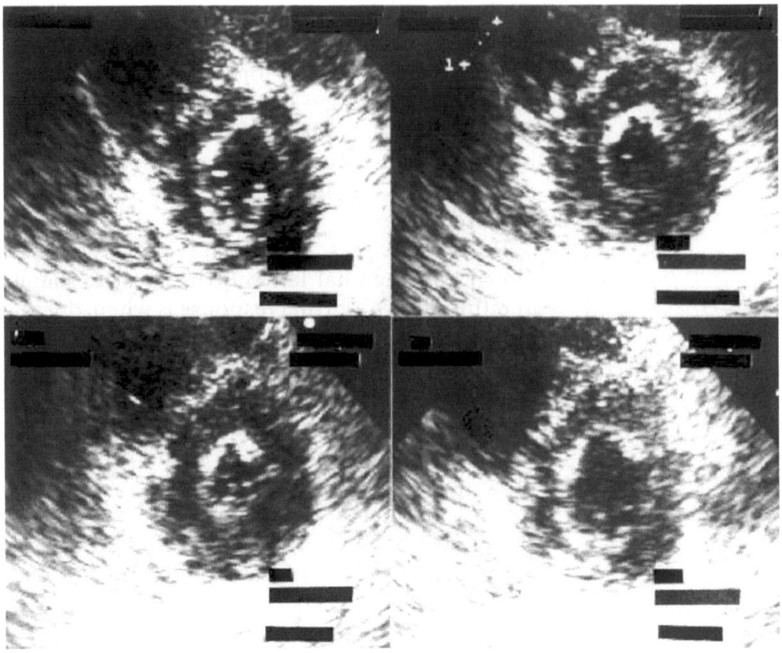

Figure 8.18. A normal left ventricular response during dobutamine stress in the short-axis view. Upper left (rest), upper right (low dose of dobutamine), lower left (high dose of dobutamine), and lower left post-stress.

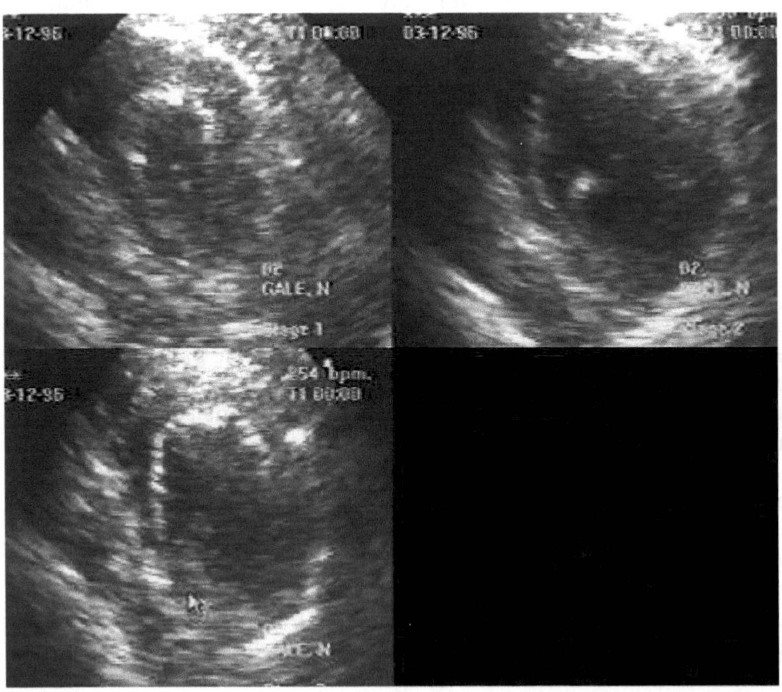

Figure 8.19. Abnormal left ventricular response during exercise. Left (rest); right (60 seconds after exercise). Left ventricle is dilated with severe systolic wall thickening abnormalities affecting septum, anterior and inferior wall, suggestive of multivessel disease.

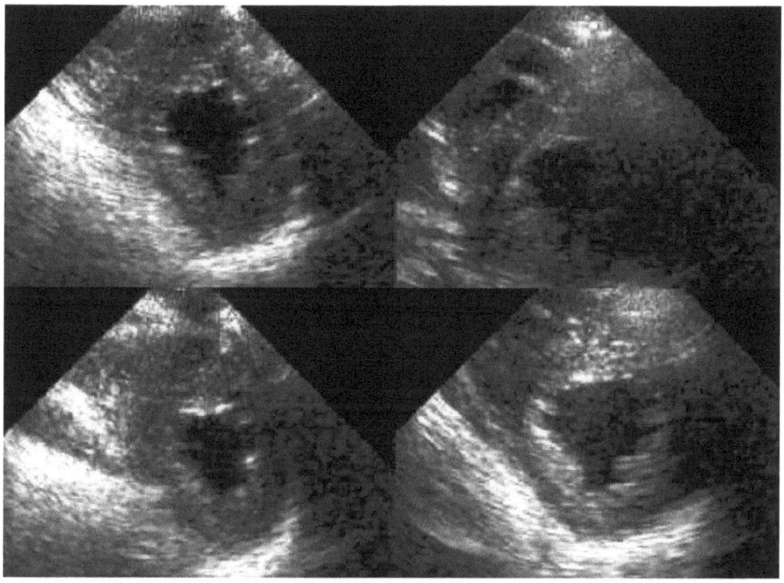

Figure 8.20. Biphasic response during dobutamine stress upper left (rest), upper right and lower left (low dose of dobutamine), and lower right (high dose of dobutamine). There was improvement of systolic wall thickness in a patient with left ventricular dysfunction with deterioration of wall thickness both anteriorly and inferiorly during high dose.

expressed as the sensitivity and specificity of the technique for the detection of angiographically demonstrated stenoses. Nonetheless, this approach has a number of limitations, which are mainly a reflection of the limitations of an angiographic cut-off for significant disease, including the variation of the physiologic effect of a stenosis based on site, length, and vessel size, as well as over- and underestimation of coronary lesion severity.[111] Therefore, it is probably more meaningful to correlate the findings of stress echo (and those of MPS and CMR) with functional and not anatomic parameters derived from coronary angiography (see above, MPS section).

Populations with a high prevalence of multivessel coronary disease and previous MI are more likely to develop ischemia in response to stress, and referral bias may also influence the recorded accuracy. Because stress echo is dependent on the induction of ischemia, the adequacy of stress has a pivotal influence on sensitivity. Finally, accuracy will be influenced by echocardiographic factors including image

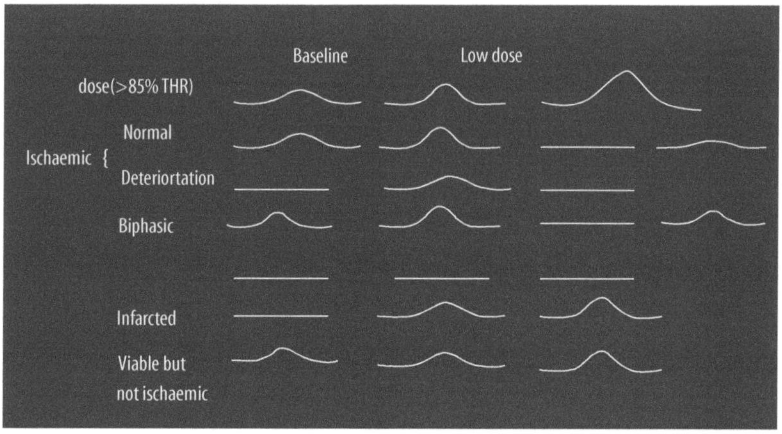

Figure 8.21. Different responses to dobutamine.

Table 8.4. Causes of false-negative and false-positive stress echocardiograms

False negatives	False positives
Inadequate stress	Over-interpretation, interpreter bias
Antianginal treatment (especially beta-blockers)	Localized basal inferior wall abnormalities
Mild stenoses	Abnormal septal motion (LBBB, post-CABG)
Left circumflex disease	Cardiomyopathies
Poor image quality	Hypertensive responses to stress
Delayed images post-stress	

LBBB, left bundle branch block; CABG, coronary artery bypass grafting.

quality and left ventricular morphology; the lateral wall is a frequent site of false negatives and the inferior wall for false positives. Causes of false-positive and -negative tests are listed in Table 8.4.

In studies of exercise echocardiography enrolling many patients (>100 patients), the sensitivity and specificity range from 74% to 97% and 64% to 86%, respectively (Figure 8.22; see color section).[112] Higher sensitivity may be obtained with bicycle exercise (because there is no loss of ischemia in the post-stress period), but this is at the cost of some impairment in specificity. Comparisons with quantitative angiography have shown stenosis diameters of 0.7–1.0 mm to be associated with ischemia.

With DSE, the sensitivity ranges from 61% to 95%, and the specificity from 51% to 95% (Figure 8.22; see color section). The increment in cardiac workload is less with dobutamine than exercise, and sensitivity can be compromised if workload is reduced by medical treatment or dose-limiting side effects. The addition of atropine augments sensitivity. Dobutamine echocardiography is a more sensitive marker of ischemia in lesions involving larger (>2.6-mm diameter) vessels than smaller vessels. The quantitative angiography parameters associated with ischemia are a lumen diameter of <1-mm diameter, percent diameter stenosis of 52%, and percent area stenosis of 75%, of which the minimal lumen diameter is most predictive of an abnormal dobutamine stress test.

The sensitivity and specificity of dipyridamole and adenosine stress echocardiography for the detection of CAD range from 61% to 81% and 90% to 94%, respectively (Figure 8.22; see color section). Some studies with these techniques have included populations with a high prevalence of extensive coronary disease or prior infarction – both of which are associated with a high sensitivity.

5.5 Comparison Between Stress Echocardiography and Radionuclide MPS

Stress echocardiography has been compared with both CMR (see above in the CMR section) and MPS in the setting of CAD. A recent meta-analysis by Geleijnse and Elhendy[113] of seven studies directly comparing exercise echocardiography and exercise MPS revealed comparable sensitivities (78% versus 83%, respectively) and specificities (91% versus 83%, respectively). In the same review, the authors also compared dobutamine echocardiography with dobutamine MPS; in eight studies, they found that dobuta-

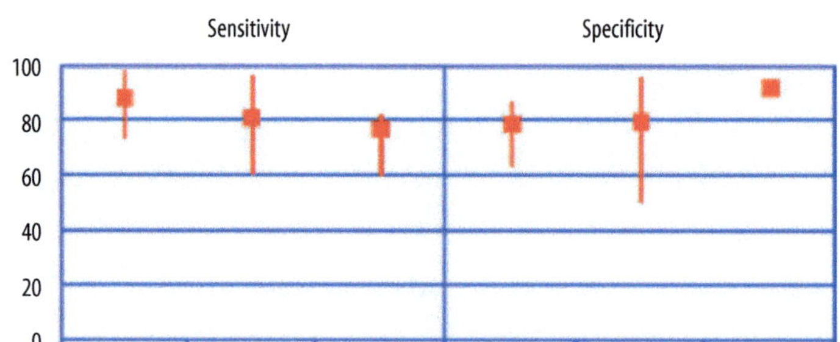

	ExE	DbE	DpyE	ExE	DbE	DpyE
Highest	97	95	81	86	95	94
Lowest	74	61	61	64	51	90
Hean	88	91	77	79	80	92

Figure 8.22. Summary of the mean, high, and low values for sensitivity and specificity in studies of >100 patients with exercise (ExE), dobutamine (DbE), and dipyridamole stress echo (DpyE).

mine echocardiography had a lower sensitivity than MPS (80% versus 86%, respectively, $P < .05$), but a higher specificity (86% versus 73%, respectively, $P < .005$).[113] The sensitivity of vasodilator echocardiography, however, was significantly lower than that of vasodilator MPS (66% versus 85%, $P < .0001$) in six studies.[113] This is not surprisingly because adenosine and dipyridamole cause blood flow heterogeneity, which is useful in MPS, but generally do not result in true myocardial ischemia, which is required for causing contractile abnormalities. Another meta-analysis by Schinkel et al.[114] examined 17 studies in which MPS was directly compared with stress echocardiography. Pooled data revealed that MPS was more sensitive than echocardiography (sensitivity 85% versus 80%, respectively, $P < .05$) but less specific (specificity 77% versus 86%, respectively, $P < .001$).

Few studies have directly compared MPS and stress echocardiography in women. One study has shown no significant difference between them,[115] whereas others have demonstrated a superior specificity of dobutamine echocardiography over dobutamine MPS in women.[116,117] It is, however, debatable whether such a comparison is appropriate and more studies are needed to assess fully the relative merits of each technique in this population. Based on the existing data (mainly from subpopulation analysis of mixed-gender studies), however, current European and American guidelines do not favor a superiority of one test over the other and accept that both stress echocardiography and gated SPECT MPS provide accurate diagnostic and prognostic information for women investigated for CAD.

Patients with generalized LVH is a group in which the specificity of MPS can be affected by perfusion defects that are caused by abnormalities in the microcirculation. Dobutamine echocardiography does not have these limitations and although some investigators have found it to be equally effective with MPS for detecting underlying CAD[118] others suggest that the former is probably the technique of choice in this clinical setting.[119]

5.5.1 Limitations in the Diagnostic Use of Stress Echocardiography

Although the presence of CAD is readily recognized in the setting of multivessel disease, and multivessel pathology is readily recognized in the presence of prior infarction ("ischemia at a distance"), the technique has a sensitivity of only 50% for the recognition of the multivessel disease pattern in normal ventricles. The development of global ventricular dysfunction (reduction of ejection fraction or left ventricular enlargement) should increase the interpreter's suspicion of multivessel disease. Clues to the presence of extensive disease despite apparently localized wall motion abnormalities include the early onset of ischemia, at a low heart rate and rate–pressure product, or at a low dose of pharmacologic stressor.

The detection of single-vessel stenoses may also be problematic, and the sensitivity of stress echo is less than that of MPS. This reflects the need for the ischemia to involve a significant area of the myocardium in order for the stress echocardiogram to be positive – which may not be fulfilled if the involved vessel is small or distal, or the stenosis is only mildly flow limiting.

Because of problems posed by identification of minor gradations of wall motion in the setting of abnormal function, the identification of ischemia within areas of resting wall motion abnormalities may be difficult. The problem is probably less significant during dobutamine stress because ischemic segments with abnormal resting function often show a biphasic response.

The last three issues reflect fundamental limitations of an ischemia-based technique,[120] which will require either a more sensitive tool for assessment of wall motion, or combination with a perfusion marker such as contrast echocardiography.

5.6 Stress Contrast Echocardiography

Myocardial contrast echocardiography is a newly developed technique that utilizes intravascular tracers, which are microbubbles (3–5 μ) that can be administered intravenously.[121] During infusion of contrast agent once steady state is reached, the contrast intensity represents microvascular blood volume.[122] During this steady state, microbubbles in the myocardium may be destroyed by a high-energy ultrasound pulse, after which microbubbles can be seen to replenish the myocardium. The rate at which the microbubbles replenish represents myocardial blood velocity.[123] The product of the myocardial blood velocity and volume represents MBF.[123] It has been shown both experimentally and clinically that flow-limiting CAD can be detected during any form of stress which includes inotropic action, when contrast intensity diminishes because of capillary derecruitment and myocardial blood velocity is slower compared with the normal vascular bed.[124,125] There are several studies that clearly showed that addition of myocardial contrast echocardiography during stress improves the diagnostic value of stress echocardiography.[126–128]

6. Recommendations for Using Noninvasive Cardiac Imaging in Patients Investigated for CAD

Many centers use a staged approach with the exercise ECG being the initial stress test and noninvasive imaging next (usually in the form of stress MPS or stress ECHO) if the likelihood of disease is indeterminate after the exercise ECG, or if further information on myocardial perfusion or function is required to assist management decisions (Figure 8.23). The choice of which test to perform depends greatly on issues of local expertise and available facilities and also on the advantages and disadvantages of each technique discussed above. Noninvasive imaging should be the initial investigation in patients who are unlikely to exercise adequately and if the exercise ECG will be uninterpretable because of resting abnormalities such as LBBB, preexcitation, LVH, or drug effects.[5] For symptomatic female patients, there is a broad consensus on the use of either stress MPS or ECHO as a first-line investigation when the resting ECG is abnormal and, although more widespread use may be justified, there is some controversy on the strength of the existing evidence for supporting the primary use of these two tests in all female patients.[20b,68] At present, there is no strong evidence to justify the use of EBCT or MS-CT for the patients discussed here. It is conceivable, however, that as these techniques become more mature, they will find their place in the management algorithm. A suggested example of potential use is the group of individuals who on the basis of symptoms and risk-factor profile are judged to have a rather low pretest probability of coronary heart disease. Such patients are usually directed to an exercise ECG which does not possess an optimal specificity value that is essential in this clinical setting (see also previous chapter).

Of course, there will always be patients with symptoms but negative results on conventional imaging, on which occasion and, depending on clinical judgment, assessment of the endothelial function or microvascular circulation may

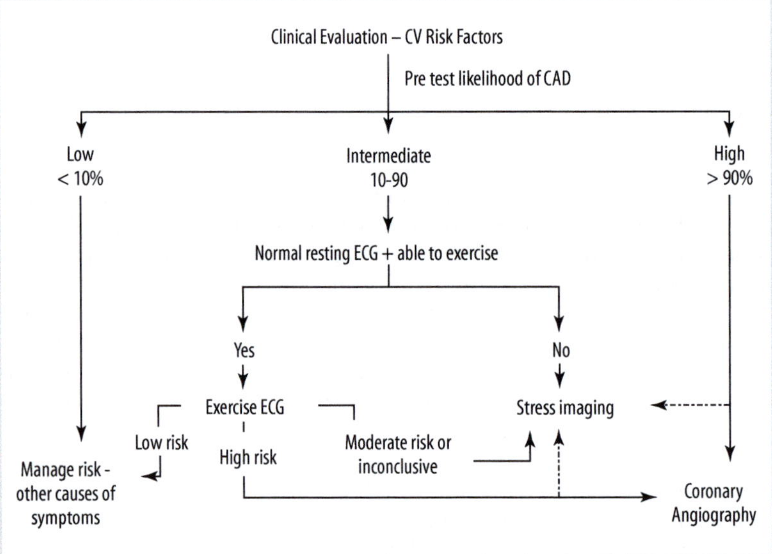

Figure 8.23. According to the ACC/AHA class I recommendations, patients should be classified into three categories based on clinical and cardiovascular risk-factors assessment: 1) low pretest likelihood of coronary artery disease (CAD) does not warrant further cardiac evaluation. Management of modifiable risk factors is recommended. 2) Patients with a high probability of CAD should be referred for coronary angiography. 3) Patients with an intermediate likelihood and a normal resting ECG who are able to exercise should undergo exercise ECG. Stress imaging is recommended in patients with an abnormal resting ECG, and in those unable to exercise adequately. Stress imaging is also indicated in patients with a moderate-risk treadmill score for further stratification, and for the assessment of the extent and severity of myocardial ischemia in patients referred for coronary angiography.

be appropriate. Brachial artery reactivity or coronary flow reserve testing (invasively by catheterization or noninvasively with special echocardiography, CMR, or PET techniques) are useful tools, and their role in this group of patients will be covered in Chapter 14.

7. Conclusions

Stress MPS, ECHO, and CMR are highly effective in diagnosing CAD. An inducible perfusion or contraction abnormality indicates impaired perfusion or contractile reserve, which in turn usually corresponds to epicardial coronary obstruction. The site and severity of the abnormality provide diagnostic and management information. Conversely, a normal result in a study that has been performed appropriately indicates the absence of coronary obstruction and hence of clinically significant disease. MPS is the most mature technique providing not only high diagnostic accuracy but also invaluable prognostic information stronger than any other technique for the management of patients investigated for CAD. Stress echocardiography has become an important counter player in this field because of its versatility and availability. In the hands of skillful operators, its diagnostic accuracy is comparable to that of MPS. CMR has been used less than the other two techniques in clinical practice, but with continuous improvements in the technology and skills of the operators and also increasing availability, it will have a more important role in the years to come. It is more versatile than MS-CT, allowing not only visualization of the coronary vessels but also assessment of perfusion, which is important for accurate assessment of the functional significance of a coronary lesion and hence for management decisions. However, combination of the latter with PET (PET/CT) offers a unique opportunity for a comprehensive imaging of cardiac morphology, perfusion, and function. It is difficult to predict the exact role of each technique in the years to come, and comparative data from good quality studies on clinical and cost effectiveness of the various imaging techniques in different subgroups of patients are still sparse. On the whole, however, it is expected that ongoing refinement of the existing techniques and introduction of new agents will allow a more accurate evaluation of different aspects of the wide spectrum of CAD and will pave the way toward molecular targeted cardiac imaging, thus increasing even further the diagnostic and prognostic value of noninvasive imaging.

References

1. Mackay J, Mensah G. Atlas of Heart Disease and Stroke. Geneva: World Health Organization;2004:1–112.
2. Ockene IS, Miller NH. Cigarette smoking, cardiovascular disease, and stroke: a statement for healthcare professionals from the American Heart Association. American Heart Association Task Force on Risk Reduction. Circulation 1997;96:3243–3247.
3. Myers RH, Kiely DK, Cupples LA, Kannel WB. Parental history is an independent risk factor for coronary artery disease: the Framingham Study. Am Heart J 1990;120:963–969.
4. Coronary Artery Surgery Study (CASS). A randomised trial of coronary artery bypass surgery. Survival data. Circulation 1983;68:939–950.
5. Gibbons RJ, Abrams J, Chatterjee K, et al. ACC/AHA 2002 guideline update for the management of patients with chronic stable angina – summary article: a report of the American College of Cardiology/American Heart Association Task Force on Practice Guidelines (Committee on the Management of Patients with Chronic Stable Angina). J Am Coll Cardiol 2003;41:159–168.
6. Diamond GA, Forrester JS. Analysis of probability as an aid in the clinical diagnosis of coronary artery disease. N Engl J Med 1979;300:1350–1358.
7. Wilson PW, D'Agostino RB, Levy D, Belanger AM, Silbershatz H, Kannel WB. Prediction of coronary heart disease using risk factor categories. Circulation 1998; 97:1837–1847.
8. Master AM, Oppenheimer ET. A simple exercise tolerance test for circulatory efficiency with standard tables for normal individuals. Am J Med Sci 1929;177:223.
9. Gibbons RJ, Balady GJ, Brocker JT, et al. ACC/AHA 2002 guideline update for exercise testing: a report of the American College of Cardiology/American Heart Association Task Force on Practice Guidelines (Committee on Exercise Testing). 2002. Available at www.acc.org/clinical/guidelines/exercise/dirIndex.htm.
10. Colby J, Hakki AH, Iskandrian AS, et al. Hemodynamic, angiographic and scintigraphic correlates of positive exercise electrocardiograms: emphasis on strongly positive exercise electrocardiograms. J Am Coll Cardiol 1983;2:21–29.
11. Fortuin NJ, Friesinger GC. Exercise-induced ST segment elevation: clinical, electrocardiographic and arteriographic studies in twelve patients. Am J Med 1970; 49:459–464.
12. Chahine RA, Raizner AE, Ishimori T. The clinical significance of exercise-induced ST-segment elevation. Circulation 1976;54:209–213.
13. Weiner DA, Ryan TJ, McCabe CH, et al. Value of exercise testing in determining the risk classification and the response to coronary artery bypass grafting in three-vessel coronary artery disease: a report from the Coronary Artery Surgery Study (CASS) registry. Am J Cardiol 1987;60:262–266.
14. Mark DB, Hlatky MA, Harrell FE Jr, Lee KL, Califf RM, Pryor DB. Exercise treadmill score for predicting prog-

nosis in coronary artery disease. Ann Intern Med 1987;106:793–800.
15. Shaw LJ, Peterson ED, Shaw LK, et al. Use of a prognostic treadmill score in identifying diagnostic coronary disease subgroups. Circulation 1998;98:1622–1630.
16. Mark DB, Shaw L, Harrell FE Jr, et al. Prognostic value of a treadmill exercise score in outpatients with suspected coronary artery disease. N Engl J Med 1991; 325:849–853.
17. Kwok Y, Kim C, Grady D, Segal M, Redberg R. Meta-analysis of exercise testing to detect coronary artery disease in women. Am J Cardiol 1999;83:660–666.
18. Kemp HG, Kronmal RA, Vlietstra RE, et al. Seven year survival of patients with normal or near normal coronary arteriograms: a CASS registry study. J Am Coll Cardiol 1986;7:479–483.
19. Sharaf BL, Pepine CJ, Kerensky RA, et al. Detailed angiographic analysis of women with suspected ischemic chest pain (pilot phase data from the NHLBI-sponsored Women's Ischemia Syndrome Evaluation [WISE] Study Angiographic Core Laboratory). Am J Cardiol 2001;87:937–941.
20a. Waters DD, Gordon D, Rossouw JE, Cannon RO, Collins P, Herrington DM. AHA/NHLBI Conference Proceedings. Women's Ischemic Syndrome Evaluation [WISE]. Current status and future research directions. Lessons from hormone replacement trials. Circulation 2004; 109:e53–e55.
20b. Mieres JH, Shaw LJ, Arai A, et al. Role of noninvasive testing in the clinical evaluation of women with suspected coronary artery disease. Consensus statement from the Cardiac Imaging Committee, Council on Clinical Cardiology, and the Cardiovascular Imaging and Intervention Committee, Council on Cardiovascular Radiology and Intervention, American Heart Association. Circulation 2005;111:682–696.
21. Wong TY, Klein R, Sharrett AR, et al. Retinal arteriolar narrowing and risk of coronary heart disease in men and women. The Atherosclerosis Risk in Communities Study. JAMA 2002;287:1153–1159.
22. Weich H, Strauss H, Pitt B. The extraction of thallium-201 by the myocardium. Circulation 1977;56:188–191.
23. Watson DD, Glover DK. Overview of kinetics and modeling. In: Zaret BL, Beller GA, eds. Nuclear Cardiology. State of the Art and Future Directions. St. Louis: Mosby; 1999:3–12.
24. Pohost GM, et al. Differentiation of transiently ischemic from infarcted myocardium by serial imaging after single dose of thallium-201. Circulation 1977;55: 294–302.
25. Dilsizian V, et al. Enhanced detection of ischemic but viable myocardium by the reinjection of thallium after stress-redistribution imaging. N Engl J Med 1990; 323:141–146.
26. Basu S, Senior R, Raval U, Lahiri A. Superiority of nitrate-enhanced Tl-201 over conventional redistribution Tl-201 imaging for prognostic evaluation after myocardial infarction and thrombolysis. Circulation 1997;96:2932–2937.
27. Loong CY, Anagnostopoulos C. Diagnosis of coronary artery disease by radionuclide myocardial perfusion imaging. Heart 2003;90(suppl V):v2–v9.
28. Glover DK, Ruiz M, Yang JY, Smith WH, Watson DD, Beller GA. Myocardial Tc-99m-tetrofosmin uptake during adenosine-induced vasodilatation with either a critical or mild coronary stenosis. Comparison with Tl-201 and regional myocardial blood flow. Circulation 1997;96:2332–2338.
29. Marshall R, Leidholt EM Jr, Zhang DY, Barnett CA. Technetium-99m-hexakis 2 methoxy-2-isobutyl isonitrile and thallium-201 extraction, washout, and retention at varying coronary flow rates in rabbit heart. Circulation 1990;82:998–1007.
30. Leon AR, Eisner RL, Martin SE, Schmarkey LS, Aaron AM, Boyers AS, et al. Comparison of single-photon emission computed tomography (SPECT) myocardial perfusion imaging with thallium-201 and technetium-99m sestamibi in dogs. J Am Coll Cardiol 1992;20: 1612–1625.
31. Hachamovitch R, Berman DS, Kiat H, et al. Exercise myocardial perfusion SPECT in patients without known coronary artery disease: incremental prognostic value and use in risk stratification. Circulation 1996;93:905–914.
32. Bateman TM, O'Keefe JH Jr, Dong VM, Barnhart C, Ligon RW. Coronary angiography rates after stress single-photon emission computed tomographic scintigraphy. J Nucl Cardiol 1995;2:217–223.
33. Iskandrian AS, Heo J, Kong B, et al. Effect of exercise level on the ability of thallium-201 tomographic imaging in detecting coronary artery disease: analysis of 461 patients. J Am Coll Cardiol 1989;14:1477–1486.
34. Anagnostopoulos C, Harbinson M, Kelion A, et al. Procedure guidelines for radionuclide myocardial perfusion imaging. Heart 2004;90(suppl I):i1–10.
35. Maddahi J, Van Train K, Pringent F, et al. Quantitative single photon emission computed thallium-201 tomography for detection and localization of coronary artery disease: optimization and prospective validation of a new technique. J Am Coll Cardiol 1989;14:1689–1699.
36. Mahmarian JJ, Boyce TM, Goldberg RK, et al. Quantitative exercise thallium-201 single photon emission computed tomography for the enhanced diagnosis of ischemic heart disease. J Am Coll Cardiol 1990;15: 318–329.
37. Chae SC, Heo J, Iskandrian AS, et al. Identification of extensive coronary artery disease in women by exercise single-photon emission computed tomographic (SPECT) thallium imaging. J Am Coll Cardiol 1993; 21:1305–1311.
38. Van Train KF, Garcia EV, Maddahi J, et al. Multicenter trial validation for quantitative analysis of same-day rest-stress technetium-99-sestamibi myocardial tomograms. J Nucl Med 1994;35:609–618.
39. Nishimura S, Mahmarian JJ, Boyce TM, et al. Equivalence between adenosine and exercise thallium-201 myocardial tomography: a multicentre, prospective, crossover trial. J Am Coll Cardiol 1992;20:265–275.
40. O'Keefe HH Jr, Bateman TM, Barnhart CS. Adenosine thallium-201 is superior to exercise thallium-201 for detecting coronary artery disease in patients with left bundle branch block. J Am Coll Cardiol 1993; 21:1332–1338.
41. Ebersole DG, Heironimus J, Toney MO, Billingsley J. Comparison of exercise and adenosine technetium-99m sestamibi myocardial scintigraphy for diagnosis of coronary artery disease in patients with left bundle branch block. Am J Cardiol 1993;71:450–453.
42. Wilson RF, Wyche K, Christensen BV, et al. Effects of adenosine on human coronary arterial circulation. Circulation 1990;82:1595–1606.

43. Chan SY, Brunken RC, Czernin J, et al. Comparison of maximal myocardial blood flow during adenosine infusion with that of intravenous dipyridamole in normal men. J Am Coll Cardiol 1992;20:979–985.
44. Akinboboye O, Idris O, Chou RL, et al. Absolute quantitation of coronary steal induced by intravenous dipyridamole. J Am Coll Cardiol 2001;37:109–116.
45. Reyes E, Wechalekar S, Loong CY, et al. Acute myocardial infarction during adenosine myocardial perfusion imaging. J Nucl Cardiol 2004;11:97–99.
46. Smits P, Lenders JW, Thien T. Caffeine and theophylline attenuate adenosine-induced vasodilation in humans. Clin Pharmacol Ther 1990;48:410–418.
47. Taillefer R, Ahlberg AW, Massod Y, et al. Acute betablockade reduces the extent and severity of myocardial perfusion defects with dipyridamole Tc-99m sestamibi SPECT imaging. J Am Coll Cardiol 2003;42:1475–1483.
48. O'Keefe JH, Bateman TM, Handlin LR, Barnhart CS. Four- versus 6-minute infusion protocol for adenosine thallium-201 single photon emission computed tomography imaging. Am Heart J 1995;129:482–487.
49. Villegas BJ, Hendel RC, Dahlberg ST, McSherry BA, Leppo JA. Comparison of a 3- versus 6-minute infusion of adenosine in thallium-201 myocardial perfusion imaging. Am Heart J 1993;126:103–107.
50. Treuth MG, Reyes GA, He XZ, Cwajg E, Mahmarian JJ, Verani MS. Tolerance and diagnostic accuracy of an abbreviated adenosine infusion for myocardial scintigraphy: a randomized prospective study. J Nucl Cardiol 2001;8:548–554.
51. Shanoudy H, Raggi P, Beller GA, et al. Comparison of technetium-99m tetrofosmin and thallium-201 single-photon emission computed tomographic imaging for detection of myocardial perfusion defects in patients with coronary artery disease. J Am Coll Cardiol 1998; 31:331–337.
52. Soman P, Taillefer R, de Puey EG, Udelson JE, Lahiri A. Enhanced detection of reversible perfusion defects by Tc-99m sestamibi compared to Tc-99m tetrofosmin during vasodilator stress SPECT imaging in mild-to-moderate coronary artery disease. J Am Coll Cardiol 2001;37:458–462.
53. Ranhosky A, Kempthorne-Rawson J. The safety of intravenous dipyridamole thallium myocardial perfusion imaging. Circulation 1990;81:1205–1209.
54. Cerqueira M, Verani M, Schwaiger M, et al. Safety profile of adenosine stress perfusion imaging: results from the Adenoscan multicentre trial registry. J Am Coll Cardiol 1994;23:384–389.
55. Pennell DJ, Mavrogeni SI, Forbat SM, et al. Adenosine combined with dynamic exercise for myocardial perfusion imaging. J Am Coll Cardiol 1995;25:1300–1309.
56. Vitola JV, Brambatti JC, Caligaris F, et al. Exercise supplementation to dipyridamole prevents hypotension, improves electrocardiogram sensitivity, and increases heart-to-liver activity ratio on Tc-99m sestamibi imaging. J Nucl Cardiol 2001;8:652–659.
57. Hurwitz GA, Saddy S, O'Donoghue P, et al. The VEX-test for myocardial scintigraphy with thallium-201 and sestamibi: effect on abdominal background activity. J Nucl Med 1995;36:914–920.
58. Samady H, Wackers FJT, Joska TM, Zaret BL, Jain D. Pharmacologic stress perfusion imaging with adenosine: role of simultaneous low-level treadmill exercise. J Nucl Cardiol 2002;9:188–196.
59. Thomas GS, Miyamoto MI. Should simultaneous exercise become the standard for adenosine myocardial perfusion imaging? Am J Cardiol 2004;94(suppl): 3D–11D.
60. Zhao G, Linke A, Xu X, et al. Comparative profile of vasodilation by CVT-3146, a novel A2a receptor agonist, and adenosine in conscious dogs. J Pharmacol Exp Ther 2003;307:182–189.
61. Hendel RC, Mahmarian JJ, Cerqueira MD, et al. Pharmacological stress SPECT myocardial perfusion imaging with a selective A2a agonist: results of a pilot study comparing adenosine with CVT-3146. Circulation 2003;108(suppl IV):636.
62. Udelson JE, Heller GV, Wackers FJ, et al. Randomised, controlled dose-ranging study of the selective adenosine A2A receptor agonist binodenoson for pharmacological stress as an adjunct to myocardial perfusion imaging. Circulation 2004;109:457–464.
63. Dubois-Randé JL, Merlet P, Duval-Moulin AM, et al. Coronary vasodilating action of dobutamine in patients with idiopathic dilated cardiomyopathy. Am Heart J 1993;125:1329–1336.
64. Germano G, Kiat H, Kavanagh PB, et al. Automatic quantification of ejection fraction from gated myocardial perfusion SPECT. J Nucl Med 1995;36:2138–2147.
65. He ZX, Cwalg E, Preslar JS, Mahmarian JJ, Verani MS. Accuracy of left ventricular ejection fraction determined by gated myocardial perfusion SPECT with Tl-201 and Tc-99m sestamibi: comparison with first-pass radionuclide angiography. J Nucl Cardiol 1999;6: 412–417.
66. Nichols K, Lefkowitz D, Faber T, et al. Echocardiographic validation of gated SPECT ventricular function measurements. J Nucl Med 2000;41:1308–1314.
67. Bax JJ, Lamb H, Dibbets P, et al. Comparison of gated single-photon emission computed tomography with magnetic resonance imaging for evaluation of left ventricular function in ischemic cardiomyopathy. Am J Cardiol 2000;86:1299–1305.
68. De Bono D. Investigation and management of stable angina: revised guidelines 1998. Heart 1999;81:546–555.
69. Klocke FJ, Baird MG, Lorell BH, et al. ACC/AHA/ASNC guidelines for the clinical use of cardiac radionuclide imaging. 2003. Available at: http://www.asnc.org.
70. Taillefer R, DePuey EG, Udelson JE, Beller GA, Latour Y, Reeves F. Comparative diagnostic accuracy of Tl-201 and Tc-99m sestamibi SPECT imaging (perfusion and ECG-gated SPECT) in detecting coronary artery disease in women. J Am Coll Cardiol 1997;29:69–77.
71. Underwood R, Godman B, Salyani S, et al. Economics of myocardial perfusion imaging in Europe – the EMPIRE Study. Eur Heart J 1999;20:157–166.
72. Shaw LJ, Hachamovitch R, Berman D, et al. The economic consequences of available diagnostic and prognostic strategies for the evaluation of stable angina patients: an observational assessment of the value of precatheterisation ischemia. J Am Coll Cardiol 1999; 33:661–669.
73. Schinkel AF, Elhendy A, Biagini E, et al. Prognostic stratification using dobutamine stress 99mmTc-tetrofosmin myocardial perfusion SPECT in elderly patients unable to perform exercise testing. J Nucl Med 2005;46:12–18.
74. National Institute for Clinical Excellence (NICE). Myocardial perfusion scintigraphy for the diagnosis

and management of angina and myocardial infarction. Technology appraisal guidance 73, November 2003. Available at: www.nice.org.uk/TA073guidance.
75. Giri S, Shaw LJ, Murthy DR, et al. Impact of diabetes on the risk stratification using stress single-photon emission computed tomography myocardial perfusion imaging in patients with symptoms suggestive of coronary artery disease. Circulation 2002;105:32–40.
76. Miller DD, Donohue TJ, Younis LT, et al. Correlation of pharmacological 99m-Tc-sestamibi myocardial perfusion imaging with poststenotic coronary flow reserve in patients with angiographically intermediate coronary artery stenoses. Circulation 1994;89:2150–2160.
77. Uren NG, Melin JA, De Bruyne B, Wijns W, Baudhuin T, Camici P. Relation between myocardial blood flow and the severity of coronary artery stenosis. N Engl J Med 1994;330:1782–1788.
78. White CW, Wright CB, Doty DB, et al. Does visual interpretation of the coronary arteriogram predict the physiologic importance of coronary stenosis? N Engl J Med 1984;310:819–824.
79. Heller LI, Cates C, Popma J, et al. and the FACTS Study Group. Intracoronary Doppler assessment of moderate coronary artery disease. Comparison with 201Tl imaging and coronary angiography. Circulation 1997; 96:484–490.
80. Zeiher AM, Drexler H, Wollschlager H, Just H. Endothelial dysfunction of the coronary microvasculature is associated with coronary blood flow regulation in patients with early atherosclerosis. Circulation 1991; 84:1984–1992.
81. Reddy KG, Nair RN, Sheehan HM, Hodgson JM. Evidence that selective endothelial dysfunction may occur in the absence of angiographic or ultrasound atherosclerosis in patients with risk factors for atherosclerosis. J Am Coll Cardiol 1994;23:833–843.
82. Picano E, Mathias W Jr, Pingitore A, Bigi R, Previtali M. Safety and tolerability of dobutamine-atropine stress echocardiography: a prospective, multicentre study: Echo Dobutamine International Cooperative Study Group. Lancet 1994;344:1190–1192.
83. Mertes H, Sawada SG, Ryan T, et al. Symptoms, adverse effects, and complications associated with dobutamine stress echocardiography: experience in 1118 patients. Circulation 1993;88:15–19.
84. Pennell DJ, Underwood SR, Manzara CC, et al. Magnetic resonance imaging during dobutamine stress in coronary artery disease. Am J Cardiol 1992;70:34–40.
85. Baer FM, Voth E, Theissen P, Schicha H, Sechtem U. Gradient-echo magnetic resonance imaging during incremental dobutamine infusion for the localization of coronary artery stenoses. Eur Heart J 1994;15:218–225.
86. van Rugge FP, van der Wall EE, de Roos A, Bruschke AV. Dobutamine stress magnetic resonance imaging for detection of coronary artery disease. J Am Coll Cardiol 1993;22:431–439.
87. Nagel E, Lehmkuhl HB, Bocksch W, et al. Noninvasive diagnosis of ischemia induced wall-motion abnormalities with the use of high-dose dobutamine stress MRI: comparison with dobutamine stress echocardiography. Circulation 1999;99:763–770.
88. Kuijpers D, Ho KY, van Dijkmann PRM, Vliegenthart R, Oudkerk M. Dobutamine cardiovascular magnetic resonance for the detection of myocardial ischemia with the use of myocardial tagging. Circulation 2003; 107:1592–1597.
89. Atkinson DJ, Burstein D, Edelman RR. First-pass cardiac perfusion: evaluation with ultrafast MR imaging. Radiology 1990;174:757–762.
90. Manning WJ, Atkinson DJ, Grossman W, Paulin S, Edelman RR. First-pass nuclear magnetic resonance imaging studies using gadolinium-DTPA in patients with coronary artery disease. J Am Coll Cardiol 1991; 18:959–965.
91. Schaefer S, van Tyen R, Saloner D. Evaluation of myocardial perfusion abnormalities with gadolinium-enhanced snapshot MR imaging in humans. Work in progress. Radiology 1992;185:795–801.
92. Wilke N, Simm C, Zhang J, et al. Contrast-enhanced first pass myocardial perfusion imaging: correlation between myocardial blood flow in dogs at rest and during hyperemia. Magn Reson Med 1993;29:485–497.
93. Wilke N, Kroll K, Merkle H, et al. Regional myocardial blood volume and flow: first-pass MR imaging with polylysine-Gd-DTPA. J Magn Reson Imaging 1995; 5:227–237.
94. Eichenberger AC, Schuiki E, Kochli VD, Amann FW, McKinnon GC, von Schulthess GK. Ischemic heart disease: assessment with gadolinium-enhanced ultrafast MR imaging and dipyridamole stress. J Magn Reson Imaging 1994;4:425–431.
95. Saeed M, Wendland MF, Sakuma H, et al. Coronary artery stenosis: detection with contrast-enhanced MR imaging in dogs. Radiology 1995;196:79–84.
96. Walsh EG, Doyle M, Lawson MA, Blackwell GG, Pohost GM. Multislice first-pass myocardial perfusion imaging on a conventional clinical scanner. Magn Reson Med 1995;34:39–47.
97. Matheijssen NA, Louwerenburg HW, van Rugge FP, et al. Comparison of ultrafast dipyridamole magnetic resonance imaging with dipyridamole SestaMIBI SPECT for detection of perfusion abnormalities in patients with one-vessel coronary artery disease: assessment by quantitative model fitting. Magn Reson Med 1996; 35:221–228.
98. Wilke N, Jerosch-Herold M, Wang Y, et al. Myocardial perfusion reserve: assessment with multisection, quantitative, first-pass MR imaging. Radiology 1997; 204:373–384.
99. Cullen JH, Horsfield MA, Reek CR, Cherryman GR, Barnett DB, Samani NJ. A myocardial perfusion reserve index in humans using first-pass contrast-enhanced magnetic resonance imaging. J Am Coll Cardiol 1999; 33:1386–1394.
100. Al-Saadi N, Nagel E, Gross M, et al. Noninvasive detection of myocardial ischemia from perfusion reserve based on cardiovascular magnetic resonance. Circulation 2000;101:1379–1383.
101. Schwitter J, Nanz D, Kneifel S, et al. Assessment of myocardial perfusion in coronary artery disease by magnetic resonance: a comparison with positron emission tomography and coronary angiography. Circulation 2001;103:2230–2235.
102. Nagel E, Klein C, Paetsch I, et al. Magnetic resonance perfusion measurements for the noninvasive detection of coronary artery disease. Circulation 2003;108: 432–437.
103. Panting JR, Gatehouse PD, Yang GZ, et al. Abnormal subendocardial perfusion in cardiac syndrome X detected by cardiovascular magnetic resonance imaging. N Engl J Med 2002;346:1948–1953.

104. Senior R, Basu S, Khattar R, Lahiri A. Independent prognostic value of the extent and severity of systolic wall thickening abnormality at infarct site after thrombolytic therapy. Am Heart J 1998;135:1093–1098.
105. Cerqueira MD, Weissman NJ, Dilsizian V, et al. Standardized myocardial segmentation and nomenclature for tomographic imaging of the heart: a statement for healthcare professionals from the Cardiac Imaging Committee of the Council on Clinical Cardiology of the American Heart Association [review]. Circulation 2002;105:539–542.
105. Kober L, Torp-Pedersen C, Carlsen J, Videbaek R, Egeblad H. An echocardiographic method for selecting high risk patients shortly after acute myocardial infarction, for inclusion in multi-centre studies (as used in the TRACE study). TRAndolapril Cardiac Evaluation. Eur Heart J 1994;15:1616–1620.
107. Kjoller E, Kober L, Jorgensen S, Torp-Pedersen C. Long-term prognostic importance of hyperkinesia following acute myocardial infarction. TRACE Study Group. TRAndolapril Cardiac Evaluation. Am J Cardiol 1999; 83:655–659.
108. Tsoukas A, Ikonomidis I, Cokkinos P, Nihoyannopoulos P. Significance of persistent left ventricular dysfunction during recovery after dobutamine stress echocardiography. J Am Coll Cardiol 1997;30:621–626.
109. Senior R, Lahiri A. Enhanced detection of myocardial ischemia by stress dobutamine echocardiography utilizing the "biphasic" response of wall thickening during low and high dose dobutamine infusion. J Am Coll Cardiol 1995;26:26–32.
110. Soman P, Lahiri A, Senior R. Vasodilator stress induces infrequent wall thickening abnormalities compared to perfusion defects in mild to moderate coronary artery disease: implications for the choice of imaging modality with vasodilator stress. Echocardiography 2004;21:307–312.
111. White CW, Wright CB, Doty DB, et al. Does visual interpretation of the coronary arteriogram predict the physiologic importance of a coronary stenosis? New Engl J Med 1984;310:819–824.
112. Marwick TH. Stress echocardiography. Heart 2003;89: 113–118.
113. Geleijnse ML, Elhendy A. Can stress echocardiography compete with perfusion scintigraphy in the detection of coronary artery disease and cardiac risk assessment? Eur J Echocardiogr 2000;1:12–21.
114. Schinkel AFL, Bax JJ, Geleijnse ML, et al. Noninvasive evaluation of ischaemic heart disease: myocardial perfusion imaging or stress echocardiography? Eur Heart J 2003;24:789–800.
115. Ho Y-L, Wu C-C, Lin L-C, et al. Assessment of coronary artery disease in women by dobutamine stress echocardiography: comparison with stress thallium-201 single-photon emission computed tomography and exercise electrocardiography. Am Heart J 1998;135:655–662.
116. Takeuchi M, Sonoda S, Miura Y, Kuroiwa A. Comparative diagnostic value of dobutamine stress echocardiography and stress thallium-201 single-photon emission computed tomography for detecting coronary artery disease in women. Coron Artery Dis 1996;7: 831–835.
117. Elhendy A, von Domburg RT, Bax JJ, et al. Non-invasive diagnosis of coronary artery stenosis in women with limited exercise capacity: comparison of dobutamine stress echocardiography and Tc-99m sestamibi single-photon emission CT. Chest 1998;114:1097–1104.
118. Elhendy A, Geleijnse ML, van Domburg RT, et al. Comparison of dobutamine stress echocardiography and technetium-99m sestamibi single-photon emission tomography for the diagnosis of coronary artery disease in hypertensive patients with and without left ventricular hypertrophy. Eur J Nucl Med 1998;25:69–78.
119. Fragasso G, Lu C, Dabrowski P, et al. Comparison of stress/rest myocardial perfusion tomography, dipyridamole and dobutamine stress echocardiography for the detection of coronary disease in hypertensive patients with chest pain and positive exercise test. J Am Coll Cardiol 1999;34:441–447.
120. O'Keefe JH Jr, Barnhart CS, Bateman TM. Comparison of stress echocardiography and stress myocardial perfusion scintigraphy for diagnosing coronary artery disease and assessing its severity. Am J Cardiol 1995;75: 25D–34D.
121. Kaul S, Force T. Assessment of myocardial perfusion with contrast two dimensional echocardiography. Am J Cardiol 1992;69:69–46H.
122. Linka AZ, Sklenar J, Wei K, et al. Spatial distribution of microbubble velocity and concentration within the myocardium insight into transmural distribution of myocardial blood flow and volume. Circulation 1998; 98:1912–1920.
123. Wei K, Jayaweera AR, Firoozan, et al. Quantification of myocardial blood flow with ultrasound-induced destruction of microbubbles administered as a continuous infusion. Circulation 1998;97:473–483.
124. Wei K, Le E, Bin JP, et al. Mechanism of reversible ^{99m}Tc-sestamibi perfusion defects during pharmacologically induced coronary vasodilation. Am J Physiol 2001;280: H1896–1904.
125. Jayaweera AR, Wei K, Coggins M, et al. Role of capillaries in determining CBF reserve: new insights using myocardial contrast echocardiography. Am J Physiol 1999;277:H2363–2372.
126. Porter TR, Xie F, Silver M, et al. Real-time perfusion imaging with low mechanical index pulse inversion Doppler imaging. J Am Coll Cardiol 2001;37:748–753.
127. Shimoni S, Zoghbi WA, Xie F, et al. Real-time assessment of myocardial perfusion and wall motion during bicycle and treadmill exercise echocardiography: comparison with single photon emission computed tomography. J Am Coll Cardiol 2001;37:741–747.
128. Senior R, Lepper W, Pasquet A, et al. Myocardial perfusion assessment in patients with medium probability of coronary artery disease and no prior myocardial infarction: comparison of myocardial contrast echocardiography with ^{99m}Tc-SPECT. Am Heart J 2004;147: 1100–1105.

9

Prognostic Assessment by Noninvasive Imaging. Part a. Clinical Decision-making in Patients with Suspected or Known Coronary Artery Disease

Rory Hachamovitch, Leslee J. Shaw, and Daniel S. Berman

Stress imaging, whether performed with combined perfusion-function imaging using myocardial perfusion scintigraphy (MPS) or with stress echocardiography, has grown both with respect to clinical use and its role in clinical decision-making. The evidence supporting the application of stress imaging for prognostication has grown at a similarly rapid pace. In this chapter, we will first review the basic concepts of risk stratification and prognostication as it applies to all testing. Subsequently, because it has a more mature literature, we will explore the prognostic literature and recent developments surrounding the use of stress MPS and stress echocardiography.

1. A Paradigm Shift: A Risk-based Approach to Patient Care

A new paradigm in management of patients without limiting symptoms who have known or suspected coronary artery disease (CAD) is that of a risk-based approach.[1] This approach reflects a basic shift in the clinical management from diagnostic strategies centered on coronary anatomy as an endpoint to prognostic strategies based on patient risk. With a risk-based approach, the focus is on identifying patients at risk for specific adverse events – cardiac death or nonfatal myocardial infarction (MI) and on post-MPS management strategies that might reduce patient risk of these outcomes. By means of this approach, coronary angiography and revascularization can be limited to those patients who may reap a survival benefit from these procedures. Hence, this approach seems better suited to the modern environment reflecting dramatic improvements in medical therapy and a recent emphasis on cost containment than the anatomic in which the patient with known or suspected disease undergoes coronary angiography, and the presence of an obstructive coronary lesion triggers revascularization irrespective of evidence regarding the impact of revascularization on subsequent patient outcome.

2. Incremental Prognostic Value

Another concept underlying prognostic utilization of stress MPS is that of incremental prognostic value.[1] Given the costs associated with newer technologies, it has become generally accepted that all diagnostic modalities must be judged by their ability to yield added or incremental information over that provided by the information known about the patient before the test (e.g., clinical, historical, and data from the nonimaging components of stress testing). This analytic approach permits us to determine the true prognostic value of a test and its actual clinical contribution. This approach was first demonstrated with planar MPS by Ladenheim et al.[2] in a cohort of patients undergoing exercise stress. Historically, incremental value was determined by demonstrating increased prognostic information with the addition of test information by means of multivariable modeling. This approach consisted of several steps initially determining the model most strongly associated with the outcome of interest, using only prestress imaging data, and subsequently assessing whether the addition of stress imaging data to this model would further enhance its prognostic value. If the stress imaging data are predictive of the endpoint after adjusting for the initial clinical data, sufficient incremental value is said to be present. The determination of incremental value and prognostic value has been made clinically more relevant by assessing the ability of stress imaging data to further enhance the risk stratification initially achieved by prestress data. Epidemiologic approaches have been employed using receiver operating characteristics (ROC) curves as well as examining improvement in misclassification rates. To date, several large studies reporting prognostic analyses of MPS in cohorts using exercise, vasodilator, or both types of stress and in various clinical settings have extended these results.[3–9] More recently, as discussed in the latter part of this chapter, similar data have also been developed with respect to the use of stress echocardiography.

3. Added Value of Gated Single Photon Emission Computed Tomography

Since gated single photon emission computed tomography (SPECT) became routine several years after ungated SPECT, there are far fewer reports of its incremental value over perfusion in assessing prognosis. Left ventricular ejection fraction (LVEF), also measured by other modalities, has been shown to risk-stratify suspected disease patients as to the risk of subsequent cardiac death. Sharir et al.,[10] demonstrated that poststress LVEF, as measured by gated SPECT, provided significant information over the extent and severity of perfusion defect in the prediction of cardiac death. Furthermore, left ventricular (LV) end-systolic volume provided added information over poststress LVEF for prediction of cardiac death.[11] Of note, Sharir et al.[11] demonstrated a relatively low cardiac death rate in patients with abnormal perfusion and normal LV function, which was subsequently shown to be the result of a referral bias in which patients with greatest ischemia by assessment of global stress perfusion abnormality using the summed stress score (SSS) were preferentially sent for early revascularization and thus censored from assessment of the prognostic value of the test.[6] The prognostic value of gated SPECT was further confirmed in other populations, including a study in a cohort from a community setting.[12–14]

4. What Is Adequate Risk Stratification?

Although the demonstration of incremental prognostic value by means of multivariable modeling provides evidence of potential utility of stress perfusion imaging, it also provides the clinician with information upon which to apply test results in daily practice. Risk stratification, however, is both conceptually important in its ability to ascertain the added value of testing and clinically important by providing a means by a basis for management decisions. In this regard, a normal stress MPS study identifies a cohort of patients as being at exceedingly low risk, for this reason unlikely to benefit from revascularization. Hence, coronary angiography is usually is not performed when normal stress perfusion is documented. However, patients with abnormal stress MPS results are at greater risk, and thus become potential candidates for intervention.[15]

5. Risk of Adverse Events after a Normal MPS Study

To date, there is an extensive literature base for examining risk after a normal stress MPS with most studies reporting rates of hard events [cardiac death or nonfatal MI] of <1% per year of follow-up,[1,16] resulting in a position statement of the American Society of Nuclear Cardiology in 1997 stating that a normal MPS study predicts a very low likelihood (<1%) of cardiac death or MI for at least 12 months, and that this level of risk is independent of gender, age, symptom status, history of CAD, presence of anatomic CAD, imaging technique, or isotope [Tl-201 or technetium (Tc)-99m sestamibi].[17] More recently, however, published prognostic studies performed in patients undergoing pharmacologic stress, a population with more comorbidities and at higher risk than patients undergoing exercise stress, have reported hard event rates of 1.3%–2.7% per year with a normal MPS, suggesting that underlying clinical risk and prior CAD may influence event rates even when the perfusion scan is normal.[18–23] Key higher-risk subsets have been defined such as those with known CAD or its risk equivalent, which include diabetic patients as well as those with a clustering of risk factors (e.g., metabolic syndrome), noncardiac atherosclerotic disease (e.g., peripheral artery disease or cerebrovascular disease or high-risk subclinical disease), or those with extensive comorbidity and/or functional disability.

Along these lines, a recent study reported a series of 7376 patients with normal stress MPS, addressing the predictors and temporal characteristics of risk.[24] This study identified a number of variables – the use of pharmacologic stress, the presence of known CAD, diabetes mellitus (in particular, female diabetics), and advanced age as markers of increased risk and shortened time to risk (e.g., risk in the first year of follow-up was less than in the second year). Although confirming that, as a whole, patients with normal MPS are at very low risk, several additional insights were revealed by this article. First, baseline patient risk after a normal MPS varied widely as a function of the patient's clinical characteristics, as described above. In certain patients, for example elderly patients who were unable to exercise with known CAD or diabetes mellitus, risk of cardiac death or MI exceeded 1% even in the first year of follow-up. This study also showed that in patients with known CAD who had normal MPS, the temporal component of risk increased rapidly, as shown in Figure 9a.1.

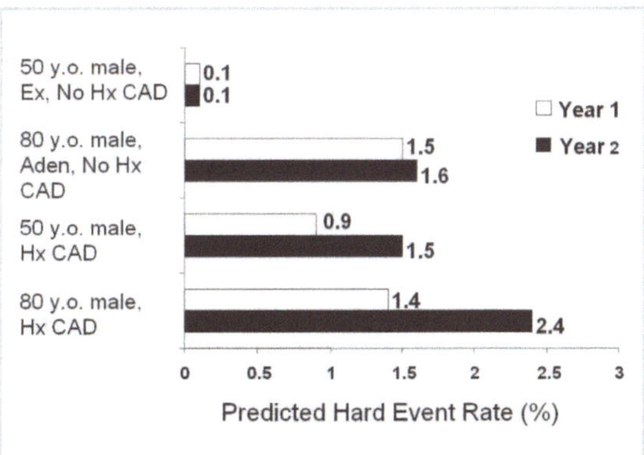

Figure 9a.1. Examples of predicted event rates in the first and second years after a normal stress MPS study. The top pair of bars represents first- and second-year event rates in a 50-year-old man with no known CAD undergoing exercise stress. In comparison, an 80-year-old man with no known CAD undergoing adenosine stress would have significantly greater first- and second-year event rates. Of note, although the risk increases, the rates in the first and second years are not different. However, the counterparts of these two patients with CAD, as shown in the bottom two pairs of bars, would have significantly greater risk; the rate in the second year would exceed that in the first year and the change in risk between years one and two would increase as a function of age in the setting of known CAD (adapted with permission from JACC[24]).

Hence, even patients who had low risk in the first year after normal MPS, may no longer be at low risk in the second year. Little is known regarding this concept of accelerated risk over time, and further studies are needed to further delineate this "warranty period" after a normal MPS in various patient subsets. Thus, to date, there is little information currently available to guide the need for and timing of retesting after a normal scan.

6. Expressing the Extent and Severity of Perfusion Results

6.1 Summed Scores

To glean the full prognostic information from MPS, it is essential that scans not be simply interpreted as normal or abnormal, but that the extent and severity of perfusion abnormalities be taken into account. To this end, we initially described a summed segmental scoring approach using 20 segments.[3,4] Recently, committees of the American College of Cardiology (ACC) and American Heart Association (AHA) have recommended a 17-segment approach[25] which provides a standardized method for LV segmentation that should facilitate comparisons between imaging modalities. With either approach, each segment is generally scored from 0 to 4, with 0 = normal, 1 = equivocal reduction, 2 = definite but moderate reduction, 3 = severe reduction of tracer uptake, and 4 = absent uptake of radioactivity. Figure 9a.2 compares the 20- and 17-segment scoring systems. With the 17-segment system, the apex is considered 1 segment and the distal short axis contains 4 segments. This system is more appropriately weighted to the amount of myocardium contained in these regions.[26]

From the scoring of the 17 or 20 segments, it is possible to derive global scores that reflect the overall extent and severity of perfusion abnormalities. These scores are to myocardial perfusion as ejection fraction is to ventricular function. The SSS, summing the scores of the 17–20 segments at stress, yields the perfusion analog of the peak ejection fraction, representing ischemic and infarcted tissue. The summed rest score is analogous to the resting ejection fraction and is related to the amount of infarcted or hibernating myocardium, and the summed difference score expresses the amount of perfusion defect reversibility. As a single overall prognostic variable, the SSS has been shown to be the single most important predictor of hard events.[5]

6.2 Percent Myocardium with Perfusion Defect

In a recent manuscript, we reported what we consider to be an improvement over the summed scores by describing and applying a system in which the visual semiquantitative summed scores is converted into % myocardium abnormal by normalizing to the maximal possible score (80 for a 5-point 20-segment system or 68 for a 5-point 17-segment system).[6] The benefits of this approach include that the % myocardium abnormal provides a measure with clinically

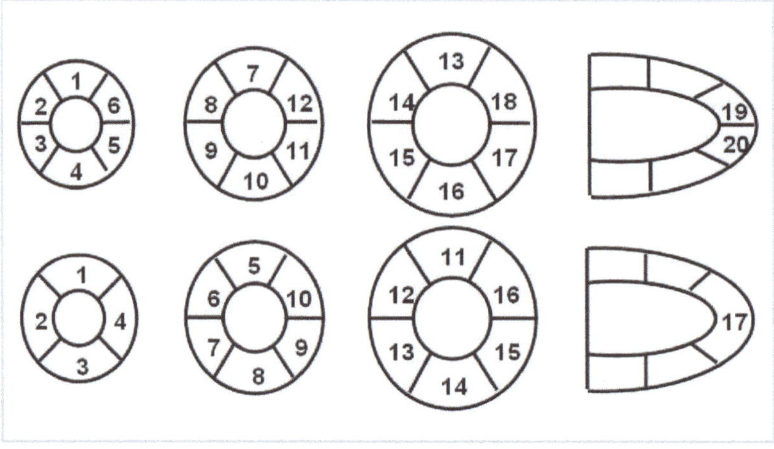

Figure 9a.2. Depiction of 17- and 20-segment models of the LV.[25]

intuitive implications not possible with the unitless summed scores, that it can easily be applied with scoring systems using varying numbers of segments [e.g., 20 (previous Cedars-Sinai system), 17 (ACC/AHA system), 14 (Mayo Clinic system), 12 (Duke University system)], and that it is applicable to quantitative methods that directly measure these abnormalities as % myocardium. We now use this % myocardium abnormal approach with all of our prognostic studies. In a large study of >16 000 patients, the 20- and 17-segment systems have been shown to perform essentially equally well when expressed as % myocardium abnormal at stress for predicting cardiac death.[26]

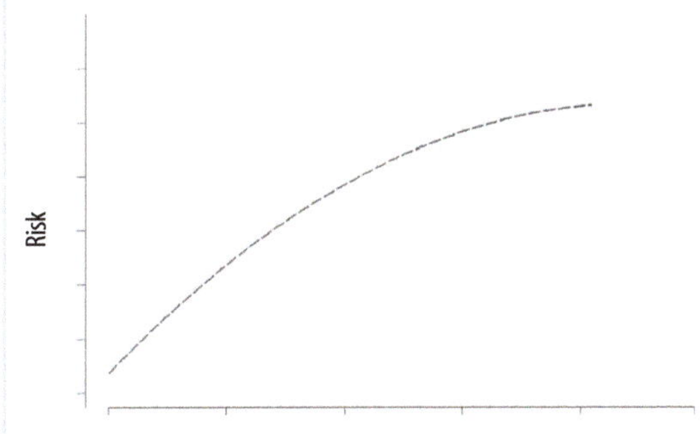

Figure 9a.3. Relationship between extent and severity of stress perfusion defects on MPS and subsequent patient risk of cardiac death or hard event (cardiac death and nonfatal MI). This depicted relationship is a generalization based on numerous studies.

6.2.1 Event Risk with Abnormal Scans

Numerous studies to date have described a direct relationship between increasing extent and severity of scan abnormality and increasing patient hard event or cardiac mortality risk.[1,2,4,5,7–10,12,13,18,22,27–29] This relationship, illustrated conceptually in Figure 9a.3, has been shown to be present irrespective of the type of stress performed, the patient cohort examined (with respect to clinical characteristics or history of CAD), or the particular radiopharmaceutical used. A decreased slope if the increase in mortality with increasing extent/severity of perfusion defect is probably primarily related to the referral of the most ischemic patients to revascularization, resulting in censoring from the prognostic evaluation of the patients at highest risk. Although the shape of this relationship between the degree of perfusion abnormality and risk seems to be the same across populations, the precise level of risk for any scan abnormality has been shown to vary with underlying clinical characteristics of the patients examined. For example, in a recent large study, for any level of defect extent and severity, risk was shown to be greater in patients with insulin-dependent diabetes mellitus than those with non-insulin-dependent diabetes mellitus, who in turn had greater risk than nondiabetics[30] (Figure 9a.4). Furthermore, the type of event likely to occur on follow-up varies as a function of the type of defect found, with MI more likely in the setting of reversible defects and cardiac death more likely in the setting of fixed defects.[31]

6.2.2 Mildly Abnormal Perfusion Scans

As shown in Figure 9a.5, an early large study evaluating risk after MPS showed patients with moderately and severely abnormal scans to be at intermediate risk for both cardiac death and MI,[5] and patients with normal scan to be at low risk for these events. However, patients with mildly abnormal scans were at intermediate risk for MI but at low risk for mortality (2.7% versus 0.8% risk per year). These findings suggested that such patients could be considered as having "flow-limiting" CAD, but unlikely to die of their disease. Because of this low mortality rate, and the observation that medical therapy, but not revascularization, has been shown to lower the risk of MI, acute ischemic syndromes, or cardiac hospitalizations, we hypothesized that, if not limited by their symptoms, these patients might be candidates for aggressive medical therapy/risk-factor modification.

However, several studies have now shown that not only does scan data provide incremental prognostic information over prescan information, but prescan data also yield incremental prognostic information over MPS results.[4,6,24,30,32] Thus, although patients with mildly abnormal MPS results are generally at low risk of cardiac death, this is not the case in patients with significant comorbidities (e.g., advanced age, prior CAD, diabetes mellitus, atrial fibrillation,[32] and pharmacologic stress). In this light, the decision whether or not to catheterize a patient with

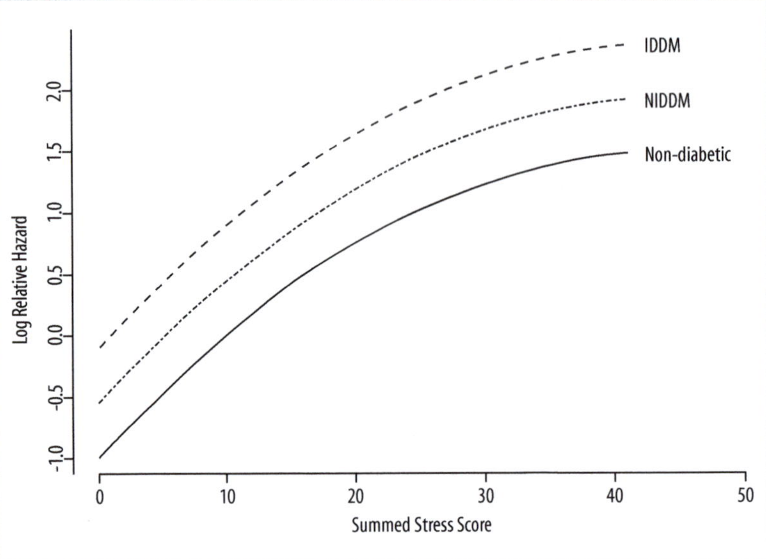

Figure 9a.4. Relationship between log relative hazard for predicted cardiac mortality and SSS in insulin-dependent diabetes mellitus (IDDM), non-insulin-dependent diabetes mellitus (NIDDM), and nondiabetics ($P < .001$). (Adapted with permission from J Am Coll Cardiol.[30])

a mildly abnormal perfusion scan becomes a function of the underlying patient condition.

6.2.3 *Moderately to Severely Abnormal Perfusion Scans*

Although both reversible and fixed stress perfusion defects are predictors of prognosis, those at highest risk of cardiac events are patients with extensive stress abnormalities. Multiple studies have described the highest event rates to be present in patients with moderately to severely abnormal perfusion defects. These results extend to both Tl-201[2,29] and Tc-99m sestamibi,[12,18] and, more recently, Tc-99m tetrofosmin,[33] as well as dual-isotope approaches.[3–5,9,22,28] Prognosis has been shown to be dependent on both the severity and extent of perfusion defects, correlates of the stenosis magnitude, and the amount of myocardium subtended by the stenosed vessels, respectively.[34] Of note, in predicting the degree of coronary stenosis, in

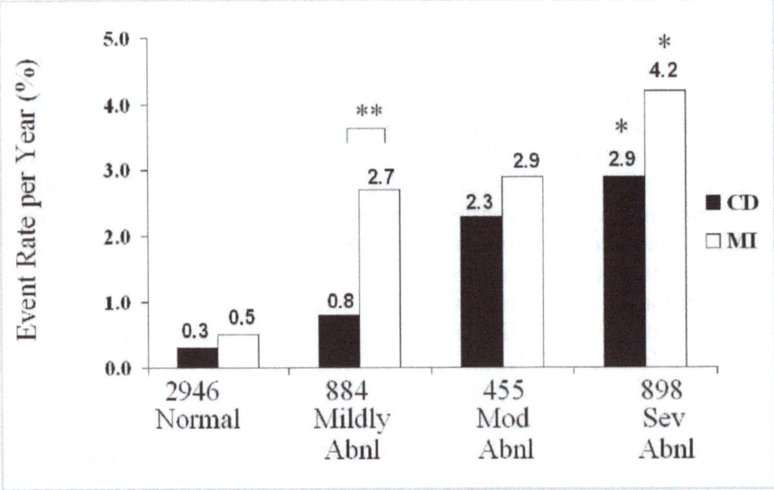

Figure 9a.5. Annualized frequencies of cardiac death (CD) and myocardial infarction (MI) as a function of scan result (normal, mildly, moderately, and severely abnormal scans). *$P < .001$ for each endpoint across scan categories; **$P < .01$ for cardiac death versus MI in mildly abnormal scans.

general, stress perfusion defects imply the presence of a >70% stenosis, and when severe perfusion defects are noted (scores 3 or 4 with the 5-point system), >90% stenosis is found angiographically in approximately 90% of patients.

7. Nonperfusion MPS Markers of Risk

7.1 Transient Ischemic Dilation of the LV

Transient ischemic dilation (TID) is considered present when the LV cavity appears to be significantly larger in the poststress images than at rest[35,36] and may actually be an apparent cavity dilation secondary to diffuse subendocardial ischemia (obscuring the endocardial border). TID is considered to represent severe and extensive ischemia, and has been shown to be highly specific for critical stenosis (>90% narrowing) in vessels supplying a large portion of the myocardium [i.e., proximal left anterior descending (LAD) or multivessel 90% lesions].[35,36] TID in the setting of vasodilator stress has been found to have similar implications as that associated with exercise,[37] although for reasons that are unclear, the threshold for TID is higher with vasodilator stress. Although TID has been known to be a marker of risk,[1] only recently has it been found to add incrementally over perfusion data for prediction of risk.[13,38] The prognostic value of TID as observed on MPS has recently been evaluated in 1560 patients with normal stress MPS (436 vasodilator and 1124 exercise) with no LV enlargement who were followed up for 2.3 years for hard and soft cardiac events.[38] In patients with otherwise completely normal MPS, TID was found to be an independent and incremental prognostic marker of total events even after adjustment for significant clinical variables – age, typical angina, and diabetes. The findings suggest that when TID is present, caution in making low-risk prognostic statements may be warranted.

7.2 Increased Lung Uptake of Perfusion Tracers

The finding of increased pulmonary uptake of Tl-201 generally reflects increased pulmonary capillary wedge pressure at the time of injection. Increased thallium lung uptake after exercise has been shown to have incremental prognostic information over myocardial perfusion defect assessment.[39] The correlation between LV TID and lung uptake is weak, even with Tl-201, suggesting that there may be different pathophysiologic mechanisms for each, and their measurements may be complementary in assessing the extent and severity of CAD for risk stratification.[40] Limited studies have examined the implications of increased pulmonary uptake of Tc-99m sestamibi with mixed results,[41–44] possibly explained by differing time between stress injection and imaging in different centers. Whereas increased lung uptake is of prognostic value with both pharmacologic and exercise thallium MPS, the finding is far less common with the Tc-99m agents, and the prognostic implications of increased lung uptake of these agents has not yet been defined for either exercise or pharmacologic stress. Increased lung uptake can occur in diffuse pulmonary inflammation without increased wedge pressure.

7.2.1 The Role of ST-segment Change in Pharmacologic Stress

A number of investigators have shown the association of ST depression during pharmacologic stress with future adverse outcomes.[45–49] Marshall and colleagues[45] found that although ST depression was infrequent – only 17% of patients had at least 1 mm of ST depression and 5.3% had at least 2 mm of ST depression – it was both a univariable and multivariable predictor of adverse outcomes in patients undergoing adenosine MPS, hence providing incremental value over perfusion data alone. Other studies, however, including larger series of patients using cardiac death as a solitary endpoint,[30] have not found ST depression during adenosine stress to be predictive of outcome.[18,20,50–52] This may be attributable to ST depression being more of a predictor of MI than cardiac death, or possibly attributable to the inclusion of patients with uninterpretable resting electrocardiograms or patients with other reasons for ST depression without ischemia (e.g., unrecognized LV hypertrophy). With respect to dobutamine stress, Calnon and colleagues,[21] as discussed above, elegantly demonstrated consideration of both ST depression and perfusion results during dobutamine stress for the optimal risk stratification of patients.

7.2.2 Clinical and Hemodynamic Responses to Vasodilator Stress

Normally, there is a mild increase in heart rate and decrease in blood pressure, particularly systolic blood pressure, with adenosine or dipyridamole infusion. However, the failure of heart rate or blood pressure to change with adenosine stress does not imply lack of myocardial perfusion response.[53] Amanullah and colleagues[53] found both a higher heart rate at rest and a blunted heart rate increase during adenosine infusion to be univariate predictors of severe or extensive CAD in women. The former was also found to be a multivariable predictor of adverse outcomes. The clinical significance and prognostic importance of different patterns of hemodynamic responses during vasodilator stress were recently described[54] in 3444 patients (53.5% women, mean age 74.0 ± 8.4 years) who underwent adenosine MPS with no additional exercise as an adjunct and were followed up for 2.0 years. During this follow-up, 224 cardiac deaths occurred (6.5%). Cox proportional hazards analysis was used to examine the prognostic implications of rest and peak adenosine stress heart rate and blood pressure after adjusting for other factors. After risk adjustment, the ratio of peak-to-rest heart rate demonstrated the strongest relationship for either observed or predicted mortality rate in both genders with the greatest risk being present in the lowest tertile of this ratio (i.e., a failure to increase heart rate during adenosine infusion is associated with a worse prognosis). Even within each category of MPS result, risk of cardiac death decreased markedly across tertiles of this ratio (Figure 9a.6). Interestingly, Cox proportional hazards analysis also revealed a significant interaction to be present between gender and peak systolic blood pressure, in which there was an increased risk associated with a low peak systolic blood pressure (<90 mm Hg) in men but not in women. Incorporating these considerations as well as findings such as TID and regional and global function responses should result in considerable improvement in the estimation of risk in patients after vasodilator stress MPS.

7.2.3 Post-MPS Patient Management and Its Prognostic Implications

To understand the relationship between MPS results and outcomes, the relationship between scan results and physician action must be understood as well as the subsequent impact on observed survival rates after MPS as a result of physician action.

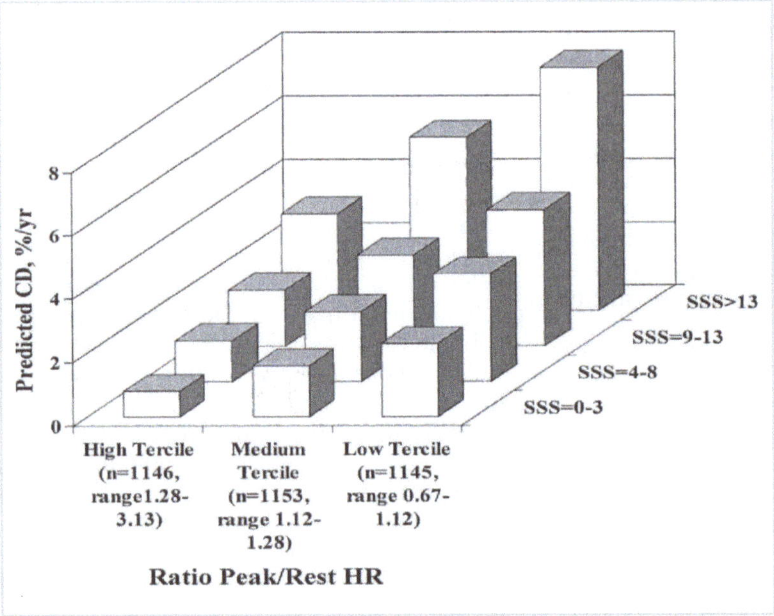

Figure 9a.6. Observed CD rate distribution terciles of peak/rest heart rate (HR) and SSS (summed stress score) categories. (Adapted from Circulation.[54])

7.3 Scan Results and Physician Action

Multiple studies to date have examined post-MPS resource utilization using referral rates to early catheterization and revascularization as measures of physician action (early defined as occurring within the first 60–90 days post-MPS.[55,56] Among patients with normal scans, only a small proportion undergo early post-MPS cardiac catheterization, usually as a result of clinical symptomatology.[3] In patients with abnormal MPS results, the extent and severity of reversible defects have been shown to be the dominant factor driving subsequent resource utilization,[4] comprising 83% of the measurable information appearing to result in myocardial revascularization by multivariable analysis. In addition, for any amount of ischemia present, a variety of clinical factors, most importantly anginal symptoms, further influence referral rates. The presence of anginal symptoms results in the highest referral rates, whereas asymptomatic patients have the lowest referral rates.[6] Thus, whereas risk is driven by stress defect extent and severity regardless of defect type, post-MPS resource utilization is driven by ischemia – i.e., the reversible defects. These results have also been reported by other investigators.[57–59] Additionally, patients undergoing revascularization procedures performed early after MPS often will have the natural history of CAD altered. It is for this reason that prognostic studies of noninvasive testing have been in large part limited to patients undergoing medical therapy after testing as patients undergoing early revascularization are censored from analyses because ischemia on noninvasive testing prompts patient referral to early revascularization.[55,56] Recent data suggest that the time chosen for this censoring depends on the practice patterns of a community or country.[59] In turn, as MPS has become increasingly used, an increasing posttest referral bias has developed, leading to an underestimation of the prognostic value of noninvasive testing because of the revascularization of the highest-risk patients.[1,60,61] That is, because the highest-risk patients are selectively revascularized, and thus removed from survival analyses, the observed event rates in these highest-risk patients are reduced and the prognostic value of the test seems to decline. This phenomenon has been recently studied and the potential reduction in event rates by early revascularization quantified.[61] Referral bias is a phenomenon that should be taken into account in future studies assessing the efficacy of MPS.

7.3.1 *Survival with Medical Therapy Versus Revascularization after Stress MPS*

A recent study of risk stratification in noninvasive imaging examined the relationship between the extent and severity of ischemia and the survival benefit associated with subsequent revascularization.[6] This study examined 10627 patients without prior MI or revascularization who underwent stress MPS and were followed up for a mean of 1.9 years (<4% lost to follow-up). Over this time period, 146 patients died of cardiovascular causes (1.4% mortality). The authors defined patient treatment on the basis of that received within 60 days post-MPS [revascularization (671 patients, 2.8% mortality) versus medical therapy (9956 patients, 1.3% mortality; $P = .0004$)] and used a risk-adjusted approach that included a propensity score to adjust for nonrandomization of treatment assignment. This propensity score was used to adjust survival analyses and was based on a logistic regression model that defined the predictors of referral to revascularization. As shown in Figure 9a.7, and confirming the discussion above, ischemia was by far the most powerful driver of referral to revascularization, with other clinical parameters such as presenting symptoms also influencing treatment.

Based on the Cox proportional hazards model most predictive of cardiac death ($\chi^2 = 539$, $P < .0001$), in the setting of no or mild ischemia, patients undergoing medical therapy as their initial treatment had superior survival to those patients referred to revascularization. However, in the setting of moderate to severe ischemia (>10% of the total myocardium ischemic) by MPS, patients undergoing revascularization had an increasing survival benefit over patients undergoing medical therapy (Figure 9a.8). As previously shown in prospective randomized clinical trials comparing medical therapy to revascularization, the absolute benefit accrued with a particular treatment varied as a function of various markers of risk.[62] Similarly, in this study, patients with characteristics associated with greater clinical risk (the elderly, women, diabetics, and patients undergoing pharmacologic stress)

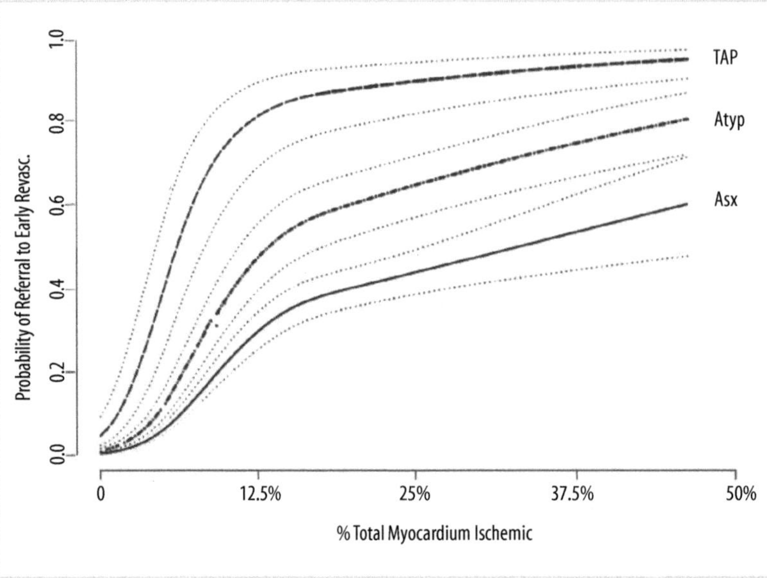

Figure 9a.7. Likelihood of referral to revascularization as a function of % myocardium ischemic based on logistic regression analysis. TAP, typical angina; Atyp, atypical angina pectoris; Asx, asymptomatic. (Adapted with permission from Circulation.[6])

were found to have the greatest increase in survival with revascularization over medical therapy in the setting of significant ischemia (Figures 9a.9–9a.11).

The analytic methodology used in this current study also provided an alternative definition of a test's clinical incremental prognostic value – *the ability to identify patients who for a given test result will benefit from a particular therapeutic approach as opposed to another.* The advantages of this approach are two-fold. It is less subject to posttest referral bias, a problem previously discussed, because it incorporates all patients. Also, it is defined in a more clinically applicable manner than simple assessment of prognosis with medical therapy alone by providing prediction of benefit associated with a therapeutic option.

These results were extended to include data from gated SPECT results and were presented in

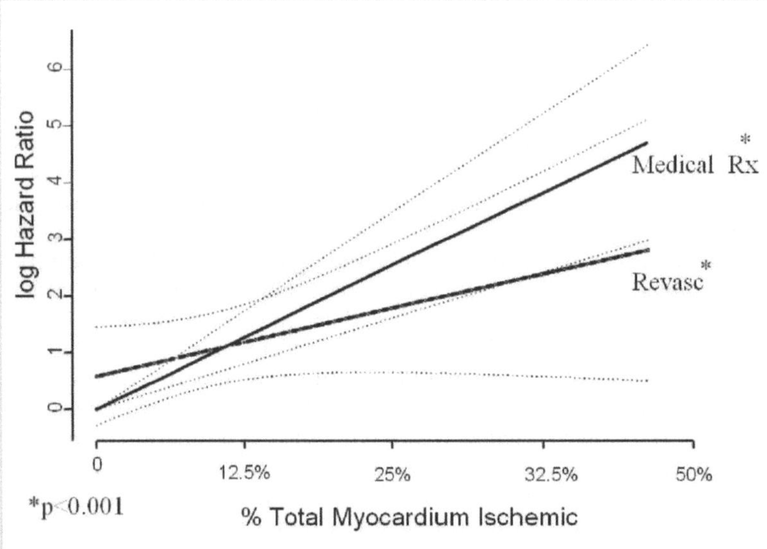

Figure 9a.8. Log hazard ratio for revascularization versus medical therapy as a function of % myocardium ischemic based on final Cox proportional hazards model. Revasc, revascularization. Model $P < .0001$, interaction $P = .0305$. (Adapted from Circulation.[6])

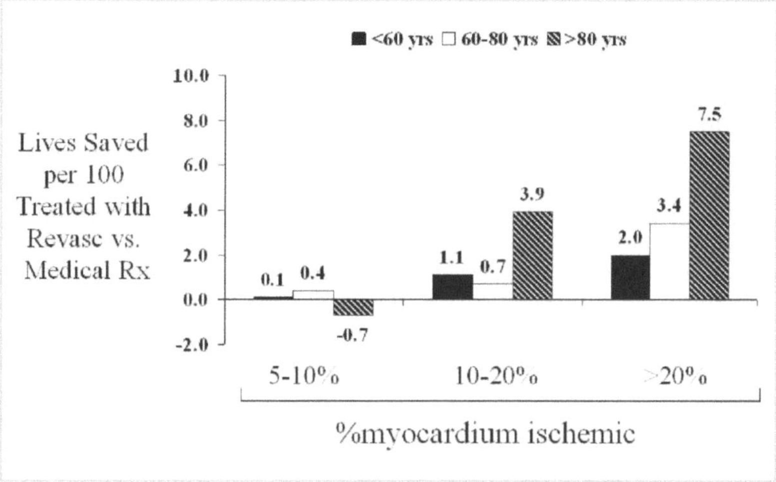

Figure 9a.9. Lives saved per 100 treated with revascularization versus medical therapy in patients by age category (<60 years: black bars; 60–80 years: clear bars; >80 years: cross-hatched bars) as a function of % myocardium ischemic (5%–10%, 10%–20%, >20%). Revasc, revascularization. Results based on Cox proportional hazards model. Statistical significance as per model. (Adapted from Circulation.[6])

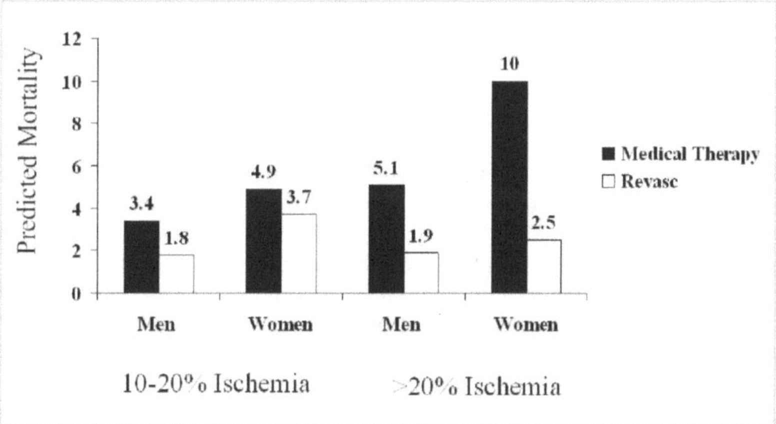

Figure 9a.10. Lives saved per 100 treated with revascularization versus medical therapy in men and women without diabetes mellitus as a function of % myocardium ischemic. Black bars: medical therapy; clear bars: revascularization. Revasc, revascularization. Results based on Cox proportional hazards model. Statistical significance as per model ($P < .0001$). (Adapted from Circulation.[6])

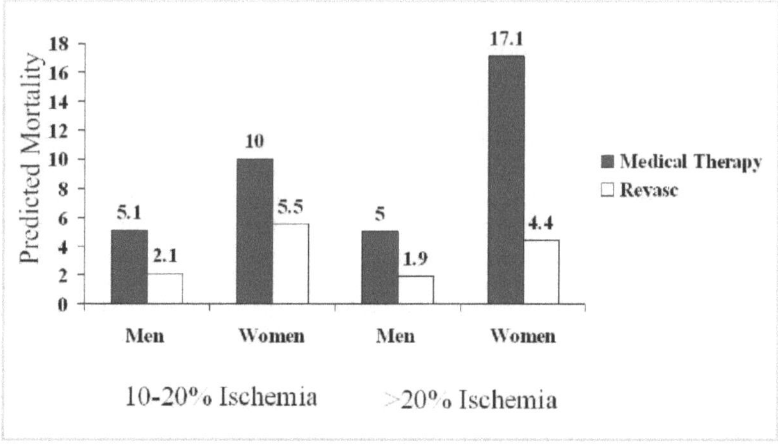

Figure 9a.11. Lives saved per 100 treated with revascularization versus medical therapy in men and women with diabetes mellitus as a function of % myocardium ischemic. Revasc, revascularization. Results based on Cox proportional hazards model. Statistical significance as per model ($P < .0001$). (Adapted from Circulation.[6])

preliminary form.[28] In this study, gated SPECT ejection fraction (EF) and ischemia were added incrementally to each other for prediction of cardiac death and assessment of potential benefit from revascularization. Although EF was found to be a superior predictor of cardiac death, only inducible ischemia identified which patients experienced a short-term benefit from revascularization. However, as described above, the absolute benefit associated with revascularization varied with patient risk. Hence, for any degree of ischemia, the survival benefit associated with revascularization was greater in patients with reduced EF.

8. A Paradigm Shift: Identification of Potential Risk Versus the Identification of Potential Benefit

8.1 Treatment Algorithms Based on Risk

It was previously suggested that from the standpoint of MPS results, post-MPS treatment recommendations should be based on the extent and severity of stress perfusion defects – the SPECT data most predictive of adverse outcomes.[5] The underlying principle of this approach was to manage patients on the basis of risk, referring patients at intermediate to high risk of cardiac death to catheterization with possible revascularization, and those at low risk of cardiac death to medial management. In general, patients with normal MPS are at exceedingly low risk; it has been recommended that they be treated with aggressive risk-factor modification. Patients with moderate to severely abnormal scans are at intermediate to high risk of adverse events, and it is recommended that they be referred to catheterization, with an eye to possible revascularization if suitable anatomy is found. In patients with mildly abnormal scans, we previously recommended medical management, because their risk for cardiac death was low, and their intermediate risk for MI could be best addressed with aggressive risk-factor modification and medical therapy. In those patients with mildly abnormal scans in whom quality of life, symptomatology, or compromise of functional status is an issue, catheterization would be justified as a means to alleviate these nonprognostic factors. More recently, we have recommended that nonperfusion abnormalities be taken into account in determining the need for coronary angiography – such as TID,[38,63] lung uptake, ischemic ST-segment changes, and gated SPECT wall motion abnormalities.[12,64,65] It may be advisable to pursue a more aggressive course of clinical action in these patients because the perfusion MPS results alone may underrepresent the amount of CAD and accompanying risk the patient faces. These recommendations were further altered in the face of gated SPECT outcomes data, because the presence of a normal gated SPECT EF was associated with a very low risk of cardiac death, hence the possibility that even in the setting of significant ischemia, perhaps catheterization and revascularization were not needed. Conversely, in the setting of compromised LV function, a more aggressive course with referral to catheterization may be indicated despite relatively smaller amounts of inducible ischemia.

8.2 Treatment Algorithms Based on Potential Benefit

Given the recently published data[66] cited above that demonstrate the close relationship between inducible ischemia and a survival benefit with revascularization, the focus of management algorithms might be shifted from decision-making based on risk to decision-making based on potential benefit. In this regard, the component of the MPS study that is most important is the extent and severity of ischemia, rather than the total stress defect size.

Using this approach (Figure 9a.12), as described above, patients with normal scans would still generally be managed medically and with risk-factor modification, because no potential survival benefit could be accrued with revascularization. In patients without prior CAD who have >10%–15% of their myocardium ischemic, the recommendation can be made to define coronary anatomy with an eye to revascularization because these patients have significantly enhanced survival with this approach compared with medical therapy. Patients with mild to moderate amounts of inducible ischemia by MPS – clearcut reversible defects but involving <10%–15% of the total myocardium – would generally undergo medical therapy because there is insufficient ischemia for revascularization to achieve a survival benefit compared with medical management alone. As above, because

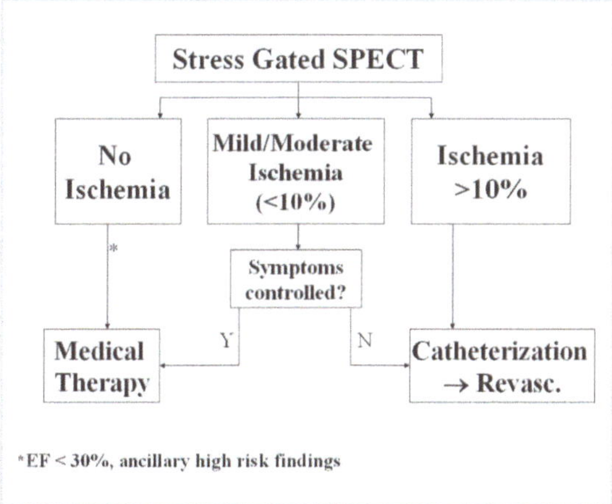

Figure 9a.12. Schema for management of patients after stress gated MPS. Patients without inducible ischemia are referred to medical therapy. The exceptions to this, as noted by the asterisk, would be patients with low ejection fractions (EF) or with ancillary high-risk findings such as TID, lung uptake, or poststress wall motion abnormalities. Patients with significant ischemia (>10% myocardium ischemic) are referred to catheterization for evaluation as revascularization candidates. Patients with mild to moderate amounts of ischemia are referred to catheterization if issues are present regarding quality of life, functional status, or symptoms. However, if patients with small amounts of ischemia have no such issues, they can be managed with medical therapy and aggressive risk-factor modification.

these recommendations are made on the grounds of potential survival benefit with revascularization versus medical therapy, patients in whom quality of life, recurring symptoms, or functional status is an issue may justify catheterization and revascularization despite insufficient ischemia to otherwise justify intervention. Also, as noted above, the presence of ancillary markers indicative of severe or extensive underlying CAD, particularly in the setting of normal or near-normal stress perfusion, would merit consideration for intervention. Finally, many other factors relating to the patient's clinical state, beyond the question of disabling symptoms, have an important role in determining the need to consider revascularization.

8.3 Can We Prognosticate in Reports? A Future Direction of Survival Analyses

There will always be a need to combine careful clinical observations with objective test results in guiding patient management. With the ongoing development of stress MPS, increasing numbers of variables are identified as being important prognosticators, and with the development of improving software, more information is being collected that may also be important for prognostication. The greatest challenge facing clinicians attempting to apply MPS results to patient care is to distill all information reported after MPS – clinical, historical, stress test, perfusion, and function data– into an estimate of likelihood of CAD or risk of adverse events for an individual patient. Ideally, the process of estimation of patient risk should be incorporated into the stress MPS report. Validated scores will be developed incorporating all available sources of information, including expressing MPS results in a manner independent of the scoring system used (e.g., percent of total myocardium abnormal at stress). Hence, by deriving the equivalent of the Duke treadmill score[67] for MPS results, accurate and reliable estimates of CAD likelihood or risk could be incorporated into MPS reporting. In light of recent data comparing survival benefits with different treatments, it may well be possible that formulas or scores to estimate risk may permit separate estimates for survival with different post-MPS treatment approaches. As noted above, it must always be recognized, however, that clinical judgment is paramount in the application of these approaches because of imperfections in the data derived from populations in defining all of the variables that might be operative in determining the risk of an individual patient.

9. Current Evidence on Stress Echocardiography

9.1 Diagnostic Accuracy

Several excellent reviews and meta-analyses are available that synthesized the existing evidence on the diagnostic accuracy of stress echo.[68–74] Of note, echocardiographic visualization of LV performance during stress results in clear improvement in diagnostic accuracy compared with the evaluation of ST-segment changes alone[69–74]; diagnostic sensitivity and specificity for exercise echocardiography are 83% and 84%, rates that are approximately 20% more sensitive than for exercise electrocardiography (ECG) alone (Table 9a.1). Similarly, for dobutamine stress echo, sensitivity and specificity measurements from 13 studies performed in 436 patients are 75%

Table 9a.1. A compilation of meta-analyses and reviews on the diagnostic accuracy of contemporary noninvasive stress testing including exercise electrocardiography (ECG) and stress echocardiography

	Ex ECG		Stress Echo	
	Sensitivity (%)	Specificity (%)	Sensitivity (%)	Specificity (%)
Fleischmann et al., 1998[87]	–	–	85	77
Kwok et al., 1999[73]	61	70	86	79
Marwick[86]			81	73

The diagnostic sensitivity and specificity values presented are uncorrected for verification bias. The most recent analysis put forth from the Agency for Health Related Quality notes an equivalent diagnostic accuracy between stress echocardiography and SPECT imaging.

and 83%. In a recent head-to-head comparison, stress echo resulted in improved risk stratification and incremental cost effectiveness compared with the exercise ECG testing.[68]

10. Risk Stratification

Although there is a larger literature base documenting the prognostic value of SPECT imaging, there is a rapidly developing broad knowledge base on risk stratification with stress echocardiography.[68,75–84] Stress echocardiography is a newer technique, and the prognostic data have been published most recently within the last decade. Large outcome series for prognosis generally include >1000 patients, and require intense efforts and resources on the part of clinical investigators with initial database development and ongoing evaluation over several years.[83] Using a compilation of published evidence from clinical guidelines or expert consensus evidence from the ACC/AHA stable angina guidelines, meta-analyses, and larger observational series, the prognostic value of stress echo is plotted using a Forest plot in Figure 9a.13. This prognostic data reports on 32 739 patients undergoing stress echo. Also for stress echo, several large outcome data registries, including the Echo Persantine International Cooperative (EPIC) study and American Society of Echocardiography (ASE) outcome registries in 7333 and 11 132 patients, have recently been published.[76,78] In the setting of a low-risk or normal exercise echo, the annual rates of cardiac death or MI averaged 0.5% and increased to 2.6% for high-risk studies defined as >1 inducible wall motion abnormality. However, for dobutamine stress echo, higher event rates have been reported and have been attributed to greater comorbidity of patients undergoing dobutamine stress compared with exercise. There is also a developing body of evidence as to the prognostic value of stress echo in key patient subsets.[80] For example, a recent meta-analysis reported that the relative risk ratio was elevated >10-fold for women with an abnormal stress echo.[80] These data included 5971 women with a normal stress echo whose annual risk of major adverse cardiac events was 0.5%. This event rate increased to approximately 6% for the 1425 women with a moderately to severely abnormal study. An example of long-term

	Death or MI Rate (%/yr) in High Risk	Death or MI Rate (%/yr) in Low Risk	N Total	p Value
Stress Echocardiography	7.0%	1.2%	32,739	<0.0001
Exercise	2.6%	0.5%	11,517	<0.0001
Dobutamine Stress	4.8%	1.7%	4,018	<0.0001
Summary Relative Risk	6.9% (n=27,170)	0.7% (n=62,097)	89,267	<0.0001

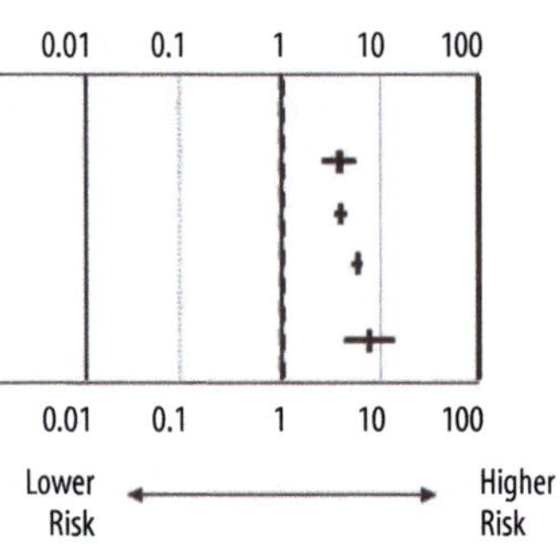

Figure 9a.13. Meta-analysis on the prognostic value of stress echocardiography as compared with other imaging modalities (e.g., SPECT and cardiac magnetic resonance).

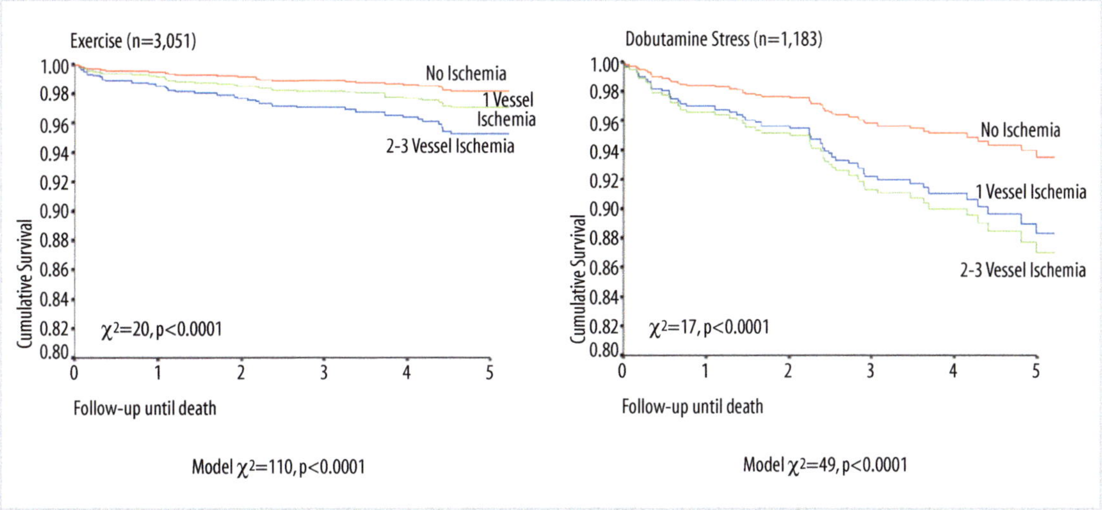

Figure 9a.14. Five-year survival by exercise and dobutamine stress echocardiography in women.[80]

survival by the extent of wall motion abnormalities in women and men is plotted in Figures 9a.14 and 9a.15 (see color section).[80]

10.1 Candidates for Cardiac Catheterization

From a synopsis of this evidence, when an inducible wall motion abnormality is found on stress echo in appropriately referred diagnostic patient subsets, the diagnosis of CAD is likely, and anti-ischemic therapies and aggressive risk-factor modification is initiated. Additionally, consideration is given to referral to coronary angiography. These considerations closely parallel those that have been described for MPS above. As with SPECT, referral to coronary angiography is dependent on the extent and severity of the inducible wall motion abnormalities as well as on the integration of this infor-

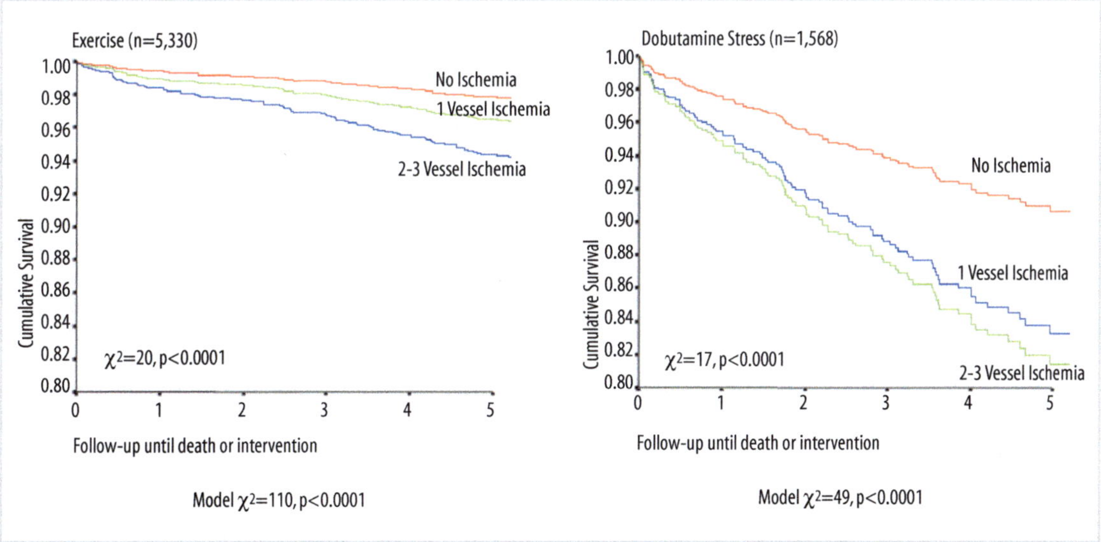

Figure 9a.15. Five-year survival by exercise and dobutamine stress echocardiography in men.[80]

mation with the patient's history and clinical presentation. In a manner similar to that used with SPECT, clinicians may prefer to treat patients medically if only small discrete areas of induced wall motion abnormality are noted, particularly if they are associated with a high level of stress. Angiography, however, is generally advised in patients with evidence of a high-risk study (Table 9a.2) indicated by multivessel wall motion abnormalities, global LV dysfunction with stress, or extensive hypocontractility or akinesis or dyskinesis across the anterior myocardium suggesting the presence of proximal LAD disease. In a recent report by Elhendy et al.,[84] patients with abnormalities in the LAD distribution had a markedly increased event rate compared with those abnormalities confined to other arterial segments (10.8% versus 2.1% at 5 years; $P = .009$). These authors further noted that this risk was independent of the resting LV function as well as extent, per se, of exertional wall motion abnormalities.

Several reports have noted that stress echo, with only a modest increase in cost compared with exercise ECG testing, can result in cost-effective testing as a result of improved detection of disease.[68,85,86] Lorenzoni et al.[85] evaluated the clinical and economic outcomes of 527 patients referred for several types of testing strategies that included coronary angiography after a positive exercise ECG alone a positive pharmacologic stress echocardiogram alone, or the combination of a positive pharmacologic stress echocardiogram and a positive exercise ECG. Both strategies using stress echo were more accurate than exercise ECG alone (approximately 91% versus 78%). For each of these strategies, the cost per correct identification was $1572, $1097, and $1081 for exercise ECG and for each of the two pharmacologic stress strategies,[85] respectively. In a more comprehensive review of the cost effectiveness of exercise echo versus ECG testing in 7656 patients, Marwick and colleagues[68] noted that imaging identified more patients as low (51% versus 24%, $P < .0001$) and high (22% versus 4%, $P < .0001$) risk. Despite having a higher initial procedural cost, imaging with echo was associated with improvements in life expectancy, averaging 0.2 added life years per patient. Interestingly, echo was also associated with a lower use of additional diagnostic procedures compared with exercise ECG alone. These authors summarized that stress echo was more cost effective than exercise ECG testing at $2615 per life year saved, substantially below the threshold for economic efficiency set at <$50,000 per life year saved.

Table 9a.2. Low- to high-risk noninvasive stress testing markers from the ACC/AHA stable angina guidelines[88]

High risk (>3% annual mortality rate or >5% annual cardiac death or nonfatal MI rate)
1. Severe resting LV dysfunction (LVEF <35%)
2. High-risk Duke treadmill score (score ≤–11)
3. Severe exercise LV dysfunction (exercise LVEF <35%)
4. Stress-induced large perfusion defect (particularly, if anterior)
5. Stress-induced multiple perfusion defects of moderate size
6. Large, fixed perfusion defect with LV dilation or increased lung uptake (thallium-201 only)
7. Stress-induced moderate perfusion defect with LV dilation or increased lung uptake (thallium-201 only)
8. Echocardiographic wall motion abnormality (involving >2 segments) developing at low dose of dobutamine (≤10 mg/kg/min) or low heart rate (<120 beats/min)
9. Stress echocardiographic evidence of extensive ischemia
Intermediate risk (1%–3% annual mortality rate or 3%–5% annual death or MI rate)
1. Mild/moderate resting LV dysfunction (LVEF = 35%–49%)
2. Intermediate risk Duke treadmill score (–11 < score < 5)
3. Stress-induced moderate perfusion defect without LV dilation or increased lung uptake (thallium-201)
4. Limited stress echocardiographic ischemia with a wall motion abnormality only at higher doses of dobutamine involving ≤2 segments
Low risk (<1% annual mortality rate or <1% annual death or MI rate)
1. Low-risk Duke treadmill score (score ≥5)
2. Normal or small myocardial perfusion defect at rest or with stress*
3. Normal stress echocardiographic wall motion or no change of limited resting wall motion abnormalities during stress*

11. Conclusions

The considerations of this review reveal that both stress nuclear and stress echo procedures are effective tools in defining a risk-based approach to the patient with known or suspected CAD. Current guidelines suggest that the choice of which of these modalities to apply in a given patient depends more on local expertise than on intrinsic differences between the modalities.[88] When used appropriately, these modalities are likely to improve patient outcomes in a cost-effective manner. How the modalities will be used in the future depends on the technological advances in each as well as those that will occur in other modalities. Of note, in this regard, the applications of both cardiac computed tomography and cardiac magnetic resonance are rapidly expanding and soon will also be supported by prognostic databases similar to those reported for stress nuclear and echo approaches.

References

1. Berman DS, Hachamovitch R, Shaw LJ, Hayes SW, Germano G. Nuclear cardiology. In: Fuster VAR, O'Rourke RA, Roberts R, King SB, Wellens HJJ, eds. Hurst's The Heart. 11th ed. New York: McGraw-Hill; 2004.
2. Ladenheim ML, Kotler TS, Pollock BH, Berman DS, Diamond GA. Incremental prognostic power of clinical history, exercise electrocardiography and myocardial perfusion scintigraphy in suspected coronary artery disease. Am J Cardiol 1987;59:270–277.
3. Berman DS, Hachamovitch R, Kiat H, et al. Incremental value of prognostic testing in patients with known or suspected ischemic heart disease: a basis for optimal utilization of exercise technetium-99m sestamibi myocardial perfusion single-photon emission computed tomography. J Am Coll Cardiol 1995;26:639–647 [published erratum appears in J Am Coll Cardiol 1996;27(3):756].
4. Hachamovitch R, Berman DS, Kiat H, et al. Exercise myocardial perfusion SPECT in patients without known coronary artery disease: incremental prognostic value and use in risk stratification. Circulation 1996;93:905–914.
5. Hachamovitch R, Berman DS, Shaw LJ, et al. Incremental prognostic value of myocardial perfusion single photon emission computed tomography for the prediction of cardiac death: differential stratification for risk of cardiac death and myocardial infarction. Circulation 1998;97:535–543.
6. Hachamovitch R, Hayes SW, Friedman JD, Cohen I, Berman DS. Comparison of the short-term survival benefit associated with revascularization compared with medical therapy in patients with no prior coronary artery disease undergoing stress myocardial perfusion single photon emission computed tomography. Circulation 2003;107:2900–2907.
7. Marwick TH, Shaw LJ, Lauer MS, et al. The noninvasive prediction of cardiac mortality in men and women with known or suspected coronary artery disease. Economics of Noninvasive Diagnosis (END) Study Group. Am J Med 1999;106:172–178.
8. Sharir T, Germano G, Kang XP, Cohen I, Friedman JD, Berman DS. Prognostic value of post-stress left ventricular volume and ejection fraction by gated myocardial perfusion single photon emission computed tomography in women: gender related differences in normal limits and outcome [abstract]. Circulation 2002;106:II-523.
9. Zellweger MJ, Lewin HC, Lai S, et al. When to stress patients after coronary artery bypass surgery? Risk stratification in patients early and late post-CABG using stress myocardial perfusion SPECT: implications of appropriate clinical strategies. J Am Coll Cardiol 2001;37:144–152.
10. Sharir T, Germano G, Kang X, et al. Prediction of myocardial infarction versus cardiac death by gated myocardial perfusion SPECT: risk stratification by the amount of stress-induced ischemia and the poststress ejection fraction. J Nucl Med 2001;42:831–837.
11. Sharir T, Berman DS, Lewin HC, et al. Incremental prognostic value of rest-redistribution Tl-201 single-photon emission computed tomography. Circulation 1999;100: 1964–1970.
12. Travin MI, Heller GV, Johnson LL, et al. The prognostic value of ECG-gated SPECT imaging in patients undergoing stress Tc-99m sestamibi myocardial perfusion imaging. J Nucl Cardiol 2004;11:253–262.
13. Thomas GS, Miyamoto MI, Morello AP, et al. Technetium99m based myocardial perfusion imaging predicts clinical outcome in the community outpatient setting: the nuclear utility in the community ("nuc") study. J Am Coll Cardiol 2004;43:213–223.
14. Moir S, Haluska BA, Jenkins C, Fathi R, Marwick TH. Incremental benefit of myocardial contrast to combined dipyridamole-exercise stress echocardiography for the assessment of coronary artery disease. Circulation 2004;110:1108–1113.
15. Hachamovitch R, Schnipper J, Young-Xu Y. Are patients with known or suspected coronary artery disease and normal stress imaging studies at low risk for adverse outcomes? Meta-analysis of stress echocardiography and SPECT. J Am Coll Cardiol 2000.
16. Klocke FJ, Baird MG, Lorell BH, et al. ACC/AHA/ASNC guidelines for the clinical use of cardiac radionuclide imaging – executive summary. A report of the American College of Cardiology/American Heart Association Task Force on Practice Guidelines (ACC/AHA/ASNC committee to revise the 1995 guidelines for the clinical use of cardiac radionuclide imaging). Circulation 2003; 108:1404–1418.
17. Bateman TM. Clinical relevance of a normal myocardial perfusion scintigraphic study. American Society of Nuclear Cardiology. J Nucl Cardiol 1997;4:172–173.
18. Heller GV, Herman SD, Travin MI, Baron JI, Santos-Ocampo C, McClellan JR. Independent prognostic value of intravenous dipyridamole with technetium-99m sestamibi tomographic imaging in predicting cardiac events and cardiac-related hospital admissions. J Am Coll Cardiol 1995;26:1202–1208.
19. Shaw L, Chaitman BR, Hilton TC, et al. Prognostic value of dipyridamole thallium-201 imaging in elderly patients [comment]. J Am Coll Cardiol 1992;19:1390–1398.
20. Stratmann HG, Tamesis BR, Younis LT, Wittry MD, Miller DD. Prognostic value of dipyridamole technetium-99m sestamibi myocardial tomography in patients with stable chest pain who are unable to exercise. Am J Cardiol 1994;73:647–652.
21. Calnon DA, McGrath PD, Doss AL, Harrell FE Jr, Watson DD, Beller GA. Prognostic value of dobutamine stress technetium-99m-sestamibi single-photon emission computed tomography myocardial perfusion imaging: stratification of a high-risk population [comment]. J Am Coll Cardiol 2001;38:1511–1517.
22. Kang X, Berman DS, Lewin HC, et al. Incremental prognostic value of myocardial perfusion single photon emission computed tomography in patients with diabetes mellitus. Am Heart J 1999;138:1025–1032.
23. Amanullah AM, Kiat H, Friedman JD, Berman DS. Adenosine technetium-99m sestamibi myocardial perfusion SPECT in women: diagnostic efficacy in

detection of coronary artery disease. J Am Coll Cardiol 1996;27:803–809.

24. Hachamovitch R, Hayes S, Friedman JD, et al. Determinants of risk and its temporal variation in patients with normal stress myocardial perfusion scans: what is the warranty period of a normal scan? J Am Coll Cardiol 2003;41:1329–1340.
25. Cerqueira MD, Weissman NJ, Dilsizian V, et al. Standardized myocardial segmentation and nomenclature for tomographic imaging of the heart: a statement for healthcare professionals from the Cardiac Imaging Committee of the Council on Clinical Cardiology of the American Heart Association. Circulation 2002;105:539–542.
26. Berman DS, Abidov A, Kang X, et al. Prognostic validation of a 17-segment score derived from a 20-segment score for myocardial perfusion SPECT interpretation. J Nucl Cardiol 2004;11:414–423.
27. Giri S, Shaw LJ, Murthy DR, et al. Impact of diabetes on the risk stratification using stress single-photon emission computed tomography myocardial perfusion imaging in patients with symptoms suggestive of coronary artery disease. Circulation 2002;105:32–40.
28. Hachamovitch R, Berman DS, Kiat H, Cohen I, Friedman JD, Shaw LJ. Value of stress myocardial perfusion single photon emission computed tomography in patients with normal resting electrocardiograms: an evaluation of incremental prognostic value and cost-effectiveness. Circulation 2002;105:823–829.
29. Vanzetto G, Ormezzano O, Fagret D, Comet M, Denis B, Machecourt J. Long-term additive prognostic value of thallium-201 myocardial perfusion imaging over clinical and exercise stress test in low to intermediate risk patients: study in 1137 patients with 6-year follow-up. Circulation 1999;100:1521–1527.
30. Berman DS, Kang X, Hayes SW, et al. Adenosine myocardial perfusion single-photon emission computed tomography in women compared with men. Impact of diabetes mellitus on incremental prognostic value and effect on patient management. J Am Coll Cardiol 2003;41:1125–1133.
31. Iskander S, Iskandrian AE. Risk assessment using single-photon emission computed tomographic technetium-99m sestamibi imaging. J Am Coll Cardiol 1998;32:57–62.
32. Abidov A, Hachamovitch R, Rozanski A, et al. Prognostic implications of atrial fibrillation in patients undergoing myocardial perfusion single-photon emission computed tomography. J Am Coll Cardiol 2004;44:1062–1070.
33. Shaw LJ, Hendel RC, Borges-Neto S, et al. Prognostic value of normal exercise and adenosine (99m)Tc-tetrofosmin SPECT imaging: results from the multicenter registry of 4,728 patients. J Nucl Med 2003;44:134–139.
34. Albro PC, Gould KL, Westcott RJ, Hamilton GW, Ritchie JL, Williams DL. Noninvasive assessment of coronary stenoses by myocardial imaging during pharmacologic coronary vasodilatation. III. Clinical trial. Am J Cardiol 1978;42:751–760.
35. Weiss AT, Berman DS, Lew AS, et al. Transient ischemic dilation of the left ventricle on stress thallium-201 scintigraphy: a marker of severe and extensive coronary artery disease. J Am Coll Cardiol 1987;9:752–759.
36. Mazzanti M, Germano G, Kiat H, et al. Identification of severe and extensive coronary artery disease by automatic measurement of transient ischemic dilation of the left ventricle in dual-isotope myocardial perfusion SPECT. J Am Coll Cardiol 1996;27:1612–1620.
37. Chouraqui P, Rodrigues EA, Berman DS, Maddahi J. Significance of dipyridamole-induced transient dilation of the left ventricle during thallium-201 scintigraphy in suspected coronary artery disease. Am J Cardiol 1990;66:689–694.
38. Abidov A, Bax JJ, Hayes SW, et al. Transient ischemic dilation ratio of the left ventricle is a significant predictor of future cardiac events in patients with otherwise normal myocardial perfusion SPECT. J Am Coll Cardiol 2003;42:1818–1825.
39. Gill JB, Ruddy TD, Newell JB, et al. Prognostic importance of thallium uptake by the lungs during exercise in coronary artery disease. N Engl J Med 1987;317:1486–1489.
40. Hansen CL, Sangrigoli R, Nkadi E, et al. Comparison of pulmonary uptake with transient cavity dilation after exercise thallium-201 perfusion imaging. J Am Coll Cardiol 1999;33:1323–1327.
41. Giubbini R, Campini R, Milan E, et al. Evaluation of technetium-99m-sestamibi lung uptake: correlation with left ventricular function. J Nucl Med 1995;36:58–63.
42. Hurwitz GA, Fox SP, Driedger AA, Willems C, Powe JE. Pulmonary uptake of sestamibi on early post-stress images: angiographic relationships, incidence and kinetics. Nucl Med Commun 1993;14:15–22.
43. Hurwitz GA, Ghali SK, Husni M, et al. Pulmonary uptake of technetium-99m-sestamibi induced by dipyridamole-based stress or exercise. J Nucl Med 1998;39:339–345.
44. Bacher-Stier C, Kavanagh PB, Sharir T, et al. Post-exercise Tc-99m sestamibi lung uptake determined by a new automatic technique [abstract]. J Nucl Med 1998;39:104P.
45. Marshall ES, Raichlen JS, Kim SM, et al. Prognostic significance of ST-segment depression during adenosine perfusion imaging. Am Heart J 1995;130:58–66.
46. Hachamovitch R, Berman DS, Kiat H, et al. Incremental prognostic value of adenosine stress myocardial perfusion single-photon emission computed tomography and impact on subsequent management in patients with or suspected of having myocardial ischemia. Am J Cardiol 1997;80:426–433.
47. Chikamori T, Doi YL, Yamada M, Takata J, Yonezawa Y, Ozawa T. Prognostic value of dipyridamole thallium scintigraphy in patients with coronary artery disease treated medically. Jpn Circ J 1993;57:851–861.
48. Abbott BG, Afshar M, Berger AK, Wackers FJ. Prognostic significance of ischemic electrocardiographic changes during adenosine infusion in patients with normal myocardial perfusion imaging. J Nucl Cardiol 2003;10:9–16.
49. Klodas E, Miller TD, Christian TF, Hodge DO, Gibbons RJ. Prognostic significance of ischemic electrocardiographic changes during vasodilator stress testing in patients with normal SPECT images. J Nucl Cardiol 2003;10:4–8.
50. Lette J, Bertrand C, Gossard D, et al. Long-term risk stratification with dipyridamole imaging. Am Heart J 1995;129:880–886.
51. Amanullah AM, Berman DS, Erel J, et al. Incremental prognostic value of adenosine myocardial perfusion single-photon emission computed tomography in

women with suspected coronary artery disease. Am J Cardiol 1998;82:725–730.
52. Stratmann HG, Younis LT, Kong B. Prognostic value of dipyridamole thallium-201 scintigraphy in patients with stable chest pain. Am Heart J 1992;123:317–323.
53. Amanullah AM, Berman DS, Kiat H, Friedman JD. Usefulness of hemodynamic changes during adenosine infusion in predicting the diagnostic accuracy of adenosine technetium-99m sestamibi single-photon emission computed tomography (SPECT). Am J Cardiol 1997;79:1319–1322.
54. Abidov A, Hachamovitch R, Hayes SW, et al. Prognostic impact of hemodynamic response to adenosine in patients older than age 55 years undergoing vasodilator stress myocardial perfusion study. Circulation 2003;107:2894–2899.
55. Staniloff HM, Forrester JS, Berman DS, Swan HJ. Prediction of death, myocardial infarction, and worsening chest pain using thallium scintigraphy and exercise electrocardiography. J Nucl Med 1986;27:1842–1848.
56. Pryor DB, Harrell FE Jr, Lee KL, et al. Prognostic indicators from radionuclide angiography in medically treated patients with coronary artery disease. Am J Cardiol 1984;53:18–22.
57. Nallamothu N, Pancholy SB, Lee KR, Heo J, Iskandrian AS. Impact on exercise single-photon emission computed tomographic thallium imaging on patient management and outcome. J Nucl Cardiol 1995;2:334–338.
58. Bateman TM, O'Keefe JH Jr, Dong VM, et al. Coronary angiographic rates after stress single-photon emission computed tomographic scintigraphy. J Nucl Cardiol 1995;2:217–223.
59. Hachamovitch R, Johnson JR, Barrett RJ, Udelson JE. International patterns of referral to revascularization early after pharmacologic stress SPECT: results from a prospective multicenter registry trial [abstract]. Circulation 2004;110:III684.
60. Hachamovitch R, Shaw L, Berman DS. Methodological considerations in the assessment of noninvasive testing using outcomes research: pitfalls and limitations. Prog Cardiovasc Dis 2000;43:215–230.
61. Hachamovitch R, Hayes SW, Friedman JD, Cohen I, Berman DS. Stress myocardial perfusion SPECT is clinically effective and cost-effective in risk-stratification of patients with a high likelihood of CAD but no known CAD. J Am Coll Cardiol 2004;43:200–208.
62. Yusuf S, Zucker D, Peduzzi P, et al. Effect of coronary artery bypass graft surgery on survival: overview of 10-year results from randomised trials by the Coronary Artery Bypass Graft Surgery Trialists Collaboration. Lancet 1994;344:563–570.
63. Abidov A, Bax JJ, Hayes SW, et al. Integration of automatically measured transient ischemic dilation ratio into interpretation of adenosine stress myocardial perfusion SPECT for detection of severe and extensive CAD. J Nucl Med 2004;45(12):1999–2007.
64. Sharir T, Berman DS, Waechter PB, et al. Quantitative analysis of regional motion and thickening by gated myocardial perfusion SPECT: normal heterogeneity and criteria for abnormality. J Nucl Med 2001;42:1630–1638.
65. Lima RS WD, Goode AR, Siadaty MS, Ragosta M, Beller GA, Samady H. Incremental value of combined perfusion and function over perfusion alone by gated SPECT myocardial perfusion imaging for detection of severe three-vessel coronary artery disease. J Am Coll Cardiol 2003;42:64–70.
66. Hachamovitch R, Hayes SW, Friedman JD, et al. Is there a referral bias against revascularization of patients with reduced LV ejection fraction? Influence of ejection fraction and inducible ischemia on post-SPECT management of patients without history of CAD. J Am Coll Cardiol 2003;42:1286–1294.
67. Mark DB, Shaw L, Harrell FE, et al. Prognostic value of a treadmill exercise score in outpatients with suspected coronary artery disease. N Engl J Med 1991;325:849–853.
68. Marwick TH, Shaw L, Case C, Vasey C, Thomas JD. Clinical and economic impact of exercise electrocardiography and exercise echocardiography in clinical practice. Eur Heart J 2003;24:1153–1163.
69. Kim C, Kwok YS, Saha S, Redberg RF. Diagnosis of suspected coronary artery disease in women: a cost-effectiveness analysis. Am Heart J 1999;137:1019–1027.
70. Imran MB, Khan MA, Aslam MN, Irfanullah J. Diagnosis of coronary artery disease by stress echocardiography and perfusion scintigraphy. J Coll Physicians Surg Pak 2003;13:465–470.
71. Kuntz KM, Fleischmann KE, Hunink MG, Douglas PS. Cost-effectiveness of diagnostic strategies for patients with chest pain. Ann Intern Med 1999;130:709–718.
72. Kim C, Kwok YS, Heagerty P, Redberg R. Pharmacologic stress testing for coronary disease diagnosis: a meta-analysis. Am Heart J 2001;142:934–944.
73. Kwok Y, Kim C, Grady D, Segal M, Redberg R. Meta-analysis of exercise testing to detect coronary artery disease in women. Am J Cardiol 1999;83:660–666.
74. Diagnosis and treatment of coronary heart disease in women: systematic reviews of evidence on selected topics. Summary, evidence report/technology assessment: Number 81. Rockville MD: AHRQ Publication; 2003:No. 03-E036.
75. Results of systematic review of research on diagnosis and treatment of coronary heart disease in women. Summary, evidence report/technology assessment: Number 80. Rockville MD: AHRQ Publication; 2003:No. 03-E034.
76. Marwick TH, Case C, Vasey C, Allen S, Short L, Thomas JD. Prediction of mortality by exercise echocardiography: a strategy for combination with the Duke treadmill score. Circulation 2001;103:2566–2571.
77. Chuah SC, Pellikka PA, Roger VL, McCully RB, Seward JB. Role of dobutamine stress echocardiography in predicting outcome in 860 patients with known or suspected coronary artery disease. Circulation 1998;97:1474–1480.
78. Sicari R, Pasanisi E, Venneri L, Landi P, Cortigiani L, Picano E. Stress echo results predict mortality: a large-scale multicenter prospective international study. J Am Coll Cardiol 2003;41:589–595.
79. Cortigiani L, Picano E, Landi P, et al. Value of pharmacologic stress echocardiography in risk stratification of patients with single-vessel disease: a report from the Echo-Persantine and Echo-Dobutamine International Cooperative Studies. J Am Coll Cardiol 1998;32:69–74.
80. Shaw LJ, Vasey C, Sawada S, Rimmerman C, Mariwck TH. Impact of gender on risk stratification by exercise and dobutamine stress echocardiography: long term mortality in 4234 women and 6898 men. Eur Heart J 2005;26(5):447–456.

81. Gibbons RJ, Balady GJ, Bricker JT, et al. ACC/AHA 2002 guideline update for exercise testing: summary article: a report of the American College of Cardiology/American Heart Association Task Force on Practice Guidelines (Committee to Update the 1997 Exercise Testing Guidelines). Circulation 2002;106:1883–1892.
82. Chung G, Krishnamani R, Senior R. Prognostic value of normal stress echocardiogram in patients with suspected coronary artery disease: a British general hospital experience. Int J Cardiol 2004;94:181–186.
83. Yao SS, Qureshi E, Sherrid MV, Chaudhry FA. Practical applications in stress echocardiography: risk stratification and prognosis in patients with known or suspected ischemic heart disease. J Am Coll Cardiol 2003;42:1084–1090.
84. Elhendy A, Mahoney DW, Khandheria BK, Paterick TE, Burger KN, Pellikka PA. Prognostic significance of the location of wall motion abnormalities during exercise echocardiography. J Am Coll Cardiol 2002;40:1623–1629.
85. Lorenzoni R, Cortigiani L, Magnani M, et al. Cost-effectiveness analysis of noninvasive strategies to evaluate patients with chest pain. J Am Soc Echocardiogr 2003;16:1287–1291.
86. Marwick TH, Anderson T, Williams MJ, et al. Exercise echocardiography is an accurate and cost-efficient technique for detection of coronary artery disease in women. J Am Coll Cardiol 1995;26:335–341.
87. Fleischmann KE, Hunink MG, Kuntz KM, Douglas PS. Exercise echocardiography or exercise SPECT imaging? A meta-analysis of diagnostic test performance. JAMA 1998;280:913–920.
88. Gibbons RJ, Abrams J, Chatterjee K, et al. ACC/AHA 2002 guideline update for the management of patients with chronic stable angina – summary article: a report of the American College of Cardiology/American Heart Association Task Force on Practice Guidelines (Committee on the Management of Patients With Chronic Stable Angina). Circulation 2003;107:149–158.

9

Prognostic Assessment by Noninvasive Imaging. Part b. Risk Assessment Before Noncardiac Surgery by Noninvasive Imaging

Olaf Schouten, Miklos D. Kertai, and Don Poldermans

Cardiovascular complications are the major cause of perioperative and late mortality and morbidity. The majority of these complications occur during the first week after surgery. Important causes for perioperative cardiac events such as myocardial infarction (MI) and death are myocardial ischemia, left ventricular (LV) dysfunction, and aortic valve stenosis. Coronary artery disease (CAD) may be asymptomatic because of reduced exercise capacity caused by noncardiac diseases such as stroke, arthritis, or claudication. To reduce perioperative cardiac mortality and morbidity, preoperative cardiac screening is of paramount importance in patients with risk factors or known CAD. This chapter discusses the role of noninvasive imaging tests in this setting with an emphasis on the assessment of risk before vascular noncardiac surgery.

1. The Clinical Problem

Of all surgical procedures, peripheral vascular surgery carries the highest mortality rate, because of the high incidence of underlying CAD (Figure 9b.1). Therefore, preoperative cardiac risk assessment and perioperative management studies are frequently analyzed in patients undergoing peripheral vascular surgery. In a landmark study by Hertzer et al.,[1] hemodynamically significant CAD was reported in 36% of patients with abdominal aortic aneurysms and in 28% of patients with lower limb ischemia. Importantly, in 94% of all cases, i.e., symptomatic and asymptomatic vascular surgery patients, abnormalities were detected during coronary angiography. Results of perioperative management are then extrapolated from high-risk patients to the general surgical population. Patients undergoing liver or renal transplantation are other important groups and these will be discussed separately in Chapter 7b.

Peripheral vascular disease (PVD) is an increasing problem in Europe and in North America. For example, between 1980 and 1995 in the Netherlands, the number of patients admitted to hospital because of PVD has increased from 17 511 to 29 346. This is an increase of 36% after correction for demographic factors.[2] The high incidence of PVD was confirmed in a recent

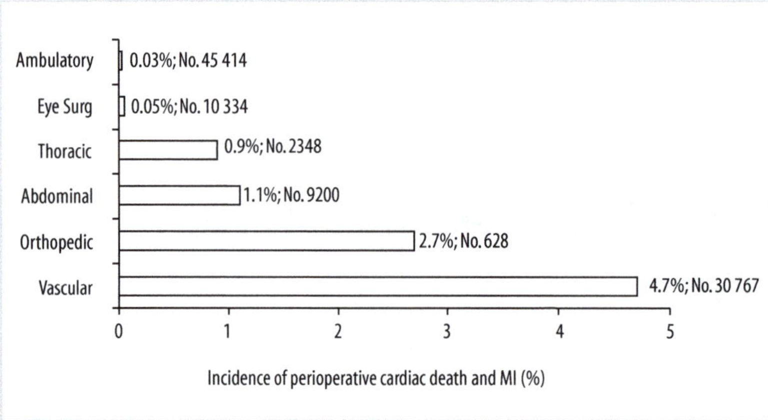

Figure 9b.1. Risk of perioperative cardiac death and MI for different types of surgery based on a study of 108 593 patients operated at Erasmus MC between 1991 and 2000 (MI, myocardial infarction; eye surg, eye surgery).

study from the United Kingdom; the study used ultrasound screening to show that between 1.5% and 3% of men older than 60 years had an occult aortic aneurysm of between 40- and 59-mm diameter.[3] Many of these patients require surgery with an associated 30-day operative mortality of 5%–6% and 5-year mortality of 45%, both of which arise principally from cardiac events.[4] This high perioperative mortality was confirmed in a study by Krupski et al.[5] who reported a similar cardiac event rate after infrainguinal procedures as after aortic operations (9% versus 7%, respectively).

Although most physicians focus on perioperative management, patients should live long enough to enjoy the benefits of surgery. The 5-year mortality rate of patients with PVD ranges between 20% and 40% because of late cardiac events.[6–8] Therefore, the preoperative cardiac evaluation and cardioprotective therapies, including lifestyle changes and medical therapy, should be continued after surgery. To optimize medical care, not only perioperatively but also the long-term postoperative care, it is mandatory that the treating physician evaluates the presence and extent of CAD as well as risk factors, such as hypertension and hypercholesterolemia that will determine long-term survival after surgery.

2. Pathophysiology

Cardiac events are mainly caused by myocardial ischemia. Myocardial ischemia may arise either from an increased myocardial oxygen demand or a reduced supply. In the perioperative period, patients with suspected or known CAD are at a higher risk for an event during the operation because factors such as increased heart rate or elevated blood pressure resulting from surgical stress, pain, or the use of sympathomimetic drugs increase further myocardial oxygen demand. Decreased supply may be the result of hypotension, vasospasm, anemia, and hypoxia.

The location of a perioperative MI is not always related to the location of the culprit coronary lesion. In a study by Dawood et al.,[9] evaluating the pathophysiology of perioperative fatal cardiac events, evidence of plaque rupture was identified in 55% of patients. After examining the location of severe lesions, the investigators found that preoperative prediction of the site of infarction based on the severity of the underlying CAD would have been unsuccessful in almost half of the cases. The unpredictable progression of an (in)significant coronary lesion reduces the predictive value for tests that aim to detect the culprit lesion, such as pharmacologic stress testing, and reinforces the importance of appropriate medical therapy that reduces coronary plaque instability.

Other important causes of perioperative cardiac events are aortic valve stenosis and LV dysfunction. For proper identification of aortic valve stenosis, echocardiography is mandatory. Long-term cardiac complications are more common in the presence of LV dysfunction.[10] Aortic valve stenosis also is an increasing problem because 6% of the population older than 80 years of age have aortic valve stenosis and an increasing number of elderly are scheduled for surgery.[11] The presence of aortic valve stenosis increases the incidence of perioperative cardiac death or MI four-fold, and also has important consequences for the type of anesthesia, e.g., general versus locoregional.[12]

3. Perioperative Care

3.1 Step One: Selection of Patients at Risk

Risk stratification begins with a careful clinical history and knowledge of the surgical procedure to be performed. A number of methods of quantifying risk have been used, the most common being the Goldman cardiac operative risk index, the Detsky modified multifactorial risk index, and Eagle's risk factors,[13–15] and these allow stratification into low, intermediate, or high risk (Table 9b.1). These indices, although in general are helpful to identify high-risk individuals, tend to underestimate the risk at the lower end of the spectrum and have a suboptimal negative predictive value. In response to this drawback, the American College of Cardiology (ACC)/American Heart Association (AHA) have proposed a classification of clinical predictors into major, intermediate, and minor (Table 9b.2).[16] More recently, Lee et al.[17] have reviewed the predictive value of several clinical risk factors in patients scheduled for noncardiac surgery. Six factors, i.e., high-risk surgery, stroke, diabetes mellitus, renal failure, heart failure, and ischemic heart disease, were identified in a study population of 2893 patients and later validated in a population of 1422 patients. The rate of major perioperative complications in the presence of 0, 1, 2, or 3 risk factors was 0.4%, 0.9%, 7%, and 11%, respectively, but a limitation of the findings for assessing patients undergoing vascular surgery was that only 110 of 2893 patients (3.8%) had abdominal aortic surgery.

The importance of common clinical cardiac risk factors was recently confirmed by Boersma et al.[18] In a study population of 108 593 patients, the combination of risk factors such as age, gender, type of surgery, and risk factors for CAD stratified patients into low, intermediate, and high risk for perioperative death (Figure 9b.2). For a more refined classification, however, noninvasive testing is also required and this will be discussed below.

3.2 Step Two: Additional Testing

Additional testing should only be performed if the results will change perioperative management. Therefore, pharmacologic stress testing should be reserved for those patients in whom the detection of CAD will lead to a change in anesthetic or surgical management or to preoperative coronary revascularization. Referral to angiography and subsequently to coronary revascularization should only be considered in a minority of patients. The CASS (Coronary Artery Surgery Study) registry showed that patients who underwent coronary revascularization before low-risk surgery were at the same risk of perioperative death or MI (2%) as those who were not revascularized.[19] Although there are few (nonrandomized) studies to evaluate the protective effect of preoperative myocardial revascularization, most studies indicate that revascularization should be performed if it would have been indicated in any case (Table 9b.3 and Table 9b.4).[20] This would include patients with unstable coronary syndromes or those with extensive coronary disease or ischemia. In addition, cardioprotective therapy such as beta-blockers and statins may reduce the need for additional testing, because the perioperative cardiac event rate is further reduced and patients are unlikely to benefit from coronary revascularization (Figure 9b.3).

There is widespread consensus that additional noninvasive testing is required in patients with at least one cardiac risk factor (angina pectoris, previous MI, diabetes mellitus, congestive heart failure, cardiac arrhythmias, age >70 years) or a reduced exercise capacity undergoing high-risk surgical procedures. The ACC/AHA algorithm for preoperative risk assessment considers initially the urgency for surgery, its inherent cardiac risk (Table 9b.5), the patient's risk factors, and exercise tolerance. Patients with only minor clinical predictors [advanced age, abnormal resting electrocardiogram (ECG), previous stroke, or hypertension] who require low- to moderate-risk surgery are at low risk and do not require further investigation. Patients with intermediate clinical predictors (mild angina, prior infarction, treated heart failure, or diabetes) or with minor predictors and reduced exercise tolerance need further assessment before moderate- or high-risk surgery.[20] Patients with major predictors may be considered for cancellation of

Table 9b.1. Commonly used indices of cardiac risk

	Original		Detsky et al.		Larsen et al.	
	Definition	No. of points	Definition	No. of point	Definition	No. of points
Ischemic heart disease	MI within 6 mo	10	MI within 6 mo	10	MI within 3 mo	1
			MI > 6 mo earlier	5	No MI within 3 mo, but pervious MI, angina pectoris, or both	
			CCS class III angina	10		
			CCS class IV angina	20		
			Unstable angina with 6 mo	10		
Congestive heart failure	S_3 gallop or regular venous distention	11	Pulmonary edema		Persistent pulmonary congestion	12
			Within 1 wk	10	No pulmonary congestion, but previous pulmonary edema	8
			Ever	5	Neither pulmonary congestion nor pervious pulmonary edema, but previous heart failure	4
Cardiac rhythm	Rhythm other than sinus or PACs on last preoperative ECG	7	Rhythm other than sinus or sinus plus PACs on last preoperative ECG	5	–	
	>5 PVCs/min at any time before surgery	7	>5 PVCs/min at any time before surgery	5		
Valvular heart disease	Important aortic stenosis	3	Suspected critical aortic stenosis	20	–	
General medical status	$Po_2 < 60$ mm Hg or $Pco_2 > 50$ mm Hg, potassium <3.0 mmol/L or bicarbonate <20 mmol/L; BUN > 50 mg/dL (18 mmol/L) or creatinine >3.0 mg/dL (260 μmol/L); abnormal AST signs of chronic liver disease or patient bedridden from Non-cardiac causes	3	Same as for original index	5	Serum creatinine > 1.5 mg/dL (130 μmol/L)	2
					Diabetes mellitus	3
Age	>70 yr	5	>70 yr	5	–	
Type of surgery	Intraperitoneal, intrathoracic, or nortic operation	3	Emergency operation	10	Emergency operation	3
	Emergency operation	4			Aortic operation	5
					Other intraperitoneal or pleural operation	3

MI, myocardial infarction; CCS, PAC, premature atrial contraction; PVC, premature ventricular contraction.

Table 9b.2. Clinical predictors of increased perioperative cardiac risk (ACC/AHA guidelines 2002)

Major	
	Unstable coronary syndromes
	Decompensated CHF
	Severe valvular disease
	Significant arrhythmias (high-grade AV block, symptomatic ventricular arrhythmias, SVT with uncontrolled ventr. rate
Intermediate	
	Mild angina pectoris
	Prior MI
	Compensated or prior CHF
	Diabetes mellitus
Minor	
	Advanced age
	Abnormal ECG
	Rhythm other than sinus
	Low functional capacity
	History of stroke
	Uncontrolled HTN

ACC, American College of Cardiology; AHA, American Heart Association; CHF, Chronic heart failure; AV, atrio-ventricular; SVT, sustained ventricular tochycardia; HTN, hypertension.

Table 9b.3. Indications for coronary angiography

Class I	
	Evidence for high risk or adverse outcomes based on noninvasive test results
	Angina unresponsive to medical treatment
	Unstable angina
	Nondiagnostic noninvasive tests in patients with high clinical risk of CHD who are undergoing high-risk surgery
Class IIa	
	Moderate to large ischemic areas but with preserved LVF
	Nondiagnostic noninvasive tests in patients with intermediate clinical risk of CHD who are undergoing high-risk surgery
	Urgent noncardiac surgery in patients recovering from an acute MI

CHD: Coronan heart disease; ACC/AHA guidelines* see text, page 211.

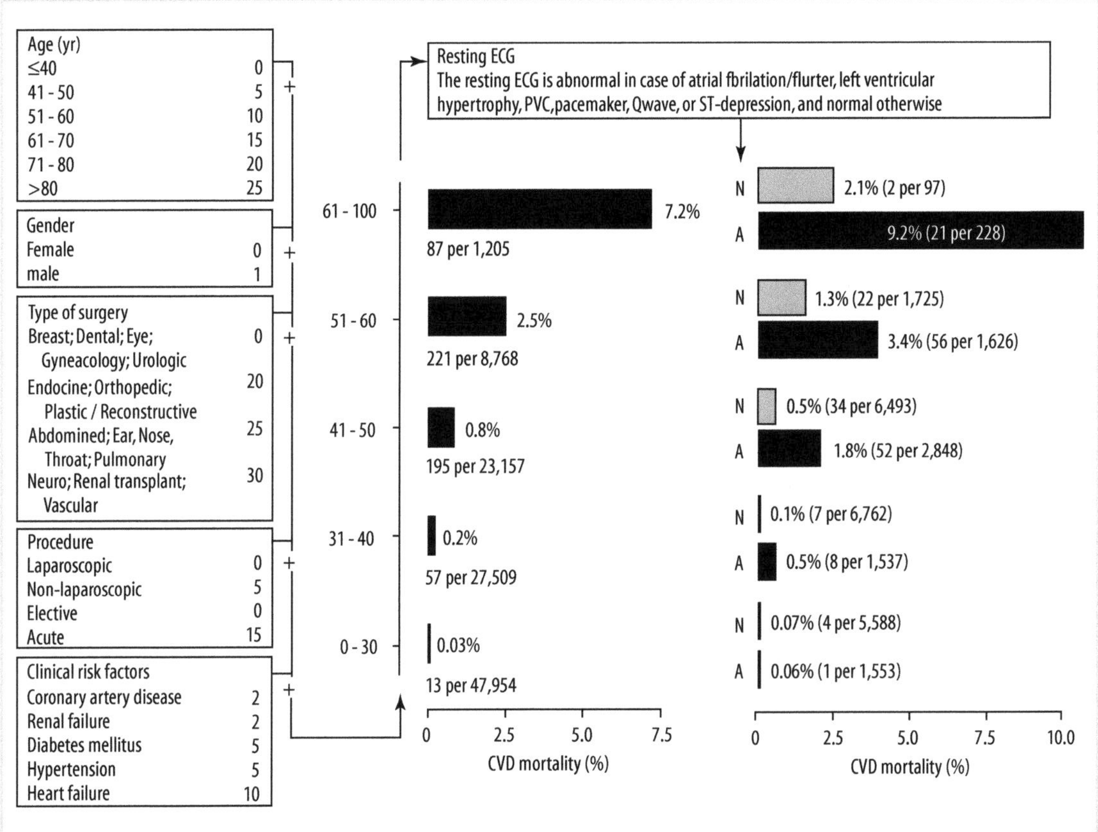

Figure 9b.2. Risk score developed by Boersma et al.[18] in which ECG and stress echocardiography can be incorporated. Points for risk factors in the left boxes are added and subsequently the risk on cardiovascular mortality can be quantified with or without further differentiation by ECG. CVD, cardiovascular disease; PVC, premature ventricular contraction.

Table 9b.4. Risk of procedure

Is the noncardiac operation necessary?
If yes, medical therapy or revascularize?
Revascularize only if otherwise indicated
No studies to demonstrate prognostic benefit of PCI
No studies of staged or simultaneous revascularization if peripheral or carotid vascular surgery
Preoperative coronary angioplasty
No randomized clinical trials documenting decreased incidence of perioperative cardiac events
No prospective studies to determine optimal period of delay
Medical therapy
Beta-blockade for hypertension, angina, or tachyarrhythmia
Peri-operative nitrates reduce ischemia but no effect on postoperative events
Preoperative intensive care for heart failure
Anesthetic considerations (hypotension)
Management of pain, fluid balance, coagulation

PCI, percutaneous coronary intervention.
ACC/AHA algorithm

Table 9b.5. Risk of procedure

High > 5%	Emergency surgery, especially in elderly Aortic/major vascular Peripheral vascular Prolonged surgery 5 h
Intermediate 1%–5%	Carotid endarterectomy Head and neck Intraperitoneal/intrathoracic Orthopedic Prostate
Low < 1%	Endoscopic procedures Superficial procedure Cataract Breast

ACC/AHA guideline for perioperative cardiovascular evaluation

the operation and risk-factor modification or for coronary angiography.

Myocardial perfusion scintigraphy (MPS) can provide useful information about cardiac risk in patients requiring noncardiac surgery. Numerous studies[21–47] have been performed in this setting and, in a meta-analysis of 3718 patients undergoing vascular and other surgery, the positive predictive value of inducible ischemia for perioperative death or infarction was 12.9% compared with a negative predictive value of 98.6%, a risk ratio of 9.1 (Table 9b.6).

Several studies of dobutamine stress echocardiography (DSE) for preoperative risk stratification[50–56] have also been performed showing comparable positive and negative predictive values with MPS.

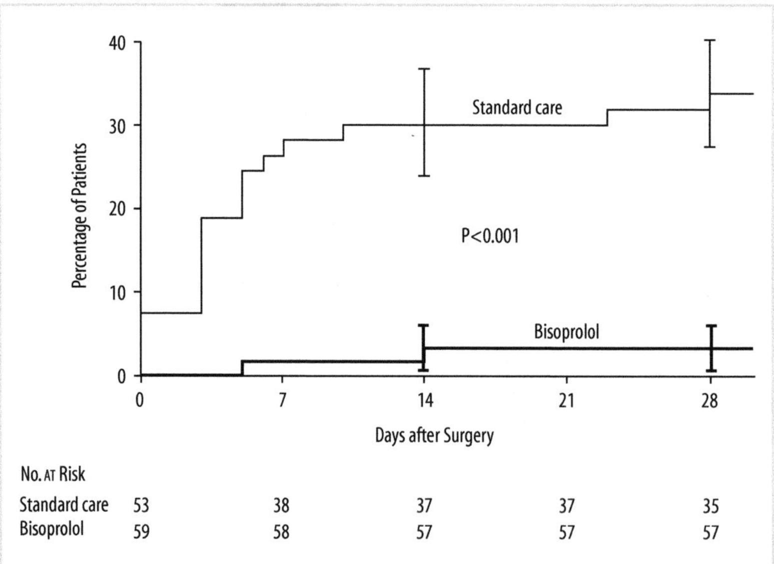

Figure 9b.3. The effect of bisoprolol on perioperative mortality and MI in high-risk patients undergoing vascular surgery. There was a 10-fold increase in event rate in the standard group.

Table 9b.6. MPS for preoperative assessment of cardiac risk

Year	Author	n	Inducible ischemia, n (%)	MI/death, n (%)	PPV	NPV
Vascular surgery						
1985	Boucher	48	16 (33)	3 (6)	19% (3/16)	100% (32/32)
1987	Cutler	116	54 (47)	11 (10)	20% (11/54)	100% (60/60)
1988	Fletcher	67	15 (22)	3 (4)	20% (3/15)	100% (56/56)
1988	Sachs	46	14 (31)	2 (4)	14% (2/14)	100% (24/24)
1989	Eagle	200	82 (41)	15 (8)	16% (13/82)	98% (61/62)
1990	McEnroe	95	34 (36)	7 (7)	9% (3/34)	96% (44/46)
1990	Younis	111	40 (36)	8 (7)	15% (6/40)	100% (51/51)
1991	Mangano	60	22 (37)	3 (5)	5% (1/22)	95% (19/20)
1991	Strawn	68	n/a	4 (6)	n/a	100% (21/21)
1991	Watters	26	15 (58)	3 (12)	20% (3/15)	100% (11/11)
1992	Hendel	327	167 (51)	28 (9)	14% (23/167)	99% (97/98)
1992	Lette	355	161 (45)	30 (8)	17% (28/161)	99% (160/162)
1992	Madsen	65	45 (69)	5 (8)	11% (5/45)	100% (20/20)
1993	Brown	231	77 (33)	12 (5)	13% (10/77)	99% (120/121)
1993	Kresowik	170	67 (39)	5 (3)	4% (3/67)	98% (64/65)
1994	Baron	457	160 (35)	22 (5)	4% (7/160)	96% (195/203)
1994	Bry	237	110 (46)	17 (7)	11% (12/110)	100% (97/97)
1995	Koutelou	106	47 (44)	3 (3)	6% (3/47)	100% (49/49)
1995	Marshall	117	55 (47)	12 (10)	16% (9/55)	97% (33/34)
1997	Van Damme	142	48 (34)	3 (2)	n/a	n/a
Nonvascular surgery						
1990	Camp	40	9 (23)	6 (15)	67% (6/9)	100% (23/23)
1991	Iqbal	31	11 (41)	3 (11)	27% (3/11)	100% (20/20)
1992	Coley	100	36 (36)	4 (4)	8% (3/36)	98% (63/64)
1992	Shaw	60	28 (47)	6 (10)	21% (6/28)	100% (19/19)
1993	Takase	53	15 (28)	6 (11)	27% (4/15)	100% (32/32)
1994	Younis	161	50 (31)	15 (9)	18% (9/50)	98% (87/89)
1996	Stratmann	229	67 (29)	10 (4)	6% (4/67)	99% (91/92)
Weighted average		3718		246 (7)	12.1% (186/1397)	98.6% (1549/1571)

NPV, negative predictive value; PPV, positive predictive value.

4. Comparison of MPS and Echocardiography

Unfortunately, there has been no direct comparison of these techniques in perioperative risk assessment. The meta-analysis of Shaw et al.[57] compares dipyridamole perfusion imaging and DSE, although not in the same patients. Both tests had comparable predictive accuracy although the summed odds ratios for cardiac death and MI were greater for DSE than for dipyridamole perfusion imaging. However, the confidence intervals for the echocardiography figures were large because of the smaller number of patients. The results of this analysis show that reversible perfusion defects or inducible wall motion abnormalities [Table 9b.7 and Figure 9b.4 (see color section)] predict adverse outcomes during the perioperative period. The prognostic power increases with semiquantitative image analysis (severity of the abnormalities assessed by segmental analysis) and for any amount of ischemia, the presence of comorbidity (e.g., prior CAD, diabetes mellitus, atrial fibrillation) increases further the risk for a hard event. In addition, fixed defects or impaired ventricular function (Tables 9b.7 & 9b.8) were found

Table 9b.7. Prognostic indicators in MPI

Reversible perfusion defects
Extent
Depth
Transient LV dilation
Fixed defects
Increased lung uptake
LVEF (gated SPECT)

MPI, myocardial perfusion imaging; LVEF, left ventricular ejection fraction.

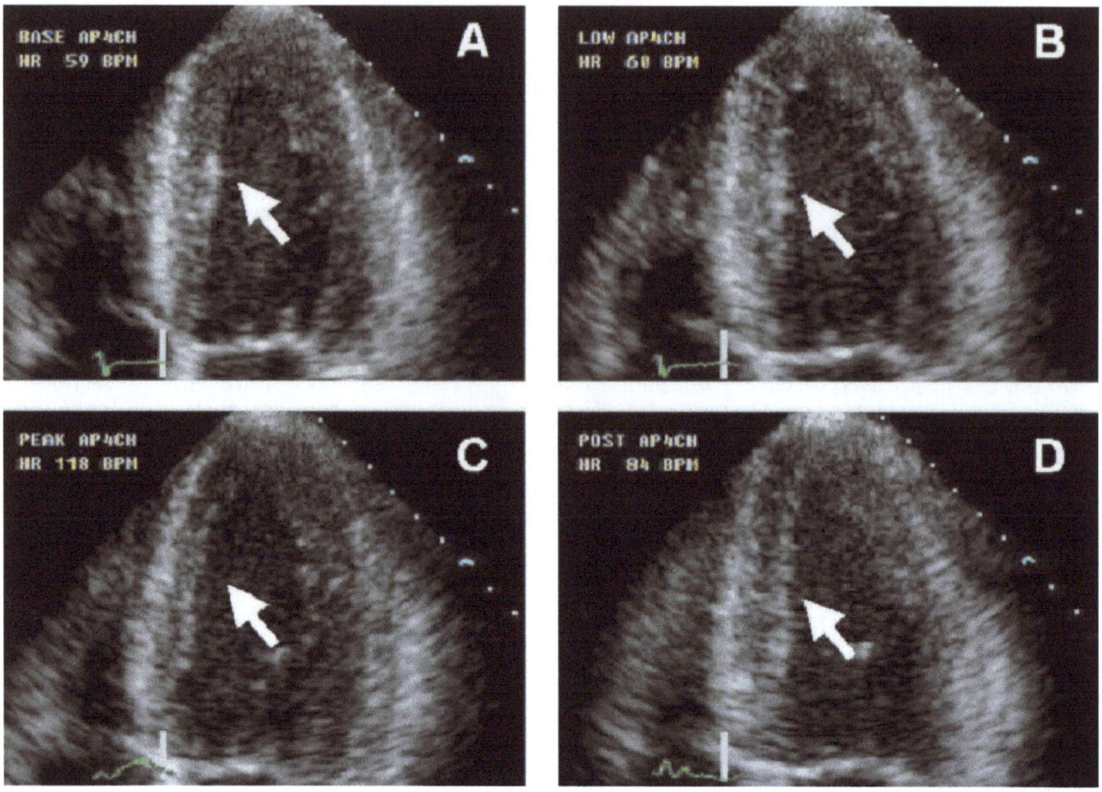

Figure 9b.4. Abnormal DSE. **A** Rest echocardiography. **B** Low-dose stress echocardiography, i.e., 10 μg/kg. **C** Peak stress echocardiography, i.e., 40 μg/kg. **D** Echocardiography at recovery. The white arrow indicates the abnormality. At rest and also at a low dose, the contraction is normal whereas the wall is dyskinetic (moving outside instead of contracting) at peak stress.

Table 9b.8. Further investigation

Resting LV function
Predicator of perioperative CHF, but not MI or ischemia and long-term mortality
High risk if LVEF <35%
Recommended for symptomatic CHF, prior CHF, or dyspnea of unknown origin

LV, left ventricular; LVEF, left ventricular ejection fraction; CHF, chronic heart failure.

to be predictors of long-term events with an accuracy similar to that of the inducible abnormalities for the perioperative period.

5. Conclusions

1. Preoperative cardiac evaluation of patients undergoing surgery offers the possibility of reducing cardiac risk by treating myocardial ischemia, hypertension, and hyperlipidemia. This will reduce perioperative risk and improve long-term outcome.

2. Patients without predictors of cardiac events are at low risk even if undergoing intermediate- or high-risk surgery. Patients with one or more predictors (e.g., angina pectoris class I or II, previous MI, diabetes mellitus, compensated or prior congestive heart failure, important cardiac arrhythmias) who are undergoing low- or intermediate-risk surgery do not benefit from additional investigation (unless their functional capacity is poor), because the risk of perioperative events is low. However, both groups will benefit from beta-blockade.

3. Noninvasive imaging should further assess the perioperative risk in patients with multiple predictors undergoing high-risk surgery. MPS and dobutamine echocardiography have comparable accuracy and the choice of test should be that in which the center has the most experience.

Accurate assessment of the ischemic burden is helpful to predict perioperative risk but simultaneous assessment of the LV function, by means of ECG gated SPECT in the case of MPS, could be helpful in the long-term evaluation of the cardiac risk.

4. Patients with mild to moderate inducible ischemia should be managed as they would be in the absence of peripheral vascular surgery, and they should receive beta-blockers before, during, and after surgery. In patients with extensive inducible ischemia, the cardioprotective effect of beta-blockers is probably insufficient and referral to coronary angiography should be considered.

References

1. Hertzer NR, Beven EG, Young JR, et al. Coronary artery disease in peripheral vascular patients. A classification of 1000 coronary angiograms and results of surgical management. Ann Surg 1984;199:223–233.
2. Hart-en vaatziekten in Nederland. Dutch Heart Foundation; 1997.
3. The UK Small Aneurysm Trial Participants. Mortality results for randomised controlled trial of early elective surgery or ultrasonographic surveillance for small aortic aneurysms. Lancet 1998;352:1649–1655.
4. Mangano DT. Perioperative cardiac morbidity. Anaesthesiology1990;72:153–184.
5. Krupski W, Layug E, Reilly L, et al. Comparison of cardiac morbidity rates between aortic and infrainguinal operations: two-year follow-up. J Vasc Surg 1993; 18:609–617.
6. Kertai MD, Boersma E, Westerhout CM, et al. Association between long-term statin use and mortality after successful abdominal aortic aneurysm surgery. Am J Med 2004;116:96–103.
7. Krupski WC. Update on perioperative evaluation and management of cardiac disease in vascular surgery patients. J Vasc Surg 2002;36:1292–1308.
8. L'Italien GJ, Cambria RP, Cutler BS, et al. Comparative early and late cardiac morbidity among patients requiring different vascular surgery procedures. J Vasc Surg 1995;21:935–944.
9. Dawood MM, Gupta DK, Southern J, et al. Pathology of fatal perioperative myocardial infarction: implications regarding pathophysiology and prevention. Int J Cardiol 1996;57:37–44.
10. Kazmers A, Cerqueira MD, Zierler RE. The role of preoperative radionuclide ejection fraction in direct abdominal aortic aneurysm repair. J Vasc Surg 1988;8: 128–136.
11. Lindroos M, Kupari M, Heikkila J, et al. Prevalence of aortic valve abnormalities in the elderly: an echocardiographic study of a random population sample. J Am Coll Cardiol 1993;21:1220–1225.
12. Kertai MD, Bountioukos M, Boersma E, et al. Aortic stenosis: an underestimated risk factor for perioperative complications in patients undergoing noncardiac surgery. Am J Med 2004;116:8–13.
13. Goldman L, Caldera DL, Nussbaum SR, et al. Multifactorial index of cardiac risk in noncardiac surgical procedures. N Engl J Med 1977;297:845–850.
14. Detsky AS, Abrams HB, Forbath N, et al. Cardiac assessment for patients undergoing noncardiac surgery. A multifactorial clinical risk index. Arch Intern Med 1986;146:2131–2134.
15. Eagle KA, Coley CM, Newell JB, et al. Combining clinical and thallium data optimizes preoperative assessment of cardiac risk before major vascular surgery. Ann Intern Med 1989;110:859–866.
16. ACC/AHA task force report. Guidelines for perioperative cardiovascular evaluation for noncardiac surgery. J Am Coll Cardiol 1996;27:910–948.
17. Lee T, Marcantonio ER, Mangione CM, et al. Derivation and prospective validation of a simple index for prediction of cardiac risk of major noncardiac surgery. Circulation 1999;100:1043–1049.
18. Boersma E, Kertai MD, Bax JJ, et al. A risk model to assess perioperative cardiovascular mortality, developed in 108,593 patients undergoing non-cardiac surgery. Circulation 2003;108(suppl IV):652.
19. Foster ED, Davis KB, Carpenter JA, et al. Risk of noncardiac operation in patients with defined coronary artery disease: the Coronary Artery Surgery Study (CASS) registry experience. Ann Thorac Surg 1986;41: 42–50.
20. Eagle KA, Berger PB, Calkins H, et al. ACC/AHA guideline update for perioperative cardiovascular evaluation for noncardiac surgery. Circulation 2002;105:1257–1267.
21. Boucher CA, Brewster DC, Darling C, Okada R, Strauss HW. Determination of cardiac risk by dipyridamole-thallium imaging before peripheral vascular surgery. N Engl J Med 1985;312:389–394.
22. Cutler BS, Leppo JA. Dipyridamole thallium 201 scintigraphy to detect coronary artery disease before abdominal aortic surgery. J Vasc Surg 1987;5:91–100.
23. Fletcher JP, Antico VF, Gruenewald S, Kershaw LZ. Dipyridamole-thallium scan for screening of coronary artery disease prior to vascular surgery. J Cardiovasc Surg (Torino) 1988;29:666–669.
24. Sachs RN, Tellier P, Larmignat P, et al. Assessment by dipyridamole-thallium-201 myocardial scintigraphy of coronary risk before peripheral vascular surgery. Surgery 1988;103:584–587.
25. Eagle KA, Coley CM, Newell JB, et al. Combining clinical and thallium data optimizes preoperative assessment of cardiac risk before major vascular surgery. Ann Intern Med 1989;110:859–866.
26. McEnroe CS, O'Donnell RF Jr, Yeager A, Konstam M, Mackey WC. Comparison of ejection fraction and Goldman risk factor analysis of dipyridamole-thallium-201 studies in the evaluation of cardiac morbidity after aortic aneurysm surgery. J Vasc Surg 1990;11:497–504.
27. Younis LT, Aguirre F, Byers S, et al. Perioperative and long-term prognostic value of intravenous dipyridamole thallium scintigraphy in patients with peripheral vascular disease. Am Heart J 1990;119: 1287–1292.
28. Mangano DT, London MJ, Tubau JF, et al. Dipyridamole thallium-201 scintigraphy as a preoperative screening test. A reexamination of its predictive potential. Study

of Perioperative Ischemia Research Group. Circulation 1991;84:493–502.
29. Strawn DJ, Guernsey JM. Dipyridamole thallium scanning in the evaluation of coronary artery disease in elective abdominal aortic surgery. Arch Surg 1991; 126:880–884.
30. Watters TA, Botvinick EH, Dae MW, et al. Comparison of the findings on preoperative dipyridamole perfusion scintigraphy and intraoperative transesophageal echocardiography: implications regarding the identification of myocardium at ischemic risk. J Am Coll Cardiol 1991;18:93–100.
31. Hendel RC, Whitfield SS, Villegas BJ, Cutler BS, Leppo JA. Prediction of late cardiac events by dipyridamole thallium imaging in patients undergoing elective vascular surgery. Am J Cardiol 1992;70:1243–1249.
32. Lette J, Waters D, Cerino M, Picard M, Champagne P, Lapointe J. Preoperative coronary artery disease risk stratification based on dipyridamole imaging and a simple three-step, three-segment model for patients undergoing noncardiac vascular surgery or major general surgery. Am J Cardiol 1992;69:1553–1558.
33. Madsen PV, Vissing M, Munck O, Kelbaek H. A comparison of dipyridamole thallium 201 scintigraphy and clinical examination in the determination of cardiac risk before arterial reconstruction. Angiology 1992;43: 306–311.
34. Brown KA, Rowen M. Extent of jeopardized viable myocardium determined by myocardial perfusion imaging best predicts perioperative cardiac events in patients undergoing noncardiac surgery. J Am Coll Cardiol 1993;21:325–330.
35. Kresowik TF, Bower TR, Garner SA, et al. Dipyridamole thallium imaging in patients being considered for vascular procedures. Arch Surg 1993;128:299–302.
36. Baron JF, Mundler O, Bertrand M, et al. Dipyridamole-thallium scintigraphy and gated radionuclide angiography to assess cardiac risk before abdominal aortic surgery. N Engl J Med 1994;330:663–669.
37. Bry JD, Belkin M, O'Donnell TF Jr, et al. An assessment of the positive predictive value and cost-effectiveness of dipyridamole myocardial scintigraphy in patients undergoing vascular surgery. J Vasc Surg 1994;19: 112–121.
38. Koutelou MG, Asimacopoulos PJ, Mahmarian JJ, Kimball KT, Verani MS. Preoperative risk stratification by adenosine thallium 201 single-photon emission computed tomography in patients undergoing vascular surgery. J Nucl Cardiol 1995;2:389–394.
39. Marshall ES, Raichlen JS, Forman S, Heyrich GP, Keen WD, Weitz HH. Adenosine radionuclide perfusion imaging in the preoperative evaluation of patients undergoing peripheral vascular surgery. Am J Cardiol 1995;76:817–821.
40. Van Damme H, Pierard L, Gillain D, Benoit T, Rigo P, Limet R. Cardiac risk assessment before vascular surgery: a prospective study comparing clinical evaluation, dobutamine stress echocardiography, and dobutamine Tc-99m sestamibi tomoscintigraphy. Cardiovasc Surg 1997;5:54–64.
41. Camp AD, Garvin PJ, Hoff J, Marsh J, Byers S, Chaitman BR. Prognostic value of intravenous dipyridamole thallium imaging in patients with diabetes mellitus considered for renal transplantation. Am J Cardiol 1990;65:1459–1463.
42. Iqbal A, Gibbons RJ, McGoon MD, Steiroff S, Frohnert P, Velosa JA. Noninvasive assessment of cardiac risk in insulin-dependent diabetic patients being evaluated for pancreatic transplantation using thallium-201 myocardial perfusion scintigraphy. Transplant Proc 1991; 23:1690–1691.
43. Coley CM, Field TS, Abraham SA, Boucher CA, Eagle KA. Usefulness of dipyridamole-thallium scanning for preoperative evaluation of cardiac risk for nonvascular surgery. Am J Cardiol 1992;69:1280–1285.
44. Shaw L, Miller DD, Kong BA, et al. Determination of perioperative cardiac risk by adenosine thallium-201 myocardial imaging. Am Heart J 1992;124:861–869.
45. Takase B, Younis LT, Byers SL, et al. Comparative prognostic value of clinical risk indexes, resting two-dimensional echocardiography, and dipyridamole stress thallium-201 myocardial imaging for perioperative cardiac events in major nonvascular surgery patients. Am Heart J 1993;126:1099–1106.
46. Younis L, Stratmann H, Takase B, Byers S, Chaitman BR, Miller DD. Preoperative clinical assessment and dipyridamole thallium-201 scintigraphy for prediction and prevention of cardiac events in patients having major noncardiovascular surgery and known or suspected coronary artery disease. Am J Cardiol 1994;74:311–317.
47. Stratmann HG, Younis LT, Wittry MD, Amato M, Miller DD. Dipyridamole technetium-99m sestamibi myocardial tomography in patients evaluated for elective vascular surgery: prognostic value for perioperative and late cardiac events. Am Heart J 1996;131:923–929.
48. Poldermans D, Arnese M, Fioretti PM, Thomson IR, Boersma E, van Urk H. Improved cardiac risk stratification in major vascular surgery with dobutamine-atropine stress echocardiography. J Am Coll Cardiol 1995;26:1197–1202.
49. Davila-Roman VG, Waggoner AD, Sicard GA, Geltman EM, Schechtman KB, Perez JE. Dobutamine stress echocardiography predicts surgical outcome in patients with an aortic aneurysm and peripheral vascular disease. J Am Coll Cardiol 1993;21:957–963.
50. Eichelberger J, Schnarz K, Black E, Green R, Ouriel K. Medical value of dobutamine echocardiography before vascular surgery. Circulation 1992;86(suppl I): I-789.
51. Lalka SG, Sawada SG, Dalsing MC, et al. Dobutamine stress echocardiography as a predictor of cardiac events associated with aortic surgery. J Vasc Surg 1992;15: 831–842.
52. Lane RT, Sawada SG, Segar DS, et al. Dobutamine stress echocardiography as predictor of perioperative cardiac events. Am J Cardiol 1991;68:976–977.
53. Williams MJ, O'Gorman D, Shan K, Pietrolungo J, Cooklin M, Marwick T. Dobutamine vs dipyridamole echo for risk stratification before vascular surgery. J Am Soc Echocardiogr 1995;8:406.
54. Xie T, Tavackoli S, Adams M, Esquivel JG, Ahmad M. Value of dobutamine stress echocardiography in risk stratification of patients with clinical predictors of "intermediate to high risk" for peripheral vascular surgery [abstract]. Circulation 1998;98(suppl S1): 390.
55. Langan EM, Youky JR, Franklin DP, Elmore JR, Costello JM, Nassef LA. Dobutamine stress echocardiography for cardiac risk assessment before aortic surgery. J Vasc Surg 1993;18:905–913.

56. Poldermans D, Fioretti PM, Forster T, et al. Dobutamine stress echocardiography for the assessment of perioperative cardiac risk in patients undergoing major non cardiac vascular surgery. Circulation 1993;87:1506–1512.

57. Shaw LJ, Eagle KA, Gersh BJ, et al. Meta-analysis of intravenous dipyidamole-thallium-201 imaging (1985–1994) and dobutamine echocardiography (1991–1994) for risk stratification before vascular surgery. J Am Coll Cardiol 1996;27:787–789.

10

Imaging in the Emergency Department or Chest Pain Unit

Prem Soman and James E. Udelson

Chest pain is a common cause of emergency department (ED) presentations worldwide. In the United States (US) alone, this symptom brings five to seven million people annually to the ED.[1,2] However, only a minority, approximately a third, of these patients have symptoms of cardiac origin.[3,4] Although the economic consequences of unnecessary hospital admissions for suspected acute coronary syndrome (ACS) impose a huge burden on health care systems (five to eight billion dollars annually in the US),[5] approximately 4%–7% of patients with true ACI are inadvertently sent home, including 2%–4% of patients with acute myocardial infarction (AMI).[6–8] Therefore, the triage of chest pain patients is a significant challenge to the ED physician, requiring unique considerations of patient safety, cost containment, and potential malpractice litigation.

1. Limitations of the 12-lead Electrocardiogram and Symptom Assessment

The 12-lead surface electrocardiogram (ECG) has become a routinely used tool for the diagnosis of myocardial ischemia, and the diagnostic standard for ST-segment elevation myocardial infarction (MI). However, its utility in the ED diagnosis of ACI is limited by a low sensitivity. In a study of 45 hospitalized patients with suspected ACS, simultaneous ECG and technetium (Tc)-99m sestamibi imaging during a spontaneous episode of chest pain showed a sensitivity of only 35% for the ECG diagnosis of angiographic coronary artery disease (CAD).[9] Even in patients subsequently proven to have an AMI, the sensitivity of the presenting ECG for the diagnosis of AMI is low, in the range of 45%.[10–12] Various studies have reported sensitivities of 65%–88% for the ECG diagnosis of ACS in the ED.[3,13–15] In addition to the low sensitivity, the resting ECG often has baseline abnormalities such as left ventricular hypertrophy and conduction defects that confound the interpretation of ischemic changes.[11] Whereas a *completely* normal ECG in ED patients with chest pain is generally indicative of a benign prognosis (despite a low *diagnostic* sensitivity), less than 20% of patients presenting to the ED with suspected ACS fit this criteria.[3] Similar considerations apply to the risk stratification of ED patients based on chest pain characteristics.[16] These findings have driven the literature on methodologies to improve the evaluation process for such patients.

2. Attributes of an Ideal Triaging Strategy for Chest Pain Patients

Screening techniques for ACS should err on the side of sensitivity to avoid the potentially dire consequences of missing this diagnosis. Because sensitivity and specificity generally vary inversely, this will generally mean some compromise on specificity.

The ED physician facing a triage decision (admit or not) is interested in the identification of patients with ACS, which includes both AMI and unstable angina. However, many reviews of ED triage strategies have concentrated on the separation of patients with AMI from those with other etiologies for chest pain, a distinction that is often not emphasized in the literature. Thus, tests dependent on the presence of myocardial necrosis, such as cardiac enzyme subfraction analysis or biomarker analysis, are less useful for the physician because they do not detect patients with unstable angina without myocardial necrosis.

Many patients presenting to the ED with chest pain arrive after their symptoms have begun to abate. A test in which sensitivity is dependent on the presence of active symptoms at the time it is performed may be less useful than one in which abnormalities indicative of ischemia are detectable when the test is performed even after the resolution of acute symptoms.

3. Rationale for Using Noninvasive Imaging for the ED Assessment of Patients with Chest Pain

The ischemic cascade describes the sequence of events that occurs when myocardial oxygen demand progressively increases beyond supply. Regional coronary flow heterogeneity detectable by perfusion imaging is the first discernible abnormality to manifest, followed by abnormalities in diastolic and regional systolic function seen on echocardiography. ECG changes and chest pain are the last to occur in this sequence.[17,18] Therefore, radionuclide myocardial perfusion imaging (MPI) and echocardiography should theoretically demonstrate abnormalities before ECG changes or symptoms occur. As a corollary to this fact, a normal myocardial perfusion scan or echocardiogram in the presence of chest pain makes cardiac ischemia an unlikely etiology for the chest pain. Furthermore, in patients with acute coronary ischemia, myocardial perfusion abnormalities may persist for several hours after symptom resolution.[19] Thus, the early occurrence and persistence of abnormalities in relation to the onset of symptoms give MPI and echocardiography a significant advantage for use in clinical decision-making for patients in the ED.

4. Radionuclide MPI

4.1 Evolution of Studies Examining the Use of MPI for Diagnosis of ACS in the ED

Early studies evaluating the use of radionuclide MPI for ED imaging utilized thallium-201, at that time the most widely used agent for MPI. In 1976, Wackers et al.[20] showed thallium-201 defects in 100% of patients with AMI who were studied within 6 hours of the onset of symptoms. The sensitivity for detecting ischemia diminished beyond 6 hours from symptom onset. In a later study involving patients with unstable angina, Wackers and coworkers[21] found planar thallium-201 scintigraphy to have 76% sensitivity and 67% specificity for predicting MI or severe CAD. In addition, in the presence of an abnormal baseline ECG with transient changes, the sensitivity for a positive thallium-201 scan increased to 94%, but with a specificity of only 46%.

Thallium-201 has several disadvantages for use in the ED setting, among them the property of redistribution with time into myocardial areas of initial low uptake. This necessitates image acquisition shortly after trace injection and introduces logistic problems when patients have to be transported to the gamma camera for image acquisition. Additionally, thallium-201 requires a cyclotron for its production, which is usually situated offsite, and thus rapid availability of the tracer is more problematic. Both these disadvantages have been overcome with the introduction of the Tc-99m-based perfusion tracers. These agents show minimal myocardial redistribution over time, thus allowing delayed image acquisition several hours after injection, and special kits for onsite preparation of the tracer are available. The higher photon energy of these agents (140 KeV) compared with thallium-201 (60–80 KeV) results in a lower propensity for attenuation artifacts and improved specificity, and their shorter half-life permits more optimal patient dosimetry.

The clinical basis for the use of Tc-99m agents in patients with suspected ACS was initially reported in a study by Bilodeau et al.[9] evaluating 45 patients already hospitalized with suspected unstable angina. Coronary angiography revealed significant CAD in 26 patients. Tc-99m sestamibi was injected during a spontaneous episode of chest pain, and single photon emission computed tomography (SPECT) imaging demonstrated 96% sensitivity and 79% specificity for the detection of angiographic CAD, whereas the predictive value of a negative scan to exclude CAD was 94%. This study was performed in patients already admitted to the hospital with suspected unstable angina, and the results of the imaging were blinded from the treating physicians, thus prospective testing of this modality to reduce the need for admission or catheterization was not analyzed. Importantly, however, this seminal study showed that the injection of sestamibi during an episode of chest pain was very sensitive for detecting ischemia caused by coronary disease, and had a strong negative predictive value for excluding significant coronary disease.

After this initial study, a substantial body of evidence documenting the feasibility of using radionuclide MPI in the ED has now accrued (Table 10.1). Christian and colleagues[22] initially evaluated the use of sestamibi imaging in ED patients without clear ST-segment elevation, by documenting perfusion defects in 13 of 14 patients presenting with chest pain and nondiagnostic ECGs, who were eventually diagnosed to have had an AMI. This study also

Table 10.1. Myocardial perfusion imaging in acute chest pain: diagnostic studies

Study	n	Sens (%)	Spec (%)	PPV (%)	NPV (%)	Endpoint
Wackers 1976	203	100	63	55	100	MI
Bilodeau 1991	45	96	79	86	94	CAD by angiography
Varetto 1993	64	100	67	43	100	MI
		100	92	90	100	CAD
Hilton 1994	102	100	78	38	99	MI
		94	83	44	99	All events
Tatum 1997	438	100	78	7	100	MI
		82	83	32	98	MI, revascularization
Kontos 1997	532	93	71	15	99	MI
		81	76	40	95	MI, revascularization
Heller 1998	357	90	60	12	99	MI
Duca 1999	75	100	73	33	100	MI
		73	93	89	81	CAD
Kosnik 1999	69	71	92	50	97	MI, revascularization, cardiac death

Sens, sensitivity; Spec, specificity; PPV, positive predictive value; NPV, negative predictive value; MI, myocardial infarction; CAD, objective evidence for coronary artery disease.

demonstrated that AMI without ECG changes did not necessarily reflect a small MI, as quantitative analysis demonstrated that the sestamibi infarct size averaged 20% ± 15% (range 2%–53%) of the left ventricle.

In the first study of a broader ED population, Varetto et al.[23] performed resting Tc-99m sestamibi SPECT imaging in 64 patients presenting to the ED with suspected ACS and nondiagnostic ECGs. Thirty-four patients had normal scans, none of whom were subsequently found to have significant CAD by coronary angiography or stress testing. Of the 30 patients with perfusion defects, 13 were found to have had an AMI (by enzyme or electrocardiographic criteria), 14 were found to have significant CAD by angiography, and the remaining 3 patients were considered to have false-positive findings. Overall, the sensitivity and specificity for the detection of AMI or significant CAD was 100% and 92%, respectively, whereas the predictive value of a negative scan to exclude CAD or a subsequent cardiac event was 100%.

Several subsequent studies in larger numbers of patients, using Tc-99m sestamibi or Tc-99m tetrofosmin have reported similar results in that the use of MPI in this setting significantly improved the sensitivity of identifying patients with chest pain attributed to acute cardiac ischemia, beyond that obtained by history and ECG alone[24–26] (Table 10.1). Put together, these studies establish that the negative predictive value of MPI for ruling out an MI in the ED is more than 99%, and the negative predictive value for future adverse cardiac events is more than 97% (Figures 10.1 and 10.2; see color section).

4.2 A Diagnostic Versus Prognostic Construct for Evaluating Chest Pain in the ED

Radionuclide MPI can also be used in the ED setting for risk stratification of patients presenting with chest pain, and decision-making on further management is informed by the

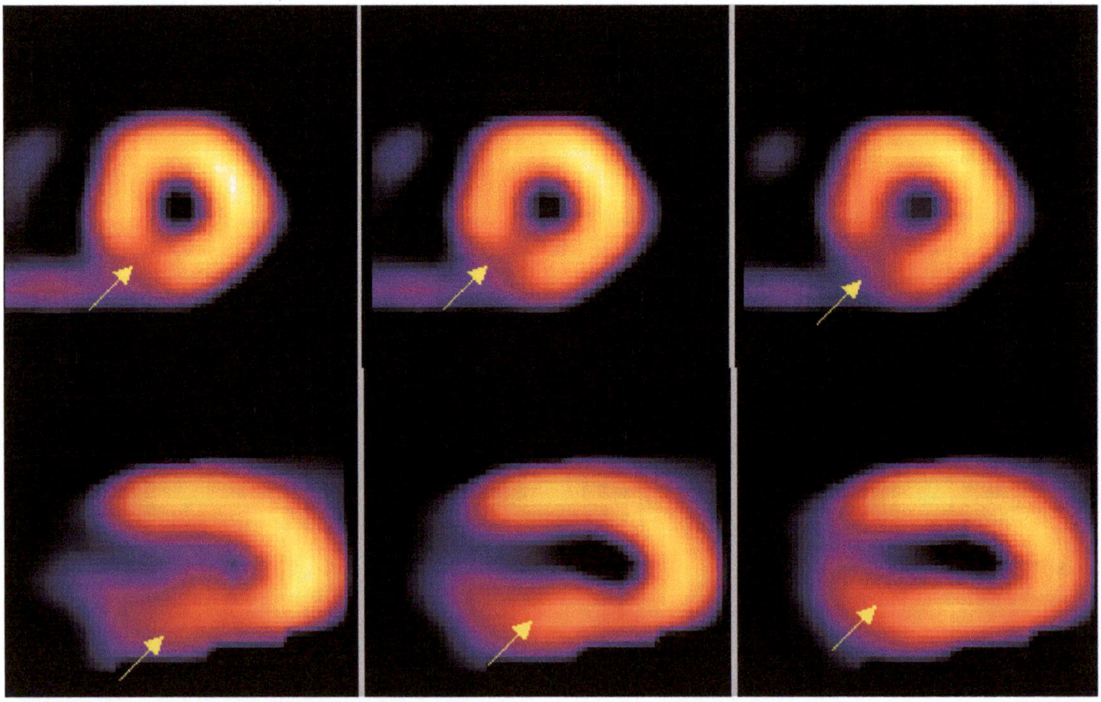

Figure 10.1. Representative short-axis (top) and vertical long-axis slices (bottom) from a Tc-99m sestamibi rest scan with an inferoseptal defect (arrows), indicative of either acute ischemia or infarction. The patient presented with chest pain and a nondiagnostic ECG, and was subsequently found to have a severe stenosis in his right coronary artery.

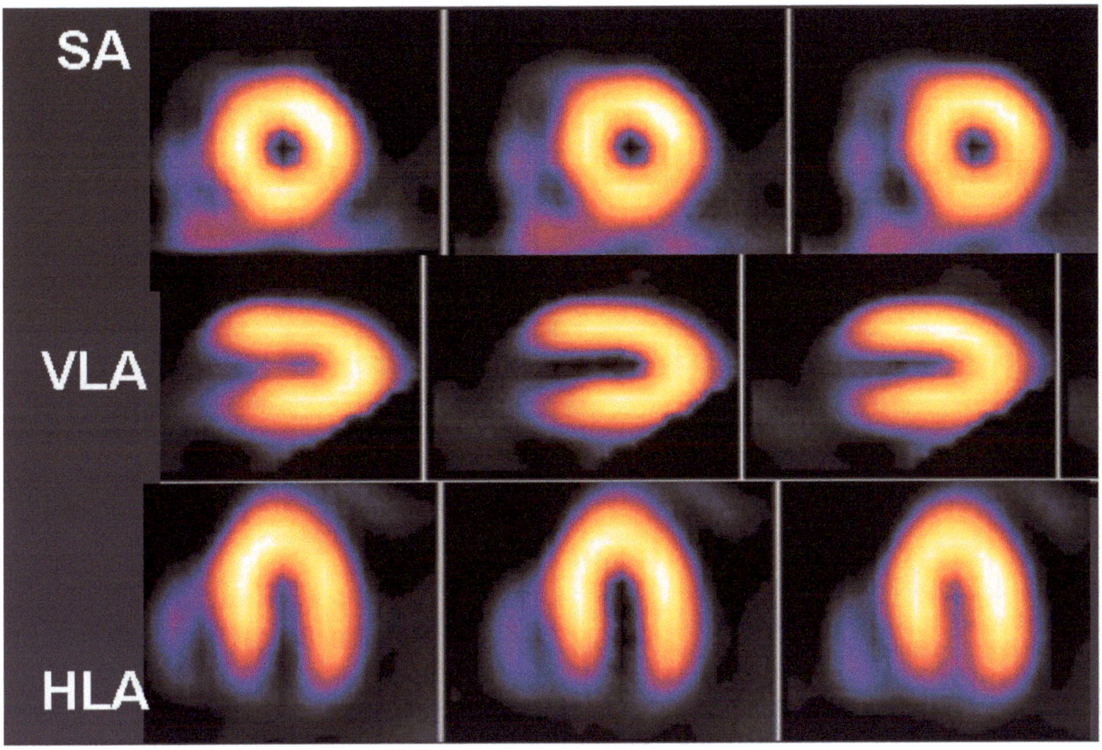

Figure 10.2. Representative short-axis (SA), vertical long-axis (VLA), and horizontal long-axis (HLA) images from a normal Tc-99m sestamibi resting scan performed during chest pain. Based on numerous studies, the negative predictive value for ruling out an MI is approximately 99%.

identified risk of subsequent adverse cardiac events. This approach is in contrast to the use of MPI for *diagnosis of CAD*, evaluated in the studies noted above, and has gained increasing popularity in recent years because diagnostic performance may vary depending on the gold standard used. Varetto and coworkers,[23] in their series of 64 ED patients, were the first to report longer-term outcomes after MPI in the ED. Among the patients with normal rest ED MPI studies, *no cardiac events occurred over 18 months of follow-up*. That is, the negative predictive value for events was 100%. Hilton and coworkers[27] also looked specifically at the prognostic significance of sestamibi myocardial perfusion images obtained in ED patients with chest pain. Only one cardiac event (defined as cardiac death, nonfatal MI, or need for acute coronary intervention) occurred during short-term hospital follow-up among 70 patients with normal scans. In a multivariable analysis using clinical and demographic variables, the presence of an abnormal sestamibi scan was the only independent predictor of a cardiac event. These investigators subsequently reported 3-month follow-up data on these patients showing no adverse cardiac events after discharge in patients with a normal ED scan.[28] Tatum and colleagues[26] reported similar data in one of the largest studies, with more than 12 months of follow-up.

The *incremental value* of ED MPI for identifying cardiac events over demographic, clinical, and enzyme data was reported by Heller and colleagues[24] from a multicenter observational study. Adding data from a resting SPECT tetrofosmin ED MPI study significantly enhanced the risk stratification information even after accounting for all of the clinical and enzyme data (Figure 10.3).

These studies, summarized in Table 10.2, provide quite concordant data in that when patient presenting to the ED with suspected ACS have a normal MPI, the risk of adverse cardiac events is very low, in the short-to-mid term. This finding suggests that such patients could be considered for early ED discharge, without the need

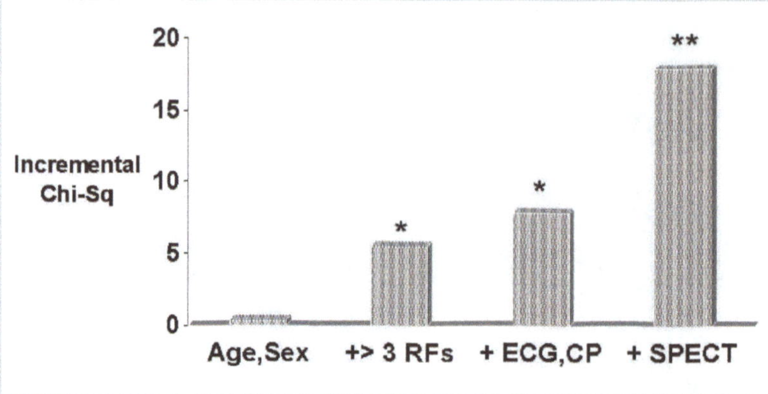

Figure 10.3. Analysis of the incremental value of resting perfusion imaging data to predict cardiac events in ED patients with suspected ischemia. The incremental chi-square value (y-axis) measures the strength of the association between individual factors added to the knowledge base in incremental manner (x-axis) and unfavorable cardiac events. Addition of SPECT perfusion imaging data (SPECT) adds highly statistically significant value even with knowledge of age, sex, risk factors for CAD (RFs), ECG changes, and presence/absence of chest pain (CP). (Adapted from Heller et al, with permission from the American College of Cardiology Foundation.)

for prolonged observation or serial biomarker analysis.

Soman et al.[29] performed a subgroup analysis of the Emergency Room Assessment of Sestamibi for the Evaluation of Chest Pain (ERASE Chest Pain) trial[30] (described below), and showed that in patients who present to the ED with suspected ACS and have a normal rest MPI, follow-up stress testing at a mean of 2 weeks in patients with no ischemic events in the intervening period demonstrated ischemia in 9%. In a stepwise regression model, age and previous CAD were independently predictive of ischemia on follow-up stress testing. Gender, presence of chest pain during tracer injection for the ED scan, presence of symptoms in the ED, and diabetes mellitus were *not* predictive of an abnormal follow-up stress test. Thus, in a small proportion of ED patients with suspected ACS and a negative rest MPI, inducible ischemia is present and may influence long-term prognosis.

4.3 Efficacy Versus Effectiveness: Randomized Trials of ED MPI to Improve Outcomes and Decision-making

It is important to note, however, that the above studies did *not prospectively assess the actual impact of utilizing MPI in the ED setting on the triage decision-making process.* Many tests are reported to have diagnostic or prognostic value in the literature when evaluated by experts, known as the "efficacy" of a test. Whether or not that test translates in real use to favorable effects on decision-making or outcomes - known as "effectiveness" - needs to be addressed by randomized trials.

Table 10.2. Myocardial perfusion imaging for acute chest pain: prognostic data

Study	n	Duration of f/u	Endpoint	Normal scan	Event rate (%) equivocal scan	Abnormal scan
Varetto 1993	64	18 mo	Death, MI, revasc	0	N/A	20
Hilton 1994	102	3 mo	Death, MI, revasc	1.4	13	71
Tatum 1997	1187	12 mo	MI	0	N/A	11
			Death	0		8
Heller 1998	357	In-hospital	AMI	0.9	N/A	12
			Cath	19		33
			CAD	7		23
			Revasc	5		16
Udelson 2002	1215	30 d	MI	0.6	0.8	10.3
			MI, death, revasc	3	6.1	20.5

MI, myocardial infarction; revasc, revascularization; CAD, coronary artery disease.

There have been two reported trials in which patients have been randomly assigned to have imaging or not to have imaging data influence subsequent management. These two randomized studies evaluated the benefit of using this modality on reducing health care costs, length of hospital stay, and for its ability to influence ED physicians' triage decision-making.

Stowers and colleague[31] evaluated 46 patients presenting to the ED with ongoing chest pain and a nondiagnostic ECG, who underwent Tc-99m tetrofosmin imaging before being randomly assigned to a conventional arm (physicians blinded from imaging results) or perfusion imaging-guided arm (imaging results were unblinded to the physician). The study's primary analyses focused on assessing the differences in total in-hospital costs and average lengths of stay between the two study arms. These investigators found that the median hospital costs were $1843 less for patients with the perfusion-guided strategy compared with costs with conventional management. In addition to these cost differences, the conventional arm had a 2.0-day-longer median hospital stay and 1.0-day-longer median intensive care unit stay. This study also demonstrated that physicians provided with imaging results ordered fewer cardiac catheterizations without any difference in outcomes by hospital discharge or by 30 days of follow-up. Thus, although the study population was small, there seems to be a cost benefit and shorter lengths of stay for intermediate-risk chest pain patients admitted from the ED when rest MPI results are made available as part of the diagnostic strategy. Clinicians were provided a suggested management strategy per protocol based on the imaging results; thus, this study did not fully evaluate how physicians would react to the MPI information on their own.

A larger prospective, randomized study, the ERASE Chest Pain trial,[30] evaluated the role of rest MPI on the triage decision made by ED physicians. The investigators enrolled 2475 patients with chest pain or any other symptoms suggestive of acute cardiac ischemia and a normal or nondiagnostic ECG. Patients were randomly assigned to either the usual ED evaluation strategy or the usual strategy supplemented by information from acute resting Tc-99m sestamibi SPECT imaging. Clinicians were given the imaging information, but not specifically directed as to how to use it, beyond initial education about the literature on ED MPI before the start of the study. Thus, this study was the first to truly evaluate how ED clinicians would incorporate MPI information into their decision-making process.

The study found that there were no differences in the ED triage decision between the two arms for those patients with either an AMI or with unstable angina. However, for those patients *without* acute cardiac ischemia, hospitalization was reduced from 52% with usual care to 42% with sestamibi imaging ($P < .001$). In this study, the median time from ED presentation to admission or discharge home was 4.7 hours in the usual care arm and 5.3 hours in the sestamibi imaging arm, thus the imaging added an average of only approximately 30 minutes to the evaluation. On 30-day follow-up, there were no differences in outcomes between the usual care and sestamibi imaging groups. Therefore, this study showed that the incorporation of sestamibi imaging into the triage decision-making provided a clear benefit in reducing unnecessary hospital admissions in patients *without* ischemia, without reducing appropriate admission for patients *with* acute ischemia. All prospectively identified subgroups benefited in terms of reduced unnecessary admissions from SPECT MPI, including those based on gender, age, presence/absence of a formal chest pain unit, and whether or not the site had prior experience with ED MPI.

These two prospective, randomized trials have shown that acute rest SPECT MPI in patients presenting to the ED with low- to intermediate-risk chest pain and nondiagnostic ECGs can significantly improve the overall clinical effectiveness of the ED triage process. Given evidence from two prospective randomized trials as well as numerous observational studies (Tables 10.1 and 10.2), the use of rest SPECT MPI in the ED setting has attained a class I, level A indication in the 2003 ACC/AHA/ASNC Guidelines for the Clinical Use of Cardiac Radionuclide Imaging document,[32] the highest indication based on strong evidence.

4.4 Is Risk Stratification of ED Patients with Chest Pain Using MPI Cost Effective?

Several observational and one randomized study have examined whether the potential reduction of inappropriate hospital admissions will offset the additional cost of an MPI study. Weissman et al.,[33] using a survey method of physicians' decision-making before and then again after being given MPI results, found that 68% of the physicians' decisions were affected by the perfusion imaging results and estimated a potential cost savings of $786 per patient.

Kontos et al.[34] prospectively performed Tc-99m sestamibi rest imaging in ED patients with low-to-moderate probability of ACS and demonstrated significant cost savings, a lower angiography rate, and shorter length of stay compared with a control population retrospectively risk stratified using identical criteria. Knott and colleagues[35] injected Tc-99m sestamibi during chest pain in 120 hospitalized or ED patients and demonstrated, based on physicians' questionnaires inquiring about impact of MPI results on management decisions, a 34% reduction in total admissions and a 59% reduction in planned admissions to the coronary care unit based on the MPI results. Conversely, coronary care management was instituted in 17 patients and discharges canceled in 7, based on abnormal MPI. In a subgroup of patients, coronary angiography was avoided in 40%.

Radensky and colleagues[36] used a decision model comparing a scan strategy versus no-scan strategy and calculated potential cost savings of $796 per patient for patients evaluated by SPECT MPI. In a report by Ziffer et al.[37] of several thousand patients evaluated in a chest pain center, after the incorporation of perfusion imaging into the algorithm, the "missed MI" rate (that is, the proportion of patients sent directly home from the ED but who were actually having an MI) decreased from 1.8% to 0.1%, and unnecessary hospital admissions were also reduced. These investigators estimated savings (charges) of approximately $1900 per patient.

The prospective, randomized study by Stowers et al.[31] assessed differences in hospital cost between a conventional and perfusion imaging-guided strategy. They found that the median hospital costs per patient were $1843 lower in the perfusion imaging-guided arm compared with the conventional arm. Heller and coworkers[24] estimated savings in a similar range. In contrast, an observational study by Kosnik and colleagues[38] evaluated 69 patients already being admitted to the hospital and estimated that the use of sestamibi imaging would hypothetically lead to more appropriate triage in 42% of patients but at an additional cost of $307 per patient.

Overall, the majority of studies, including the only prospective, randomized study, point to a potential cost savings by incorporating the routine use of acute rest MPI in patients with low- to moderate-risk chest pain and nondiagnostic ECGs. When this saving is extrapolated to the 5–7 million patients who present yearly to EDs with chest pain, the yearly potential cost savings for this group would be substantial.

4.5 Other Considerations: Presence or Absence of Symptoms

In a substantial proportion of patients presenting to the ED with suspected ACS, symptoms would have begun to resolve by the time the initial assessment has been completed and decisions regarding further testing made. In the study by Wackers et al., the sensitivity for detecting ischemia diminished as time increased beyond 6 hours from the onset of symptoms. Bilodeau and colleagues[9] found perfusion abnormalities in 65% of patients injected more than 4 hours after the episode of chest pain. Similarly, Varetto et al.[23] reported that the diagnostic sensitivity of MPI was maintained when Tc-99m sestamibi injection was delayed for up to 3–4 hours after symptom resolution. In a subgroup analysis of the ERASE Chest Pain trial, Hendel et al.[39] found no association between the presence or absence (<3 hours after resolution) of chest pain during Tc-99m sestamibi injection and the prognostic value of normal MPI, or influence on triage decisions.

Experimental support for the concept that perfusion images may remain abnormal for a substantial period of time after resolution of ischemia comes from a study of patients undergoing percutaneous coronary intervention as a model of "supply" type ischemia consistent with what occurs in ACS. Fram and coworkers[19] studied patients undergoing coronary angioplasty and demonstrated perfusion defects in all patients injected with Tc-99m sestamibi during balloon inflation and in 70%, 37%, and 19% of patients reinjected 15 minutes, 1–3 hours, and 24 hours after balloon deflation, respectively.

Therefore, the available data that address this issue seem to suggest that, after an episode of transient myocardial ischemia, perfusion abnormalities may persist for several hours after symptom resolution. Nevertheless, for practical purposes of ED triaging, tracer injection should be performed as early after the patient presents as possible, and it must be borne in mind that the sensitivity of the technique tends to diminish with time after symptom resolution.

4.6 Dealing with Imaging Artifacts

Attempts to distinguish true perfusion defects from artifacts have included the use of attenuation correction and prone imaging. Unlike stress-rest imaging in which preserved regional function on ECG-gated SPECT imaging may be used to differentiate true fixed perfusion defects from artifacts, gating may be less useful for this purpose in the ED setting where abnormalities of regional function associated with transient ischemia may have resolved by the time of image acquisition. Hendel and colleagues[40] examined the ERASE Chest Pain trial database in which some centers routinely used attenuation correction and gated SPECT imaging. In 319 patients, the use of both attenuation correction and gating reduced the number of equivocal scans and increased reader confidence in interpretation. Segmental scores were more normal in patients ultimately found to not have an acute ischemic syndrome, by both methods. However, attenuation correction slightly reduced the scores of patients with an acute ischemic syndrome (inappropriately). From these data, it seems that either method has the potential to be useful, although gating perhaps more so. The comparative usefulness of these modalities will need to be reevaluated as attenuation correction techniques continue to evolve.

Prone imaging can also be used to assist in the determination of the presence or absence of a true abnormality in the inferior wall, discriminating from diaphragmatic attenuation.[26,41] Although this has not been systematically studied in the ED setting, the experience in our laboratory has been that in selected situations prone imaging may be quite effective in this regard (Figure 10.4; see color section).

Given this problem of differentiating artifact from real defects in some patients, it is important to remember that the goal of perfusion scintigraphy in the ED setting is the *optimal identification of patients with acute cardiac ischemia*. Therefore, when a study appears to be equivocal, one should err on the side of interpreting it as abnormal so as to obtain a high sensitivity for the detection of cardiac ischemia. In the study by Hilton and colleagues,[27] which reported the prognostic significance of resting perfusion imaging in ED patients with typical angina and a nondiagnostic ECG, patients with studies interpreted as equivocal had a prognosis that was *intermediate* between patients with a normal scan and those with an abnormal scan. Whereas patients with a normal scan had an

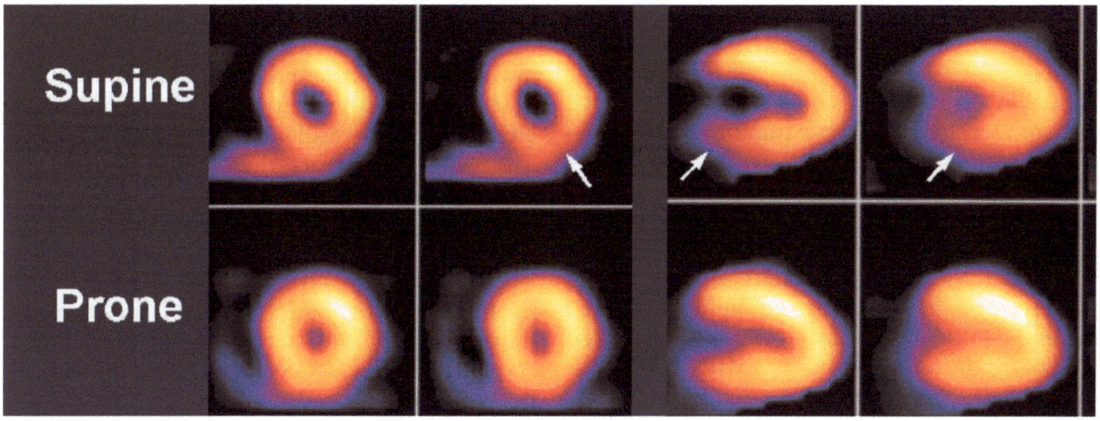

Figure 10.4. In a patient who presented to the ED with symptoms suspicious for ischemia but a nondiagnostic ECG, initial resting Tc-99m sestamibi imaging (top row, supine) demonstrated a possible inferobasal defect (arrow), consistent with either acute ischemia in that territory or diaphragmatic attenuation artifact. Prone imaging (bottom row) was performed, and inferobasal perfusion appeared normal, suggesting that the initial study represented diaphragmatic attenuation artifact and not ischemia.

extremely low (1 event in 70) rate of cardiac events defined as predischarge cardiac death, nonfatal MI, or the need for immediate coronary intervention, patients with an equivocal or abnormal scan had higher event rates of 13% and 71%, respectively. In the ERASE Chest Pain trial, whereas the risk of AMI was 0.6%, 0.8%, and 10.3% for normal, equivocal, and abnormal Tc-99m sestamibi rest scans, respectively, the risk of the combined endpoint of AMI, death, or revascularization was 3%, 6.1%, and 20.5%, respectively. Given these results, interpretation of perfusion images in this setting should be "aggressive," in order to optimize sensitivity for detecting acute ischemia.

4.7 Comparison of the Utility of MPI, Biomarkers, and Serum Markers of Inflammation in the ED

The serial measurement cardiac specific markers in the blood has emerged as a valuable clinical tool for the diagnosis of ACS and risk stratification of patients presenting to the ED with chest pain. The cardiac specific troponins T and I are extremely sensitive indicators of minute amounts of myocardial necrosis, and also elevated in 20% to 30% of patients with a clinical syndrome consistent with unstable angina. In the latter group, they predict an adverse prognosis and benefit from glycoprotein IIbIIIA inhibitors. However, analysis of biomarkers has two inherent disadvantages when used in the ED setting: the need for serial sampling to obtain maximum sensitivity, and the fact that when significant myocardial ischemia occurs without necrosis, it remains undetected by this technique.

Several studies have compared the utility of MPI and serial biomarker estimation in the evaluation of chest pain patients in the ED. Kontos et al.[42] studied 620 such patients and found a 92% sensitivity of early rest MPI for detecting acute MI. Whereas serial troponin I estimations over 24 hours provided similar sensitivity, the *initial* troponin value, drawn at an approximately similar time point as isotope injection, was poorly sensitive (39% for MI). These data demonstrate that a major potential advantage of MPI is that of *early* diagnosis in the ED, as biomarkers take time to achieve maximum sensitivity, whereas MPI is abnormal as soon as a flow abnormality is present.

Swinburn and colleagues[43] studied 80 patients within 6 hours of chest pain onset using rest gated Tc-99m sestamibi imaging and serial troponin T and I estimation. MI was the presenting event in 13 patients (16%), and 23 (34%) of those without index MI sustained a cardiovascular event during follow-up. MIBI, troponins T and I, and the ECG had similar negative predictive values for the index MI (97%, 97%, 95%, and 97%, respectively). However, only MIBI had a high negative predictive value (86%) for the prediction of subsequent events during follow-up (Figure 10.5). Of note, these authors found no utility for the inflammatory markers C-reactive protein, interleukin-6, and tumor necrosis factor-α in this setting. Duca et al., in a similar study, showed 100% sensitivity of rest Tc-99m sestamibi/tetrofosmin MPI for the diagnosis of AMI and, as with the other studies, the *initial* troponin values had low sensitivity for the same endpoint.

Following the recent recommendation by the American College of Cardiology/European Society of Cardiology joint committee for a renewed definition of AMI based on detectable troponin levels, Kontos et al.[44] examined the sensitivity of rest Tc-99m sestamibi imaging for identifying patients with elevated troponin I among those presenting to the ED with suspected ACS. Of 319 such patients who eventually demonstrated an elevation in troponin I, 76% had a positive MPI, defined as a discrete perfusion abnormality with a matched abnormality in regional function. In the subgroup of patients who underwent coronary arteriography, 32% with elevated troponin I and a negative MPI had significant CAD. However, patients with positive MPI had greater elevations in CPK-MB, and lower ejection fractions. The authors speculate that patients with negative MPIs have only small amounts of myocardial damage because at least 3%–5% of the myocardium must be ischemic before the MPI becomes positive.[45] The ultimate test of this hypothesis would be follow-up prognostic data, which was not a focus of this report.

Recent studies have also examined the diagnostic and prognostic utility of other serum markers of inflammation including CD40 ligand, myeloperoxidase, and placental growth factor in patients presenting to the ED with suspected ACS, and suggest a promising role for these markers for prognostication especially in patients who are troponin negative.[46–49] However, comparative studies with MPI and echocardiog-

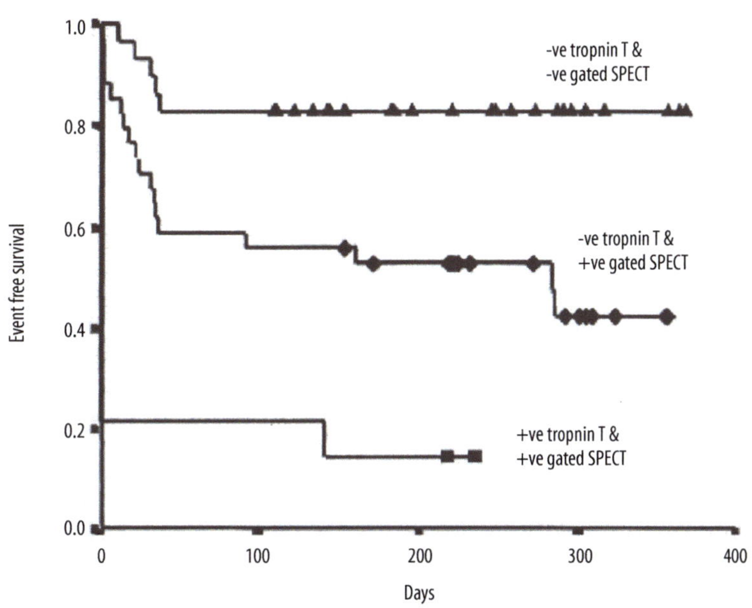

Figure 10.5. First event-free survival curves in 80 ED chest pain patients demonstrating the increased risk associated with an abnormal gated SPECT scan and/or increased troponin T on serial estimation. All troponin-positive patients had abnormal gated SPECT scans. Whereas both gated SPECT and troponin had a high negative predictive value for MI at presentation, only a normal gated SPECT had a high negative predictive value for subsequent adverse events. (Adapted from Swinburn et al.[43])

raphy have not been performed, and routine use of these markers beyond the research setting is not currently available.

5. Echocardiography

The occurrence of regional wall motion abnormalities (RWMA) in the ischemic bed within seconds of coronary occlusion has been known since Tennant and Wiggers' initial observation in 1935.[50] In the ischemic cascade, RWMA quickly succeeds flow heterogeneity and occurs before ECG changes and symptoms,[17] making its assessment a sensitive and specific indicator of myocardial ischemia. In addition, the portability, universal availability, and range of information provided make echocardiography attractive for use in the ED setting. A few studies have examined the utility of bedside echocardiography in the ED for the assessment of patients with suspected ACS. In a small study, Peels et al.[51] found echocardiography to be highly sensitive for the detection of AMI as well as acute ischemia in the ED setting (92% and 88%, respectively). However, this high sensitivity was importantly dependent on the presence of symptoms *during the echocardiographic study*. The specificity of this approach was limited, at 53% and 78% for infarction and ischemia, respectively. Sasaki et al.[52] demonstrated similar results, in that the sensitivity of this technique was low in the absence of ongoing symptoms. In another study, Sabia and coworkers[53] reported a sensitivity of 93% for echocardiographically detected RWMA to correctly identify acute ischemic heart disease presenting as AMI. These investigators estimated that the use of echocardiography in the ED could result in a 32% reduction in hospital admissions, although this procedure was not demonstrated to do so in a prospective manner. This study again demonstrated a modest specificity (57%) and was also limited by the requirement of ongoing symptoms at the time of study, as well as the lack of wall motion abnormalities in a small subset of patients ultimately diagnosed as having non-Q wave infarction. Other investigators have also observed these false-negative findings,[54,55] which may be attributed to the fact that RWMA occur only when the infarct involves greater than 20% of the transmural thickness of the myocardium and 12% of the left ventricular circumference.[56,57]

In a more contemporary study, Kontos et al.[58] showed a high negative predictive value of a normal echocardiogram in patients with chest pain, which correlated with a benign prognosis at 10 months. Trippi and colleagues[59] have demonstrated the possible role of dobutamine stress tele-echocardiography for the evaluation of ED patients with chest pain, reporting a sensitivity of 90% and a specificity of 89%. This technology, however, is not currently in widespread use.

Thus, although these studies demonstrated the feasibility of using echocardiography in the ED setting, they were concordant in demonstrating that optimal sensitivity for this approach seems to require ongoing symptoms during the study. In addition, in previous studies, 7%–23% of patients had to be excluded for suboptimal images,[54,58] although these studies did not use contemporary modalities such as harmonic imaging or contrast echocardiography (the latter can also be used to assess microvascular function post-thrombolysis or percutaneous coronary intervention) to enhance endocardial visualization. No study has evaluated the actual impact of the use of echocardiography on triage from the ED, and the body of literature pertaining to the use of echocardiography for the evaluation of chest pain in the ED is smaller than the analogous data available for radionuclide MPI.

5.1 Prognostic Utility of ED Echocardiography and Comparison with Biomarkers

Swinburn and colleagues compared ED echocardiography using tissue harmonic imaging and serial estimation of troponins T and I in 80 patients presenting with non-ST-segment elevation chest pain. Twelve patients had an MI as the presenting event; 29 had adverse cardiac events during follow-up for a mean of 224 days. Echocardiography (97%), troponin I (97%), and troponin T (98%) all had similar negative predictive values for excluding an MI as the presenting event. Echocardiography was not independently predictive of MI as the presenting event, but was the only independent predictor of subsequent adverse cardiac events. In an earlier study of 100 similar patients, Mohler and colleagues[60] demonstrated that a combination of admission troponin T and echocardiography yielded a positive predictive value of 84% and a negative predictive value of 90% for future adverse cardiac events.

6. Future Directions

A potential future approach to risk stratification in ED patients is the use of fatty acid metabolism in the aftermath of acute ischemic symptoms to image "ischemic memory." After an ischemic insult, fatty acid metabolism may be abnormal for a prolonged time period (possibly days), far beyond the time when flow returns to normal and signs and symptoms of regional ischemia have resolved. Thus, there is potential for imaging the ongoing abnormality in fatty acid metabolism as a signal of "ischemic memory."

A radiolabeled iodinated fatty acid analog, 15-(p-[iodine-123] iodophenyl)-3-(R,S) methylpentadecanoic acid (BMIPP) has been used to assess fatty acid utilization in the myocardium. This has been studied by Kawai and colleagues,[61] who reported data on 111 patients presenting with symptoms of ACS but no MI. BMIPP SPECT imaging, performed 1–5 days after presentation, was more sensitive than rest perfusion imaging (performed within 24 hours of presentation) in identifying the presence and site of the culprit coronary stenosis or spasm (74 versus 38% respectively, $P < .05$) at similar high specificity. Preliminary data from development of this agent in the US also supports this concept.[62] Further studies will evaluate the use of BMIPP imaging in this setting, which would be particularly attractive for patients whose ischemic insult may have occurred hours before their presentation to the ED.

7. Conclusions

The assessment and triage of ED patients with suspected ACS is a process that requires considerations of clinical risk, patient safety, and cost-effectiveness. The strategies used should be highly sensitive to minimize the chances of missing the diagnosis of ACS. The noninvasive modalities of MPI and echocardiography have suitable characteristics. Data on MPI predominate in the literature, with prospective, randomized studies demonstrating applicability, safety, and cost-effectiveness, such that ED MPI for evaluation of suspected ACS has attained a class I, level A indication in the US. In the future, imaging of ischemic memory using fatty acid analogs such as BMIPP may further enhance the utility of radionuclide imaging in this setting.

References

1. Selker HP, Zalenski RJ, Antman EM, et al. An evaluation of technologies for identifying acute cardiac ischemia in the emergency department: executive summary of a National Heart Attack Alert Program Working Group Report. Ann Emerg Med 1997;29:1–12.
2. Pozen MW, D'Agostino RB, Selker HP, Sytkowski PA, Hood WBJ. A predictive instrument to improve coronary-care-unit admission practices in acute ischemic heart disease. A prospective multicenter clinical trial. N Engl J Med 1984;310:1273–1278.
3. Lee TH, Cook EF, Weisberg M, Sargent RK, Wilson C, Goldman L. Acute chest pain in the emergency room. Identification and examination of low-risk patients. Arch Intern Med 1985;145:65–69.
4. Short D. The earliest electrocardiographic evidence of myocardial infarction. Br Heart J 1970;32:6–15.
5. Fineberg HV, Scadden D, Goldman L. Care of patients with a low probability of acute myocardial infarction. Cost effectiveness of alternatives to coronary-care-unit admission. N Engl J Med 1984;310:1301–1307.
6. Lee TH, Rouan GW, Weisberg MC, et al. Clinical characteristics and natural history of patients with acute myocardial infarction sent home from the emergency room. Am J Cardiol 1987;60:219–224.
7. Pope JH, Aufderheide TP, Ruthazer R, et al. Missed diagnoses of acute cardiac ischemia in the emergency department. N Engl J Med 2000;342:1163–1170.
8. Schor S, Behar S, Modan B, Barell V, Drory J, Kariv I. Disposition of presumed coronary patients from an emergency room. A follow-up study. JAMA 1976;236: 941–943.
9. Bilodeau L, Theroux P, Gregoire J, Gagnon D, Arsenault A. Technetium-99m sestamibi tomography in patients with spontaneous chest pain: correlations with clinical, electrocardiographic and angiographic findings. J Am Coll Cardiol 1991;18:1684–1691.
10. McGuinness JB, Begg TB, Semple T. First electrocardiogram in recent myocardial infarction. Br Med J 1976;2:449–451.
11. Lee TH, Rouan GW, Weisberg MC, et al. Sensitivity of routine clinical criteria for diagnosing myocardial infarction within 24 hours of hospitalization. Ann Intern Med 1987;106:181–186.
12. Goldman L, Weinberg M, Weisberg M, et al. A computer-derived protocol to aid in the diagnosis of emergency room patients with acute chest pain. N Engl J Med 1982; 307:588–596.
13. Behar S, Schor S, Kariv I, Barell V, Modan B. Evaluation of electrocardiogram in emergency room as a decision-making tool. Chest 1977;71:486–491.
14. Goldman L, Cook EF, Brand DA, et al. A computer protocol to predict myocardial infarction in emergency department patients with chest pain. N Engl J Med 1988;318:797–803.
15. Rude RE, Poole WK, Muller JE, et al. Electrocardiographic and clinical criteria for recognition of acute myocardial infarction based on analysis of 3,697 patients. Am J Cardiol 1983;52:936–942.
16. Tierney WM, Roth BJ, Psaty B, et al. Predictors of myocardial infarction in emergency room patients. Crit Care Med 1985;13:526–531.
17. Nesto RW, Kowalchuk GJ. The ischemic cascade: temporal sequence of hemodynamic, electrocardiographic and symptomatic expressions of ischemia. Am J Cardiol 1987;59:23C–30C.
18. Kerber RE, Marcus ML, Ehrhardt J, Wilson R, Abboud FM. Correlation between echocardiographically demonstrated segmental dyskinesis and regional myocardial perfusion. Circulation 1975;52:1097–1104.
19. Fram DB, Azar RR, Ahlberg AW, et al. Duration of abnormal SPECT myocardial perfusion imaging following resolution of acute ischemia: an angioplasty model. J Am Coll Cardiol 2003;41:452–459.
20. Wackers FJ, Sokole EB, Samson G, et al. Value and limitations of thallium-201 scintigraphy in the acute phase of myocardial infarction. N Engl J Med 1976;295:1–5.
21. Wackers FJ, Lie KI, Liem KL, et al. Thallium-201 scintigraphy in unstable angina pectoris. Circulation 1978;57:738–742.
22. Christian TF, Clements IP, Gibbons RJ. Noninvasive identification of myocardium at risk in patients with acute myocardial infarction and nondiagnostic electrocardiograms with technetium-99m-sestamibi. Circulation 1991;83:1615–1620.
23. Varetto T, Cantalupi D, Altieri A, Orlandi C. Emergency room technetium-99m sestamibi imaging to rule out acute myocardial ischemic events in patients with nondiagnostic electrocardiograms. J Am Coll Cardiol 1993; 22:1804–1808.
24. Heller GV, Stowers SA, Hendel RC, et al. Clinical value of acute rest technetium-99m tetrofosmin tomographic myocardial perfusion imaging in patients with acute chest pain and nondiagnostic electrocardiograms. J Am Coll Cardiol 1998;31:1011–1017.
25. Kosnik JW, Zalenski RJ, Shamsa F, et al. Resting sestamibi imaging for the prognosis of low-risk chest pain. Acad Emerg Med 1999;6:998–1004.
26. Tatum JL, Jesse RL, Kontos MC, et al. Comprehensive strategy for the evaluation and triage of the chest pain patient. Ann Emerg Med 1997;29:116–125.
27. Hilton TC, Thompson RC, Williams HJ, Saylors R, Fulmer H, Stowers SA. Technetium-99m sestamibi myocardial perfusion imaging in the emergency room evaluation of chest pain. J Am Coll Cardiol 1994; 23:1016–1022.
28. Hilton TC, Fulmer H, Abuan T, Thompson RC, Stowers SA. Ninety-day follow-up of patients in the emergency department with chest pain who undergo initial single-photon emission computed tomographic perfusion scintigraphy with technetium 99m-labeled sestamibi. J Nucl Cardiol 1996;3:308–311.
29. Soman P, Beshansky JR, Ruthazer R, et al. Is there value in follow-up stress testing for emergency department patients with chest pain and normal rest SPECT myocardial perfusion? [abstract] J Am Coll Cardiol 2004;43:232A.
30. Udelson JE, Beshansky JR, Ballin DS, et al. Myocardial perfusion imaging for evaluation and triage of patients with suspected acute cardiac ischemia: a randomized controlled trial. JAMA 2002;288:2693–2700.
31. Stowers SA, Eisenstein EL, Wackers FJ, et al. An economic analysis of an aggressive diagnostic strategy with single photon emission computed tomography myocardial perfusion imaging and early exercise stress testing in emergency department patients who present with chest pain but nondiagnostic electrocardiograms: results from a randomized trial. Ann Emerg Med 2000;35:17–25.

32. Klocke FJ, Baird MG, Lorell BH, et al. ACC/AHA/ASNC guidelines for the clinical use of cardiac radionuclide imaging – executive summary: a report of the American College of Cardiology/American Heart Association Task Force on Practice Guidelines (ACC/AHA/ASNC Committee to Revise the 1995 Guidelines for the Clinical Use of Cardiac Radionuclide Imaging). Circulation 2003;108:1404–1418.
33. Weissman IA, Dickinson CZ, Dworkin HJ, O'Neill WW, Juni JE. Cost-effectiveness of myocardial perfusion imaging with SPECT in the emergency department evaluation of patients with unexplained chest pain. Radiology 1996;199:353–357.
34. Kontos MC, Schmidt KL, McCue M, et al. A comprehensive strategy for the evaluation and triage of the chest pain patient: a cost comparison study. J Nucl Cardiol 2003;10:284–290.
35. Knott JC, Baldey AC, Grigg LE, Cameron PA, Lichtenstein M, Better N. Impact of acute chest pain Tc-99m sestamibi myocardial perfusion imaging on clinical management. J Nucl Cardiol 2002;9:257–262.
36. Radensky PW, Hilton TC, Fulmer H, McLaughlin BA, Stowers SA. Potential cost effectiveness of initial myocardial perfusion imaging for assessment of emergency department patients with chest pain. Am J Cardiol 1997;79:595–599.
37. Ziffer ZA, Nateman DR, Janowitz WR, Williams K, Shaw L. Improved patient outcomes and cost effectiveness of utilizing nuclear cardiology protocols in an emergency department chest pain center: two year results in 6548 patients [abstract]. J Nucl Med 1998;39:139P.
38. Kosnik JW, Zalenski RJ, Grzybowski M, Huang R, Sweeny PJ, Welch RD. Impact of technetium-99m sestamibi imaging on the emergency department management and costs in the evaluation of low-risk chest pain. Acad Emerg Med 2001;8:315–323.
39. Hendel RC, Udelson JE, Ruthazer R, et al. Does the absence of active chest pain at the time of Tc-99m sestamibi injection affect the value of rest Tc-99m sestamibi imaging for emergency department patients with acute chest pain? [abstract] Circulation 2000; 102:II-543.
40. Hendel RC, Selker HP, Heller GV, et al. The impact of attenuation correction and gating on SPECT perfusion imaging in patients presenting to the emergency department with chest pain [abstract]. Circulation 2000;102:II-543.
41. Kiat H, Van T, Friedman JD, et al. Quantitative stress-redistribution thallium-201 SPECT using prone imaging: methodologic development and validation. J Nucl Med 1992;33:1509–1515.
42. Kontos MC, Jesse RL, Anderson FP, Schmidt KL, Ornato JP, Tatum JL. Comparison of myocardial perfusion imaging and cardiac troponin I in patients admitted to the emergency department with chest pain. Circulation 1999;99:2073–2078.
43. Swinburn JM, Stubbs P, Soman P, et al. Rapid assessment of patients with non-ST-segment elevation acute chest pain: troponins, inflammatory markers, or perfusion imaging? J Nucl Cardiol 2002;9:491–499.
44. Kontos MC, Shah R, Fritz LM, et al. Implication of different cardiac troponin I levels for clinical outcomes and prognosis of acute chest pain patients. J Am Coll Cardiol 2004;43:958–965.
45. Verani MS, Jeroudi MO, Mahmarian JJ, et al. Quantification of myocardial infarction during coronary occlusion and myocardial salvage after reperfusion using cardiac imaging with technetium-99m hexakis 2-methoxyisobutyl isonitrile. J Am Coll Cardiol 1988; 12:1573–1581.
46. Aukrust P, Muller F, Ueland T, et al. Enhanced levels of soluble and membrane-bound CD40 ligand in patients with unstable angina. Possible reflection of T lymphocyte and platelet involvement in the pathogenesis of acute coronary syndromes. Circulation 1999;100:614–620.
47. Heeschen C, Dimmeler S, Hamm CW, et al., for the CAPTURE Study Investigators. Soluble CD40 ligand in acute coronary syndromes. N Engl J Med 2003;348: 1104–1111.
48. Baldus S, Heeschen C, Meinertz T, et al., CAPTURE Investigators. Myeloperoxidase serum levels predict risk in patients with acute coronary syndromes. Circulation 2003;108:1440–1445.
49. Heeschen C, Dimmeler S, Fichtlsherer S, et al., for the CAPTURE Investigators. Prognostic value of placental growth factor in patients with acute chest pain. JAMA 2004;291:435–441.
50. Tennant R, Wiggers CJ. The effect of coronary occlusion on myocardial contractions. Am J Physiol 1935;112: 351.
51. Peels CH, Visser CA, Kupper AJ, Visser FC, Roos JP. Usefulness of two-dimensional echocardiography for immediate detection of myocardial ischemia in the emergency room. Am J Cardiol 1990;65:687–691.
52. Sasaki H, Charuzi Y, Beeder C, Sugiki Y, Lew AS. Utility of echocardiography for the early assessment of patients with nondiagnostic chest pain. Am Heart J 1986;112:494–497.
53. Sabia P, Afrookteh A, Touchstone DA, Keller MW, Esquivel L, Kaul S. Value of regional wall motion abnormality in the emergency room diagnosis of acute myocardial infarction. A prospective study using two-dimensional echocardiography. Circulation 1991; 84:I85–I92.
54. Loh IK, Charuzi Y, Beeder C, Marshall LA, Ginsburg JH. Early diagnosis of nontransmural myocardial infarction by two-dimensional echocardiography. Am Heart J 1982;104:963–968.
55. Horowitz RS, Morganroth J, Parrotto C, Chen CC, Soffer J, Pauletto FJ. Immediate diagnosis of acute myocardial infarction by two-dimensional echocardiography. Circulation 1982;65:323–329.
56. Lieberman AN, Weiss JL, Jugdutt BI, et al. Two-dimensional echocardiography and infarct size: relationship of regional wall motion and thickening to the extent of myocardial infarction in the dog. Circulation 1981;63:739–746.
57. Kaul S, Pandian NG, Gillam LD, Newell JB, Okada RD, Weyman AE. Contrast echocardiography in acute myocardial ischemia. III. An in vivo comparison of the extent of abnormal wall motion with the area at risk for necrosis. J Am Coll Cardiol 1986;7:383–392.
58. Kontos MC, Arrowood JA, Paulsen WH, Nixon JV. Early echocardiography can predict cardiac events in emergency department patients with chest pain. Ann Emerg Med 1998;31:550–557.
59. Trippi JA, Lee KS, Kopp G, Nelson DR, Yee KG, Cordell WH. Dobutamine stress tele-echocardiography for evaluation of emergency department patients with chest pain. J Am Coll Cardiol 1997;30: 627–632.

60. Mohler ER, Ryan T, Segar DS, et al. Clinical utility of troponin T levels and echocardiography in the emergency department. Am Heart J 1998;135:253–260.
61. Kawai Y, Tsukamoto E, Nozaki Y, Morita K, Sakurai M, Tamaki N. Significance of reduced uptake of iodinated fatty acid analogue for the evaluation of patients with acute chest pain. J Am Coll Cardiol 2001;38:1888–1894.
62. Udelson JE, Bateman TM, Bergmann SR, et al. Proof of principle study of beta-methyl-p-[1231]-iodophenyl-pentadecanoic acid (BMIPP) for ischemic memory following demand ischemia [abstract]. Circulation 2003;108:IV-405.

11

Risk Stratification after Acute Coronary Syndromes

George A. Beller

The major determinants of prognosis after acute coronary syndromes (ACSs) are the degree of left ventricular (LV) dysfunction, the extent of residual jeopardized myocardium, particularly in the setting of multivessel coronary artery disease (CAD), and the manifestation of nonsustained ventricular tachycardia. Certain high-risk clinical variables have been identified that are associated with an increased risk of subsequent cardiac death or reinfarction after hospitalization with an acute myocardial infarction (MI). They include age ≥70 years, prior MI, anterior MI, congestive heart failure during admission, hypotension and sinus tachycardia in the early phase of hospitalization, female gender, diabetes, ineligibility for early exercise testing, postinfarction angina, or history of previous coronary artery bypass graft surgery.

Noninvasive imaging, at rest and/or during exercise or pharmacologic stress, provides additional useful information in the risk stratification process in stable patients who have survived the acute phase of hospitalization for an ACS.[1] Certainly, patients who are seen in the early hours of an acute ST-segment elevation (STEMI) should undergo reperfusion strategies as rapidly as possible. Pooled data from the literature suggest that primary percutaneous coronary intervention (PCI) offers enhanced survival over thrombolytic therapy in patients presenting with symptoms and signs of an STEMI, especially within the first 6 hours after onset of symptoms.[2] With coronary angiography for primary PCI, the overall extent of underlying CAD can be ascertained. Additionally, LV function can be accurately measured by ventriculography. With successful reperfusion and absence of the no-reflow phenomenon, LV function will improve over time when the period of postischemic stunning is resolved.

In this chapter, the role of noninvasive imaging for detection of residual jeopardized myocardium in intermediate- or low-risk patients will be discussed. Even in high-risk patients who have undergone early invasive strategies, resting imaging with either radionuclide agents, echocardiography, or cardiac magnetic resonance (CMR) imaging can be used to evaluate the extent of myocardial viability and infarct size. Patients with a severe reduction in viability and an extensive zone of myocardial necrosis will have a higher probability of developing LV remodeling, a higher probability of heart failure, and a higher risk of cardiac death, compared with patients who have preserved viability after reperfusion of the infarct zone.[3] Stress imaging may be useful in patients who have undergone early coronary angiography for the purposes of reperfusion to evaluate the functional significance of intermediate remote coronary artery stenoses. Patients with multivessel disease and an acute STEMI should not undergo multivessel PCI at the time of primary PCI. Only the infarct vessel should be opened, with subsequent revascularization performed if the noninfarct stenotic lesions are ischemia producing. This can be easily determined by low-level exercise or pharmacologic stress imaging with any of the noninvasive modalities previously cited.

Table 11.1. High-risk myocardial perfusion imaging variables in patients undergoing stress imaging after acute myocardial infarction

1) Reversible defects within the zone of infarction.
2) A multivessel disease scan pattern.
3) A large nonreversible defect indicative of a large infarct size or cumulative zone of nonviability (new and old infarction).
4) Transient left ventricular cavity dilation from stress to rest imaging.
5) Multiple regional wall motion or systolic thickening abnormalities on the poststress images.
6) A resting ejection fraction of <40% on gated single photon emission computed tomography.

1. Radionuclide Techniques for Detecting Ischemia in High-risk Patients after Uncomplicated ACSs

Stress radionuclide myocardial perfusion imaging (MPI) may be clinically useful in the evaluation of patients who have survived an acute MI in that myocardial ischemia within and/or remote from the infarct zone identifies patients with an increased risk of cardiac events.[1] This application for risk assessment can be undertaken with either exercise or pharmacologic stress. High-risk MPI variables in patients undergoing stress imaging after acute MI are listed in Table 11.1.

1.1 Exercise MPI

A pooled analysis performed by Shaw et al.[4] combining studies relevant to exercise stress MPI after MI showed the mortality rate to be 7.1% of patients with a stress-induced reversible defect compared with 1.6% in those without a reversible defect. Similarly, patients with multiple defects in more than one coronary supply region had a 16.7% combined death or MI rate, compared with a 2% event rate in patients without a multivessel disease scan pattern.

Gibson et al.,[5] using submaximal exercise thallium-201 (^{201}Tl) planar scintigraphy performed before hospital discharge, demonstrated that approximately 50% of patients with an uncomplicated STEMI or non-STEMI who had a high-risk scan experienced either subsequent cardiac death, nonfatal infarction, or rehospitalization for class III–IV angina. In contrast, the event rate was only 6% in patients with a low-risk scan reflected by a nonreversible defect confined solely to the infarct zone. In that study, perfusion scan variables separated high- and low-risk subgroups better than did the exercise electrocardiographic (ECG) stress test variables. In fact, scintigraphic variables separated low- and high-risk patients better than did exercise ECG stress test or coronary angiographic variables (Figure 11.1). In the Veterans Affairs Non–Q-Wave

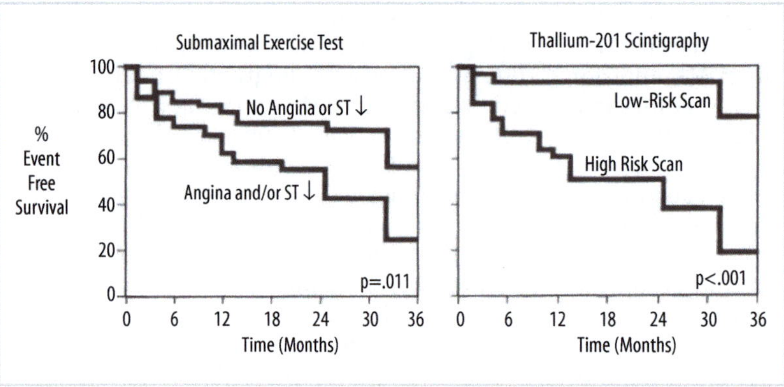

Figure 11.1. Survival free of cardiac death, nonfatal infarction, or hospitalization for unstable angina in post-myocardial infarction patients who underwent submaximal exercise electrocardiographic stress testing and thallium-201 scintigraphy. Note that the low-risk patient was better identified by thallium-201 scintigraphic variables. Patients without angina or inducible ST-segment depression had a significantly worse event-free survival than patients whose thallium scan did not show defect reversibility, a multivessel disease scan pattern, or increased lung thallium-201 uptake. (Adapted from Gibson et al.[5] with permission.)

Infarction Strategies in Hospital (VANQWISH) trial,[6] 36% of patients in the conservative group had reversible thallium defects on stress planar imaging without ST-segment changes, whereas only 8% had ST-segment changes without reversible ^{201}Tl defects.

A pooled analysis by Shaw et al.[4] demonstrated that exercise ECG testing alone identified fewer high-risk patients than did exercise MPI. The cardiac death or MI rate was 15.7% during follow-up in patients demonstrating ischemic ST-segment depression on the exercise ECG stress tests, compared with a 9.9% event rate in patients with no inducible ST-segment depression. This 9.9% event rate in the low-risk group was considerably higher than the 5.1% event rate in patients without reversible perfusion abnormalities compared with the 2% event rate in patients without multiple defects.

Exercise MPI performed with ^{201}Tl single photon emission computed tomography (SPECT) in patients who received thrombolytic therapy also has proven to be of significant incremental prognostic value.[7] In that study, coronary angiography did not further improve the model that comprised clinical, ejection fraction (EF), and ^{201}Tl SPECT variables (Figure 11.2). Patients with defects of <20% of the left ventricle had a low subsequent cardiac event rate, and the separation of high- and low-risk subgroups using this cutoff was comparable to that achieved with coronary angiography in which patients with single-vessel disease were identified as a low-risk group and those with multivessel disease were designated as the high-risk group.

Exercise technetium-99m (^{99m}Tc)-sestamibi SPECT has now emerged as an effective alternative to ^{201}Tl stress scintigraphy for risk stratification after MI. Not only is image quality superior with the ^{99m}Tc-labeled radiopharmaceutical agents for perfusion imaging, but the ease of gating the images permits the assessment of regional and global LV function. Thus, the variable of EF, which is such a powerful predictor of outcome, can be quantified at one noninvasive study. Similarly, poststress regional thickening abnormalities enhances the detection of multivessel disease and provides incremental value for identifying three-vessel disease compared with the assessment of perfusion imaging variables alone.[8]

Travin et al.[9] reported that the presence of either ischemia seen on ^{99m}Tc-sestamibi SPECT images or defects seen in multiple coronary supply regions, identified 92% of patients who subsequently experienced an event after hospital discharge. Cox regression analysis of clinical, ECG stress tests, and imaging variables showed that the number of ischemic defects on ^{99m}Tc-sestamibi scans was the only significant correlate of future events. Patients with more than three ^{99m}Tc-sestamibi reversible defects had an event rate of 38% in that study (Figure 11.3).

The EF performed at the time of gated SPECT was shown to provide significant independent

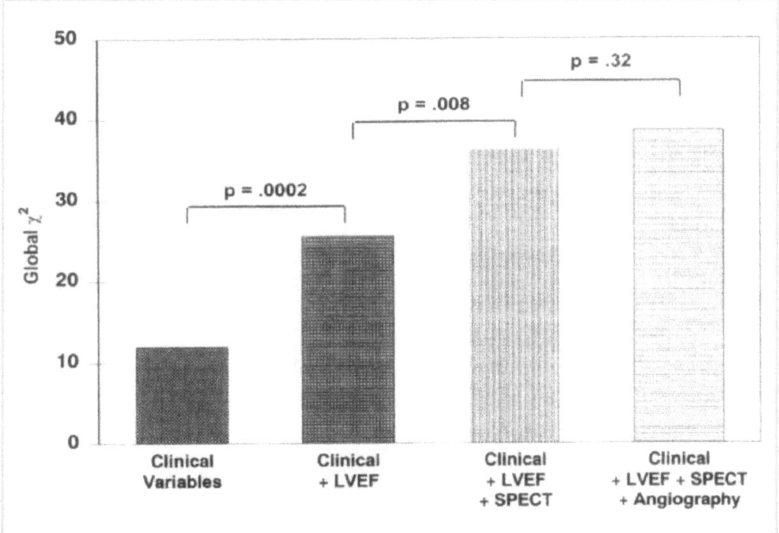

Figure 11.2. Incremental prognostic value of the left ventricular ejection fraction (LVEF) and thallium-201 single photon emission computed tomographic (SPECT) variables in post-myocardial infarction patients treated with thrombolytic therapy. Note that the addition of angiographic variables do not increase the cumulative prognostic information in this model over clinical variables, the LVEF, and SPECT variables. (Reprinted from Dakik et al.[7] with permission.)

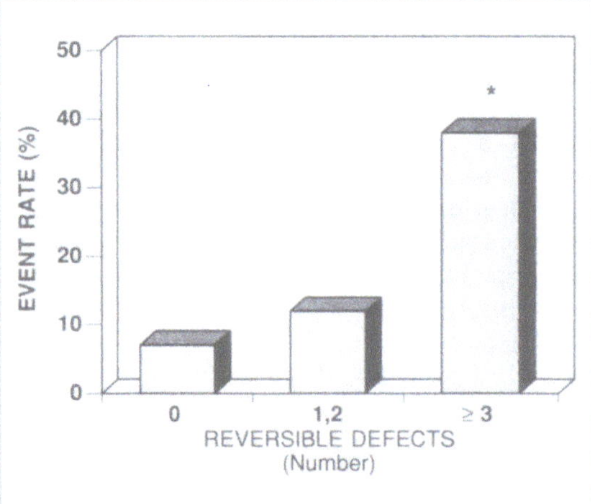

Figure 11.3. Cardiac event rate in relation to the number of reversible technetium-99m-sestamibi defects (*P = .017) compared with patients with no reversible defects. All patients had an acute myocardial infarction and were followed up for an average of 15 ± 10 months. (Reprinted from Travin et al.,[9] Copyright 1995, with permission from Excerpta Medica.)

prognostic value in 124 patients who underwent predischarge gated ^{99m}Tc-sestamibi SPECT after acute MI and did not undergo subsequent revascularization.[10] The cardiac death or recurrent MI rate was 38.1% in patients with a LVEF of <40% versus 9.4% in those with LVEF of >40%.

Basu et al.[11] determined the prognostic role of ^{201}Tl compared with exercise ECG testing in patients with acute MI who were treated with thrombolytic therapy. They found that reversible ischemia on ^{201}Tl scintigraphy predicted adverse cardiac events (death, reinfarction, unstable angina, and congestive heart failure) in 33 of 37 patients with such events during follow-up (hazard ratio 8.1; $P < .001$). Exercise ECG showed reversible ischemia in 33 patients, of whom 13 had subsequent events, and failed to predict events in 24 patients (hazard ratio 1.1; $P = .8$). The authors concluded that ^{201}Tl imaging was a sensitive predictor of subsequent events in patients who received thrombolytic therapy after acute MI, whereas exercise ECG failed to predict outcome.

1.2 Pharmacologic Stress MPI

Vasodilator stress MPI can be easily substituted for exercise scintigraphy in postinfarction patients undergoing predischarge risk stratification.[1] The test is safe and can be performed as early as 48 hours after admission, as long as such patients have had an uncomplicated course. A large multicenter trial[12] in which dipyridamole ^{99m}Tc-sestamibi imaging was performed 2–4 days after admission for acute MI showed that the extent and severity of defect reversibility had significant incremental prognostic value when added to clinical stress-test variables for predicting subsequent cardiac events. The annual cardiac death or MI rates as a function of the summed difference score for a given summed stress score are shown in Figure 11.4. The summed difference scores were derived

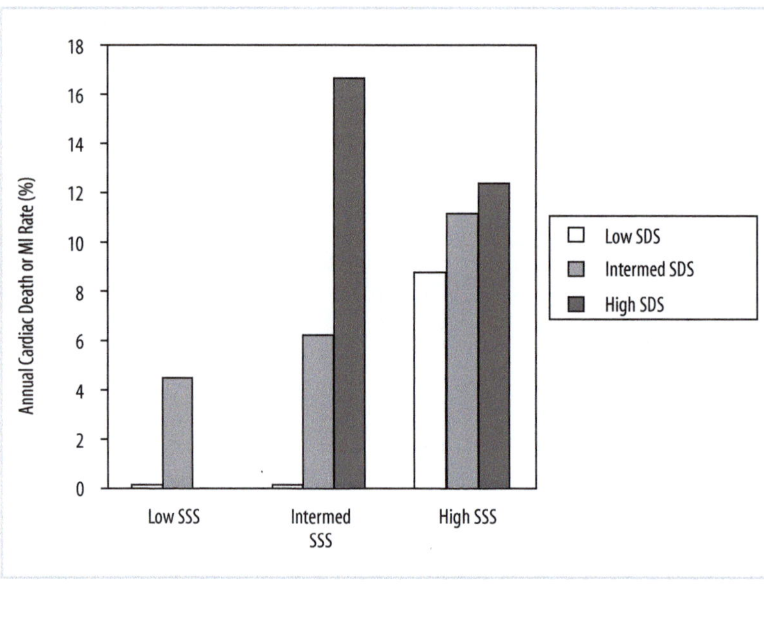

Figure 11.4. Annual cardiac death or myocardial infarction (MI) rate as a function of the summed stress score (SSS) and the extent of ischemia characterized by the summed difference score (SDS) in post-MI patients undergoing dipyridamole technetium-99m-sestamibi imaging 2–4 days after admission. For any given SSS, the interaction of reversibility score further improved the predictive value. In this study, dipyridamole perfusion imaging showed better risk stratification than submaximal exercise myocardial perfusion imaging. Intermed = intermediate. (Reprinted from Brown et al.[12] with permission.)

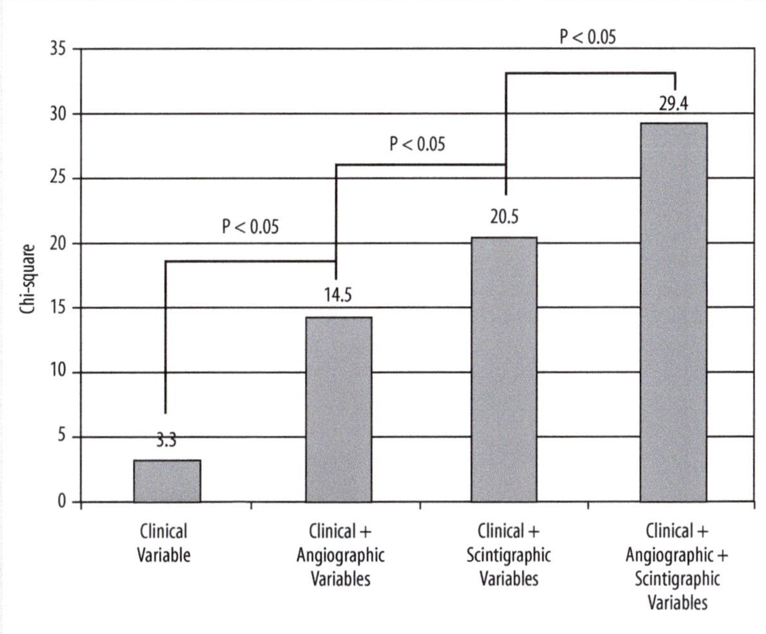

Figure 11.5. Incremental prognostic power of angiographic and scintigraphic variables over clinical variables in predicting cardiac events after acute myocardial infarction in patients who underwent rest thallium and dipyridamole technetium-99m-sestamibi single photon emission computed tomography 3–21 days after infarction. After multivariate analysis, the presence of any scintigraphic reversibility, had the strongest correlation with clinical events, with better predictive value than angiographic multivessel stenoses. (Reprinted from Chiamvimonvat et al.[13] with permission.)

using a 17-segment model in which segmental tracer uptake was graded by a five-point scoring system ranging from 0, indicative of normal, to 4, indicative of absence of tracer activity. Note that for each of the subgroups demarcated by the extent and severity of the poststress defect (SSS), the cardiac event rate increased as the extent of defect reversibility increased. This effect was greatest in the intermediate defect size group. In this study, the cardiac event rate at 2 years was <2% per year in patients with a low-risk dipyridamole SPECT ^{99m}Tc-sestamibi scan.

Chiamvimonvat et al.[13] also determined the prognostic worth of dipyridamole ^{99m}Tc-sestamibi SPECT imaging in stable postinfarction patients and compared scintigraphic variables with clinical and angiographic variables. In this study, on multivariate analysis, the presence of any scintigraphic reversibility had the strongest correlation with clinical events, with better predictive value than angiographic multivessel stenoses. The extent of scintigraphic reversibility was directly correlated with clinical events. Figure 11.5 shows the incremental prognostic power of scintigraphic variables over just clinical and angiographic variables.[13]

2. Echocardiographic Techniques for Detecting Ischemia in High-risk Patients after Uncomplicated ACSs

Rest and stress echocardiography is an alternative to rest and stress MPI for risk assessment after an ACS. In one multicenter trial comprising 759 inpatients with an uncomplicated MI, stress echocardiography provided stronger prognostic information than clinical and exercise ECG stress variables.[14] In this study, patients with a negative pharmacologic stress echocardiogram had a 94.7% event-free survival compared with 74.8% with those with positive tests. When all variables were analyzed in this study, the difference between wall motion score index at rest and peak stress, and exercise duration were independent predictors of future spontaneous events. It appears that dobutamine echocardiography and exercise ECG have a similar high negative predictive value for both events following a first uncomplicated MI as well as for only hard events. However, a positive dobutamine echocardiography, but not a positive exercise ECG stress test, identified a group of patients at higher risk for subsequent cardiac events.[15] Carlos et al.[16] also reported that

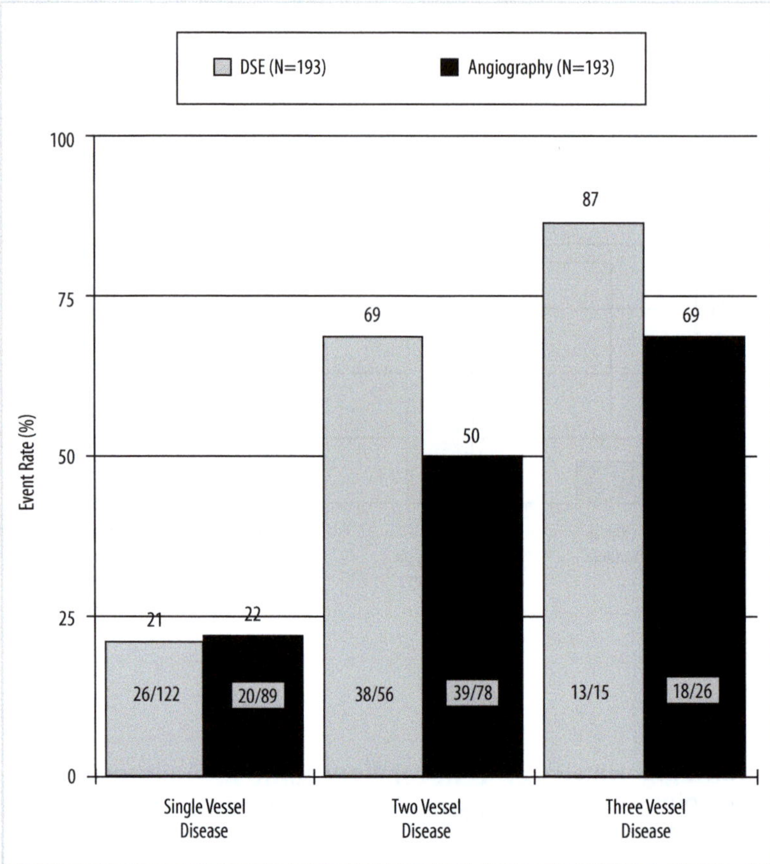

Figure 11.6. Comparison of the incidence of cardiac events according to extent of coronary artery disease indicated by dobutamine stress echocardiography (DSE) and coronary angiography in 214 patients who underwent testing at 2–7 days after infarction. Multivessel disease identified through DSE was more predictive of adverse outcome than was angiographically determined multivessel disease. (Reprinted from Carlos et al.[16] with permission.)

multivessel disease identified by dobutamine stress echocardiography was more predictive of an adverse outcome in patients with acute MI than was angiographically determined multivessel CAD. This is similar to what has been reported for vasodilator stress MPI in which a multivessel disease scan pattern is more predictive than multivessel angiographic disease for predicting subsequent cardiac events in patients with uncomplicated MI. In the study by Carlos et al.,[16] significant predictors of an adverse outcome included prior MI, anterior infarction, multivessel CAD, global resting LV motion score index, and infarction zone nonviability based on akinesis unresponsive to low-dose dobutamine and ischemia/infarction at a distance. Figure 11.6 shows the comparison of incidence of cardiac events according to extent of CAD as reflected by dobutamine stress echocardiography and coronary angiography.[16]

3. Medical Versus Interventional Therapy in Coronary Syndromes: Recent Trials, Future Directions, and Are We Under-utilizing Medical Therapy?

Considerable controversy exists regarding whether a medical or an invasive strategy should be undertaken for risk stratification in patients who have survived the early phase of an acute STEMI or an ACS. There are four major multicenter randomized studies that have been reported, that address this controversy.

The first was the Thrombolysis in Myocardial Infarction (TIMI)-IIIB trial, which randomized patients to a medical strategy or angioplasty, who had unstable angina or a non-STEMI.[17] In this particular study, there was no difference in either early or 1-year outcomes in patients randomized to either group. However, there was a more than 55% crossover of patients from the medical group to the intervention group. This study has been criticized because of the high rate of crossover and the fact that stents were not yet available for PCI when this study was undertaken.

A second study was the VANQWISH study, which randomized patients with non-STEMI to a medical or early interventional/coronary bypass strategy.[6] Similar to the TIMI-IIIB study, no difference in subsequent MI or death at 1 year was observed between the two groups. In fact, the medical-treated group seemed to do better. This study was criticized because of the 10% mortality rate in the patients who underwent early coronary bypass surgery predominantly for multivessel CAD in the invasive group. Also, this study was done in a rather high-risk population because the patients were from Veterans' Hospitals who have a high prevalence of comorbidities. In fact, the VANQWISH trial showed an extremely low mortality rate for patients randomized to early angioplasty in the invasive arm. At 2 years of follow-up, the mortality rate was comparable for patients with a spontaneous non-Q wave MI randomized to invasive or noninvasive strategies.

The third major study to be reported was the FRagmin during InStability in Coronary artery disease (FRISC) study, which randomized patients 5 days after medical therapy to invasive or noninvasive strategies.[18,19] In this study, patients who were randomized to the invasive arm actually had a better outcome. This study has been criticized because only treadmill testing was done to identify patients with myocardial ischemia. If an imaging technology had been performed, then more patients with inducible ischemia might have been identified, and they would have crossed over to an invasive strategy. Also, patients were not permitted to cross over from the medical to the invasive study group unless they had ≥3.0 mm of ST depression on exercise stress testing.[20] Patients with 1.0–2.0 mm of ST depression had a high prevalence of multivessel disease in the FRISC trial.

Perhaps the most relevant trial dealing with early invasive versus conservative therapy is the Treat Angina with Aggrastat and determine Cost of Therapy with Invasive or Conservative Strategy (TACTICS) trial in which 2220 patients with unstable angina and non-STEMI were treated with aspirin, heparin, and the glycoprotein IIb/IIIa antagonist, tirofiban.[21] Patients were then randomized to either an early invasive strategy (catheterization within 4–48 hours) or a more conservative therapy (selective catheterization: objective evidence of ischemia or a positive stress test). Imaging techniques were used in conjunction with stress testing in this trial. At 6 months, 15.9% of patients in the early invasive group experienced death, nonfatal MI, or rehospitalization for an ACS, compared with 19.4% in the group undergoing the conservative strategy. Death or MI was similarly reduced. Fifty-four percent of the patients in the entire study cohort had an elevated troponin T. Fifty-one percent of patients in the conservative group had cardiac catheterization and 24% a PCI versus 97% and 41%, respectively, in the invasive group. Figure 11.7 shows the cumulative incidence of death, nonfatal MI, or rehospitalization for ACS during the 6-month follow-up period.[21]

In the TACTICS trial,[21] patients with an ACS and no elevation of troponin T did *not* benefit from an invasive strategy. Conversely, the event rate was 24.2% with conservative therapy versus 14.3% with invasive therapy ($P < .001$ or: .52) in the subgroup with a troponin elevation. The benefit of the invasive strategy was even evident in patients with minor elevations of troponin I or T (e.g., 0.1–0.4 ng/mL of troponin I). Also, patients with a low TIMI risk score did not benefit from an invasive strategy. Patients with ST depression on the admission ECG benefited more from the invasive strategy.

When compared with the FRISC II trial,[18] more than 50% of patients crossed over from the

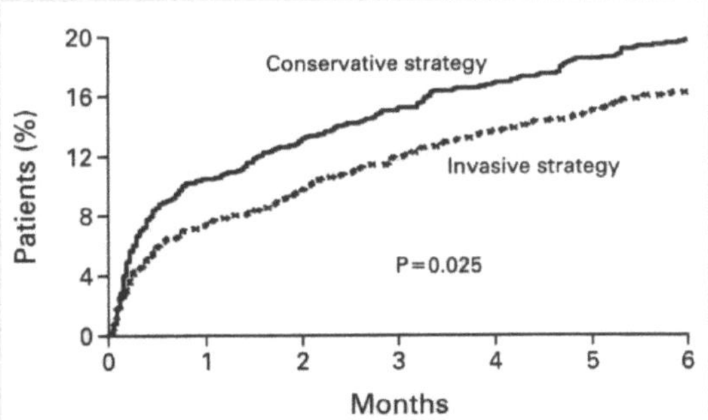

Figure 11.7. Cumulative incidence of the primary endpoint of death, nonfatal infarction, or rehospitalization for an acute coronary syndrome during a 6-month follow-up period in patients randomized to an invasive strategy versus a conservative strategy. All patients had an acute coronary syndrome without ST-segment elevation. (Reprinted from Cannon et al.,[21] Copyright 2001, Massachusetts Medical Society. All rights reserved.)

conservative to the invasive strategy based on ischemia seen on stress testing (>1.0 mm of ST depression and/or ischemia by nuclear or echocardiographic testing). In FRISC II, only 10% crossed over.

Medical therapy has improved considerably in the treatment of patients with ACS. In the Myocardial Ischemia Reduction with Aggressive Cholesterol Lowering (MIRACL) study,[22] in-hospital treatment with atorvastatin (80 mg/day) resulted in a reduction in subsequent hospitalizations for recurrent ischemia. The primary endpoint of death, nonfatal MI, cardiac arrest with resuscitation, or recurrent symptomatic ischemia requiring hospitalization was reduced by 16% in the atorvastatin group at 16 weeks.

Patients with elevated C-reactive protein levels who have been recently discharged after an episode of unstable angina are at higher risk for recurrent ischemic events.[23] Such patients may particularly benefit from the antiinflammatory effect of statin drugs.

The addition of clopidogrel to aspirin in patients with an ACS without ST-segment elevation was evaluated in the Clopidogrel in Unstable angina to prevent Recurrent ischemic Events (CURE) trial,[24] which showed a 20% reduction in cardiovascular death, nonfatal MI, or stroke (9.3% vs 11.4%; $P < .001$) in the clopidogrel plus aspirin group compared with aspirin alone. Major bleeding, however, was higher in the clopidogrel group (3.7% vs 2.7%; RR 1.38).

Other recommendations regarding medical therapy after an ACS include: 1) the value of combining niacin with a statin in patients with a high density lipoprotein of <40; 2) the use of angiotensin-converting enzyme inhibitors in all patients with ACS who can tolerate the drug; 3) the use of beta-blockers early and after discharge in ACS patients; 4) continuing clopidogrel indefinitely (at least 9 months) in patients with ACS not undergoing PCI; and 5) not using antioxidant vitamins.

The perfusion defect size and the size of ischemic defects are reduced with either medical therapy or invasive PCI. Dakik et al.[25] showed that post-MI patients whose defect size decreased by ≥9% had fewer cardiac events during follow-up compared with patients whose defect size decreased by <9% with either type of therapy. Figure 11.8 depicts these differences.

4. Conclusion

From the above discussion we conclude that, patients who are judged to be at high risk with an acute ischemic syndrome should be triaged to an invasive strategy. Such patients have significant ECG changes with pain and have an elevation of a serum marker such as troponin I or T. The issue with this group of patients relates to the timing of cardiac catheterization. Should such patients be medically stabilized first with

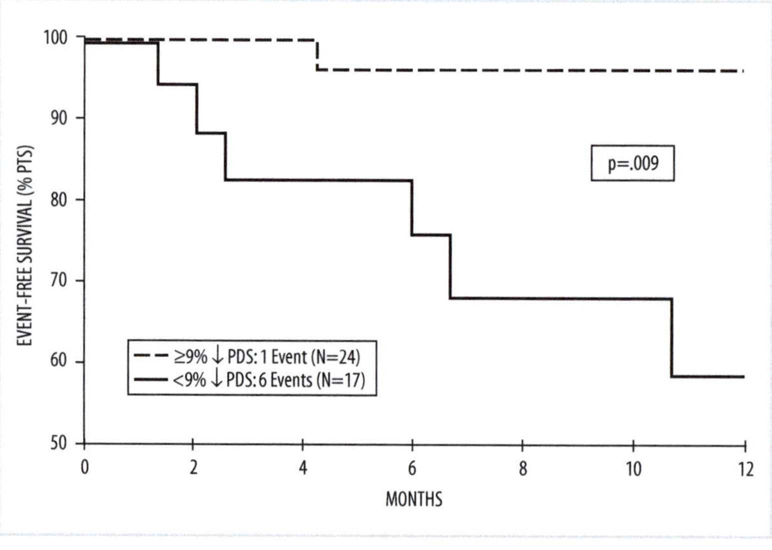

Figure 11.8. Event-free survival based on changes in the perfusion defect size (PDS) after anti-ischemic therapy in patients with an acute myocardial infarction who underwent pre- and posttreatment adenosine thallium-201 single photon emission computed tomography. (Reprinted from Dakik et al.[25] with permission.)

aspirin, low weight heparin, and/or IIb/IIIa glycoprotein platelet inhibitor, before going to catheterization? Should such patients be immediately referred for angiography? Patients judged not to be at high risk can easily undergo a noninvasive strategy without any significant increased risk of ischemic events compared with an initial invasive strategy. Such patients with a suspected or documented acute ischemic syndrome who have no elevation of a serum marker can undergo treadmill testing or pharmacologic stress testing with an imaging technique. The latter is recommended over submaximal ECG treadmill testing because it increases sensitivity for detecting ischemia in postinfarction patients.

References

1. Mahmarian JJ, Dwivedi G, Lahiri T, et al. Role of nuclear cardiac imaging in myocardial infarction: postinfarction risk stratification. J Nucl Cardiol 2004;11:186–209.
2. Keeley EC, Boura JA, Grines CL. Primary angioplasty versus intravenous thrombolytic therapy for acute myocardial infarction: a quantitative review of 23 randomised trials. Lancet 2003;361(9351):13–20.
3. Bolognese L, Cerisano G, Buonamici P, et al. Influence of infarct-zone viability on left ventricular remodeling after acute myocardial infarction. Circulation 1997;96: 3353–3359.
4. Shaw LJ, Peterson ED, Kesler K, et al. A metaanalysis of predischarge risk stratification after acute myocardial infarction with stress electrocardiographic, myocardial perfusion, and ventricular function imaging. Am J Cardiol 1996;78:1327–1337.
5. Gibson RS, Watson DD, Craddock GB, et al. Prediction of cardiac events after uncomplicated myocardial infarction: a prospective study comparing predischarge exercise thallium-201 scintigraphy and coronary angiography. Circulation 1983;68:321–336.
6. Boden WE, O'Rourke RA, Crawford MH, et al. Outcomes in patients with acute non-Q-wave myocardial infarction randomly assigned to an invasive as compared with a conservative management strategy. Veterans Affairs Non-Q-Wave Infarction Strategies in Hospital (VANQWISH) Trial Investigators [erratum in: N Engl J Med 1998;339:1091]. N Engl J Med 1998;338: 1785–1792.
7. Dakik HA, Mahmarian JJ, Kimball KT, et al. Prognostic value of exercise ^{201}Tl tomography in patients treated with thrombolytic therapy during acute myocardial infarction. Circulation 1996;94:2735–2742.
8. Lima RSL, Watson DD, Goode AR, et al. Incremental value of combined perfusion and function over perfusion alone by gated SPECT MPI for detection of severe three-vessel coronary artery disease. J Am Coll Cardiol 2003;42:64–70.
9. Travin MI, Dessouki A, Cameron T, et al. Use of exercise technetium-99m sestamibi SPECT imaging to detect residual ischemia and for risk stratification after acute myocardial infarction. Am J Cardiol 1995;75:665–669.
10. Kroll D, Farah W, McKendall GR, et al. Prognostic value of stress-gated Tc-99m sestamibi SPECT after acute myocardial infarction. Am J Cardiol 2001;87:381–386.
11. Basu S, Senior R, Dore C, et al. Value of thallium-201 imaging in detecting adverse cardiac events after myocardial infarction and thrombolysis: a follow up of 100 consecutive patients. BMJ 1996;313(7061):844–848.
12. Brown KA, Heller GV, Landin RS, et al. Early dipyridamole ^{99m}Tc-sestamibi single photon emission computed tomographic imaging 2 to 4 days after acute myocardial infarction predicts in-hospital and postdischarge cardiac events: comparison with submaximal exercise imaging. Circulation 1999;100:2060–2066.
13. Chiamvimonvat V, Goodman SG, Langer A, et al. Prognostic value of dipyridamole SPECT imaging in low-risk patients after myocardial infarction. J Nucl Cardiol 2001;8:136–143.
14. Sicari R, Landi P, Picano E, et al. EPIC (Echo Persantine International Cooperative); EDIC (Echo Dobutamine International Cooperative) Study Group. Exercise-electrocardiography and/or pharmacological stress echocardiography for non-invasive risk stratification early after uncomplicated myocardial infarction. A prospective international large scale multicentre study. Eur Heart J 2002;23:1030–1037.
15. Greco CA, Salustri A, Seccareccia F, et al. Prognostic value of dobutamine echocardiography early after uncomplicated acute myocardial infarction: a comparison with exercise electrocardiography. J Am Coll Cardiol 1997;29:261–267.
16. Carlos ME, Smart SC, Wynsen JC, et al. Dobutamine stress echocardiography for risk stratification after myocardial infarction. Circulation 1997;95:1402–1410.
17. The TIMI IIIB Investigators. Effects of tissue plasminogen activator and a comparison of early invasive and conservative strategies in unstable angina and non-Q-wave myocardial infarction: results of the TIMI IIIB trial. Thrombolysis in Myocardial Infarction. Circulation 1994;89:1545–1556.
18. FRagmin and Fast Revascularisation during InStability in Coronary artery disease (FRISC II) Investigators. Invasive compared with non-invasive treatment in unstable coronary-artery disease: FRISC II prospective randomised multicenter study. Lancet 1999;354(9180): 708–715.
19. Wallentin L, Lagerqvist B, Husted S, et al. Outcome at 1 year after an invasive compared with a non-invasive strategy in unstable coronary-artery disease: the FRISC II invasive randomized trial. FRISC Investigators. Lancet 2000;356:9–16.
20. Goyal A, Samaha FF, Boden WE, et al. Stress test criteria used in the conservative arm of the FRISC-II trial underdetects surgical coronary artery disease when applied to patients in the VANQWISH trial. J Am Coll Cardiol 2002;39:1601–1607.
21. Cannon CP, Weintraub WS, Demopoulos LA, et al. TACTICS (Treat Angina with Aggrastat and determine Cost of Therapy with an Invasive or Conservative Strategy) – Thrombolysis in Myocardial Infarction 18 Investigators. Comparison of early invasive and conservative strategies in patients with unstable coronary syndromes treated with the glycoprotein IIb/IIIa inhibitor tirofiban. N Engl J Med 2001;344:1879–1887.
22. Schwartz GG, Olsson AG, Ezekowitz MD, et al. Myocardial Ischemia Reduction with Aggressive Cholesterol

Lowering (MIRACL) Study Investigators. Effects of atorvastatin on early recurrent ischemic events in acute coronary syndromes: the MIRACL study: a randomized controlled trial [erratum in: JAMA 2001;286:536]. JAMA 2001;285:1711–1718.
23. Biasucci LM, Liuzzo G, Grillo RL, et al. Elevated levels of C-reactive protein at discharge in patients with unstable angina predict recurrent instability. Circulation 1999;99:855–860.
24. Yusuf S, Zhao F, Mehta SR, et al., Clopidogrel in Unstable Angina to Prevent Recurrent Events (CURE) Trial Investigators. Effects of clopidogrel in addition to aspirin in patients with acute coronary syndromes without ST-segment elevation [erratum in: N Engl J Med 2001;345:1716 and N Engl J Med 2001;345:1506]. N Engl J Med 2001;345:494–502.
25. Dakik HA, Kleiman NS, Farmer JA, et al. Intensive medical therapy versus coronary angioplasty for suppression of myocardial ischemia in survivors of acute myocardial infarction: a prospective, randomized pilot study. Circulation 1998;98:2017–2023.

12

Role of Stress Imaging Techniques in Evaluation of Patients Before and after Myocardial Revascularization

Abdou Elhendy

Stress imaging techniques have a pivotal role in the evaluation of patients before and after myocardial revascularization. Stress echocardiography and myocardial perfusion imaging are useful in identifying high-risk patients who are likely to benefit from revascularization. The advantages of these techniques include ability to assess patients unable to exercise, high diagnostic accuracy, quantification and localization of ischemia, evaluation of global and regional function, evaluation of myocardial viability, and determination of physiologic significance of coronary artery disease (CAD). Despite the technical advances in percutaneous interventions, restenosis occurs in a significant number of patients. Stress imaging techniques are useful in detection of in stent stenosis, coronary artery bypass grafting (CABG) stenosis or occlusion, and progression of native CAD. The extent and severity of wall motion and perfusion abnormalities were shown to predict cardiac events in patients with previous revascularization. The current guidelines recommend the use of stress testing only in symptomatic patients. However, there is growing evidence that the adverse outcome of myocardial ischemia observed on stress imaging techniques is not related to symptoms. Prospective studies are required to assess whether reinterventions can improve outcome in patients with ischemia on stress imaging techniques after revascularization.

1. Evaluation of Patients Before Myocardial Revascularization

1.1 Identification of Patients Who Will Benefit from Revascularization

Stress echocardiography and myocardial perfusion imaging have pivotal roles in selecting high-risk patients for revascularization.[1–16] Both techniques were shown to provide a higher sensitivity for diagnosis of CAD in conjunction with exercise stress test compared with the electrocardiogram.[1–4] Other advantages include the assessment of myocardial function, quantification of ischemia, localization of CAD, and the ability to evaluate patients with limited exercise capacity by pharmacologic stress.[1–4] The high sensitivity of stress echocardiography and myocardial perfusion imaging techniques for the diagnosis of CAD and the low incidence of mortality and hard cardiac events after a normal stress test eliminate the need for further diagnostic workup in patients with a normal stress echocardiogram or perfusion scan during the following 1–3 years unless a change in clinical status occurs.[8,9,16] Observational studies have shown that early coronary angiography in patients with normal stress myocardial perfusion imaging is associated with a trend to increased cardiac events.[5]

The improved outcome with myocardial revascularization is mostly observed among high-risk patients. In a meta-analysis of seven randomized studies comparing medical treatment to CABG, the improvement of survival was more evident among patients with left main disease, multivessel disease, left ventricular systolic dysfunction, and abnormal stress test.[17] Stress echocardiography and myocardial perfusion imaging provide accurate assessment of left ventricular function. Additionally, the extent of perfusion and wall motion abnormalities parallel the extent and severity of angiographic CAD.[18] Therefore, data obtained by these techniques can guide the physician in determining which patient may benefit from revascularization compared with medical treatment (Table 12.1). Observational studies have shown that the extent and severity of myocardial perfusion abnormalities on exercise or vasodilator stress determines the benefit of early referral for coronary angiography and subsequent revascularization.[5] Patients with severe or moderate to severe perfusion abnormalities had better outcome with early angiography and intervention than with medical treatment alone. In patients with mild or mild to moderate abnormalities, there was no difference in outcome between medical treatment versus early catheterization, and the management decision in these patients should be individualized.

Table 12.1. Indications for noninvasive imaging before revascularization

Detection, localization, and quantification of ischemia as a cause of symptoms
Detection of silent ischemia
Risk stratification and prognostication
Detection and quantification of viable/hibernating myocardium

There is increasing evidence that revascularization has a pivotal role in the management of patients with acute coronary syndromes; however, even in this setting, noninvasive imaging can also be helpful in certain lower-risk patients for management decisions (for a more detailed description, see discussion in previous chapter).

1.2 Comparison of Different Management Strategies

The pretest probability of CAD is related to gender, age, and chest pain characteristics.[19] Most patients with typical angina are considered to have a high probability of CAD. In clinical practice, many of these patients are referred directly for coronary angiography without prior stress testing, even in the presence of stable symptoms. Shaw et al.[6] enrolled 11 372 consecutive stable angina patients who were referred for stress myocardial perfusion tomography or cardiac catheterization. Stress imaging patients were matched by their pretest clinical risk of coronary disease to a series of patients referred to cardiac catheterization. Composite 3-year costs of care were compared for two patients' management strategies: 1) direct cardiac catheterization (aggressive), and 2) initial stress myocardial perfusion tomography and selective catheterization of high-risk patients (conservative). Observational comparisons of aggressive compared with conservative testing strategies revealed that costs of care were higher for direct cardiac catheterization in all clinical risk subsets (range: $2878 to $4579), compared with stress myocardial perfusion imaging plus selective catheterization (range: \$2387 to \$3010, $P < 0.0001$). Coronary revascularization rates were higher for low-, intermediate-, and high-risk direct catheterization patients compared with the initial stress perfusion imaging cohort (13% to 50%, $P < 0.0001$); cardiac death or myocardial infarction rates were similar. It was concluded that stable chest pain patients who undergo a more aggressive diagnostic strategy have higher diagnostic costs and greater rates of intervention and follow-up costs. Cost differences may reflect a diminished necessity for resource consumption for patients with normal test results.

Elhendy et al.[20] demonstrated that, among patients with classic angina, exercise echocardiogram was normal in approximately 50% of patients. These patients had a low event rate during 2 years after the stress test. A multivessel pattern of wall motion abnormalities was incremental to clinical and exercise stress data in predicting hard cardiac events.[20] Therefore, a strategy of performing stress echocardiography or myocardial perfusion imaging in patients with chronic stable angina, with referral for coronary angiography and possible revascularization procedures based on presence and severity of abnormalities can result in lowering the cost of health care, reducing the need for invasive and interventional procedures without increase of the risk of mortality or hard cardiac events compared with a strategy of direct cardiac catheterization in these patients.

1.3 Role of Stress Imaging in Patients with Known Coronary Angiographic Data

In clinical practice, many patients are referred for noninvasive stress imaging techniques after performing the coronary angiogram because the data obtained by coronary angiography are not sufficient to make a decision regarding the subsequent management.

1.3.1 Evaluation of Functional Significance of Coronary Stenosis

Although coronary angiography is considered a golden standard against which the accuracy of stress imaging techniques is weighed, the technique provides mostly anatomic information by imaging the silhouette of the coronary artery lumen. In the presence of diffuse CAD, a reference healthy segment may be lacking and, therefore, the percentage diameter coronary artery stenosis will underestimate the actual severity of coronary stenosis. Additionally, conventional coronary angiography does not provide physiologic data on whether a given stenosis is associated with flow limitation under stress conditions. Finally, coronary angiography does not characterize the atherosclerotic plaque. The latter may determine the ischemic response in the related myocardial segments. Therefore, stress echocardiography and myocardial perfusion imaging can be useful in determining the functional significance of a given coronary stenosis. Patients without inducible ischemia should continue medical treatment and aggressive risk-factor modification unless they have a change in symptoms or with failure of medical treatment to relief their angina. Exercise stress test is the preferred method if the patient is able to exercise, because it provides additional information regarding the future risk of cardiac events such as heart rate and systolic blood pressure response and exercise tolerance.[21] These data are useful in addition to perfusion and functional data in determining the anticipated risk in a given patient. According to current guidelines, percutaneous coronary intervention (PCI) can be considered the initial mode of revascularization for most patients with objective evidence of clinically important inducible ischemia. CABG is indicated in patients with unprotected left main CAD, and those with multivessel disease particularly if they are diabetics or present with left ventricular dysfunction.[22]

1.4 Evaluation of Myocardial Viability

Patients with CAD can exhibit segmental and global left ventricular systolic dysfunction, which can be reversible after revascularization.[23,24] Patients with heart failure and those with advanced left ventricular systolic dysfunction are at greater risk for complications during or after CABG and PCI. Therefore, selection of patients in whom the benefit of revascularization outweighs the risk is very important to improve patients' outcome. Evaluation of myocardial viability requires identification of the extent and severity of left ventricular dysfunction in the first place. Diabetic patients and those with manifest or occult renal disease are at a high risk of contrast nephropathy. The ability to evaluate global and regional function accurately by echocardiography or gated single photon emission computed tomography (SPECT) obviates the need for left ventriculography in these patients and this can help minimize the dose of contrast agents and reduce the risk of contrast nephropathy. In patients with total occlusion, the presence and the grade of angiographic collaterals cannot determine the presence of viable myocardium.[25,26] Dobutamine stress echocardiography or CMR and radionuclide imaging provided more accurate assessment of myocardial viability in these regions.

Stress imaging techniques can also help the physician in determining the type of revascularization in a given patient with known angiographic anatomy. For example, a patient with high-grade left anterior descending (LAD) CAD, a kinetic inferior wall, and total occlusion of the right coronary artery (RCA) that is not amenable to PCI can be managed by PCI for LAD alone if there is no ischemia or viable myocardium in the akinetic inferior wall. However, the same patient may be considered a candidate for CABG of both LAD and RCA if she/he demonstrated a sizable amount of viability and ischemia in the inferior wall, because, in this condition, revascularization will not be complete with PCI only.

The diagnosis of myocardial viability by stress radionuclide imaging is based on the presence of a reversible perfusion abnormality, or a mild to moderate fixed defect in a severely dyssynergic myocardium.[23] The diagnosis of viability by dobutamine stress echocardiography (DSE) is based on eliciting contractile reserve at low-dose dobutamine (5–10 μg/kg/min). The biphasic response which is characterized by improvement at a low dose and worsening at a higher dose is a specific marker of potential functional improvement in an akinetic area after revascularization. Improvement of function is related to the extent of myocardial viability.[24,25] The relative merits of various imaging techniques for diagnosis of myocardial viability and prediction of functional recovery and prognosis after revascularization are described in the next chapter.

2. Role of Stress Imaging Techniques after Revascularization

2.1 Evaluation of Myocardial Function, Contractile Reserve, and Functional Capacity

Coronary revascularization procedures have several aims in the appropriate patients. These include amelioration of angina, improvement of heart failure symptoms if these were present before revascularization, improvement of functional capacity, improvement of global and regional systolic function, and reducing the incidence of mortality and cardiac events.[27–31]

Stress imaging techniques can provide an objective evidence of beneficial effect of revascularization in an individual patient. These data are easier to interpret if the patient had the same stress study before revascularization. In patients who are able to exercise, exercise echocardiography or myocardial perfusion imaging can document improvement of exercise tolerance. All stress imaging techniques can demonstrate amelioration or significant reduction of ischemic burden, manifested as inducible wall motion or perfusion abnormalities after revascularization, and therefore provide a physiologic clue to the patency of revascularized arteries and completeness of revascularization.

Among patients with left ventricular dysfunction and viable myocardium, stress imaging with echocardiography or gated SPECT can demonstrate improvement of regional and global left ventricular function. These changes have been initially observed 1–3 months after revascularization. However, the time required for dysfunctioning viable myocardium to recover after revascularization varies from patient to patient and there are recent data to indicate that functional recovery may take up to 1 year after revascularization particularly in the presence of hibernating myocardium which is thought to require a longer time for recovery compared with the stunned myocardium.[29] For a more detailed discussion, see also the next chapter.

2.2 Evaluation of Patency of Grafts, Revascularized Coronary Arteries, and Progression of Native CAD

Despite the potential benefits of myocardial revascularization procedures, myocardial perfusion can be compromised by restenosis after PCI, bypass graft occlusion or stenosis, and progression of native CAD.[32–36] This may involve coronary arteries that had minimal angiographic disease at the time of revascularization as well as arterial segments distal to the grafts or the stent placement. The improved outcome with the use of stents and the implementation of new antiplatelet agents has resulted in a significant increase in the number of PCI procedures over the last decade. As a result, the use of, and indications for, PCI have greatly expanded to include patients with acute coronary syndromes and patients with anatomically difficult stenoses such as those with complex lesions, small-diameter vessels, chronic total occlusions, multivessel disease, and diseased bypass grafts. It is estimated that more than one million PCI procedures were performed in the United States in 2000. Nevertheless, restenosis remains a major clinical problem. When restenosis does occur, it usually happens within 3–9 months.[32,33]

The greatest incidence of graft occlusion occurs between 5 and 8 years after surgery. Analysis of pooled data from previous studies have shown that serial saphenous vein graft patency was 95% at 1 week, 84% at 1 year, 80% at 3 years, and 69% at 6 years. The serial data for internal mammary grafts are 99%, 95%, 93%, and 87% at each of the same time points.[35,36] Approximately 50% of patients remain asymptomatic when restenosis or graft disease occurs. Conversely, many patients developing chest pain after revascularization do not have angiographic stenosis.[37] Routine coronary angiography is not recommended because of the associated risk and cost and the lack of functional information (in most centers) regarding the observed angiographic abnormalities. This demonstrates the need of an objective and accurate noninvasive method to detect jeopardized myocardium in these patients.

In general, it is not recommended to repeat the stress testing shortly after revascularization to evaluate patency of revascularized artery, unless there is a clinical suspicion of graft or stent closure (Table 12.2).[38] Patients with unstable symptoms or significant elevation of cardiac enzymes should not receive stress testing. A baseline echocardiogram or a resting perfusion study can usually document extension of abnormalities compared with a previous study and direct the physician for the need to revise the revascularization results invasively.

Table 12.2. Indications for noninvasive imaging after revascularization

After percutaneous coronary intervention
Suboptimal results
Recurrence of symptoms or suspected restenosis
Multivessel disease with incomplete revascularization
Procedural complications
Assessing the effects of intervention if required for occupational reasons
After coronary artery bypass grafting
Incomplete revascularization or poor distal vessels
Recurrence of symptoms or suspected graft occlusion
Procedural complications
Assessing the effects of intervention if required for occupational reasons

2.3 Diagnosis of Ischemia after Interventions

Exercise electrocardiography has low accuracy in detecting restenosis or graft occlusion.[39] In contrast, the sensitivity and specificity of myocardial perfusion imaging, performed at varying times after PCI, range from 39% to 100% and 46% to 100%, respectively, improving with time after revascularization.[40–47]

Giedd and Bergmann[32] pooled data from eight studies involving 640 patients, in which stress SPECT and coronary angiography were performed within 2 to 48 months of PCI. The overall sensitivity and specificity of SPECT for detecting myocardial ischemia 2 or more months after PCI were both 79%, and similar in all three vascular territories.

Takeuchi et al.[48] compared dobutamine thallium with echocardiography in 53 patients after percutaneous transluminal coronary angioplasty (PTCA). The sensitivities of echocardiography and myocardial perfusion SPECT for detecting restenosis were 78% and 74%, respectively; specificities were both 93% and accuracies were 87% and 85%, respectively.

2.4 Myocardial Perfusion Imaging Early after PCI

Myocardial perfusion imaging depends on regional difference in tracer uptake during hyperemia and microvascular function as well. Regional hypoperfusion can occur in the absence of coronary obstruction if absolute myocardial flow reserve is impaired. Early after PCI, absolute coronary flow reserve is diminished; thus, even in the presence of patent vessel, regional perfusion can be affected by endothelial dysfunction and injury at the treated site and/or abnormal microvascular and resistive vessel function distal to the site. As a result of this, it is prudent to interpret the results of stress imaging techniques with caution, within the first 4–6 weeks after PCI.[32]

This phenomenon was noted after PTCA, and shortly after coronary stenting. Bachmann et al.[49] observed reversible perfusion defects in the treated vascular territory within 48 hours of successful PCI in 54% of patients after PTCA or atherectomy, and in 43% of patients after stenting. Although such defects were associated with greater residual stenoses and higher plaque burdens, there was significant overlap of residual stenosis values between patients with and those without perfusion defects observed with intravascular ultrasound. The authors concluded that there are "additional mechanisms capable of impairing myocardial blood flow" and cited endothelial dysfunction as a possible cause of perfusion defects after PCI.

3. Diagnosis of Graft Disease

3.1 Myocardial Perfusion Scintigraphy

Stress myocardial perfusion scintigraphy (MPS) is a useful tool for the diagnosis of CABG disease.[50–67] Lakkis et al.[68] studied 50 patients, 51 ± 47 months after CABG. There were 119 grafts, of which 48 had >50% stenosis by angiography. Thallium-201 SPECT detected 40 of these 48 (83%) stenosed grafts. The sensitivity of thallium-201 SPECT for detecting any graft stenosis was higher than that of the exercise electrocardiogram in patients with typical recurrent angina (84% vs 24%), as well as in those with atypical symptoms (70% vs 50%). The sensitivity of thallium-201 SPECT for correctly localizing the graft stenosis site was 82% for the left anterior descending, 92% for the right coronary, and 75% for the circumflex coronary artery.

Khoury et al.[69] studied 109 patients who underwent both adenosine thallium-201 SPECT and coronary angiography at 6.7 ± 4.8 years after CABG surgery. Significant graft stenoses were present in 68 patients, 65 of whom had a corresponding perfusion defect as shown by quantitative myocardial perfusion SPECT (sensitivity 96%). Significant stenoses were present in 107 (38%) of 283 grafts. The overall specificity by quantitative myocardial perfusion SPECT was 61%. Seventy percent of the apparently false-positive perfusion defects were related to disease in ungrafted native vessels or to the presence of fixed defects in patients with previous myocardial infarction.

Elhendy et al.[70] assessed the accuracy of dobutamine stress myocardial perfusion SPECT for the diagnosis of vascular stenosis in 71 patients 3.7 ±3.5 years after CABG. Global sensitivity, specificity, and accuracy values were 81%, 79%, and 80%, respectively, whereas the same parameters for regional vascular stenosis were 66%, 83%, and 74%, respectively. Patients with multivessel stenosis had a higher number of ischemic segments and ischemic perfusion score than patients with single-vessel stenosis, respectively.[70]

3.2 Stress Echocardiography

Sawada et al.[54] reported a sensitivity of 94% for the detection of "nonrevascularized" vessels, with a specificity of 83%. In this study, the majority of patients (35 of 42) had nonrevascularized vessels, and most of these patients (n = 20) had inadequate revascularization in multiple vascular territories. The graft patency rate was not reported in this study. Crouse et al.[55] reported a sensitivity of exercise echocardiography of 98%, with a specificity of 92% for detecting "compromised regional vascular supply." In this study, most patients (112 of 125 patients) had compromised vascular supply. The graft patency rate and number of patients with a previous myocardial infarction and rest wall motion abnormalities were not reported.

Kafka et al.[56] studied 182 patients after coronary bypass grafting. These investigators found a positive predictive value of 85% and negative predictive value of 81% for exercise echocardiography. Chirillo et al.[57] studied 110 patients with previous CABG by dipyridamole stress echocardiography and Doppler evaluation of flow reserve of each CABG. Stress echocardiography showed 67% sensitivity, 91% specificity, and 71% accuracy for identification of 50% to 100% stenosis in the graft or in the recipient coronary vessel. There was a fair agreement with angiography (κ = 0.60). Identification of impaired flow reserve in a graft by Doppler had 91% sensitivity, 88% specificity, and 89% accuracy. There was good agreement with angiographic findings (κ = 0.77). The combination of the two techniques achieved 93% sensitivity, specificity, and accuracy, showing a very good agreement with the patency status of the grafts as evaluated at angiography. Elhendy et al.[58] studied 50 patients 5.1 ± 5.4 years after CABG by DSE. Graft disease or native ungrafted disease was detected in 32 patients. Sensitivity, specificity, and accuracy of DSE were 78%, 89%, and 82%, respectively.

3.3 Alternative Noninvasive Diagnostic Techniques for the Assessment of Graft Stenosis

Cardiac computed tomography started more than 10 years ago to assess CABG noninvasively using electron beam tomography. Several studies investigated the patency of grafts. Sensitivity and specificity values varied between 80% to 98% and 82% to 91%, respectively.[59] Cardiovascular Magnetic Resonance (CMR) has also been recently used for the evaluation of coronary bypass grafts. Three-dimensional MR angiography techniques, such as gadolinium-enhanced breathhold MR angiography sequence and navigator-gated MR angiography with 1-mm resolution, proved to be feasible in assessing graft patency over a longer course.[60–66] The overall sensitivity and specificity of these techniques in detecting patent grafts varied from 88% to 98% and 72% to 100%, respectively. Langerak et al.[62] studied patients with vein grafts using high-resolution MR angiography sequence, which allowed the identification of vein graft occlusion with a good sensitivity (83%) and specificity (98%–100%), respectively.

CMR with flow velocity mapping is a new noninvasive technique to assess coronary flow velocity reserve, and evaluate the functional significance of angiographic disease. Recently, the value of CMR with velocity mapping in the detection of stenoses in bypass grafts and recipient vessels was demonstrated. A sensitivity of 94% with a specificity of 63% for the detection of angiographically significant stenoses in single-vein grafts has been reported (Langerak et al.). In another study, CMR with velocity mapping yielded a sensitivity and specificity of 78% and 80% for detecting vein grafts with a significant stenosis.[60]

Salm et al.[66] compared SPECT and CMR to evaluate hemodynamic significance of angiographic findings in 46 arterial and vein grafts. There was good agreement between SPECT and CMR for functional evaluation of bypass grafts. The authors concluded that CMR may offer an alternative method to SPECT for functional characterization of angiographic lesions.

Positron emission tomography has been used predominantly in the evaluation of myocardial viability before revascularization, but not in the prediction of graft patency status after bypass surgery, although perfusion studies with this technique could conceivably be used for this purpose.

4. Risk Stratification after Myocardial Revascularization

4.1 The Role of Myocardial Perfusion Scintigraphy

Current American Heart Association guidelines recommend radionuclide studies only in symptomatic patients.[27] Various studies have demonstrated the prognostic value of stress myocardial perfusion imaging after revascularization.[67,71–79]

Lauer et al.[67] studied 873 symptom-free patients with previous CABG with the use of exercise Tl-201 SPECT. During a mean follow-up period of 3 years, there were 57 deaths and 27 patients had experienced a myocardial infarction. Tl-201 perfusion defects were predictive of death and major events after adjustment for clinical variables. Acampa et al.[79] studied 206 patients with exercise technetium-99m sestamibi SPECT between 12 and 18 months after PCI. During a mean follow-up of 37 months, 24 patients had events. The occurrence of cardiac events was higher in the presence of ischemia at SPECT in symptomatic and symptom-free patients.

Zellweger et al.[71] studied 1544 patients at a mean of 7.1 years after CABG who underwent dual-isotope SPECT imaging. During follow-up, 53 cardiac deaths occurred. A multivariate analysis identified age, ischemia, and infarct size as independent predictors of cardiac death. The authors concluded that symptomatic patients may benefit from testing at 5 years or less after

CABG and all patients may benefit from testing more than 5 years after CABG.

Miller et al.[72] studied 411 patients within 2 years after CABG by exercise Tl-201 scintigraphy. The number of abnormal Tl-201 segments was independently associated with the follow-up endpoints. Nallamothu et al.[76] studied 255 patients who underwent coronary angiography and stress Tl-201 at a mean of 5 years after CABG. During a mean follow-up period of 41 months, there were 24 cardiac deaths and 10 nonfatal myocardial infarctions. The SPECT variables of multivessel perfusion abnormality, perfusion deficit size, and increased lung thallium uptake were independent predictors of death and total events. Palmas et al.[77] studied 294 patients at a minimum of 5 years after CABG with exercise thallium SPECT. There were 20 cardiac deaths and 21 nonfatal myocardial infarctions during a mean follow-up of 31 months. The Tl-201 summed reversibility score and the presence of increased lung uptake of Tl-201 added incremental prognostic information.

Elhendy et al.[73] studied 381 patients 4.5 ± 3.2 years after myocardial revascularization (CABG in 201 patients and PCI in 180 patients), who underwent exercise or dobutamine stress tetrofosmin SPECT. Events during a mean follow-up period of 3.5 ± 1.4 years were cardiac death in 22 patients, nonfatal myocardial infarction in 11 patients, and late revascularization in 50 patients. There was no incidence of hard cardiac events (myocardial infarction or death) in the 100 patients with normal perfusion. Hard cardiac events occurred in 19% of patients with reversible perfusion abnormalities and in 4% of patients without them ($P < 0.01$). The incidence of hard cardiac events was similar in patients with and without angina before stress testing (8.6% versus 8.7%). Reversible perfusion abnormalities were independently associated with the composite endpoints of cardiac death, nonfatal myocardial infarction, and late revascularization. In an incremental multivariate analysis model, an abnormal scan offered additive value to clinical data in the prediction of hard cardiac events.

Alazraki et al.[75] studied 336 patients 1 year after revascularization (CABG or PCI) by stress Tl-201 SPECT. The incidence of composite cardiac events (death, infarction, late myocardial revascularization) was higher in patients with reversible perfusion abnormalities than in those without them (19% vs 6%).

Cottin et al.[78] studied 152 patients 5 months after coronary stenting with stress Tl-201 imaging. The relative risk of major cardiac events for patients with significant ischemia was 10.5 compared with nonischemic patients. Ho et al.[74] studied 211 patients who underwent exercise Tl-201, 1 to 3 years after PCI. Two thirds of the patients were symptomatic. The summed stress score exhibited a significant univariate association ($P = 0.047$) with the endpoint of cardiac death or myocardial infarction.

4.2 Risk Stratification after Revascularization with Stress Echocardiography

Bountioukos et al.[80] studied the prognostic value of DSE in 331 patients with previous percutaneous or surgical coronary revascularization. During a mean follow-up of 24 months, 37 patients (13%) died and 89 (30%) had at least one cardiac event (21 cardiac deaths, 11 nonfatal myocardial infarctions, and 68 late revascularizations). In multivariate analysis of clinical data, independent predictors of late cardiac events were hypertension and congestive heart failure. Ischemia on DSE was incrementally predictive of cardiac events.

Arruda et al.[81] studied the value of exercise echocardiography in predicting outcome of 718 patients who were studied at a mean of 5.7 years after CABG. During a median follow-up period of 2.9 years, cardiac events included cardiac death in 36 patients and nonfatal myocardial infarction in 40 patients. The addition of the exercise echocardiographic variables, abnormal left ventricular end-systolic volume response and exercise ejection fraction to the clinical, resting echocardiographic, and exercise electrocardiographic model provided incremental information in predicting cardiac events.

5. Conclusions

Stress echocardiography and MPS are clinically useful tools for selection of patients with known or suspected CAD who are likely to benefit from revascularization. Both imaging modalities are the mainstay tests for the diagnosis of in-stent stenosis and graft disease and are integral parts of the investigative strategies recommended by both European and American guidelines. However, CMR and multislice computed tomography are increasingly used for this purpose in centers with access to these techniques. Myocardial perfusion and wall motion abnormalities after myocardial revascularization are predictive of cardiac events and the risk associated with these abnormalities is not related to symptoms.

References

1. Cheitlin MD, Armstrong WF, Aurigemma GP, et al. ACC/AHA/ASE 2003 guideline update for the clinical application of echocardiography: summary article. A report of the American College of Cardiology/American Heart Association Task Force on Practice Guidelines (ACC/AHA/ASE Committee to Update the 1997 Guidelines for the Clinical Application of Echocardiography. J Am Soc Echocardiogr 2003;16:1091–1110.
2. Klocke FJ, Baird MG, Lorell BH, et al. American College of Cardiology; American Heart Association; American Society for Nuclear Cardiology. ACC/AHA/ASNC guidelines for the clinical use of cardiac radionuclide imaging – executive summary: a report of the American College of Cardiology/American Heart Association Task Force on Practice Guidelines (ACC/AHA/ASNC Committee to Revise the 1995 Guidelines for the Clinical Use of Cardiac Radionuclide Imaging). J Am Coll Cardiol 2003;42:1318–1333.
3. Elhendy A, Bax JJ, Poldermans D. Dobutamine stress myocardial perfusion imaging in coronary artery disease. J Nucl Med 2002;43:1634–1646.
4. Beller GA, Zaret BL. Contributions of nuclear cardiology to diagnosis and prognosis of patients with coronary artery disease. Circulation 2000;101:1465–1478.
5. Hachamovitch R, Hayes SW, Friedman JD, Cohen I, Berman DS. Comparison of the short-term survival benefit associated with revascularization compared with medical therapy in patients with no prior coronary artery disease undergoing stress myocardial perfusion single photon emission computed tomography. Circulation 2003;107:2900–2907.
6. Shaw LJ, Hachamovitch R, Heller GV, et al. Noninvasive strategies for the estimation of cardiac risk in stable chest pain patients. The Economics of Noninvasive Diagnosis (END) Study Group. Am J Cardiol 2000; 86:1–7.
7. Shaw LJ, Heller GV, Travin MI, et al. Cost analysis of diagnostic testing for coronary artery disease in women with stable chest pain. Economics of Noninvasive Diagnosis (END) Study Group. J Nucl Cardiol 1999;6: 559–569.
8. Elhendy A, Schinkel A, Bax JJ, Van Domburg RT, Poldermans D. Long-term prognosis after a normal exercise stress Tc-99m sestamibi SPECT study. J Nucl Cardiol 2003;10:261–266.
9. Hachamovitch R, Hayes S, Friedman JD, et al. Determinants of risk and its temporal variation in patients with normal stress myocardial perfusion scans: what is the warranty period of a normal scan? J Am Coll Cardiol 2003;41:1329–1340.
10. Poldermans D, Fioretti PM, Boersma E, et al. Long-term prognostic value of dobutamine-atropine stress echocardiography in 1737 patients with known or suspected coronary artery disease: a single-center experience. Circulation 1999;99:757–762.
11. Chuah SC, Pellikka PA, Roger VL, McCully RB, Seward JB. Role of dobutamine stress echocardiography in predicting outcome in 860 patients with known or suspected coronary artery disease. Circulation 1998; 97:1474–1480.
12. Marcovitz PA. Prognostic issues in stress echocardiography. Prog Cardiovasc Dis 1997;39:533–542.
13. Krivokapich J, Child JS, Walter DO, Garfinkel A. Prognostic value of dobutamine stress echocardiography in predicting cardiac events in patients with known or suspected coronary artery disease. J Am Coll Cardiol 1999;33:708–716.
14. Biagini E, Elhendy A, Bax JJ, et al. Seven-year follow-up after dobutamine stress echocardiography impact of gender on prognosis. J Am Coll Cardiol 2005;45:93–97.
15. Elhendy A, Schinkel AF, Bax JJ, Van Domburg RT, Poldermans D. Prognostic value of dobutamine stress echocardiography in patients with normal left ventricular systolic function. J Am Soc Echocardiogr 2004;17:739–743.
16. Sozzi FB, Elhendy A, Roelandt JR, et al. Long-term prognosis after normal dobutamine stress echocardiography. Am J Cardiol 2003;92:1267–1270.
17. Yusuf S, Zucker D, Peduzzi P, et al. Effect of coronary artery bypass graft surgery on survival: overview of 10-year results from randomised trials by the Coronary Artery Bypass Graft Surgery Trialists. Lancet 1994;344: 563–570.
18. Elhendy A, Schinkel AF, Van Domburg RT, Bax JJ, Valkema R, Poldermans D. Prognostic value of stress Tc-99m tetrofosmin SPECT in patients with previous myocardial infarction: impact of scintigraphic extent of coronary artery disease. J Nucl Cardiol 2004; 11:704–709.
19. Diamond GA, Forrester JS. Analysis of probability as an aid in the clinical diagnosis of coronary-artery disease. N Engl J Med 1979;300:1350–1358.
20. Elhendy A, Mahoney DW, Burger KN, McCully RB, Pellikka PA. Prognostic value of exercise echocardiography in patients with classic angina pectoris. Am J Cardiol 2004;94:559–563.
21. Gibbons RJ, Balady GJ, Beasley JW, et al. ACC/AHA guidelines for exercise testing. A report of the American College of Cardiology/American Heart Association Task Force on Practice Guidelines (Committee on Exercise Testing). J Am Coll Cardiol 1997;30:260–311.
22. Silber S, Albertsson P, Aviles FF, et al. Guidelines for percutaneous coronary interventions: the task force for percutaneous coronary interventions of the European Society of Cardiology. Eur Heart J 2005;26(8):804–847.
23. Bax JJ, Poldermans D, Elhendy A, Boersma E, Rahimtoola SH. Sensitivity, specificity, and predictive accuracies of various noninvasive techniques for detecting hibernating myocardium. Curr Probl Cardiol 2001;26:141–186.
24. Cornel JH, Bax JJ, Elhendy A, et al. Biphasic response to dobutamine predicts improvement of global left ventricular function after surgical revascularization in patients with stable coronary artery disease: implications of time course of recovery on diagnostic accuracy. J Am Coll Cardiol 1998;31:1002–1010.
25. Elhendy A, Cornel JH, Roelandt JR, et al. Impact of severity of coronary artery stenosis and the collateral circulation on the functional outcome of dyssynergic

myocardium after revascularization in patients with healed myocardial infarction and chronic left ventricular dysfunction. Am J Cardiol 1997;79:883–888.
26. Di Carli M, Sherman T, Khanna S, et al. Myocardial viability in asynergic regions subtended by occluded coronary arteries: relation to the status of collateral flow in patients with chronic coronary artery disease. J Am Coll Cardiol 1994;23:860–868.
27. Smith SC Jr, Dove JT, Jacobs AK, et al. ACC/AHA guidelines of percutaneous coronary interventions (revision of the 1993 PTCA guidelines) – executive summary. A report of the American College of Cardiology/American Heart Association Task Force on Practice Guidelines committee to revise the 1993 guidelines for percutaneous transluminal coronary angioplasty). J Am Coll Cardiol 2001;37:2215–2239.
28. Bax JJ, Poldermans D, Schinkel AF, et al. Perfusion and contractile reserve in chronic dysfunctional myocardium: relation to functional outcome after surgical revascularization. Circulation 2002;106:I14–18.
29. Bax JJ, Poldermans D, Elhendy A, et al. Improvement of left ventricular ejection fraction, heart failure symptoms and prognosis after revascularization in patients with chronic coronary artery disease and viable myocardium detected by dobutamine stress echocardiography. J Am Coll Cardiol 1999;34:163–169.
30. Senior R, Kaul S, Lahiri A. Myocardial viability on echocardiography predicts long-term survival after revascularization in patients with ischemic congestive heart failure. J Am Coll Cardiol 1999;33:1848–1854.
31. Pagley PR, Beller GA, Watson DD, et al. Improved outcome after coronary bypass surgery in patients with ischemic cardiomyopathy and residual myocardial viability. Circulation 1997;96:793–800.
32. Giedd KN, Bergmann SR. Myocardial perfusion imaging following percutaneous coronary intervention: the importance of restenosis, disease progression, and directed reintervention. J Am Coll Cardiol 2004;43:328–336.
33. Anderson HV, Shaw RE, Brindis RG, et al. A contemporary overview of percutaneous coronary interventions: the American College of Cardiology–National Cardiovascular Data Registry (ACC-NCDR). J Am Coll Cardiol 2000;39;1096–1103.
34. Lowe HC, Oesterle SN, Khachigian LM. Coronary in-stent restenosis: current status and future strategies. J Am Coll Cardiol 2002;39:183–193.
35. Goldman S, Zadina K, Moritz T, et al. VA Cooperative Study Group. Long-term patency of saphenous vein and left internal mammary artery grafts after coronary artery bypass surgery: results from a Department of Veterans Affairs Cooperative Study. J Am Coll Cardiol 2004;44:2149–2156.
36. Fitz GM, Gibbon LR, Henryk P, et al. Coronary bypass graft fate and patient outcome: angiographic follow-up of 5,065 grafts related to survival and reoperation in 1,388 patients during 25 years. J Am Coll Cardiol 1996;28:616–626.
37. Pfisterer M, Rickenbacher P, Kiowski W, Muller-Brand J, Burkart F. Silent ischemia after percutaneous transluminal coronary angioplasty: incidence and prognostic significance. J Am Coll Cardiol 1993;22:1446–1454.
38. Krone RJ, Hardison RM, Chaitman BR, et al. Risk stratification after successful coronary revascularization: the lack of a role for routine exercise testing. J Am Coll Cardiol 2001;38:136–142.
39. Legrand V, Raskinet B, Laarman G, Danchin N, Morel MA, Serruys PW. Diagnostic value of exercise electrocardiography and angina after coronary artery stenting. Am Heart J 1997;133:240–248.
40. Hecht HS, Shaw RE, Chin HL, et al. Silent ischemia after coronary angioplasty: evaluation of restenosis and extent of ischemia in asymptomatic patients by tomographic thallium-201 exercise imaging and comparison with symptomatic patients. J Am Coll Cardiol 1991;17:670–677.
41. Marie PY, Danchin N, Karcher G, et al. Usefulness of exercise SPECT-thallium to detect asymptomatic restenosis in patients who had angina before coronary angioplasty. Am Heart J 1993;126:571–577.
42. Milan E, Zoccarato O, Terzi A, et al. Technetium-99m-sestamibi SPECT to detect restenosis after successful percutaneous coronary angioplasty. J Nucl Med 1996;37:1300–1305.
43. Kósa I, Blasini R, Schneider-Eicke J, et al. Myocardial perfusion scintigraphy to evaluate patients after coronary stent implantation. J Nucl Med 1998;39:1307–1311.
44. Milavetz JJ, Miller JD, Hodge DO, Holmes DR, Gibbons RJ. Accuracy of single-photon emission computed tomography myocardial perfusion imaging in patients with stents in native coronary arteries. Am J Cardiol 1998;82:857–861.
45. Beygui F, Le Feuvre C, Maunoury C, et al. Detection of coronary restenosis by exercise electrocardiography thallium-201 perfusion imaging and coronary angiography in asymptomatic patients after percutaneous transluminal coronary angioplasty. Am J Cardiol 2000;86:35–40.
46. Galassi AR, Foti R, Azzarelli S, et al. Usefulness of exercise tomographic perfusion imaging for detection of restenosis after coronary stent implantation. Am J Cardiol 2000;85:1362–1364.
47. Caner B, Oto A, Ovunc K, Kiratli P. Prediction of restenosis after successful percutaneous coronary angioplasty by dobutamine thallium-201 scintigraphy. Int J Cardiol 1998;66:175–181.
48. Takeuchi M, Miura Y, Toyokawa T, Araki M, Nakashima Y, Kuroiwa A. The comparative diagnostic value of dobutamine stress echocardiography and thallium stress tomography for detecting restenosis after coronary angioplasty. J Am Soc Echocardiogr 1995;8:696–702.
49. Bachmann R, Sechtem U, Voth E, Schroder J, Hopp HW, Schicha H. Dipyridamole scintigraphy and intravascular ultrasound after successful coronary intervention. J Nucl Med 1997;38:553–558.
50. Kureshi SA, Tamaki N, Yonekura Y, et al. Value of stress thallium-201 emission tomography for predicting improvement after coronary bypass grafting and assessing graft patency. Jpn Heart J 1989;30:287–299.
51. Pfisterer M, Emmenegger H, Schmitt HE, et al. Accuracy of serial myocardial perfusion scintigraphy with thallium-201 for prediction of graft patency early and later after coronary artery bypass surgery: a controlled, prospective study. Circulation 1982;66:1017–1024.
52. Rasmussen SL, Nielsen SL, Amtorp O, Folke K, Fritz-Hansen P. 201-Thallium imaging as an indicator of graft patency after coronary artery bypass surgery. Eur Heart J 1984;5:494–499.
53. Ritchie JL, Narahara KA, Trobaugh GB, Williams DL, Hamilton GW. Thallium-201 myocardial imaging before and after coronary revascularization: assess-

ment of regional myocardial blood flow and graft patency. Circulation 1977;56:830–836.
54. Sawada SG, Judson WE, Ryan T, Armstrong W, Feigenbaum H. Upright bicycle exercise echocardiography after coronary artery bypass grafting. Am J Cardiol 1989;64:1123–1129.
55. Crouse LJ, Vacek JL, Beauchamp GD, Porter CB, Rosamond TL, Kramer PH. Exercise echocardiography after coronary artery bypass grafting. Am J Cardiol 1992; 70:572–576.
56. Kafka H, Leach AJ, Fitzgibbon GM. Exercise echocardiography after coronary artery bypass surgery: correlation with coronary angiography. J Am Coll Cardiol 1995;25:1019–1023.
57. Chirillo F, Bruni A, De Leo A, et al. Usefulness of dipyridamole stress echocardiography for predicting graft patency after coronary artery bypass grafting. Am J Cardiol 2004;93:24–30.
58. Elhendy A, Geleijnse ML, Roelandt JR, et al. Assessment of patients after coronary artery bypass grafting by dobutamine stress echocardiography. Am J Cardiol 1996;77:1234–1236.
59. Budoff MJ, Achenbach S, Duerinckx A. Clinical utility of computed tomography and magnetic resonance techniques for noninvasive coronary angiography. J Am Coll Cardiol 2003;42:1867–1878.
60. van der Wall EE, Langerak SE. Magnetic resonance imaging for the non-invasive detection of stenosis in coronary artery bypass grafts: clinical reality? Int J Cardiovasc Imaging 2002;18:479–482.
61. Langerak SE, Vliegen HW, Jukema JW, et al. Value of magnetic resonance imaging for the noninvasive detection of stenosis in coronary artery bypass grafts and recipient coronary arteries. Circulation 2003;107: 1502–1508.
62. Langerak SE, Vliegen HW, de Roos A, et al. Detection of vein graft disease using high-resolution magnetic resonance angiography. Circulation 2002;105:328–333.
63. Wintersperger BJ, Engelmann MG, von Smekal A, et al. Patency of coronary bypass grafts: assessment with breath-hold contrast-enhanced MR angiography – value of a non-electrocardiographically triggered technique. Radiology 1998;208:345–351.
64. Vrachliotis TG, Bis KG, Aliabadi D, et al. Contrast-enhanced breath-hold MR angiography for evaluating patency of coronary artery bypass grafts. AJR Am J Roentgenol 1997;168:1073–1080.
65. Kessler W, Achenbach S, Moshage W, et al. Usefulness of respiratory gated magnetic resonance coronary angiography in assessing narrowings ≥50% in diameter in native coronary arteries and in aortocoronary bypass conduits. Am J Cardiol 1997;80:989–993.
66. Salm LP, Bax JJ, Vliegen HW, et al. Functional significance of stenoses in coronary artery bypass grafts: evaluation by single-photon emission computed tomography perfusion imaging, cardiovascular magnetic resonance, and angiography. J Am Coll Cardiol 2004;44:1877–1882.
67. Lauer MS, Lytle B, Pashkow F, Snader CE, Marwick TH. Prediction of death and myocardial infarction by screening with exercise-thallium testing after coronary-artery-bypass grafting. Lancet 1998;351:615–622.
68. Lakkis NM, Mahmarian JJ, Verani MS. Exercise thallium-201 single photon emission computed tomography for evaluation of coronary artery bypass graft patency. Am J Cardiol 1995;76:107–111.
69. Khoury AF, Rivera JM, Mahmarian JJ, Verani MS. Adenosine thallium-201 tomography in evaluation of graft patency late after coronary artery bypass graft surgery. J Am Coll Cardiol 1997;29:1290–1295.
70. Elhendy A, van Domburg RT, Bax JJ, et al. Dobutamine-atropine stress myocardial perfusion SPECT imaging in the diagnosis of graft stenosis after coronary artery bypass grafting. J Nucl Cardiol 1998;5:491–497.
71. Zellweger MJ, Lewin HC, Lai S, et al. When to stress patients after coronary artery bypass surgery? Risk stratification in patients early and late post-CABG using stress myocardial perfusion SPECT: implications of appropriate clinical strategies. J Am Coll Cardiol 2001;37:144–152.
72. Miller TD, Christian TF, Hodge DO, Mullan BP, Gibbons RJ. Prognostic value of exercise thallium-201 imaging performed within 2 years of coronary artery bypass graft surgery. J Am Coll Cardiol 1998;31:848–854.
73. Elhendy A, Schinkel AF, Van Domburg RT, Bax JJ, Valkema R, Poldermans D. Risk stratification of patients after myocardial revascularization by stress Tc-99m tetrofosmin myocardial perfusion tomography. J Nucl Cardiol 2003;10:615–622.
74. Ho KT, Miller TD, Holmes DR, Hodge DO, Gibbons RJ. Long-term prognostic value of Duke treadmill score and exercise thallium-201 imaging performed one to three years after percutaneous transluminal coronary angioplasty. Am J Cardiol 1999;84:1323–1327.
75. Alazraki NP, Krawczynska EG, Kosinski AS, et al. Prognostic value of thallium-201 single-photon emission computed tomography for patients with multivessel coronary artery disease after revascularization (the Emory Angioplasty versus Surgery Trial [EAST]). Am J Cardiol 1999;84:1369–1374.
76. Nallamothu N, Johnson JH, Bagheri B, Heo J, Iskandrian AE. Utility of stress single-photon emission computed tomography (SPECT) perfusion imaging in predicting outcome after coronary artery bypass grafting. Am J Cardiol 1997;80:1517–1521.
77. Palmas W, Bingham S, Diamond GA, et al. Incremental prognostic value of exercise thallium-201 myocardial single-photon emission computed tomography late after coronary artery bypass surgery. J Am Coll Cardiol 1995;25:403–409.
78. Cottin Y, Rezaizadeh K, Touzery C, et al. Long-term prognostic value of 201Tl single-photon emission computed tomographic myocardial perfusion imaging after coronary stenting. Am Heart J 2001;141:999–1006.
79. Acampa W, Petretta M, Florimonte L, Mattera A, Cuocolo A. Prognostic value of exercise cardiac tomography performed late after percutaneous coronary intervention in symptomatic and symptom-free patients. Am J Cardiol 2003;91:259–263.
80. Bountioukos M, Elhendy A, van Domburg RT, et al. Prognostic value of dobutamine stress echocardiography in patients with previous coronary revascularisation. Heart 2004;90:1031–1035.
81. Arruda AM, McCully RB, Oh JK, Mahoney DW, Seward JB, Pellikka PA. Prognostic value of exercise echocardiography in patients after coronary artery bypass surgery. Am J Cardiol 2001;87:1069–1073.

13

Imaging Techniques for Assessment of Viability and Hibernation

Arend F.L. Schinkel, Don Poldermans, Abdou Elhendy, and Jeroen J. Bax

The number of patients presenting with heart failure has increased exponentially over the past decade.[1] It has been estimated that 4.7 million people in the United States have chronic heart failure, with 400 000 new cases per year, resulting in 1 million hospitalizations.[1] Coronary artery disease is the most common cause of congestive heart failure. More than 70% of patients with heart failure symptoms have underlying coronary disease, whereas the majority of patients with ischemic left ventricular (LV) dysfunction had a previous myocardial infarction.[1,2] The prognosis of these patients is poor, particularly in men, and many of them need intermittent hospitalization because of decompensated heart failure. In the near future, chronic heart failure will be encountered even more often, as our population ages.[1,2] The clinical characteristics of the patient, the presence of ischemia, and severity of LV dysfunction determine the prognosis in heart failure.

In the past, ischemic LV dysfunction was considered an irreversible process. In patients with heart failure, medical therapy was regarded as the only management option. Currently, three routinely available directions of treatment are available: medical treatment, heart transplantation, and revascularization. Newer treatment

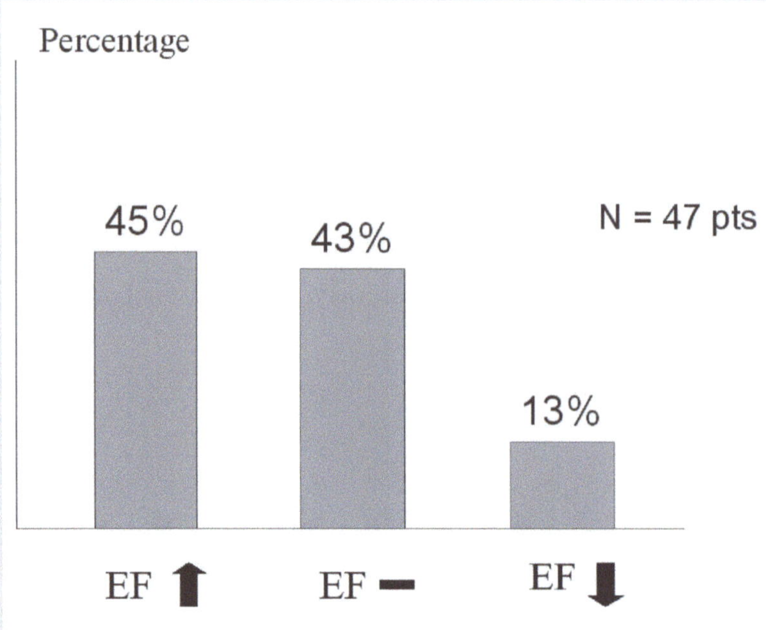

Figure 13.1. Changes in LVEF, observed in 47 patients with ischemic cardiomyopathy undergoing revascularization. Improvement in LVEF was defined as increase in LVEF ≥5% after revascularization. (Data based on Bax et al.[13])

modalities include laser treatment, advanced surgery, assist devices, and even artificial hearts,[3] and transplantation of different (progenitor) cells.[4] These options should currently be considered experimental, but may offer alternative therapies in the future. Medical therapy has improved substantially over the past years, with the introduction of angiotensin-converting enzyme inhibitors, angiotensin-II receptor blockers, and spironolactone. Four recent trials have demonstrated the value of beta-adrenergic blocking agents in the treatment of patients with heart failure.[5] Finally, amiodarone has been demonstrated to reduce sudden death in patients with heart failure.[6] Despite all of these new drugs, mortality of patients with severe heart failure remains high; Cowie et al.[7] reported that the 12-month mortality was 38%, and extrapolation of these results demonstrated 5-year mortality >70%. The second option, heart transplantation, has a fairly good long-term prognosis, but the limited number of donor hearts is largely exceeded by the demand.[8] In addition, many patients with heart failure have significant comorbidities, excluding them as candidates for heart transplantation. Revascularization is the third option in patients with heart failure. The major drawback in performing revascularization in these patients is the high peri-procedural morbidity and mortality.[9] However, a substantial survival benefit after surgical revascularization compared with medical therapy has been shown in a number of retrospective studies.[10] Also, improvement in regional contractile function and in LV ejection fraction (LVEF) was shown after revascularization.[11] Because LVEF is an important prognostic parameter,[12] improvement in LVEF may (at least in part) contribute to the improved survival. However, not all segments improve in contractile function and the LVEF does not improve in all patients. Almost only one third of segments show functional improvement and <50% of patients improve their LVEF (Figure 13.1).[13] Consequently, identification of patients with the potential of improvement in LVEF and survival is needed to justify the higher risk of surgery in this group.

1. Pathophysiology/Definition of Viable Myocardium

More than two decades ago, Diamond et al.[14] and Rahimtoola et al.[15] recognized that ischemic LV dysfunction is not always permanent and introduced the theory of myocardial hibernation. It was proposed that hibernation refers to a condition of chronic sustained abnormal contraction caused by chronic underperfusion in patients with coronary artery disease in whom revascularization causes recovery of function.[15] The presence of hibernating myocardium has become an additional motive to perform coronary revascularization. In fact, if a significant amount of hibernating myocardium is present, coronary revascularization may substantially improve regional and global contractile function in selected patients with ischemic LV dysfunction.[16]

In this group of patients, several (patho)physiologic conditions of the myocardium may coexist. Often there are areas with preserved contractile function supplied by coronary arteries without significant stenoses. However, contractile dysfunction can be observed in myocardial regions that are subtended by a stenotic or occluded coronary artery. Coronary occlusion may cause cellular death resulting in irreversibly scarred myocardium.[17] Alternatively, the reduced contractile function could be the result of impaired perfusion reserve or even of a reduction in resting blood flow. This physiologic down-regulation of contractile function, also referred to as myocardial hibernation, is probably an adaptive response to myocardial ischemia, to protect myocytes from irreversible damage. Such down-regulation of function is associated with "down-regulation" of structure. Biopsy samples obtained during coronary bypass surgery from viable dysfunctional myocardium is characterized by quite severe changes of the sarcomeres, the intracellular space and organelles, the cardiomyocytes themselves, and the extracellular matrix. There is a mixture of normal, atrophied, and hypertrophied myocytes with or without evidence of necrosis. Cells with partial or complete loss of intracellular contractile proteins are seen, sarcomeres and myofibrils are lost, and there is intracellular accumulation of glycogen and variable intercellular fibrosis. There is also new expression of proteins such as smooth muscle α-actin, titin, and cardiotin that are normally found in fetal tissue.[18]

Restoration of blood flow by coronary revascularization may result in recovery of contractile function in hibernating myocardium. The time course of functional recovery may vary considerably,[19] and depends on several factors including the duration and severity of myocardial ischemia, the time and completeness of myocardial revascularization, and the extent of ultrastructural alterations within the dysfunctional myocardium. Less severely damaged myocardium may improve within 3 months of revascularization, in contrast to severely damaged tissue, which may take more than 1 year to fully recovery in function after revascularization. Changes at cellular or subcellular level could therefore be reversible before significant structural disorders occur because long-term hibernation may lead to irreversible loss of myocardial function.

Besides hibernating myocardium, patients with ischemic LV dysfunction often have some regions that contain stunned myocardium. Myocardial stunning is characterized by a depressed contractile function in the presence of normal resting blood flow,[17] and may occur as a result of repetitive ischemic episodes. Thus, conflicting findings in terms of functional improvement in patients with LV dysfunction may result from different duration or state of chronic dysfunction, and repetitive stunning and hibernation may represent different parts of the spectrum of chronic dysfunction. However, from a clinical point of view, this differentiation may not be so important, because both repetitively stunned and hibernating myocardium probably need to be revascularized in order to improve function. Finally, chronic dysfunction can also result from a combination of nontransmural necrosis with viable (normal) myocardium. The subendocardial layer contributes significantly to contraction and subendocardial necrosis >20% of the myocardial wall results frequently in akinesia.[20] Revascularization of these regions will not improve contractile function, but may be of clinical relevance in terms of preventing remodeling.[21]

2. Methods to Assess Myocardial Viability and Hibernation

Some information on myocardial viability can be derived from the surface electrocardiogram (ECG), but imaging is more contributing in this clinical setting. Several noninvasive imaging techniques have been developed to identify dysfunctional but viable tissue: dobutamine stress echocardiography, single photon emission computed tomography (SPECT) imaging with thallium-201 or technetium-99m-labeled tracers, and positron emission tomography (PET) metabolic imaging with F18-fluorodeoxyglucose

Table 13.1. Characteristics of dysfunctional but viable myocardium

Characteristic	Technique	Signs of viability
Contractile reserve	Dobutamine echocardiography Dobutamine MRI	Improved contraction during infusion of low-dose dobutamine
Intact cell membrane	Thallium-201 SPECT	Tracer activity > 50% Redistribution (>10%)
Intact mitochondria	Technetium-99m SPECT	Tracer activity > 50% Improved tracer uptake after nitrates
Glucose metabolism	^{18}F-FDG imaging	Tracer activity > 50% Preserved perfusion/^{18}F-FDG uptake Perfusion-metabolism mismatch

Source: Schinkel et al.[85]
^{18}F-FDG, F18-fluorodeoxyglucose; MRI, magnetic resonance imaging; SPECT, single photon emission computed tomography.

(^{18}F-FDG). These techniques evaluate different characteristics of viable myocardium and can delineate irreversibly scarred from dysfunctional but viable myocardium (Table 13.1). These characteristics include intact perfusion, cell membrane integrity, intact mitochondria, preserved glucose utilization, and contractile reserve.[22] The presence or absence of the different characteristics may be related to the severity of ultrastructural damage at the myocyte level. Contractile reserve has most frequently been evaluated by echocardiography [or magnetic resonance imaging (MRI)] using dobutamine stress. In addition, it has been recently demonstrated that contractile reserve may also be evaluated by ECG-gated SPECT (using technetium-99m-labeled agents) during dobutamine infusion.[23] Perfusion can be evaluated by thallium-201 or technetium-99m-labeled tracers, cell membrane integrity can be evaluated by thallium-201, intact mitochondria can be probed by technetium-99m-labeled tracers, preserved glucose and free fatty acid metabolism can be assessed by ^{18}F-FDG and radio-labeled fatty acids, respectively.

2.1 Surface Electrocardiography

The ECG has the advantage of a widespread availability and limited costs, but there is no clear correlation between Q waves on surface electrocardiography and the presence of viable or nonviable myocardium.[24] Also, the relation between ST-segment changes (in particular ST-segment elevation) during stress testing and myocardial viability is not entirely clear. However, QT dispersion is related to the presence of myocardial viability in patients with ischemic LV dysfunction. Patients with low QT dispersion (<70 ms) are likely to have a substantial amount of viable myocardium, whereas patients with a high QT dispersion have predominantly nonviable scar tissue.[25]

2.2 Echocardiography

2.2.1 Echocardiography at Rest

From the resting images, an initial impression on myocardial viability can be derived. A marked end-diastolic wall thinning virtually excludes the presence of viable tissue.[26] In patients without a clear thinning of the dysfunctional area, low-dose dobutamine echocardiography can be performed to evaluate myocardial viability.

2.2.2 Stress Echocardiography

Stress echocardiography is a widespread and relatively inexpensive method to assess myocardial viability (Figure 13.2; see color section). Dysfunctional but viable myocardium is characterized by preserved contractile reserve during dobutamine echocardiography.[27] In hypokinetic or akinetic regions, an improvement of contraction during low-dose dobutamine infusion (5–10 μg/kg/min) is indicative of viable tissue and, if there is also inducible ischemia, then a biphasic response is seen with initial improvement of function and deterioration at higher doses. This

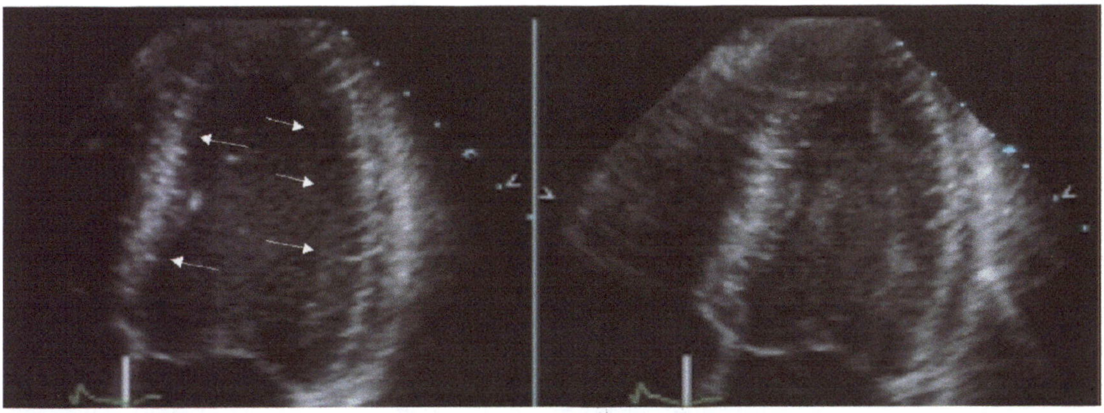

Figure 13.2. Transthoracic two-dimensional echocardiogram (apical four-chamber view, end-systolic) at rest (left panel) and during infusion of low-dose dobutamine (right panel) in a patient with ischemic cardiomyopathy and severe hypokinesia of the septum and lateral wall. The arrows indicate regions with improved contractility during low-dose dobutamine infusion. During low-dose dobutamine, improved contraction of the dysfunctional segments indicates myocardial viability. (Image reproduced from Schinkel et al.[85])

response is highly predictive of recovery of function after revascularization. Dobutamine stress echocardiography is a safe test in patients with ischemic LV dysfunction.

2.2.3 Tissue Doppler Imaging

Tissue Doppler imaging was developed to overcome the subjective nature of the echocardiographic examination. Tissue Doppler imaging allows quantification of myocardial function using the Doppler shift principle. Tissue Doppler images may be displayed as color-encoded velocity profiles in M-mode and two-dimensional (2D) imaging formats. For viability assessment, tissue Doppler echocardiography may be combined with low-dose dobutamine infusion. In dysfunctional but viable myocardium, baseline tissue velocity is impaired, and myocardial velocities increase during dobutamine infusion. The major advantage of this technique is the high spatial and temporal resolution. Rambaldi et al.[28] compared pulsed-wave tissue Doppler imaging with dobutamine stress echocardiography in 40 patients with ischemic LV dysfunction, using FDG imaging as the gold standard for viability assessment. Tissue Doppler imaging resulted in a significant increase in sensitivity of dobutamine echocardiography to detect viable myocardium.

2.2.4 Contrast Echocardiography

Two-dimensional echocardiography may be combined with intravenous contrast administration to assess both myocardial function and myocardial perfusion in real-time (Figure 13.3; see color section). A bolus of contrast is intravenously injected followed by a saline flush. Echocardiography using a low mechanical index is started before contrast injection and subsequently "flash" imaging with high mechanical index is used at peak contrast intensity to destroy the microbubbles in the myocardium, to avoid artifacts, and to visualize myocardial contrast replenishment. Because contrast echocardiography allows simultaneous assessment of function and perfusion, stunned myocardium can be distinguished from hibernation. Shimoni et al.[29] studied the accuracy of contrast echocardiography in 20 patients with coronary disease and LV dysfunction who underwent bypass surgery. Optimal identification of viable myocardium was obtained when perfusion as assessed by contrast echocardiography was analyzed quantitatively.

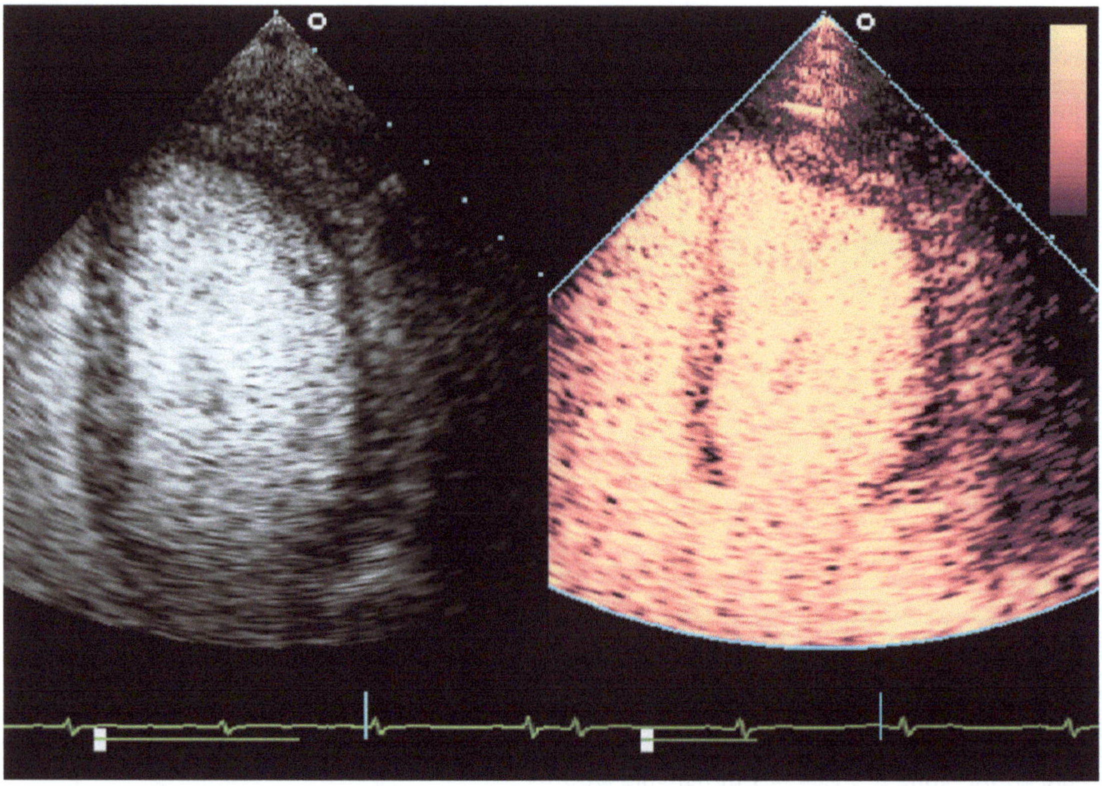

Figure 13.3. Transthoracic two-dimensional echocardiogram after intravenous injection of a contrast agent (apical four-chamber view). Opacification of the left ventricular cavity after administration of the contrast agent facilitates endocardial border delineation (left panel). Subsequently, a destruction-fill method can be used to assess myocardial perfusion. In this example, a perfusion defect was present in the hypokinetic lateral wall. (Image reproduced from Schinkel et al.[85])

2.3 Radionuclide Imaging with Single Photon Emitting Tracers

2.3.1 Thallium-201 Chloride

Thallium-201 chloride is a cation emitting mainly X-rays of energy 67–82 keV (88% abundance) and gamma photons of 135 and 167 keV (12% abundance) and is taken up by the myocardium similarly to potassium. The initial uptake of thallium-201 after injection is mainly determined by regional perfusion, whereas sustained uptake (usually imaged at 3–4 hours after injection) is dependent on cell-membrane integrity, which reflects viability.[30] Because redistribution can be slow or incomplete in regions subtended by a vessel with severe stenosis, the usual stress/redistribution protocol can underestimate myocardial viability and additional steps to ensure complete assessment of viability and hibernation are required. These include late redistribution imaging at 8–72 hours after stress injection, reinjection of tracer at rest after redistribution imaging, and a resting injection on a separate day with both early and delayed imaging or adjuncts aimed at speeding redistribution toward the pattern of viability such as ribose or nitrates.

From the above, the most frequently used protocols in the clinical setting are rest-redistribution and stress-redistribution-reinjection imaging.[30] The former provides information on perfusion at rest and viability, whereas the latter provides information on both viability and stress-induced ischemia. With rest-redistribution imaging, two sets of images are acquired: the first set of images (obtained directly after tracer injection), represents perfusion and the second set of images (obtained 3–4 hours after tracer injection) represents viability. With the stress-redistribution-reinjection protocol, the initial images are obtained after stress, the second set of images is obtained 3–4 hours thereafter (redistribution images); then, a second dose of thallium-201 is injected and usually 1 hour later, the reinjection images are acquired. The reinjection images provide information on viability whereas changes of thallium-201 uptake between stress and resting images represent inducible ischemia.

Several different features of thallium-201 scintigraphy that indicate the presence of myocardial viability have been proposed as markers of hibernation: stress-induced perfusion defects alone are not predictive of functional recovery and a number of studies have focused on the resting images. The most frequently used criterion is simply the extent of regional uptake. Activity >50% of maximum in hypokinetic/akinetic segments has been used as a criterion for hibernation but this threshold has been arbitrarily defined. The level of thallium-201 uptake is linearly related to the proportion of remaining viable myocardium, hence it should be treated as a continuous variable and not as a dichotomy distinguishing viable from nonviable tissue.[31] Receiver operating characteristic curves have therefore been used and the most accurate threshold for defining clinically significant hibernation seems to be between 55% and 60%. Redistribution after a resting injection has been reported as a marker of hibernation but it appears to be a relatively uncommon observation, although is highly predictive of hibernation when seen.

2.3.2 Technetium-99m Sestamibi or Tetrofosmin SPECT

The uptake and retention of these tracers depends on perfusion, cell membrane integrity, and mitochondrial function (membrane potential).[32] Most studies for assessment of viability have been performed with technetium-99m sestamibi, but recent studies with technetium-99m tetrofosmin have shown a comparable value of this tracer for the assessment of viability.[33,34]

Most frequently, technetium-99m-labeled tracers are injected under resting conditions.[32] In these studies, dysfunctional segments with tracer uptake >50%–60% are considered viable.[32] Because attenuation may result in lower activities, particularly in the inferior and lower septal wall, Schneider and colleagues[35] have suggested to use a cutoff value of 35% tracer uptake in these regions. A major advantage is that recent technical developments have resulted in ECG-gated imaging that allows simultaneous assessment of myocardial perfusion and contractile function. Currently, gating is performed in the majority of studies with the technetium-99m-labeled agents. ECG gating provides additional information on function and may potentially enhance accuracy to detect viable myocardium.[36] Several studies have shown that technetium-99m-labeled tracers may underestimate myocardial viability as compared with ^{18}F-FDG PET. However, more recent studies have shown that viability assessment using technetium-99m-labeled tracers can be improved by oral or intravenous administration of nitrates[37] which enhance blood flow and hence tracer uptake to myocardial regions that are subtended by severely stenosed arteries.

2.4 Radionuclide Imaging with Positron Emitting Tracers

2.4.1 ^{18}F-FDG PET and SPECT

FDG is a glucose analog (one $^{-}$OH group has been replaced by an F-18 atom) and initial transsarcolemmal uptake is identical to that of glucose. After phosphorylation, FDG-6-PO_4 remains trapped in the myocyte (physical half-life 110 min) and provides a strong signal for imaging.[38] With ^{18}F-FDG imaging, the metabolic circumstances determine tracer uptake[39]; optimal studies are performed during hyperinsulinemic euglycemic clamping (see chapter on PET), but for clinical routine oral glucose loading is frequently used.[39] For optimal identification of viable tissue, ^{18}F-FDG imaging should be combined with perfusion imaging. Dysfunctional segments with preserved perfusion and ^{18}F-FDG uptake are thought to represent (repetitively) stunned myocardium whereas segments with reduced perfusion but preserved ^{18}F-FDG uptake (perfusion-^{18}F-FDG mismatch) hibernating myocardium.[38] In contrast, segments with reduced perfusion and concordantly reduced ^{18}F-FDG uptake represent scar tissue.

Because ^{18}F-FDG is a positron emitter, ^{18}F-FDG imaging has been traditionally performed with PET cameras. PET, however, is not available in all centers; hence, FDG imaging is often performed

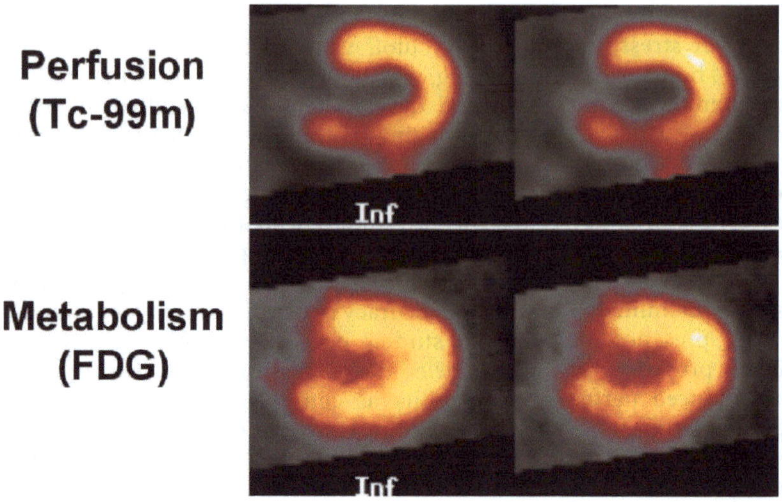

Figure 13.4. Dual-isotope simultaneous acquisition SPECT scan (vertical long-axis slices) showing a substantial perfusion-metabolism mismatch in the inferior wall, indicating viable myocardium. (Image reproduced from Schinkel et al.[85])

nowadays with conventional gamma cameras using 511-keV collimators (Figure 13.4; see color section).[38] Several studies have demonstrated that the ^{18}F-FDG gamma camera and ^{18}F-FDG PET imaging have a comparable diagnostic accuracy for assessment of myocardial viability.[38,40] More recently, gamma cameras with the option of coincidence imaging have been developed; this approach provides images of better quality, but necessitates the use of attenuation correction.[38]

2.4.2 Other PET Techniques

Besides ^{18}F-FDG imaging, PET may be combined with C11-acetate to assess residual oxidative metabolism. Clearance rates of C11-acetate from dysfunctional myocardium reflect the rate of oxidative phosphorylation. The rate of oxidative metabolism has been demonstrated to correlate closely to improvement of function after myocardial revascularization. Gropler and colleagues[41] studied 34 patients with coronary artery disease and compared C11-acetate PET with ^{18}F-FDG PET for prediction of functional recovery after revascularization. Assessment of regional oxidative metabolism by PET with C11-acetate was an accurate predictor of functional recovery with a slightly higher accuracy than ^{18}F-FDG PET.

Rubidium-82 is another PET tracer, which allows assessment of both myocardial perfusion and cell membrane integrity. Yoshida and Gould[42] evaluated a large cohort of patients with rubidium-82 and demonstrated that the prognosis of patients with chronic ischemic LV dysfunction was dependent on both the infarct size and the extent of viability assessed by the rubidium-82 images.

PET also allows noninvasive assessment of the water-perfusable tissue fraction (PTF). This parameter is derived from quantification of myocardial blood flow using ^{15}O-water. Information on the accuracy of PTF for the prediction of functional recovery is still limited. Bax et al.[43] studied 34 patients with ischemic LV dysfunction who underwent myocardial revascularization. Both ^{15}O-water and ^{18}F-FDG PET were used to compare the relative merits of myocardial blood flow, metabolic rate of glucose (absolute and relative), and PTF. High sensitivities for the prediction of improvement of LVEF after revascularization were observed for all PET indexes, whereas the specificities of the various techniques were somewhat lower.

2.5 Magnetic Resonance Imaging

MRI is another technique for assessment of myocardial viability. Currently, three techniques are being used:

- Resting MRI to measure end-diastolic wall thickness

- Dobutamine MRI to evaluate contractile reserve
- Contrast-enhanced MRI to detect the extent and transmurality of scar tissue

2.5.1 Resting MRI

Resting MRI can be used to assess end-diastolic wall thickness and contractile function at rest. Several studies have demonstrated that segments with an end-diastolic wall thickness <6 mm are likely to represent transmural scar formation and contractile function will not improve after myocardial revascularization. However, dysfunctional segments with a preserved wall thickness will not always recover after revascularization. This may be related to the presence of subendocardial scar in these segments. Therefore, additional testing is needed to predict outcome in the segments with preserved end-diastolic wall thickness.

2.5.2 Dobutamine MRI

Dobutamine MRI can be used to evaluate contractile reserve, in a similar manner to dobutamine echocardiography.[44] The major advantage of MRI over echocardiography is the increased resolution of MRI, allowing for quantitative assessment of wall thickening during dobutamine infusion, and thus avoiding the subjective analysis of echocardiography. Baer and coworkers[44] have initially demonstrated an excellent agreement between dobutamine MRI and ^{18}F-FDG PET, and in a subsequent study,[45] the authors have reported a sensitivity of 89% with a specificity of 94% to predict improvement in resting function after revascularization.

2.5.3 Contrast-enhanced MRI

When combined with gadolinium-based contrast agents, MRI allows precise detection of scar tissue. Animal experiments have demonstrated an excellent correlation between the extent and transmurality of scar tissue and contrast enhancement on MRI.[46] Because of the high spatial resolution, MRI is currently the only technique that permits evaluation of the different myocardial layers, and contrast-enhanced imaging makes detection of subendocardial scar tissue possible (Figure 13.5). Klein et al.[47] compared contrast-enhanced MRI with ^{18}F-FDG PET in 31 patients with ischemic LV dysfunction and showed an excellent agreement between the two techniques to detect scar tissue. More recently, Kim et al.[48] applied contrast-enhanced MRI in 41 patients with chronic LV dysfunction undergoing revascularization. The authors demonstrated that the likelihood of improvement in regional contractility after revascularization progressively decreased as the transmural extent of hyperenhancement increased.

2.6 Electromechanical Mapping

Electromechanical assessment of myocardial viability has been developed using the NOGA system, a catheter-based, nonfluoroscopic, 3D endocardial mapping system. Based on integrated assessment of function and electrical activity, delineation of dysfunctional but viable myocardium is possible. When a threshold amplitude of 7.5 mV was used, the sensitivity and specificity for detecting viable myocardium were 77% and 75%.[49] Electromechanical mapping is not the technique of choice to assess viability in a diagnostic setting, but may be

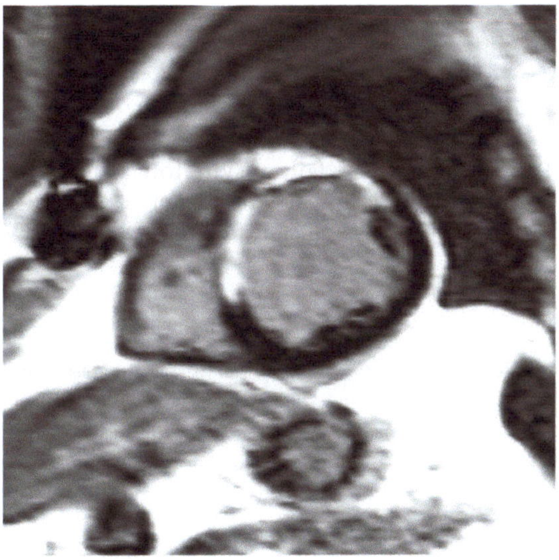

Figure 13.5. Contrast-enhanced MRI in a patient with an anterior wall infarction. The hyper-enhanced (white) region indicates infarction. (Image reproduced from Schinkel et al.[85])

useful as a platform for additional procedures. For example, electromechanical mapping may be used to assess viability and generate 3D LV reconstruction before laser revascularization, intramyocardial gene transfer, or myoblast injection.[50]

3. Clinical Importance of Viability Assessment

3.1 Incidence of Viable Myocardium

Although from a theoretical point of view, assessment of viability in patients may be of interest, the key question is how frequently is viable myocardium present in chronic dysfunctional myocardium? Various studies have reported on the incidence of viability in patients with chronic ischemic LV dysfunction (Table 13.2), with varying results. Recent studies have demonstrated that in >50% of patients with ischemic LV dysfunction, a clinically significant amount of viable myocardium is present. In these patients, revascularization may improve, and even normalize LVEF, heart failure symptoms, exercise capacity, and survival. Moreover, data from 258 consecutive patients indicated that recovery of global function could be anticipated after myocardial revascularization in almost 40% of patients with ischemic LV dysfunction.[51]

3.2 Revascularization in Patients' LV Dysfunction and Viable Myocardium

Patients with heart failure symptoms caused by coronary artery disease represent a high-risk group. In various registries of patients with LV dysfunction, the 1-year mortality rates range from 15% to 40%.[1,2] Coronary revascularization seems to be a good treatment for the subgroup of patients with a substantial amount of dysfunctional but viable myocardium.[16] These observations indicate the need of a careful analysis of patients with heart failure including assessment of viability, on a routine basis. Two-dimensional echocardiography is an excellent first step to assess regional and global contractile function and valvular function. Assessment of myocardial viability and perfusion reserve can then be performed as described above, followed by coronary angiography to assess the extent and severity of coronary artery disease and to evaluate whether the coronary anatomy is amendable to coronary revascularization. Based on the findings, therapy can then be tailored to the individual patient.

Improvement of function after revascularization is still considered the "gold standard" for viability. Pooled data from 105 viability studies, with 3003 patients, included 15045 dysfunctional segments, with 7941 (53%) improving in function after revascularization.[52] Clinically, improvement in global LV function (LVEF) may be more important than improvement in regional function. The majority of the viability studies have evaluated only improvement of regional LV function, but studies that included assessment of LVEF before and after revascularization consistently showed that patients with a substantial amount of viable tissue improved their LVEF after revascularization. It is currently unclear whether an improvement in LVEF is strictly necessary to result in an improved prognosis. Samady et al.[53] recently evaluated 135 patients with ischemic LV dysfunction (LVEF ≤30%) undergoing revascularization and 68 patients (65%) improved their LVEF by at least 5 units. Survival at 32 ± 23 months was compara-

Table 13.2. Incidence of viable myocardium in patients with ischemic cardiomyopathy

Author, year	No. of patients	LVEF (%)	Viability technique	Incidence of viability
Al-Mohammad et al.,[80] 1998	27	19 ± 6	^{18}F-FDG/N13 ammonia PET	52
Auerbach et al.,[81] 1999	283	26 ± 8	^{18}F-FDG/N13 ammonia PET	55
Schinkel et al.,[82] 2001	83	25 ± 7	DSE	57
Fox et al.,[83] 2001	27	NA	Tc-99m MIBI/TF SPECT	37
Schinkel et al.,[84] 2002	104	25 ± 7	^{18}F-FDG/Tc-99m TF SPECT	61

Source: Bax et al.[86]
DSE, dobutamine stress echocardiography; ^{18}F-FDG, F18-fluorodeoxyglucose; LVEF, left ventricular ejection fraction; MIBI, technetium-99m sestamibi; TF, tetrofosmin.

ble between patients with and without improvement in LVEF. However, viability assessment was not part of the routine workup of these patients and improvement in LVEF was assessed within 6 weeks after revascularization. This time interval is probably too short to exclude improvement in LVEF, because recovery of function may occur up to 1 year after revascularization.[54] Still, it is important to realize that besides improvement in LVEF, revascularization of viable myocardium may have a beneficial effect on prevention of remodeling, arrhythmias, and sudden cardiac death which may also improve longevity.[21]

Finally, Beanlands and colleagues[55] have demonstrated the impact of viability assessment on subsequent management of patients with ischemic LV dysfunction. The authors evaluated 67 patients with ^{18}F-FDG PET, while therapy was already established on clinical information. Thus, 11 patients were scheduled for heart transplantation, 38 for revascularization, and 18 for medical treatment. Based on the presence/absence of viability, the treatment changed in 31 patients (46%). In a different study, the same group demonstrated that once viability has been detected, revascularization should follow as soon as possible.[56] The authors evaluated 35 patients with ^{18}F-FDG PET; 18 patients underwent early revascularization (12 ± 9 days after ^{18}F-FDG PET) and 17 underwent late revascularization (145 ± 97 days after ^{18}F-FDG PET). In the early revascularization group, the preoperative mortality was lower, the LVEF improved in more patients postoperatively, and the event-free survival was higher. All these findings support the necessity and clinical relevance of viability assessment in patients with ischemic LV dysfunction.

3.2.1 *Prediction of Improvement of Function after Revascularization*

The relative merits of the techniques for prediction of functional recovery are summarized in Figure 13.6. All the aforementioned techniques have been studied extensively, although most expertise has been obtained with dobutamine stress echocardiography and nuclear imaging. In general, the nuclear imaging techniques seem to have a higher sensitivity for the prediction of functional recovery whereas stress echocardiography seems to be more specific.[52] The difference between nuclear imaging and dobutamine stress echocardiography for the prediction of functional improvement after myocardial revascularization is even more obvious when only direct comparative studies are considered.[52] Pooling of head-to-head comparisons underscores the differences in sensitivity and specificity of dobutamine stress echocardiography and radionuclide imaging (Figure 13.7). This discrepancy may be related to different levels of ultrastructural cell damage in dysfunctional myocardium. The inotropic response during dobutamine stimula-

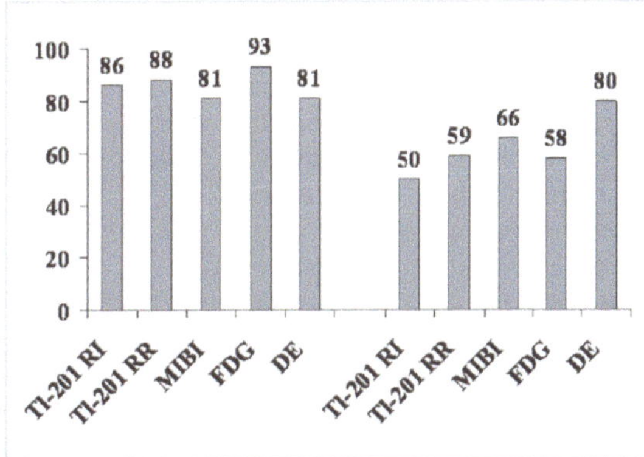

Figure 13.6. Sensitivity and specificity of the various viability techniques to predict improvement of regional LV function after revascularization. DE, dobutamine echocardiography; ^{18}F-FDG, F18-fluorodeoxyglucose; MIBI, technetium-99m sestamibi; Tl-201 RI, thallium-201 reinjection; Tl-201 RR, thallium-201 rest-redistribution. (Data based on Bax et al.[52])

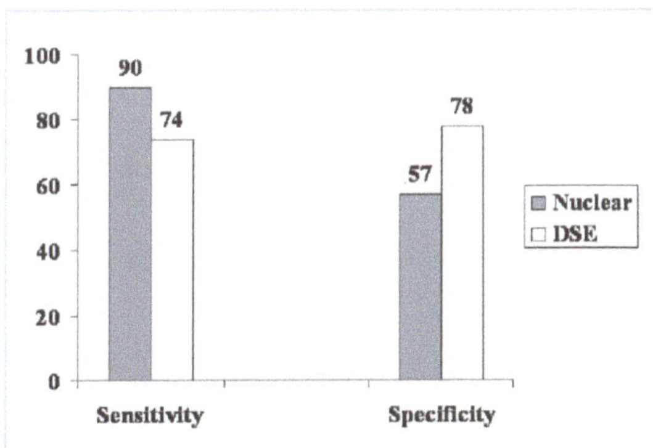

Figure 13.7. Sensitivity and specificity of dobutamine stress echocardiography (DSE) and nuclear imaging techniques [based on pooled data from 11 studies (n = 325 patients) that performed a direct comparison between dobutamine stress echocardiography and nuclear imaging to predict improvement in regional left ventricular function after revascularization]. The sensitivity of the nuclear techniques was significantly higher compared with dobutamine stress echocardiography, whereas the specificity of dobutamine stress echocardiography was significantly higher. (Data based on Bax et al.[52])

tion may no longer be intact while more basic characteristics such as cell membrane integrity and glucose utilization are still preserved. However, most of the studies had a limited follow-up with a maximum of 3–6 months post-revascularization.[52] Recent data have demonstrated that improvement of function may occur up to 1 year after revascularization[19,54] because more severely damaged myocardium might need longer time to recover in function as compared with mildly damaged myocardium. It is conceivable that more severely damaged myocardium may no longer exhibit contractile reserve, but may still have preserved perfusion, cell membrane integrity, or glucose utilization. More studies are needed to confirm these findings.

From a clinical point of view, improvement of global function is more important than improvement of regional function. A total of 29 studies, with 758 patients evaluated LVEF before and after revascularization, in relation to presence/absence of viability. The results of these studies are summarized in Table 13.3; the studies consistently showed improvement in LVEF in patients with substantial viable myocardium.

3.2.2 Amount of Viable Myocardium Needed for Improvement

An open question is the exact amount of viable myocardium that is needed to result in improvement of LVEF post-revascularization. The extent of improvement in global function is related to the extent of dysfunctional but viable tissue. Several studies have demonstrated that a certain amount of dysfunctional but viable tissue is needed for an improvement of global function after revascularization. Usually a cut-off level of ≥4 viable segments in a 16-segment model of the left ventricle is advised as a cutoff value to predict improvement of LVEF.[16] This cutoff value represents approximately 25% of the left ventricle, and may be used to identify patients who may benefit from revascularization. However, this cutoff value of viable segments is to some extent artificial, because other factors also influence recovery of function. Recent data indicate that in patients with ischemic LV dysfunction and a mixture of viable and nonviable tissue, the extent of scar tissue should also be taken into account in order to accurately predict functional recovery after revascularization.[57] In addition, remodeling and enlargement of the left ventricle should also be considered. Remodeling of the left ventricle resulting in an enlarged end-systolic volume may prevent global recovery, even in patients with substantial viability.[58] Consideration of these issues and integration into a mathematic model may further improve patient selection for revascularization. Furthermore, surgical therapeutic options are developing rapidly, and myocardial revascularization can now be combined with additional mitral valve repair to further optimize outcome. Also, resection of LV aneurysms can be considered in the presence of extensive scar formation.

3.2.3 Alternative Endpoints: Symptoms, Exercise Capacity, Remodeling

Additional endpoints besides improvement in function have been considered. Few studies have evaluated the relation between preoperative viability and postoperative improvement in symptoms and exercise capacity. Several viability studies [evaluating New York Heart Association (NYHA) class before and after revascularization] have shown that mean NYHA class

Table 13.3. Pooled data from viability studies predicting improvement of LVEF after revascularization

		Viability present		Viability absent	
Technique	No. studies/patients	LVEF pre	LVEF post	LVEF pre	LVEF post
Thallium-201	5/96	30	38	29	31
Tc-99m tracers	4/75	47	53	40	39
^{18}F-FDG PET	12/333	37	47	39	40
DSE	8/254	35	43	35	36

Source: Bax et al.[86]

"LVEF pre" and "LVEF post" indicate LVEF before and after revascularization. DSE, dobutamine stress echocardiography; ^{18}F-FDG, F18-fluorodeoxyglucose; LVEF, left ventricular ejection fraction; PET, positron emission tomography.

improved significantly in patients with viable myocardium. Individual data, however, varied significantly, and accurate prediction of improvement of symptoms in an individual patient remains difficult.[59] Few studies have demonstrated that exercise capacity improved in patients with viable myocardium.[60–62] Marwick and colleagues[60] evaluated 23 patients with ^{18}F-FDG PET before revascularization and demonstrated that patients with extensive viability improved significantly in exercise capacity post-revascularization (from 5.6 ± 2.7 to 7.5 ± 1.7 METS). Similar results were reported by DiCarli et al.[61] and Gunning et al.[62]

Moreover, the relation between preoperative assessment of viability and prevention of remodeling has been studied recently. DalleMule and coworkers[63] evaluated 50 patients with ischemic LV dysfunction with thallium-201 stress-redistribution-reinjection SPECT before revascularization. Patients with residual viability/ischemia (involving >20% of the LV) improved in LVEF (from 35% ± 6% to 43% ± 6%, $P < .001$) and actually demonstrated reversed remodeling after revascularization: LV end-systolic volume index decreased from 68 ± 16 to 52 ± 14 mL/m^2 ($P < .001$), and LV end-diastolic volume index decreased from 103 ± 21 to 91 ± 18 mL/m^2 ($P < .001$). These patients also improved in NYHA class and exhibited excellent long-term survival (100%). In contrast, patients with predominantly scar tissue failed to improve in LVEF (34% ± 4% vs 33% ± 7%, not significant), and exhibited ongoing remodeling (LV end-systolic volume index increased from 70 ± 14 to 78 ± 23 mL/m^2, $P < .001$, and LV end-diastolic volume index increased from 106 ± 19 to 116 ± 25 mL/m^2, $P < .001$), without improvement in NYHA class and worse long-term prognosis (29% event rate).

3.2.4 Prediction of Long-term Prognosis

The most important clinical issue is the prediction of long-term survival. Various studies have evaluated long-term prognosis in relation to treatment and viability; in these studies, the patients were grouped according to the presence/absence of viable tissue and treatment (medical versus revascularization). Currently, 17 prognostic studies are available (seven using ^{18}F-FDG PET, four thallium-201 imaging, and six dobutamine echocardiography).[47,48,61–75] The results of these studies are summarized in Figure 13.8.

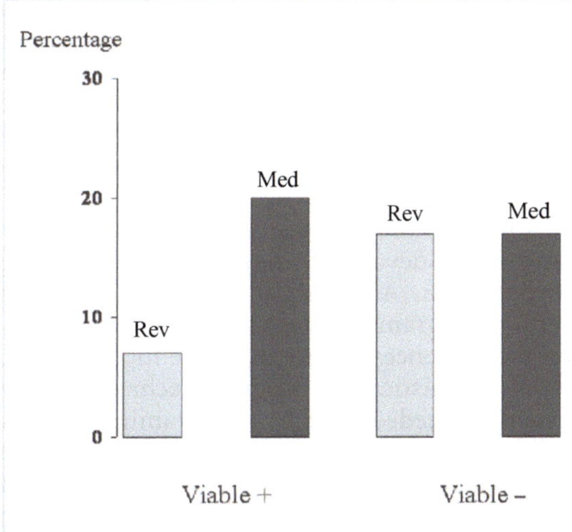

Figure 13.8. Prognostic value of the viability studies: event rate is plotted versus presence/absence of viability and treatment (medical/revascularization). The highest mortality is observed in the patients with viable myocardium who were treated medically. (Based on pooled data[16,64–79]). Med, medical treatment; Revasc, revascularization.

A high mortality rate was observed in all groups, except in the group of patients with viable myocardium who underwent revascularization. Thus, the combination of viability and revascularization seems to favorably influence long-term survival. However, all of these studies were nonrandomized, retrospective analyses, and the findings need to be confirmed in randomized, prospective trials.

4. Conclusion

Heart failure secondary to chronic coronary artery disease is an important challenge in clinical cardiology. With the increasing number of patients presenting with heart failure, assessment of myocardial viability and prediction of functional recovery after myocardial revascularization have become common clinical issues. In patients with viable myocardium, revascularization is likely to result in improvement of regional and global LV function, heart failure symptoms, and long-term prognosis.

Patients with severely depressed LVEF (<35%), secondary to chronic coronary artery disease [without a recent (<1 month) myocardial infarction] and presenting with heart failure are candidates for additional viability testing. Patients with accompanying angina or those with preserved LVF should not be referred routinely for viability testing. In addition, the precise role of viability assessment in patients with an acute myocardial infarction is open to research.

A number of noninvasive imaging techniques have been developed to identify hibernating myocardium. Although the ECG and resting echocardiogram may provide some initial clues on the presence/absence of viable myocardium, more sophisticated imaging techniques are usually needed. Both dobutamine stress echocardiography and nuclear imaging have been extensively used for the assessment of hibernating myocardium, and newer techniques such as MRI may further enhance the assessment of viability. Besides assessment of viability, additional factors need to be considered to allow precise prediction of outcome, including the presence and extent of scar tissue, the severity of remodeling of the left ventricle, and the presence of concomitant mitral regurgitation. Integrated information on all these issues will optimize patient selection for surgery, resulting in improved outcome and long-term survival after revascularization. Finally, despite the fact that a wealth of information on viability assessment in patients with ischemic LV dysfunction has been obtained over the past decade, prospective randomized trials, comparing medical therapy versus revascularization, and focusing on prognosis, are needed.

References

1. Ho KK, Pinsky JL, Kannel WB, et al. The epidemiology of heart failure: the Framingham Study. J Am Coll Cardiol 1993;22:6A–13A.
2. Gheorghiade M, Bonow RO. Chronic heart failure in the United States – a manifestation of coronary artery disease. Circulation 1998;97:282–289.
3. Westaby S, Frazier OH, Pigott DW, Saito S, Jarvik RK. Implant technique for the Jarvik 2000 Heart. Ann Thorac Surg 2002;73:1337–1340.
4. Xu C, Police S, Rao N, Carpenter MK. Characterization and enrichment of cardiomyocytes derived from human embryonic stem cells. Circ Res 2002;91:501–508.
5. Braunwald E. Expanding indications for beta-blockers in heart failure. N Engl J Med 2001;344:1711–1712.
6. Caims JA, Connolly SJ, Roberts R, Gent M, for the CAMIAT investigators. Randomized trial of outcome after myocardial infarction in patients with frequent or repetitive premature depolarizations. Lancet 1997; 349:675–682.
7. Cowie MR, Wood DA, Coats AJ, et al. Incidence and aetiology of heart failure: a population-based study. Eur Heart J 1999;20:421–428.
8. Evans RW, Manninen DL, Garrison LP, et al. Donor availability as the primary determinant of the future of heart transplantation. JAMA 1986;255:1892–1898.
9. Baker DW, Jones R, Hodges J, et al. Management of heart failure. III. The role of revascularization in treatment of patients with moderate or severe left ventricular systolic dysfunction. JAMA 1994;272:1528–1534.
10. Pigott JD, Kouchoukos NT, Oberman A, et al. Late results of surgical and medical therapy for patients with coronary artery disease and depressed left ventricular function. J Am Coll Cardiol 1985;5:1036–1045.
11. Elefteriades JA, Tolis G, Levi E, Mills LK, Zaret BL. Coronary artery bypass grafting in severe left ventricular dysfunction: excellent survival with improved ejection fraction and functional state. J Am Coll Cardiol 1993; 22:1411–1417.
12. White HD, Norris RM, Brown MA, Brandt PWT, Whitlock RML, Wild CJ. Left ventricular end-systolic volume as the major determinant of survival after recovery from myocardial infarction. Circulation 1987;76:44–51.
13. Bax JJ, Visser FC, Poldermans D, et al. Relationship between preoperative viability and postoperative improvement in LVEF and heart failure symptoms. J Nucl Med 2001;42:79–86.
14. Diamond GA, Forrester JS, deLuz PL, et al. Post-extrasystolic potentiation of ischemic myocardium by atrial stimulation. Am Heart J 1978;95:204–209.
15. Rahimtoola SH. A perspective on the three large multicenter randomized clinical trials of coronary bypass surgery for chronic stable angina. Circulation 1985; 72(suppl V):V123–135.
16. Bax JJ, Poldermans D, Elhendy A, et al. Improvement of left ventricular ejection fraction, heart failure symptoms and prognosis after revascularization in patients with chronic coronary artery disease and viable myocardium detected by dobutamine stress echocardiography. J Am Coll Cardiol 1999;34:163–169.
17. Kloner RA, Bolli R, Marban E, et al. Medical and cellular implications of stunning, hibernation, and preconditioning: an NHLBI workshop. Circulation 1998;97:1848–1867.
18. Underwood SR, Bax JJ, vom Dahl J, et al. Imaging techniques for the assessment of patients with chronic ischaemic heart failure. Eur Heart J 2004;25:815–836.
19. Vanoverschelde JL, Depre C, Gerber BL, et al. Time course of functional recovery after coronary artery bypass graft surgery in patients with chronic left ventricular ischemic dysfunction. Am J Cardiol 2000; 85:1432–1439.
20. Kaul S. There may be more to myocardial viability than meets the eye. Circulation 1995;92:2790–2793.
21. Bonow RO. Identification of viable myocardium. Circulation 1996;94:2674–2680.
22. Bax JJ, Van Eck-Smit BLF, Van der Wall EE. Assessment of tissue viability: clinical demand and problems. Eur Heart J 1998;19:847–858.
23. Leoncini M, Marcucci G, Sciagra R, et al. Nitrate-enhanced gated technetium 99m sestamibi SPECT for evaluating regional wall motion at baseline and during low-dose dobutamine infusion in patients with chronic coronary artery disease and left ventricular dysfunction: comparison with two-dimensional echocardiography. J Nucl Cardiol 2000;7:426–431.

24. Schinkel AFL, Bax JJ, Elhendy A, et al. Assessment of viable tissue in Q-wave regions by metabolic imaging using single-photon emission computed tomography in ischemic cardiomyopathy. Am J Cardiol 2002;89: 1171–1175.
25. Schinkel AFL, Bountioukos M, Poldermans D, et al. Relation between QT dispersion and myocardial viability in ischemic cardiomyopathy. Am J Cardiol 2003;92:712–715.
26. Cwajg JM, Cwajg E, Nagueh SF, et al. End-diastolic wall thickness as a predictor of recovery of function in myocardial hibernation: relation to rest-redistribution Tl-201 tomography and dobutamine stress echocardiography. J Am Coll Cardiol 2000;35: 1152–1161.
27. Cigarroa CG, deFilippi CR, Brickner E, et al. Dobutamine stress echocardiography identifies hibernating myocardium and predicts recovery of left ventricular function after coronary revascularization. Circulation 1993;88:430–436.
28. Rambaldi R, Poldermans D, Bax JJ, et al. Doppler tissue velocity sampling improves diagnostic accuracy during dobutamine stress echocardiography for the assessment of viable myocardium in patients with severe left ventricular dysfunction. Eur Heart J 2000;21: 1091–1098.
29. Shimoni S, Frangogiannis NG, Aggeli CJ, et al. Identification of hibernating myocardium with quantitative intravenous myocardial contrast echocardiography: comparison with dobutamine echocardiography and thallium-201 scintigraphy. Circulation 2003;107: 538–544.
30. Dilsizian V, Borrow RO. Current diagnostic techniques for assessing myocardial viability in patients with hibernating and stunned myocardium. Circulation 1993;87:1–20.
31. Perrone-Filardi P, Pace L, Prastaro M, et al. Assessment of myocardial viability in patients with chronic coronary artery disease. Rest-4-hour-24-hour 201Tl tomography versus dobutamine echocardiography. Circulation 1996;94:2712–2719.
32. Bonow RO, Dilsizian V. Thallium-201 and technetium-99m-sestamibi for assessing viable myocardium. J Nucl Med 1992;33:815–818.
33. Gunning MG, Anagnostopoulos A, Knight CJ, et al. Comparison of 201Tl, 99mTc-tetrofosmin, and dobutamine magnetic resonance imaging for identifying hibernating myocardium. Circulation 1998;98:1869–1874.
34. Gunning MG, Kaprielian RR, Pepper J, et al. The histology of viable and hibernating myocardium in relation to imaging characteristics. J Am Coll Cardiol 2002; 39:428–435.
35. Schneider CA, Voth E, Gawlich S, et al. Significance of rest technetium-99m sestamibi imaging for the prediction of improvement of left ventricular dysfunction after Q wave myocardial infarction: importance of infarct location adjusted thresholds. J Am Coll Cardiol 1998;32:648–654.
36. Levine MG, McGill CC, Ahlberg AW, et al. Functional assessment with electrocardiographic gated single-photon computed tomography improves the ability of technetium-99m sestamibi myocardial perfusion imaging to predict myocardial viability in patients undergoing revascularization. Am J Cardiol 1999;83: 1–5.
37. Sciagra R, Pellegri M, Pupi A, et al. Prognostic implications of Tc-99m sestamibi viability imaging and subsequent therapeutic strategy in patients with chronic coronary artery disease and left ventricular dysfunction. J Am Coll Cardiol 2000;36:739–745.
38. Bax JJ, Patton JA, Poldermans D, Elhendy A, Sandler MP. 18-Fluorodeoxyglucose imaging with PET and SPECT: cardiac applications. Semin Nucl Med 2000;30:281–298.
39. Gropler RJ. Methodology governing the assessment of myocardial glucose metabolism by positron emission tomography and fluorine 18-labeled fluorodeoxyglucose. J Nucl Cardiol 1994;1:S1–S14.
40. Sandler MP, Patton JA. Fluorine 18-labeled fluorodeoxyglucose myocardial single-photon emission computed tomography: an alternative for determining myocardial viability. J Nucl Cardiol 1996;3: 342–349.
41. Gropler RJ, Geltman EM, Sampathkumaran K, et al. Comparison of carbon-11-acetate with fluorine-18-fluorodeoxyglucose for delineating viable myocardium by positron emission tomography. J Am Coll Cardiol 1993;22:1587–1597.
42. Yoshida K, Gould KL. Quantitative relation of myocardial infarct size and myocardial viability by positron emission tomography to left ventricular ejection fraction and 3-year mortality with and without revascularization. J Am Coll Cardiol 1993;22:984–997.
43. Bax JJ, Fath-Ordoubadi F, Boersma E, et al. Accuracy of PET in predicting functional recovery after revascularisation in patients with chronic ischaemic dysfunction: head-to-head comparison between blood flow, glucose utilisation and water-perfusable tissue fraction. Eur J Nucl Med Mol Imaging 2002;29:721–727.
44. Baer FM, Voth E, Schneider CA, et al. Comparison of low-dose dobutamine-gradient-echo magnetic resonance imaging and positron emission tomography with^{18F}fluorodeoxyglucose in patients with chronic coronary artery disease. A functional and morphological approach to the detection of residual myocardial viability. Circulation 1995;91:1006–1015.
45. Baer FM, Theissen P, Schneider CA, et al. Dobutamine magnetic resonance imaging predicts contractile recovery of chronically dysfunctional myocardium after successful revascularization. J Am Coll Cardiol 1998;31:1040–1048.
46. Kim RJ, Fieno DS, Parrish TB, et al. Relationship of MRI delayed contrast enhancement to irreversible injury, infarct age, and contractile function. Circulation 1999; 100:1992–2002.
47. Klein C, Nekolla SG, Bengel FM, et al. Assessment of myocardial viability with contrast-enhanced magnetic resonance imaging: comparison with positron emission tomography. Circulation 2002;105:162–167.
48. Kim RJ, Wu E, Rafael A, et al. The use of contrast-enhanced magnetic resonance imaging to identify reversible myocardial dysfunction. N Engl J Med 2000; 343:1445–1453.
49. Koch KC, vom Dahl J, Wenderdel M, et al. Myocardial viability assessment by endocardial electroanatomic mapping: comparison with metabolic imaging and functional recovery after coronary revascularization. J Am Coll Cardiol 2001;38:91–98.
50. Strauer BE, Kornowski R. Stem cell therapy in perspective. Circulation 2003;107:929–934.
51. Schinkel AFL, Poldermans D, Vanoverschelde JL, et al. Incidence of recovery of contractile function following

revascularization in patients with ischemic left ventricular dysfunction. Am J Cardiol 2004;93:14–17.
52. Bax JJ, Poldermans D, Elhendy A, Boersma E, Rahimtoola SH. Sensitivity, specificity, and predictive accuracies of various noninvasive techniques for detecting hibernating myocardium. Curr Probl Cardiol 2001;26:142–186.
53. Samady H, Elefteriades JA, Abbott BG, Mattera JA, McPherson CA, Wackers FJ. Failure to improve left ventricular function after coronary revascularization is not associated with worse outcome. Circulation 1999;100:1298–1304.
54. Bax JJ, Visser FC, Poldermans D, et al. Time course of functional recovery of stunned and hibernating segments after surgical revascularization. Circulation 2001;104(suppl 1):I314–I318.
55. Beanlands RSB, DeKemp R, Smith S, Johansen HL, Ruddy TD. F-18-fluorodeoxyglucose PET imaging alters clinical decision making in patients with impaired ventricular function. Am J Cardiol 1997;79: 1092–1095.
56. Beanlands RSB, Hendry PJ, Masters RG, et al. Delay in revascularization is associated with increased mortality rate in patients with severe left ventricular dysfunction and viable myocardium on fluorine 18-fluorordeoxyglucose positron emission tomography. Circulation 1998;98:II-51–II-56.
57. Rizzello V, Schinkel AFL, Bax JJ, et al. Individual prediction of functional recovery after coronary revascularization in patients with ischemic cardiomyopathy: the scar-to-biphasic model. Am J Cardiol 2003;91: 1406–1409.
58. Schinkel AFL, Poldermans D, Rizzello V, et al. Why do patients with ischemic cardiomyopathy and a substantial amount of viable myocardium not always recover in function after revascularization? J Thorac Cardiovasc Surg 2004;127:385–390.
59. Tawakol A, Gewirtz H. Does CABG improve left ventricular ejection fraction in patients with ischemic cardiomyopathy and does it matter? J Nucl Med 2001;42:87–90.
60. Marwick TH, Nemec JJ, Lafont A, Salcedo EE, MacIntyre WJ. Prediction by postexercise fluoro-18 deoxyglucose positron emission tomography of improvement in exercise capacity after revascularization. Am J Cardiol 1992;69:854–859.
61. DiCarli MF, Asgarzadie F, Schelbert HR, et al. Quantitative relation between myocardial viability and improvement in heart failure symptoms after revascularization in patients with ischemic cardiomyopathy. Circulation 1995;92:3436–3444.
62. Gunning MG, Chua TP, Harrington D, et al. Hibernating myocardium: clinical and functional response to revascularisation. Eur J Cardiothorac Surg 1997;11: 1105–1112.
63. DalleMule J, Bax JJ, Zingone B, et al. The beneficial effect of revascularization on jeopardized myocardium: reverse remodeling and improved long-term prognosis. Eur J Cardiothorac Surg 2002;22:426.
64. Williams MJ, Odabashian J, Laurer MS, Thomas JD, Marwick TH. Prognostic value of dobutamine echocardiography in patients with left ventricular dysfunction. J Am Coll Cardiol 1996;27:132–139.
65. Di Carli M, Davidson M, Little R, et al. Value of metabolic imaging with positron emission tomography for evaluating prognosis in patients with coronary artery disease and left ventricular dysfunction. Am J Cardiol 1994;73:527–533.
66. Eitzman D, Al-Aouar ZR, Kanter HL, et al. Clinical outcome of patients with advanced coronary artery disease after viability studies with positron emission tomography. J Am Coll Cardiol 1992;20:559–565.
67. Vom Dahl J, ALtehoefer C, Sheehan FH, et al. Effect of myocardial viability assessed by technetium-99m-sestamibi SPECT and fluorine-18-18F-FDG PET on clinical outcome in coronary artery disease. J Nucl Med 1997;38:742–748.
68. Yoshida K, Gould KL. Quantitative relation of myocardial infarct size and myocardial viability by positron emission tomography to left ventricular ejection fraction and 3-year mortality with and without revascularization. J Am Coll Cardiol 1993;22:984–987.
69. Lee KS, Marwick TH, Cook SA, et al. Prognosis of patients with left ventricular dysfunction, with and without viable myocardium after myocardial infarction. Relative efficacy of medical therapy and revascularization. Circulation 1994;90:2687–2694.
70. Pagano D, Lewis ME, Townend JN, Davies P, Camici PG, Bonser RS. Coronary revascularization for postischemic heart failure: how myocardial viability affects survival. Heart 1999;82:684–688.
71. Tamaki N, Kawamoto M, Takahashi N, et al. Prognostic value of an increase in fluorine-18 deoxyglucose uptake in patients with myocardial infarction: comparison with stress thallium imaging. J Am Coll Cardiol 1993; 22:1621–1627.
72. Gioia G, Powers J, Heo J, Iskandrian AS. Prognostic value of rest-redistribution tomographic thallium-201 imaging in ischemic cardiomyopathy. Am J Cardiol 1995;75:759–762.
73. Pagley PR, Beller GA, Watson DD, Gimple LW, Ragosta M. Improved outcome after coronary bypass surgery in patients with ischemic cardiomyopathy and residual myocardial viability. Circulation 1997;96:793–800.
74. Zafrir N, Leppo JA, Reinhardt CP, Dahlberg ST. Thallium reinjection versus standard stress/delay redistribution imaging for prediction of cardiac events. J Am Coll Cardiol 1998;31:1280–1285.
75. Cuocolo A, Petretta M, Nicolai E, et al. Successful coronary revascularization improves prognosis in patients with previous myocardial infarction and evidence of viable myocardium at thallium-201 imaging. Eur J Nucl Med 1998;25:60–68.
76. Chaudhry FA, Tauke JT, Alessandrini RS, et al. Prognostic implications of myocardial contractile reserve in patients with coronary artery disease and left ventricular dysfunction. J Am Coll Cardiol 1999;34:730–738.
77. Senior R, Kaul S, Lahiri A. Myocardial viability on echocardiography predicts long-term survival after revascularization in patients with ischemic congestive heart failure. J Am Coll Cardiol 1999;33:1848–1854.
78. Afridi I, Grayburn PA, Panza J, Oh JK, Zoghbi WA, Marwick TH. Myocardial viability during dobutamine echocardiography predicts survival in patients with coronary artery disease and severe left ventricular systolic dysfunction. J Am Coll Cardiol 1998;32:921–926.
79. Meluzin J, Cerny J, Frelich M, et al. Prognostic value of the amount of dysfunctional but viable myocardium in revascularized patients with coronary artery disease and left ventricular dysfunction. J Am Coll Cardiol 1998;32:912–920.

80. Al-Mohammad A, Mahy IR, Norton MY, et al. Prevalence of hibernating myocardium in patients with severely impaired ischemic left ventricles. Heart 1998;80:559–564.
81. Auerbach MA, Schöder H, Gambhir SS, et al. Prevalence of myocardial viability as detected by positron emission tomography in patients with ischemic cardiomyopathy. Circulation 1999;99:2921–2926.
82. Schinkel AFL, Bax JJ, Boersma E, et al. How many patients with ischemic cardiomyopathy exhibit viable myocardium? Am J Cardiol 2001;88:561–564.
83. Fox KF, Cowie MR, Wood DA, et al. Coronary artery disease as the cause of incident heart failure in the population. Eur Heart J 2001;22:221–236.
84. Schinkel AFL, Bax JJ, Sozzi FB, et al. Prevalence of myocardial viability assessed by single photon emission computed tomography in patients with chronic ischaemic left ventricular dysfunction. Heart 2002;88:125–130.
85. Schinkel AFL, Bax JJ, Poldermans D. Clinical assessment of myocardial hibernation. Heart 2005;91:111–117.
86. Bax JJ, Poldermans D, van der Wall EE. Evaluation of hibernating myocardium. Heart 2004;90:1239–1240.

14

Myocardial Ischemia in Conditions Other Than Atheromatous Coronary Artery Disease

Eike Nagel and Roderic I. Pettigrew

1. Causes and Basic Pathophysiology

Regulation of coronary blood flow is a complex process that is determined by multiple factors. These are more fully reviewed in Chapter 1. Myocardial ischemia is generally associated with atherosclerotic coronary artery disease (CAD). However, it may be provoked under circumstances when coronary arteries are normal, or may occur when coronary vascular function is abnormal despite the absence of atherosclerosis. The former may occur when arterial oxygen-carrying capacity is insufficient (a supply problem), or when oxygen requirement is excessive (a demand problem). Myocardial oxygen supply may be insufficient in the presence of significant anemia, severe hypoxia, or carbon monoxide poisoning. If these problems are severe enough, myocardial ischemia will result, even in the absence of what would normally be considered a flow-limiting coronary stenosis. Similarly, if oxygen demand is markedly increased by, for example, a prolonged tachyarrhythmia acutely, or by increased myocardial mass (ventricular hypertrophy) chronically, then this will outstrip oxygen delivery and will result in myocardial ischemia.

Structural or functional abnormalities of the coronary arteries, which are often clinically detectable as reduced coronary flow reserve, may also cause ischemia. In healthy subjects, blood flow is down-regulated at rest allowing for an increase of flow during exercise. This down-regulation is performed by a luminal reduction of the intramural vessels. Any mechanism that reduces perfusion pressure will first induce a stimulation of the autoregulatory processes (vasodilatation of the intramural vessels)[1–6] and – if autoregulation is exceeded – lead to true myocardial ischemia. Because direct measurement of intramyocardial adenosine triphosphate fluxes is clinically not possible, true myocardial ischemia can be proven by an increase of myocardial lactate production and decreased coronary sinus oxygen saturation.

The overwhelming majority of patients with clinically recognizable chronic ischemic heart disease have atherosclerosis of the coronary arteries as the pathologic basis. However, coronary arteries may have a reduction of their lumen without atherosclerosis,[7] and this may result in myocardial ischemia. A variety of conditions such as congenital coronary anomalies, arteritis, emboli, thrombi, metabolic disorders (e.g., Hunter's and Hurler's diseases), intimal proliferation (e.g., irradiation therapy, transplantation) external compression, or Kawasaki disease may compromise the coronary lumen. Other mechanisms that cause myocardial ischemia are dynamic coronary lesions (e.g., vasospasm, thrombus formation)[8,9] which produce symptoms by reducing supply without change in demand, increase of intraventricular pressure (and thus coronary resistance), alterations of microvessels (e.g., diabetes mellitus, systemic sclerosis), or severely increased demand (e.g., caused by hypertrophy)[10] which cannot be compensated for even by normal coronary arteries. Inadequate reaction to increased demand without epicardial CAD (= inadequate flow reserve) may occur in patients with left ventricular hypertrophy,[11] diabetes, or hypercholesterolemia (see Tables 14.1 and 14.2).

A number of noncoronary disorders of the heart such as arrhythmia, aortic aneurysm, aortic dissection, pericardial disease, myocarditis, cardiomyopathy, or valvular heart disease (e.g., aortic stenosis) may induce myocardial ischemia or mimic the symptoms or signs of ischemia. In addition, many patients with anginal pain have neither signs of ischemia during noninvasive testing, nor epicardial CAD. The proportion of these patients may be approximately 15% of those with normal coronary arteries during invasive angiography. Whether these patients have ischemia below the level of detection or a reduced level of threshold for pain perception remains unclear. Whatever the mechanism, as a result of myocardial ischemia, a sequence of events occurs, including tissue acidosis, change in intracellular electrolyte concentration, release of adenosine and other metabolites, and production of bradykinin, serotonin, and histamine (see also Chapter 1). These cause anginal pain in varying degrees. In addition, development of heart failure or low cardiac output may occur because of depressed myocardial contractility.

Clinical presentation in patients with myocardial ischemia may vary strongly among patients. Especially in noncoronary ischemic heart disease, symptoms may be very unspecific, less dependent or even independent from exertion. Frequently, ischemia is manifested as dyspnea, pulmonary edema, weakness, dizziness, palpitation, arrhythmia, or syncope. Because of this variation in clinical presentation, noninvasive cardiac imaging could be helpful to prove or exclude myocardial ischemia, define the underlying disease mechanism, assess the severity and extent of disease, and determine prognosis and management.

Table 14.1. Pathophysiology and diseases

Pathophysiology	Disease
Epicardial luminal area reduction	Congenital anomalies Kawasaki disease Arteritis Emboli Thrombi
Dynamic coronary lesions	Vasospasm Thrombus formation
Increased intraventricular pressure	Arterial hypertension Aortic stenosis
Alterations of microvessels	Diabetes mellitus Systemic sclerosis
Increased demand	Left ventricular hypertrophy
Inadequate vasodilatory capacity	Left ventricular hypertrophy Diabetes mellitus Hypercholesterolemia

Table 14.2. Diseases and mechanisms for ischemia

Disease	Mechanism for ischemia
Syndrome X	Microvascular dysfunction • Microvascular spasm • Endothelial dysfunction • Estrogen deficiency • Increased sympathetic tone • Diffuse epicardial and microvascular coronary constriction • Structural abnormalities in coronary microvessels • Inadequate vasodilatory capacity Nonischemic mechanisms • Abnormal interstitial potassium release • Adenosine release • Early cardiomyopathy • Increased pain perception Myocardial metabolic abnormality • Insulin resistance
Diabetes mellitus	• Alterations of microvessels • Impaired microcirculatory coronary vasodilation
Left ventricular hypertrophy	• Increased demand • Inadequate vasodilatory capacity
Systemic lupus erythematosus	• Thrombi (hypercoagulation, antiphospholipid antibodies) • Vasospasm • Arteritis
Hypoestrogenism	• Reduced endothelial function

A special group of patients discussed in this chapter includes individuals with angina or angina-like pain but angiographically unobstructed coronary arteries and no evidence of coronary artery spasm. These are labeled as "syndrome X" patients[12] or patients with a "sensitive heart syndrome." The etiology of symptoms is not clear and they could be attributable to a variety of causes (see Table 14.2).

2. Diagnostic Testing in Noncoronary Ischemic Heart Disease

Similar to the varied definitions of syndromex, imaging techniques have also shown a wide variety of results which are probably the result of its heterogeneous pathophysiology. Whereas some authors have reported signs of ischemia during stress, including lactate production,[13] or increased transmyocardial lipoperoxide activity,[14] others found some perfusion changes at rest but not during stress.[15] Chauhan et al. reported both a reduction of flow reserve[16] and an increased sensitivity for pain.[17] The latter was also confirmed by other investigators using positron emission tomography (PET) imaging.[18,19] A recent study[20] used cardiovascular magnetic resonance (MR) perfusion imaging and reported a reduction of subendocardial flow reserve without reduction of total blood flow in patients with syndrome X in comparison to controls.

2.1 Diagnosis of Vascular Dysfunction

Several investigators using different techniques (with or without radiotracers) found a reduced coronary flow reserve in patients with angina and unobstructed coronary vessels. An impaired coronary flow reserve indicates that ischemia can be provoked under conditions of increased myocardial oxygen demand. In principle, assessment of myocardial perfusion is very sensitive for detection of myocardial ischemia, because a reduction of perfusion is the pathophysiologic substrate, which causes all the other effects of ischemia. Different groups of patients display different patterns of myocardial perfusion. Whereas stenotic disease of the epicardial coronary arteries usually results in regional localized ischemia which can be attributed to a specific coronary artery, diseases of the microcirculation, hypertrophy, or pressure overload are more likely to lead to a global reduction of perfusion usually involving the subendocardium (Figures 14.1 and 14.2). Assessment of the latter is only feasible using techniques with high spatial resolution, which allow differentiation between subendocardial and subepicardial myocardial perfusion.

2.1.1 Radionuclide Myocardial Perfusion Imaging (Single Photon Emission Computed Tomography, PET)

Currently, in most centers, single photon emission computed tomography (SPECT) with thallium-201 or technetium-99m-labeled tracers (sestamibi or tetrofosmin) is routinely used, if exercise stress testing has been inconclusive or more detailed and accurate definition of the severity of myocardial ischemia is needed. In addition, myocardial perfusion scintigraphy (MPS) provides information on the significance of a stenosis and also on myocardial viability, and when it is combined with ECG gating, it can also provide accurate assessment of global and regional left ventricular function. However, the technique has a very limited spatial resolution (approximately $1 \times 1\,cm^{25}$) and, thus, a differentiation of transmural and subendocardial ischemia is not possible in most cases. In contrast, PET has the technical ability for absolute quantification and therefore it is well suited for accurate assessment of myocardial ischemia and its metabolic consequences.[26,27] However, spatial resolution is insufficient to detect subendocardial ischemia and, thus, the disease mechanism may remain unclear despite a PET examination. Both SPECT and PET imaging have been used to demonstrate perfusion defects and hence impairment of coronary flow reserve in several of the patient groups discussed here, such as syndrome X, diabetes mellitus,[22,23] systemic lupus erythematosus,[24] and ventricular hypertrophy.[26]

Transient abnormalities of myocardial perfusion were found in up to 60% of "syndrome X" patients, suggesting that vascular dysfunction is common in this population. There are several likely causes for impairment of perfusion reserve in these patients including endothelium-dependent and -independent factors. There is ongoing research in this field but it has already been shown that exercise-induced perfusion defects in patients with chest pain and unobstructed

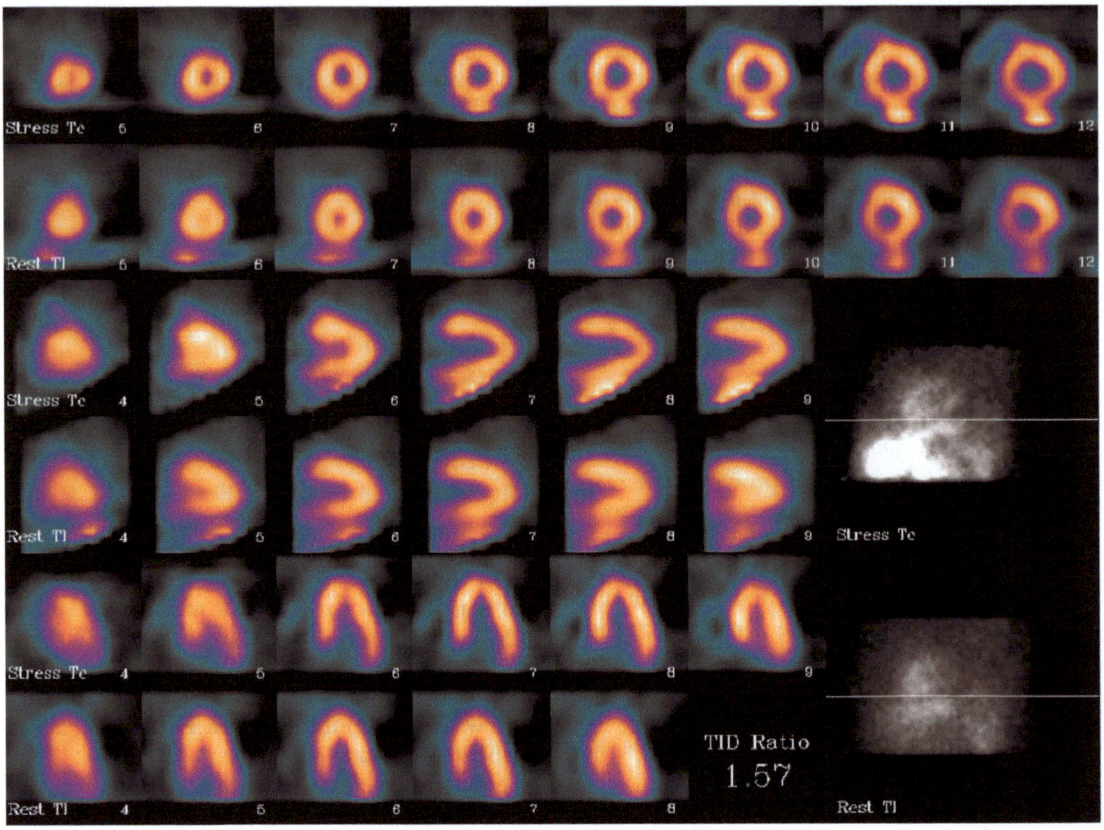

Figure 14.1. A 76-year-old woman with CAD, diabetes, hyperlipidemia. SPECT images show no defect with only increased TID (transient ischemic dilation ratio) suggestive of balanced ishaemia. Invasive angiography showed multi-vessel disease. See video of case 7.

coronary arteries are associated with decreased (endothelium-dependent) vasodilatory responses to acetylcholine.[29] Impaired vasodilator response of coronary resistance vessels to sympathetic stimulation was found in patients with diabetes mellitus and autonomic neuropathy assessed by [(11)C] hydroxyephedrine PET.[22] Moreover, patients with diabetes mellitus, normal coronary arteries but perfusion defects during MPS showed an impaired coronary artery flow during cold pressor testing in comparison to controls.[23] MPS demonstrated perfusion defects in 28% of female patients with chronic systemic lupus erythematosus and unobstructed coronary arteries, and also in patients with acute vasculitis. Similarly, perfusion defects were found in patients with progressive systemic sclerosis and have been attributed to disturbances of the microcirculation. Earlier studies have demonstrated short-term improvements with calcium antagonists[30] but more recent data suggest that they fail to ameliorate the diminished perfusion reserve.[31]

2.1.2 Nonradionuclide Techniques

Measurements of MR perfusion indexes are not yet routinely performed in many institutions but the technique is very promising for this approach (see also Chapter 3). Usually, the speed and amount of regional wash-in of a peripherally injected extracellular contrast agent is analyzed during the first pass. Myocardial perfusion can also be assessed by the alterations of signal intensities and speed of wash-in (up-slope) during vasodilation, which correlate well with alterations of myocardial perfusion[32] as shown in animal experiments with microspheres.[33] Other investigators have proposed methods for full quantification of myocardial perfusion (milliliters of blood per gram of muscle mass per time).[34]

Assessment of global perfusion in combination with the good spatial resolution of the technique (approximately 3.5 × 3.5 mm in plane) allows for differentiation between subendocardial and subepicardial perfusion, and better assessment of the amount and mechanism of malperfusion in the patients under discussion. Indeed, in patients who have received cardiac transplantation, a reduction of global perfusion reserve was found in comparison to controls, which was related to diffuse microvessel disease observed in these patients.[35] There are also similar reductions in patients with diabetic neuropathy.[36] In patients with "syndrome X," a reduction of subendocardial but not epicardial or global perfusion reserve was demonstrated.[20]

MR imaging also combines perfusion measurements with a highly sensitive method to detect fibrosis ("late enhancement"). This method demonstrates areas of cell death, fibrosis, and infiltration as foci of focal enhancement after gadolinium (Gd-DTPA) contrast-agent administration with imaging 10–20 minutes thereafter. In a study of 17 patients with severe aortic stenosis, subendocardial enhancement was found in seven patients and related to the severity of the aortic stenosis.[37] Patients with subendocardial necrosis had more clinical symptoms (history of heart failure, New York Heart Association class III–IV), a smaller aortic valve area (0.28 vs $0.38\,cm^2/m^2$), higher transvalvular pressure gradient (109 vs 68 mm Hg), and a lower ejection fraction (40% vs 59%).[37]

Even though the potential of noninvasive methods for direct measurements of coronary

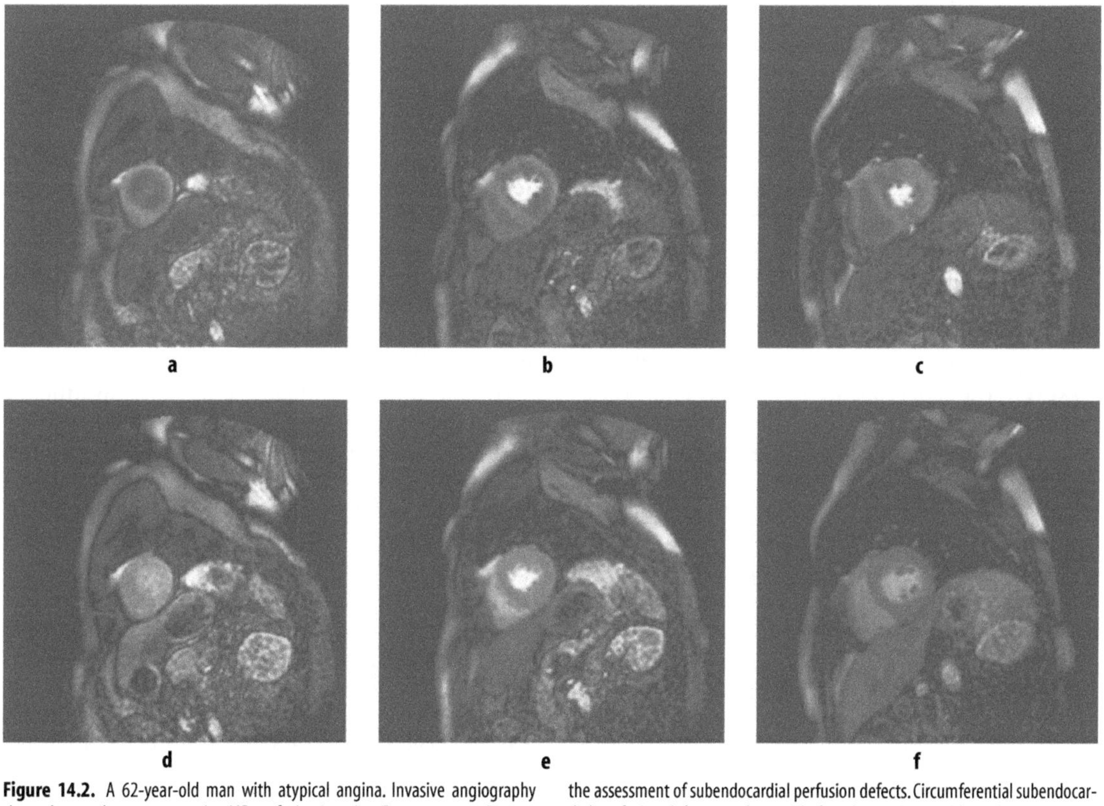

Figure 14.2. A 62-year-old man with atypical angina. Invasive angiography showed normal coronary arteries. MR perfusion imaging. Top row: stress. Bottom row: rest. From left to right: apex, mid, base. Endocardial regionally pronounced perfusion defects. The high spatial resolution of MR perfusion imaging allows for the assessment of subendocardial perfusion defects. Circumferential subendocardial perfusion defects are frequently found in patients with unobstructed coronary vessels.

artery flow velocity, flow, and flow reserve has been reported for echocardiography and MR[38,39] as well as for flow measurements of the coronary sinus and the aortic root with MR,[40] the methods seem to be not yet sufficiently robust to be applied on a routine basis (see also Chapter 3). Literature on patients with nonatherosclerotic ischemia is sparse and further research seems to be warranted.

2.2 Assessment of the Causes of Reduced Coronary Flow Reserve

There are many factors that regulate myocardial perfusion. Endothelium-independent factors include aortic pressure, extravascular compressive forces, neurohormones, and myocardial metabolism. Endothelial function is regulated by the endothelial cells (a monolayer of cells) and by the tone of the muscle cells in the vessel wall.[41] The endothelial cells release vasoactive substances, such as nitric oxide, endothelin, and prostacyclin. Vasodilation induced by activation of the endothelial cells is called "endothelium-dependent" vasorelaxation and can be induced by infusion of acetylcholine, papaverine, adenosine, or cold pressor testing as well as during reactive hyperemia. Endothelium-independent function (i.e., dilation induced by relaxation of the smooth muscle cells independent of the release of vasoactive substances from the endothelial cells) can be assessed by infusion of smooth muscle cell relaxants, e.g., nitroglycerin or sodium nitroprusside.[41] Assessment of vasomotor function can be performed centrally and peripherally[42,43]; however, the correlation of endothelial function/dysfunction between the two vascular systems is modest.[42] Endothelial function is an indicator of vascular health and recent data have shown that poor coronary endothelial function is associated with an increased risk of cardiovascular events.[43] Similarly, abnormal forearm endothelial function correlates with long-term cardiac events in patients with hypertension.[44]

Endothelial function has been assessed noninvasively with peripheral ultrasound imaging to measure dilatation of the brachial artery, either flow mediated as a marker of vascular endothelial function or nitrate-induced as a marker of endothelium-independent function.[45] Alternatively, PET, and transthoracic Doppler echocardiography have been proposed, and MR methods have been applied to determine the cross-section, rather than the diameter of a vessel.[46,47] In addition to vascular imaging techniques, a number of novel biomarkers are being explored to assess the integrity of the endothelium including cellular adhesion molecules, C-reactive protein, or metabolites of nitric oxide. However, a detailed description on this topic is well beyond the scope of this chapter (for the role and assessment of IMT, see Chapter 7b).

A significant reduction of endothelial function similar to patients with atheromatous CAD has been found in a large variety of patients without significant coronary stenoses, such as syndrome X,[48,49] hypertension, diabetes mellitus,[50] hypercholesterolemia, rheumatoid arthritis,[51] and in female postmenopausal women with low estrogen levels[52,53] using ultrasound and MR techniques.

2.3 Assessment of Metabolic Regulation

Changes in cardiac metabolism can be readily assessed with MR spectroscopy. This technique can determine absolute adenosine triphosphate (ATP) levels and the ratio of ATP/ADP (adenosine biphosphate). These measurements can determine the energy levels of the myocardium and, thus, the effect of reduced blood flow or energy allocation. Clinical applications, however, suffer from long measurement times, low spatial resolution, and the need to have both a special MR scanner, as well as a specialist operator available.

In patients with heart failure, a significant reduction of the phosphocreatine/ATP ratio has been demonstrated.[54] This reduction correlated with clinical severity of heart failure[55] and left ventricular ejection fraction.[56] The reduction of phosphocreatine/ATP ratios only in the more severe stages of heart failure suggests that changes in cardiac energetics may not be the primary causal mechanism of heart failure, but that such alterations are one factor that contributes to worsening of heart failure in advanced stages. A similar reduction of this ratio was observed in patients with longstanding left ventricular hypertrophy caused by hypertensive heart disease[57] and in the hypertrophied areas of patients with hypertrophic cardiomyopathy.[58,59] These findings could either be related to regional ischemia or to a loss of the total creatine pool in hypertrophied myocardium. In addition, a significant decrease of phosphocreatine/ATP ratios was found during exercise in female patients with syndrome X which is likely to indicate impaired myocardial microcirculation.[60] Because local imbalance between oxygen demand and supply inhibits oxidative metabolism leading into a PCr depletion and a subsequent slower decline of ATP, it is conceivable that assessment of such molecular changes may yield additional insights into the mechanism of ischemia/angina in patients with unobstructed coronary arteries.

2.4 Assessment of Myocardial Motion and Wall Thickening

Wall motion imaging allows for the identification and quantification of the consequences of ischemic heart disease by assessment of global and regional left ventricular function, wall thickness, and thickening. Demonstration of left ventricular hypertrophy may explain anginal symptoms of patients despite normal coronary arteries. Additional findings that lead to a diagnosis may be the detection of a left ventricular aneurysm, papillary muscle dysfunction, ventricular septal defect, left ventricular thrombus, transmural scar, systolic or diastolic dysfunction, and valvular or congenital abnormalities. However, imaging of wall motion at rest will neither demonstrate areas of small subendocardial necrosis, nor myocardial ischemia. The detection of myocardial ischemia usually requires stress testing (exercise or dobutamine). Even though the assessment of global and regional left ventricular function during stress has a large impact on the diagnosis of ischemic heart disease, the method is limited in its ability to determine the localization, extent, or underlying pathophysiologic disorder of myocardial ischemia. This is of special importance for the patient groups discussed in this chapter, because global subendocardial ischemia may or may not cause a wall motion defect and this may or may not be localized in a specific coronary artery territory. Recently, tissue Doppler imaging has been suggested as a new, load independent method to determine myocardial contractility.[61] This method may allow objective quantification of alterations attributed to mild ischemia.

Myocardial tagging is a new MR imaging method that allows quantification of regional wall motion, such as circumferential shortening, wall thickening, or principal strains. A highly sensitive parameter for myocardial ischemia or fibrosis is the diastolic untwisting of the heart which follows a systolic wringing motion of the ventricle. A significant prolongation and delay of diastolic untwisting was found in patients with pressure overload hypertrophy (aortic stenosis), but not in volunteers with volume overload hypertrophy.[62] This finding may explain the diastolic dysfunction frequently encountered in these patients. However, the method has not yet been specifically applied to nonatherosclerotic myocardial ischemia.

Wall motion abnormalities occur relatively late in the ischemic cascade, and thus are less sensitive for the detection of global subendocardial ischemia. This lack of sensitivity may be the major reason for not finding any abnormalities in patients with syndrome X. Specifically, studies using stress echocardiography have shown normal systolic ventricular function during stress-induced chest pain in syndrome X patients.[63,64] Whether more sensitive techniques, such as tissue Doppler, myocardial tagging, or high-resolution perfusion imaging with MR will consistently show blood flow abnormalities remains unanswered at present.

3. Conclusions and Future Directions of Noninvasive Imaging

Even though noninvasive imaging may not always allow a final diagnosis to be made, the assessment of vascular function (by nuclear techniques, and, increasingly by MR imaging) and also of endothelial function, provide important information and guide management of these patients (Figure 14.3).[65] In the near future, fast and user-independent assessment of regional wall motion including shear and stress using automated analysis of myocardial tagging may provide additional information.[66] Tissue Doppler imaging is also well suited to gain a more sophisticated insight into the underlying disease mechanisms in nonatherosclerotic myocardial ischemia.[67] The determination of the blood oxygenation level (BOLD) seems to be a promising MR imaging method that might allow measurement of the compensatory mechanisms of the heart, rather than the

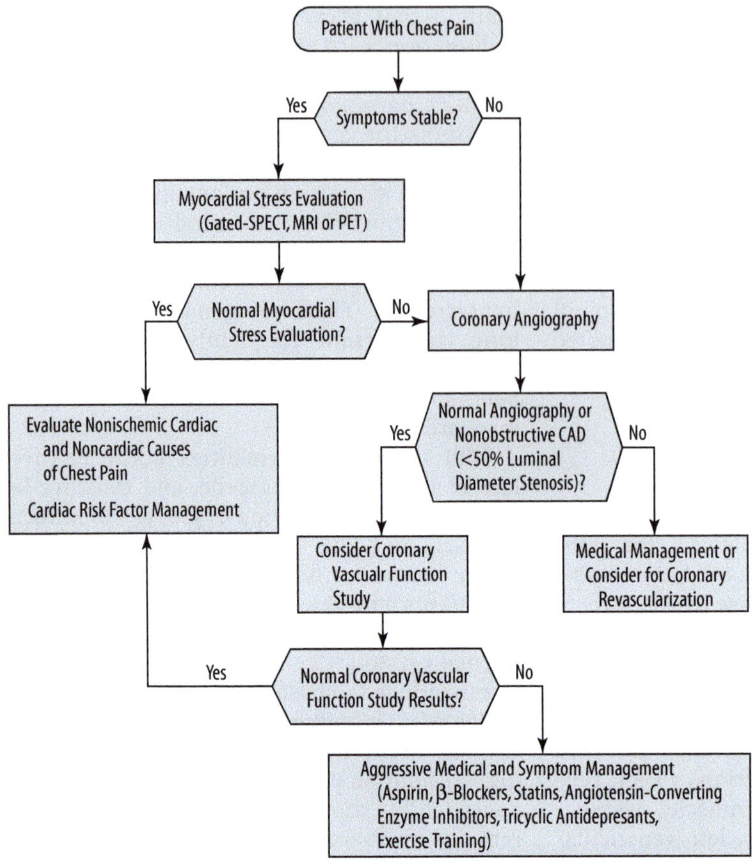

Figure 14.3. Practical algorithm for management of patients with symptoms and nonobstructive CAD.

presence of ischemia.[68] Both BOLD imaging and myocardial tagging will likely profit from the use of higher field strength (such as 3 Tesla) magnets. These stronger magnets will also facilitate the application of spectroscopy in the human heart and, thus, allow for a quantitative determination of energy-rich phosphocreatine levels.

Acknowledgment

The authors would like to thank Dr. James Gruden for supporting us with image materials (Figure 14.1 and parts of CD supplement).

References

1. Cranefield PF, Hoffman BF. The physiologic basis and clinical implications of paired pulse stimulation of the heart. Dis Chest 1966;49(6):561–567.
2. Braunwald E, Sonnenblick EH, Frommer PL, Ross J Jr. Paired electric stimulation of the heart: physiologic observations and clinical implications. Adv Intern Med 1967;13:61–96.
3. Bassenge E, Heusch G. Endothelial and neuro-humoral control of coronary blood flow in health and disease. Rev Physiol Biochem Pharmacol 1990;116:77–165.
4. Feigl EO. Coronary physiology. Physiol Rev 1983; 63(1):1–205.
5. Dole WP. Autoregulation of the coronary circulation. Prog Cardiovasc Dis 1987;29(4):293–323.
6. Hoffman JI. Transmural myocardial perfusion. Prog Cardiovasc Dis 1987;29(6):429–464.
7. Waller BF. Nonatherosclerotic coronary heart disease. In: Fuster V, Alexander RW, O'Rourke RA, eds. Hurst's the Heart. 11th ed. New York: McGraw-Hill; 2004.
8. Maseri A, L'Abbate A, Baroldi G, et al. Coronary vasospasm as a possible cause of myocardial infarction. A conclusion derived from the study of "preinfarction" angina. N Engl J Med 1978;299(23):1271–1277.
9. Lanza GA, Pedrotti P, Pasceri V, Lucente M, Crea F, Maseri A. Autonomic changes associated with spontaneous coronary spasm in patients with variant angina. J Am Coll Cardiol 1996;28(5):1249–1256.
10. Mueller TM, Tomanek RJ, Kerber RE, Marcus ML. Myocardial infarction in dogs with chronic hyperten-

sion and left ventricular hypertrophy. Am J Physiol 1980;239(6):H731–H735.
11. Bache RJ, Wright L, Laxson DD, Dai XZ. Effect of coronary stenosis on myocardial blood flow during exercise in the chronically pressure-overloaded hypertrophied left ventricle. Circulation 1990;81(6):1967–1973.
12. Cannon RO 3rd, Camici PG, Epstein SE. Pathophysiological dilemma of syndrome X. Circulation 1992; 85(3):883–892.
13. Mohri M, Koyanagi M, Egashira K, et al. Angina pectoris caused by coronary microvascular spasm. Lancet 1998;351(9110):1165–1169.
14. Buffon A, Rigattieri S, Santini SA, et al. Myocardial ischaemia reperfusion damage after pacing induced tachycardia in patients with cardiac syndrome X. Am J Physiol Heart Circ Physiol 2000;279:H2627–H2633.
15. Fragasso G, Rossetti E, Dosio F, et al. High prevalence of the thallium-201 reverse redistribution phenomenon in patients with syndrome X. Eur Heart J 1996; 17(10):1482–1487.
16. Chauhan A, Mullins PA, Taylor G, Petch MC, Schofield PM. Both endothelium-dependent and endothelium-independent function is impaired in patients with angina pectoris and normal coronary angiograms. Eur Heart J 1997;18(1):60–68.
17. Chauhan A, Mullins PA, Thuraisingham SI, Taylor G, Petch MC, Schofield PM. Abnormal cardiac pain perception in syndrome X. J Am Coll Cardiol 1994; 24(2):329–335.
18. Rosen SD, Uren NG, Kaski JC, Tousoulis D, Davies GJ, Camici PG. Coronary vasodilator reserve, pain perception, and sex in patients with syndrome X. Circulation 1994;90(1):50–60.
19. Rosen SD, Paulesu E, Wise RJ, Camici PG. Central neural contribution to the perception of chest pain in cardiac syndrome X. Heart 2002;87(6):513–519.
20. Panting JR, Gatehouse PD, Yang GZ, et al. Abnormal subendocardial perfusion in cardiac syndrome X detected by cardiovascular magnetic resonance imaging. N Engl J Med 2002;346(25):1948–1953.
21. Inobe Y, Kugiyama K, Morita E, et al. Role of adenosine in pathogenesis of syndrome X: assessment with coronary hemodynamic measurements and thallium-201 myocardial single-photon emission computed tomography. J Am Coll Cardiol 1996;28(4):890–896.
22. Di Carli MF, Bianco-Batlles D, Landa ME, et al. Effects of autonomic neuropathy on coronary blood flow in patients with diabetes mellitus. Circulation 1999; 100(8):813–819.
23. Nitenberg A, Ledoux S, Valensi P, Sachs R, Attali JR, Antony I. Impairment of coronary microvascular dilation in response to cold pressor-induced sympathetic stimulation in type 2 diabetic patients with abnormal stress thallium imaging. Diabetes 2001;50(5): 1180–1185.
24. Sella EM, Sato EI, Leite WA, Oliveira Filho JA, Barbieri A. Myocardial perfusion scintigraphy and coronary disease risk factors in systemic lupus erythematosus. Ann Rheum Dis 2003;62(11):1066–1070.
25. vom Dahl J. [Examination of myocardial perfusion with positron emission tomography: a clinically useful and valid method?] Herz 1997;22:1–15.
26. Botker HE, Sonne HS, Bagger JP, Nielsen TT. Impact of impaired coronary flow reserve and insulin resistance on myocardial energy metabolism in patients with syndrome X. Am J Cardiol 1997;79(12):1615–1622.
27. Cecchi F, Olivotto I, Gistri R, Lorenzoni R, Chiriatti G, Camici PG. Coronary microvascular dysfunction and prognosis in hypertrophic cardiomyopathy. N Engl J Med 2003;349(11):1027–1035.
28. Haley JH, Miller TD. Myocardial ischemia on thallium scintigraphy in hypertrophic cardiomyopathy: predictor of sudden cardiac death. Circulation 2001;104(13): E71–1.
29. Zeiher AM, Krause T, Schachinger V, Minners J, Moser E. Impaired endothelium-dependent vasodilation of coronary resistance vessels is associated with exercise-induced myocardial ischemia. Circulation 1995; 91(9):2345–2352.
30. Kahan A, Devaux JY, Amor B, et al. Nifedipine and thallium-201 myocardial perfusion in progressive systemic sclerosis. N Engl J Med 1986;314(22):1397–1402.
31. Sutsch G, Oechslin E, Mayer I, Hess OM. Effect of diltiazem on coronary flow reserve in patients with microvascular angina. Int J Cardiol 1995;52:135–143.
32. Nagel E, Klein C, Paetsch I, et al. Magnetic resonance perfusion measurements for the noninvasive detection of coronary artery disease. Circulation 2003;108(4): 432–437.
33. Klocke FJ, Simonetti OP, Judd RM, et al. Limits of detection of regional differences in vasodilated flow in viable myocardium by first-pass magnetic resonance perfusion imaging. Circulation 2001;104(20):2412–2416.
34. Wilke N, Jerosch-Herold M, Wand Y, et al. Myocardial perfusion reserve: assessment with multisection, quantitative, first-pass MR imaging. Radiology 1997;204: 373–384.
35. Muehling OM, Wilke NM, Panse P, et al. Reduced myocardial perfusion reserve and transmural perfusion gradient in heart transplant arteriopathy assessed by magnetic resonance imaging. J Am Coll Cardiol 2003;42(6):1054–1060.
36. Taskiran M, Fritz-Hansen T, Rasmussen V, Larsson HB, Hilsted J. Decreased myocardial perfusion reserve in diabetic autonomic neuropathy. Diabetes 2002;51: 3306–3310.
37. Ochiai K, Ishibashi Y, Shimada T, Murakami Y, Inoue S, Sano K. Subendocardial enhancement in gadolinium-diethylene-triamine-pentaacetic acid-enhanced magnetic resonance imaging in aortic stenosis. Am J Cardiol 1999;83(10):1443–1446.
38. Hundley W, Hamilton C, Clarke G, et al. Visualization and functional assessment of proximal and middle left anterior descending coronary stenoses in humans with magnetic resonance imaging. Circulation 1999;99: 3248–3254.
39. Nagel E, Bornstedt A, Hug J, Schnackenburg B, Wellnhofer E, Fleck E. Noninvasive determination of coronary blood flow velocity with magnetic resonance imaging: comparison of breath-hold and navigator techniques with intravascular ultrasound. Magn Reson Med 1999;41(3):544–549.
40. Schwitter J, DeMarco T, Kneifel S, et al. Magnetic resonance-based assessment of global coronary flow and flow reserve and its relation to left ventricular functional parameters. A comparison with positron emission tomography. Circulation 2000;101:2696–2702.
41. Kuvin JT, Karas RH. Clinical utility of endothelial function testing: ready for prime time? Circulation 2003; 107(25):3243–3247.

42. Anderson TJ, Uehata A, Gerhard MD, et al. Close relation of endothelial function in human coronary and peripheral circulation. J Am Coll Cadiol 1995;26: 1235–1241.
43. Schachinger V, Britten MB, Zeiher AM. Prognostic impact of coronary vasodilator dysfunction on adverse long-term outcome of coronary heart disease. Circulation 2000;101(16):1899–1906.
44. Perticone F, Ceravolo R, Pujia A, et al. Prognostic significance of endothelial dysfunction in hypertensive patients. Circulation 2001;104(2):191–196.
45. Corretti MC, Plotnick GD, Vogel RA. Technical aspects of evaluating brachial artery vasodilatation using high-frequency ultrasound. Am J Physiol 1995;268(4 pt 2): H1397–H1404.
46. Dimitrow PP. Transthoracic Doppler echocardiography: noninvasive diagnostic window for coronary flow reserve assessment. Cardiovasc Ultrasound 2003;1:4.
47. Silber HA, Bluemke DA, Ouyang P, Du YP, Post WS, Lima JA. The relationship between vascular wall shear stress and flow-mediated dilation: endothelial function assessed by phase-contrast magnetic resonance angiography. J Am Coll Cardiol 2001;38(7):1859–1865.
48. Egashira K, Inou T, Hirooka Y, Yamada A, Urabe Y, Takeshita A. Evidence of impaired endothelium-dependent coronary vasodilatation in patients with angina pectoris and normal coronary angiograms. N Engl J Med 1993;328(23):1659–1664.
49. Opherk D, Zebe H, Schuler G, Weihe E, Mall G, Kubler W. Reduced coronary reserve and abnormal exercise left ventricular reserve in patients with syndrome X. Arch Mal Coeur Vaiss 1983;76(spec no):231–235.
50. Jarvisalo MJ, Raitakari M, Toikka JO, et al. Endothelial dysfunction and increased arterial intima-media thickness in children with type 1 diabetes. Circulation 2004;109(14):1750–1755. 51. Vaudo G, Marchesi S, Gerli R, et al. Endothelial dysfunction in young patients with rheumatoid arthritis and low disease activity. Ann Rheum Dis 2004;63(1):31–35.
52. Rosano GM, Collins P, Kaski JC, Lindsay DC, Sarrel PM, Poole-Wilson PA. Syndrome X in women is associated with oestrogen deficiency. Eur Heart J 1995;16(5): 610–614.
53. Sorensen MB, Collins P, Ong PJ, et al. Long-term use of contraceptive depot medroxyprogesterone acetate in young women impairs arterial endothelial function assessed by cardiovascular magnetic resonance. Circulation 2002;106(13):1646–1651.
54. Hardy CJ, Weiss RG, Bottomley PA, Gerstenblith G. Altered myocardial high-energy phosphate metabolites in patients with dilated cardiomyopathy. Am Heart J 1991;122(3 pt 1):795–801.
55. Neubauer S, Krahe T, Schindler R, et al. 31P magnetic resonance spectroscopy in dilated cardiomyopathy and coronary artery disease. Altered cardiac high-energy phosphate metabolism in heart failure. Circulation 1992;86(6):1810–1818.
56. Neubauer S, Horn M, Cramer M, et al. Myocardial phosphocreatine-to-ATP ratio is a predictor of mortality in patients with dilated cardiomyopathy. Circulation 1997;96(7):2190–2196.
57. Lamb HJ, Beyerbacht HP, van der Laarse A, et al. Diastolic dysfunction in hypertensive heart disease is associated with altered myocardial metabolism. Circulation 1999;99(17):2261–2267.
58. Jung WI, Sieverding L, Breuer J, et al. 31P NMR spectroscopy detects metabolic abnormalities in asymptomatic patients with hypertrophic cardiomyopathy. Circulation 1998;97(25):2536–2542.
59. Rajagopalan B, Blackledge MJ, McKenna WJ, Bolas N, Radda GK. Measurement of phosphocreatine to ATP ratio in normal and diseased human heart by 31P magnetic resonance spectroscopy using the rotating frame-depth selection technique. Ann NY Acad Sci 1987;508:321–332.
60. Buchthal SD, den Hollander JA, Merz CN, et al. Abnormal myocardial phosphorus-31 nuclear magnetic resonance spectroscopy in women with chest pain but normal coronary angiograms. N Engl J Med 2000;342(12):829–835.
61. Greenberg NL, Firstenberg MS, Castro PL, et al. Doppler-derived myocardial systolic strain rate is a strong index of left ventricular contractility. Circulation 2002;105(1):99–105.
62. Stuber M, Scheidegger MB, Fischer SE, et al. Alterations in the local myocardial motion pattern in patients suffering from pressure overload due to aortic stenosis. Circulation 1999;100(4):361–368.
63. Panza JA, Laurienzo JM, Curiel RV, et al. Investigation of the mechanism of chest pain in patients with angiographically normal coronary arteries using transesophageal dobutamine stress echocardiography. J Am Coll Cardiol 1997;29(2):293–301.
64. Nihoyannopoulos P, Kaski JC, Crake T, Maseri A. Absence of myocardial dysfunction during stress in patients with syndrome X. J Am Coll Cardiol 1991; 18(6):1463–1470.
65. Bugiardini R, Bairey Merz CN. Angina with "normal" coronary arteries A changing philosophy, JAMA; 293: 477–484.
66. Osman NF, McVeigh ER, Prince JL. Imaging heart motion using harmonic phase MRI. IEEE Trans Med Imaging 2000;19(3):186–202.
67. Korinek J, Anagnostopoulos P, Pislaru C, et al. Both systolic and diastolic dysfunction characterize nonischemic inhibition of myocardial energy metabolism: an experimental strain rate echocardiographic study. J Am Soc Echocardiogr 2004;(17):1239–1244.
68. Wacker CM, Hartlep AW, Pfleger S, Schad LR, Ertl G, Bauer WR. Susceptibility-sensitive magnetic resonance imaging detects human myocardium supplied by a stenotic coronary artery without a contrast agent. J Am Coll Cardiol 2003;41(5):834–840.

15

Myocardial Ischemia in Congenital Heart Disease: The Role of Noninvasive Imaging

J.L. Tan, C.Y. Loong, A. Anagnostopoulos-Tzifa, P.J. Kilner, W. Li, and M.A. Gatzoulis

Patients with congenital heart disease (CHD) are not only surviving into adulthood, but are also living longer and growing older.[1] This is attributed to major achievements in their diagnosis, medical management, surgical repair, and postoperative treatment in the last three to four decades.

Ever-increasing numbers of patients with CHD are encountered in our everyday practice. It is therefore timely and appropriate to start addressing the somewhat-neglected issue of myocardial ischemia in this patient population.

1. The Size of the Problem

The true prevalence of CHD in the adult population is unknown.[1,2] It is estimated that there were nearly 140 000 patients with simple congenital lesions and nearly 12 000 patients with complex congenital lesions, in the United Kingdom alone, in the year 2000.[3] This figure is estimated to increase to 170 000 and 17 000, respectively, by the year 2010. There are no published data on the incidence and prevalence of ischemic heart disease (IHD) in the adult CHD (ACHD) population. One could assume that the prevalence and incidence of IHD in those patients with simple surgically corrected cardiac lesions [e.g., atrial septal defect (ASD), ventricular septal defect (VSD)] would mirror that of the general population. Likewise, those with complex unoperated or significant residual lesions and also patients with single ventricle physiology, whose survival decreases dramatically after the fourth decade of life, may not live long enough to experience the full effects of atherosclerosis. Nevertheless, there remains a subgroup of ACHD patients who are at increased risk of developing myocardial ischemia or premature coronary artery disease (CAD) as the result of: a) congenital coronary artery abnormalities (e.g., anomalous origin and course of coronary arteries, myocardial bridging, coronary artery fistulas); b) previous surgery [e.g., arterial switch operation for transposition of the great arteries (TGA) and surgical coarctation repair]; and c) myocardial ischemia not related directly to coronary artery anomalies but presenting after the atrial switch procedure for TGA (Mustard, Senning) and also in patients with congenitally corrected TGA (ccTGA). In these conditions, the right ventricle supports the systemic circulation and can become dilated and hypertrophied with time. Once ventricular dilatation and hypertrophy settle in, the blood supply through a normal right coronary artery can become insufficient to meet the increased metabolic demands of the systemic right ventricle,[4,5] leading to further ventricular dysfunction. The latter may also have a deleterious effect on left ventricular perfusion, ultimately leading to left ventricular dysfunction.[5] d) Lastly, nonatherosclerotic coronary events have been described in patients who had Kawasaki disease in childhood, secondary to the development of coronary aneurysms and coronary stenoses.

2. Optimal Imaging Modality for Detection of Ischemia in CHD

The utilization of any imaging modality for assessment of myocardial ischemia in CHD has to be carefully thought through or otherwise the information acquired may at best still be incomplete or at worse misinterpreted. Studies should only be undertaken when there is a clear understanding of the underlying congenital heart defect. Attention should be given to the original cardiac anatomy, previous surgical or transcatheter interventions, and residual cardiac shunts. However, of paramount importance is the understanding of the current physiology (biventricular or univentricular) and the effect that exercise and stress may have on the patient's hemodynamic status. This knowledge in combination with an understanding of the inherent strengths and limitations of each imaging modality will help the physician not only in choosing the optimal imaging method but more importantly in the correct interpretation of the results.

3. Specific Considerations in CHD Patients

Patients with CHD surviving into adulthood represent a heterogeneous group ranging from those with simple cardiac lesions, who may have had a complete repair, to those with complex lesions, either unoperated or with previous cardiac procedures. Therefore, when choosing the optimal mode of imaging for the detection of myocardial ischemia in ACHD patients, one should consider the various issues and aspects that are inherently unique to different subgroups of ACHD population (Figure 15.1).

3.1 Simple Lesions

Patients with simple congenital lesions [e.g., ASD, VSD, atrioventricular septal defect (AVSD)] who had uncomplicated surgical repair in their childhood or those with small restrictive shunts can be treated in the same category as the general population. However, interventricular septum (IVS) motion abnormalities and perfusion defects can be normally present in patients who have had patch repair of a VSD or AVSD.

When a residual left to right shunt is present, exercise or pharmacologic stress during cardiac imaging will result in increased cardiac output and greater left to right shunting. This is generally well tolerated if the shunt is small ($Qp/Qs < 1.5$). Patients with significant shunts ($Qp/Qs > 2.0$) would usually need a full workup including cardiac catheterization and coronary angiography for consideration of operative or transcatheter closure and hence noninvasive imaging for myocardial ischemia in this group is usually not indicated. Patients with large unrestrictive shunts and elevated pulmonary artery pressures with Eisenmenger physiology can become profoundly cyanosed during exercise as a result of right to left shunting; therefore, they

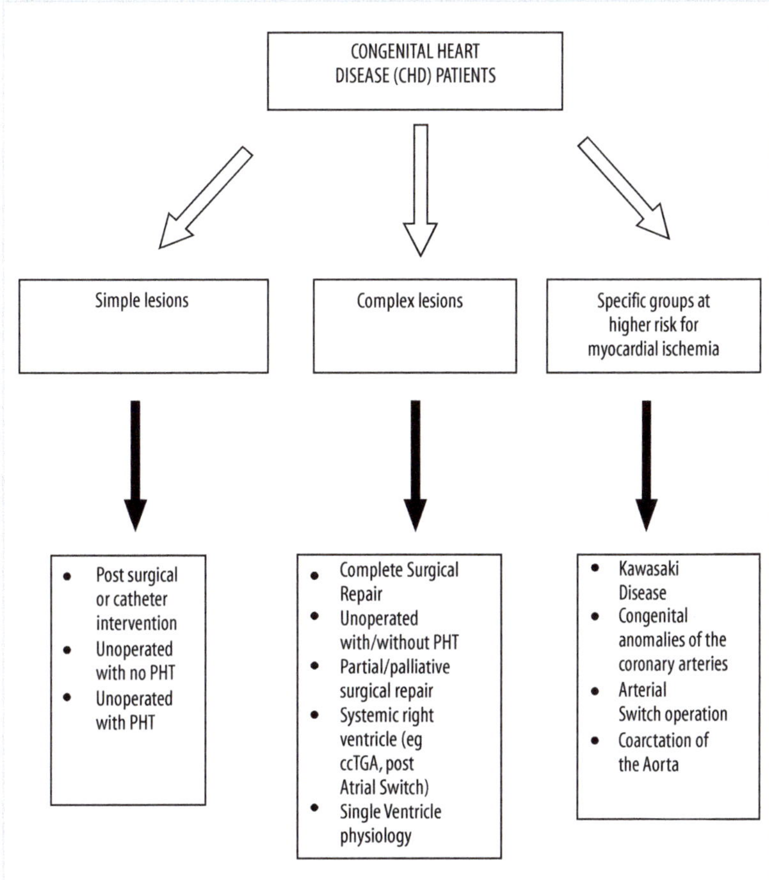

Figure 15.1. Imaging for myocardial ischemia in congenital heart disease (CHD) patients. Specific issues to consider for different CHD subgroups. PHT, pulmonary hypertension; TGA, transposition of the great arteries; ccTGA, congenitally corrected transposition of the great arteries.

may not tolerate the level of exercise or pharmacologic stress required during imaging for myocardial ischemia.

3.2 Complex Lesions

The subgroups of patients in this category are extremely heterogeneous and a detailed discussion on each group is beyond the scope of this chapter. The following issues should be considered when evaluating the patient's ability to undergo exercise/pharmacologic stress imaging and in interpreting the imaging results.

- Patients who had complete surgical repair may still have residual lesions or imaging abnormalities (perfusion defects or wall motion abnormalities):
  - Scarring and dyskinesia of the right ventricular outflow tract may result after repair of tetralogy of Fallot accounting for abnormal wall motion abnormalities and perfusion defects. IVS motion abnormalities and perfusion defects can also coexist at the region of the VSD patch.
  - Other repaired complex conditions where a VSD patch has been used for the repair [e.g., pulmonary atresia/VSD, TGA/VSD] can lead to septal dyskinesia and IVS perfusion defects.

  These patients would be suitable to undergo stress imaging provided that their residual lesions (i.e., outflow tract obstruction) are hemodynamically insignificant.
- Patients with systemic right ventricle
  - Patients in this category are most often those with ccTGA and after atrial switch operation (Senning or Mustard) for TGA.

  For this patient group, an imaging modality should be chosen that best assesses the right ventricle. Perfusion defects and regional wall motion abnormalities (RWMA) do not necessarily indicate coexisting CAD and may merely reflect an imbalance in supply and demand of systemic right ventricular perfusion.[4,5]

- Patients with single ventricle physiology
  - This category includes all entities of CHD in which the heart – for different reasons – cannot be septated in order to achieve biventricular repair. This can be due to: a) absent left or right atrioventricular connection, b) underdeveloped right or left ventricle (i.e., pulmonary atresia with intact ventricular septum, hypoplastic left heart syndrome, unbalanced AVSD, double inlet left ventricle) and c) straddling and overriding of atrioventricular valves.

Palliation of such patients was previously achieved by inserting aortopulmonary shunts, PA bands, etc. In more recent years, a staged palliation is attempted. In the final stage of the palliation (the so-called "Fontan procedure" or "total cavopulmonary connection"), the systemic venous blood flow is directed straight to the lungs (superior vena cava and inferior vena cava anastomosis to right pulmonary artery), while leaving one outlet (aorta) off the single ventricle physiology heart.

Patients with single ventricle physiology have reduced cardiac reserve and often have other associated cardiac lesions (e.g., ventricular septal defects, stenotic semilunar valves, regurgitant atrioventricular valves, surgical shunts). There is little indication for routine stress imaging, which may be hazardous and may not be well tolerated in this group of complex patients, whose natural lifespan is already reduced.

4 Specific Groups at Increased Risk of Myocardial Ischemia

Patients in the following groups are at a higher risk for the development of myocardial ischemia:

- Congenital anomalies of the coronary arteries.
- Myocardial bridging
- Post-arterial switch operation for TGA
- Post-surgical repair for aortic coarctation
- Post-Kawasaki disease

4.1 Congenital Anomalies of the Coronary Arteries

These anomalies mostly include: a) anomalous origin of one or more of the coronary arteries from the aorta or b) the pulmonary trunk (Figure 15.2a and b), c) unusual coronary epicardial course, d) high take-off coronary ostia or ostial atresia, and e) coronary artery fistulas.

Anomalous origin of a coronary artery from the aorta does not necessarily imply perfusion abnormality unless there is associated anatomic or functional coronary artery obstruction.[6] However, when both right and left coronary arteries arise from the same sinus of Valsalva, functional obstruction may be induced during exercise in the vessel that runs between the aortic and pulmonary trunk.

Adult patients with anomalous coronary artery from the pulmonary artery (ALCAPA) are mostly those who have had surgical intervention during childhood, as survival into adulthood without surgical correction is less than 10%. Myocardial ischemia can result from diseased grafts, stenotic conduits, or stenotic origin of the reimplanted coronary arteries and may manifest as ischemic mitral regurgitation. Indeed, Harpaz et al.[7] reported the use of dobutamine stress echo (DSE) in assessing the relative contribution of ischemic mitral regurgitation and mitral valve prolapse to the severity of mitral regurgitation in a young woman with ALCAPA syndrome. The DSE suggested that ischemia was the predominant cause of the mitral regurgitation and as a result appropriate revascularization surgery with sparing of the mitral valve was performed.

In patients with unusual epicardial course of coronary arteries, ischemia may be induced during exercise, in the territory of the coronary artery that runs between the great artery trunks secondary to compression of their lumen from the dilated great vessels. Similarly, functional obstruction may be observed in coronary arteries that have an intramural course within the vessel wall before they emerge onto the epicardial surface. High take-off coronary ostia located in the tubular portion of the aorta may be associated with decreased coronary perfusion.[8]

Lastly, coronary artery fistulae, most frequently occurring between a coronary artery and a cardiac chamber or a major vessel (vena cava, coronary sinus, pulmonary artery), can be responsible for myocardial ischemia and perfu-

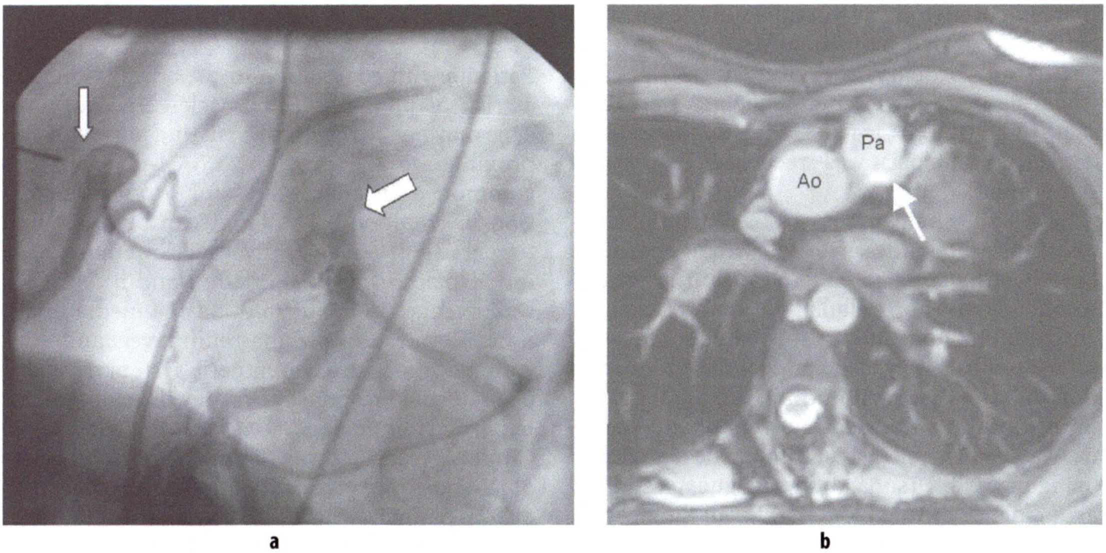

Figure 15.2. **a** Coronary angiogram showing anomalous left coronary artery from the pulmonary artery (ALCAPA). Thin arrow, catheter at aortic sinus of right coronary artery which fills the left anterior descending (LAD) and left circumflex (LCx) retrogradely; thick arrow, left main opens into the pulmonary artery (backfill of contrast into PA). **b** Magnetic resonance imaging showing the left coronary artery arising from the pulmonary artery. Ao, aorta; Pa, pulmonary artery.

sion defects at the area distal to the fistula (coronary steal phenomenon).

4.2 Myocardial Bridging

Myocardial bridging by definition occurs when a coronary artery segment runs through an intramyocardial course with overlying myocardial fibers bridging the segment, resulting in systolic compression of the intramyocardial segment by the surrounding myocardium. There is an association between myocardial bridging and hypertrophic cardiomyopathy, although a recent series[9] from Mayo Clinic did not show any observed increased risk of sudden death and overall survival. The usual site is in the middle segment of the left anterior descending artery.[10] The intramyocardial segment of the artery is often free of atherosclerosis although there may be atherosclerotic plaques without any significant stenosis just proximal to the myocardial bridging.[11] The exact mechanism of ischemia is unclear but delayed diastolic relaxation after systolic compression may be an important factor.[11] Perfusion defects may be absent as reported by Greenspan et al.[12] in a series of seven patients with myocardial bridging who underwent exercise thallium scanning.

4.3 Arterial Switch Operation for TGA

The arterial switch operation was first described by Jatene et al.[13] in 1975, although it started gaining wide acceptance in the early 1980s. Patients that first underwent this type of operation for correction of TGA are still young individuals in their twenties. In a prospective angiographic study of 165 arterial switch patients,[14] coronary artery abnormalities were detected in 18% of these patients, of whom 12% had either coronary occlusions or major stenosis. When Tanel and colleagues[15] reviewed the patency of the coronary arteries in 366 patients who had undergone the arterial switch operation, it was found that a subgroup of 3% had coronary arterial abnormalities despite being asymptomatic. Routine postoperative diagnostic studies had shown no evidence of myocardial ischemia or systolic dysfunction. In the group of patients reported by Cohen M et al.,[20] the frequency of coronary arterial stenosis was 40% when signs of myocardial ischemia were present, but also 7% when signs were absent. A dangerous stenosis was recorded in 29% of symptomatic patients.

Several mechanisms of coronary arterial complications after the arterial switch operation have been postulated. Late occlusion is usually secondary to fibrocellular intimal thickening and resultant formation of thrombus.[17] Coronary artery stenosis may also be secondary to formation of scars that surround the proximal part of the surgically mobilized and reimplanted coronary artery, the ultrastructure of the vessel wall being normal.[18] Tsuda and colleagues[17] reported an incidence of 10% of late deaths in their series. The usual cause of these deaths was subendocardial infarction resulting from stenosis of the coronary trunk. All patients had concentric, as compared with nonconcentric stenosis in the case of atherosclerotic changes, and fibrocellular intimal proliferation of both the left and right coronary trunk, resulting in segmental stenosis of both main coronary arteries. The stenosis involved primarily the coronary orifices, but no intimal thickening at the coronary button in the aortic wall was found. The histopathologic mechanism of intimal thickening remains unknown. The clinical significance of the concentric intimal proliferation should be related to the size and patency of the coronary arteries. This could explain why most of the sudden deaths occur within the first 6 months after surgery. The rarity of late deaths after 1 year of age could be attributed to the fact that the process of fibrocellular intimal proliferation has subsided, or the stenosing process has been overcome by the growth of the coronary vessels.[17]

Patients with severe coronary arterial stenosis, or complete arterial occlusion, can develop collateral circulation if left untreated. Because the aorta has been transected, along with the sensory nervous supply to the heart, the heart is effectively denervated. This means that the sensation of angina may not be apparent in these patients. A detailed clinical history should always be obtained. The clinical examination may range from normal to frank heart failure and cardiogenic shock. The wide clinical spectrum depends on the rate of progression of the coronary arterial stenosis, and the development of collateral circulation.[19]

4.4 Coarctation of the Aorta Repair

Patients with coarctation of the aorta (CoA) are at risk of premature atherosclerosis and CAD. This may be the result of persisting hypertension proximal to the previous CoA site, which is common even after successful surgical correction in childhood. The latter can be attributed to persistent vascular dysfunction due to: a) impairment of arterial dilation and b) vascular wall changes in the form of intima media thickness. Elevation of plasma renin levels and activation of the neurosympathetic system have also been deemed responsible for the development of hypertension postoperatively. In the 1989 Mayo Clinic series, CAD was the most common cause of late postoperative death after CoA repair in 32 of 571 patients who had long-term follow-up.[20] Of interest is that paradoxical hypertension has only rarely been described in patients who have undergone transcatheter treatment for aortic coarctation with either balloon dilation of the lesion or stent implantation.

4.5 Kawasaki Disease

Kawasaki disease, an acute childhood systemic inflammatory disease with acute vasculitis affecting small and medium-sized arteries including coronary arteries (Figure 15.3a) may lead to CAD in young adults and require long-term monitoring. In a 10- to 21-year follow-up of 594 patients post-Kawasaki disease, Kato et al.[21] have reported the incidence of coronary artery aneurysm in acute Kawasaki to be 25%, of which 55% showed regression after 2 years with development of IHD and myocardial infarction in 4.7% and 1.9% of the cohort, respectively. The long-term cardiac sequelae of Kawasaki disease in the adult population includes aneurysmal formation of the coronary arteries with subsequent thrombotic occlusion and premature atherosclerosis from systemic arteritis. Most of these patients are asymptomatic with the silent ischemia detected only during functional stress testing.[22]

5. Detection of Myocardial Ischemia in CHD

5.1 The Role of Echocardiography

Echocardiography is the predominant imaging modality used for the diagnosis and manage-

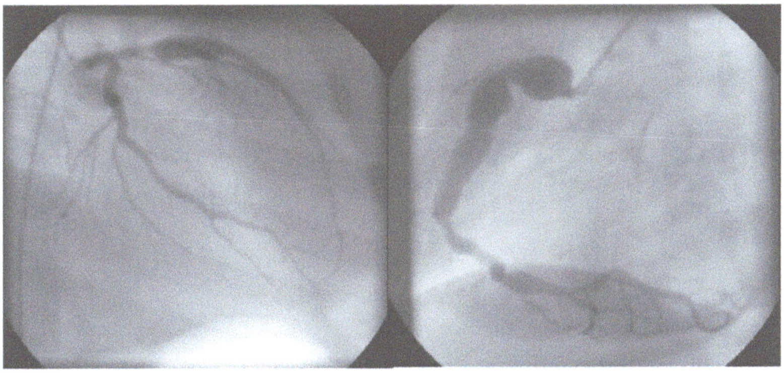

a

Figure 15.3a. Coronary angiography of a 2-year-old boy with Kawasaki disease presenting with acute posterior myocardial infarction. Coronary angiography revealed coronary arterial dilatation affecting the right coronary artery (RCA) more than the left coronary artery (LCA). Left, left coronary artery (right anterior oblique caudal view); right, right coronary artery (left anterior oblique cranial view).

ment of CHD because of its widespread availability, ease of use, real-time imaging and cost effectiveness. The role of echocardiography specifically for the detection of myocardial ischemia in the ACHD population is less well established. Published data on the use of exercise or pharmacologic stress echo in this patient population are scanty (Table 15.1) and limited to a few specific conditions such as Kawasaki disease,[22–26] postatrial switch (Mustard) repair,[27] and congenital anomalies of coronary arteries.[7] As the ACHD population grows older and the need to exclude myocardial ischemia arises, there will no doubt be a renewed interest in the use of stress echo in this patient group. Furthermore, the indications and clinical applications of other newer echo techniques such as tissue Doppler imaging, strain and strain rate imaging, contrast and real-time three-dimensional (3D) echocardiography to detect myocardial ischemia will need to be determined in these patients.

5.2 Stress Echocardiography in Patients with CHD

Exercise stress echo and pharmacologic stress echo using dobutamine are well established tools in the evaluation of IHD. Their feasibility, safety, sensitivity, specificity, and prognostic values in the general population have been extensively discussed elsewhere. Very little published data exist on the use of stress echo for the detection of myocardial ischemia in the setting of CHD; however, as a guide to the general cardiologist contemplating stress echo in this group of patients, we suggest the following stepwise approach:

1. Assess the underlying anatomy, physiology, and associated technical problems
   - Examine the patient. Locate the cardiac apical impulse, feel the femoral arteries, and auscultate the heart and chest.
   - Obtain clear understanding of the underlying congenital defects, cardiac situs and position, previous surgical corrections, morphology, and position of the systemic ventricle and current hemodynamic status.
   - Search for nonstandard transthoracic echo windows in patients with limited echo windows secondary to chest wall deformity, abnormal heart position as in dextrocardia and in patients with abnormal systemic ventricular position as in situs inversus (mirror image heart).
   - Decide whether the image quality acquired is good enough for assessment of global and RWMA. If not, consider evaluating other parameters such as long-axis function using M-mode, myocardial tissue Doppler velocities, strain-rate and strain derivatives, or the usage of contrast echocardiography for additional confirmation.
2. Choosing the optimal form of stress
   - The decision whether to choose exercise or pharmacologic stress to assess ischemia may depend on the patient's ability to perform adequate exercise, which is usually defined as achieving at least 85% of predicted heart rate, based on resting heart rate and age. It is debatable whether 85% is

Table 15.1. Study groups, congenital lesions, and parameters evaluated

Study Group	Congenital lesions	Patients, n (age)	Stress modality	Parameters evaluated	Results	Complications
Ogawa et al.[20]	Kawasaki disease	76 (10 mo to 18 yr)	Dobutamine Echo	LV wall motion	8 of 76 patients with coronary stenosis >25% had positive DSE (silent ischemia)	None reported
Noto et al.[23]	Kawasaki disease	50 (3–16 yr)	Dobutamine Echo	LV wall motion	Sensitivity 90%, specificity 100% (cath correlated)	10 self-limiting side effects
Henein et al.[24]	Kawasaki disease	17 (6.6 ± 2 yr)	Exercise Echo	M-mode long axis function	Decreased LV long-axis function in Kawasaki patients	None reported
Pahl et al.[25]	Kawasaki disease	28 (6–16 yr)	Exercise Echo	Left ventricle wall motion	2 of the 28 had new RWMA, cardiac cath – critical stenosis	None reported
Dahdah et al.[26]	Kawasaki disease	13 (1.8–14.3 yr)	Exercise Echo correlated with SPECT MIBI	LV wall motion + myocardial perfusion	Enhanced perfusion (MIBI) does not always correspond to improved contractility (DSE)	None reported
Hiraishi et al.[29] CFVR	Kawasaki disease	49 (3–24 yr)	Dipyridamole Infusion Transthoracic echo	Coronary flow velocity reserve	Peak and mean CFVR >2 predicts significant stenosis (cath correlated)	None reported
Li et al.[27]	Post-Mustard operation for TGA	27 (29 ± 7 yr)	Dobutamine Echo	RV and LV long-axis function and tissue Doppler	Systemic RV function depressed and correlated with exercise capacity	None reported
Harpaz et al.[7]	Anomalous origin of left coronary artery from pulmonary artery (ALCAPA) and mitral valve prolapse (MVP)	Case report (34-yr-old woman)	Dobutamine Echo	Contribution of left ventricle wall motion and MVP to severity of mitral regurgitation	Positive for ischemia and worsening of MR with LV dilatation. Conclusion: ischemic MR > MVP in contribution of MR	Transient chest pain and dyspnea

LV, left ventricle; RV, right ventricle.

too high a target to achieve for some ACHD patients with complex anatomy and already reduced cardiac reserve.

- The pharmacologic agent most often used in stress echo is dobutamine. Atropine is occasionally administered if peak heart rate achieved is less than 85% of predicted. The effects of dobutamine vary at different concentrations; at low dose its effect is predominantly inotropic and at higher doses of more than 20 µg/kg/min, dobutamine increases the heart rate and causes vasodilatation. These effects should be borne in mind when working out the physiologic response of patients with complex anatomy and shunts to the administered stressor agents.

3. Safety issues and special precautions
   - There were no reported serious complications in the few published studies of DSE in children and teenagers with Kawasaki disease[22–26] and in adult patients post-Mustard operation.[27]
   - Special precautions such as good aseptic technique during venepuncture and insertion of an intravenous line for dobutamine infusion should be taken, as infective endocarditis carries both a high mortality and morbidity in this patient group. The use of special filters for air bubbles in patients with cardiac shunts should also be considered. Nausea and vomiting, which are relatively common during high-dose dobutamine infusion, can result in right to left shunting and subsequent desaturation caused by transient elevation in right-sided pressures.
   - Patients with CHD who had previous cardiac surgery with resultant atrial or ventricular scarring and those with dilated atria or ventricles from abnormal hemody-

namics and physiology have an elevated baseline risk for development of atrial or ventricular arrhythmias. The risk of precipitating these arrhythmias during exercise or dobutamine infusion should be considered.

4. Problems with interpretation and limitations of stress echo in CHD
   - Detection of ischemia in the right ventricle
     - The assessment of right ventricular ischemia is important in many groups of CHD patients. Those with systemic right ventricle in the setting of ccTGA or postatrial switch operation for TGA are typical examples. Unlike the left ventricle where one can divide echocardiographically into 16 segments to specifically look for segmental RWMA, similar approach does not apply to the right ventricle. The complex geometry of the right ventricle, which essentially comprises three portions – inlet, trabecular, and an outlet portion – does not make this any easier as the standard 2D echo views used for left ventricle assessment are unhelpful. Because the right ventricle is solely supplied by the right coronary artery most of the time except in left circumflex dominant system, it would make sense to assess the global rather than regional right ventricular function during stress. In addition, RWMA after Mustard operation for TGA are common. Redington et al.[28] reported that segmental hypokinesia and dyskinesia were common in the systemic right ventricle in 18 asymptomatic patients 10 years after their Mustard operation. The cause of the RWMA is unknown but interestingly some of the RWMA had been present before surgery suggesting that some degree of myocardial damage may have occurred preoperatively in the systemic right ventricle of these patients. Li et al.[27] have shown that global assessment of the right ventricle using M-mode systemic right ventricular long-axis amplitude at rest and during stress in 27 adults who had undergone Mustard repair for TGA, correlated well with exercise capacity in these patients. Longer follow-up data are required to assess its potential predictive value.
   - Detection of ischemia in right-sided systemic left ventricle
     - Right-sided systemic left ventricle is found in patients with double switch operation (atrial and arterial switch) for ccTGA and also in patients with situs inversus. It is extremely challenging to visualize and obtain good quality images of all the myocardial walls, let alone attempt to analyze RWMA of the left ventricle on the right side.
   - Detection of ischemia in other abnormally positioned hearts
     - Patients with dextrocardia (cardiac apex pointing to the right) or mesocardia (cardiac apex pointing to the middle) may have a left or right-sided systemic left or right ventricle. Often the echo windows are limited in these patients, making it technically impossible to obtain all segmental regions. Additional other imaging modalities will be required.

5. Newer technologies
   - Tissue Doppler imaging
     - Motion estimation techniques including tissue Doppler imaging, myocardial strain rate and strain analysis which use regional myocardial velocity estimates and velocity gradients of the myocardium, respectively, are exciting developments in echocardiography. They will no doubt find greater clinical applications and usage in the CHD population. The fact that echo assessment of regional function during stress can be made more quantitative with these technologies without relying on high-quality 2D echo pictures would be particularly applicable to CHD patients with abnormal heart positions and poor acoustic windows.
   - Contrast echocardiography
     - Contrast echocardiography using intravenous microbubbles not only improves endocardial border delineation for better assessment of RWMA but more importantly allows real-time perfusion imaging for detection of myocardial ischemia. This could technically be extremely useful in detection of myocardial ischemia in both the systemic as well as the subpulmonary ventricle in the ACHD population.
   - Coronary flow velocity reserve
     - Coronary flow velocity reserve (CFVR), which is the ratio of hyperemic to basal

coronary flow velocity, may be useful for noninvasive assessment of coronary artery stenosis particularly in patients with Kawasaki disease. Hiraishi et al.[29] have shown the feasibility of CFVR measurements by transthoracic echocardiography in 49 patients (age range 3–24 years) with Kawasaki disease (Table 15.1). The limitations of CFVR lie mainly in the difficulty encountered in some patients to visualize and obtain a good parallel alignment with the coronary flow and at present this technique only allows interrogation of the left anterior descending artery and the posterior descending artery, the latter usually arising from the right coronary artery.

- Live 3D echocardiography
  - Live 3D transthoracic echocardiography has great diagnostic potential as it is capable of providing unique imaging planes and projections. Nevertheless, its clinical application and usage in the detection of myocardial ischemia is still in its infancy. Its application in CHD patients may be limited in patients with poor acoustic windows particularly for assessing the right ventricle in the systemic and pulmonary circulation.

5.3 The Role of Nuclear Imaging Techniques

Two forms of nuclear imaging techniques – single photon computed emission tomography (SPECT) and positron emission tomography (PET) – can be used to detect hemodynamically significant CAD. Both techniques involve intravenous administration of a perfusion tracer (such as thallium-201 or technetium-99m sestamibi for SPECT, and oxygen-15-water Rubidium-82 or nitrogen-13-ammonia for PET) to evaluate regional coronary perfusion after stress and at rest. Stress may be performed by dynamic exercise or with pharmacologic agents (adenosine, dipyridamole, or dobutamine). Comparison of the stress and resting images permits comment on the presence or absence of inducible ischemia and/or infarction, and hence on the likely presence or absence of flow-limiting coronary lesions. The incorporation of electrocardiogram-gating provides additional information regarding regional and global ventricular function, as well as enhances image interpretation. Furthermore, regional perfusion can be quantified (in terms of milliliter/minute/gram) and perfusion reserve calculated with dynamic PET.

9.3.1 Technical Considerations: Stress Techniques, Image Acquisition, and Image Interpretation

1. Choosing the optimal form of stress

   In patients with congenital defects, all studies have used dynamic exercise as the stress method for single photon myocardial perfusion imaging, typically on a treadmill or bicycle ergometer. Certainly, this is the most physiologic form of stress and provides additional useful information such as exercise capacity and hemodynamic changes. However, sudden death is associated with some congenital anomalies, especially during exercise – this has been particularly documented for anomalous origin of the left main coronary artery from the right aortic sinus and anomalous origin of the right coronary artery from the left aortic sinus (as the vessel can be compressed between the great vessels secondary to an exercise-induced increase in cardiac output).[30] Although there is potentially legitimate concern with exercising such patients, there has been no reported mortality in the literature.[31,32] Indeed, these patients may be safely exercised if stress is terminated at the onset of symptoms consistent with ischemia and the radiopharmaceutical injected. With PET studies, adenosine has been used to induce coronary hyperemia.[33,34] Pharmacologic stress is more convenient in PET studies because of the need for rapid image acquisition once a (short-living) perfusion radiopharmaceutical has been administered.

2. Technical considerations

   Dextrocardia, if present, should be noted as the acquisition arc should be changed to start at 45° right posterior oblique and end at 45° left anterior oblique (instead of the usual 45° right anterior oblique to 45° left posterior oblique rotation). Even in the absence of dextrocardia, many patients with CHD have a rotated heart, and the arc of acquisition may be changed accordingly to permit optimal myocardial count registration. Children may require light sedation during image acquisition to reduce motion. Finally, it should be noted that nuclear imaging techniques may be of limited value in the assessment of young infants (weighing < 9 kg) with small hearts because of the relatively poor resolution of the gamma camera.[35]

3. Problems with interpretation

   The interpretation of myocardial perfusion images in patients with CHD is in principle no different from that of patients without congenital defects. Indeed, image interpretation in patients with simple congenital defects, such as isolated congenital coronary anomaly or a small septal defect, is relatively straightforward. However, image interpretation in patients with complex congenital defects who have gross distortion of cardiac anatomy may be extremely difficult. This is partly related to the limited resolution of the gamma camera, and difficulties in axis and slice selection and stress-rest comparison (particularly if transient perfusion abnormalities are also present), but is also related to the unpredictable effect of surgery and underlying myocardial disease on regional tracer uptake. Literature review in this respect has not been helpful because there are no published studies examining the diagnostic accuracy of nuclear imaging techniques in the detection of myocardial ischemia in these patients, unlike the adult noncongenital population.

4. Nuclear imaging techniques in specific forms of CHD

   - *Congenital coronary artery anomalies*

Congenital coronary artery anomalies include a wide range of pathologic manifestations and are associated with a full spectrum of clinical presentations.[36] Early studies have demonstrated that planar resting thallium imaging can be used to diagnose myocardial infarction in patients with anomalous origin of the left coronary artery and single-trunk anomalous origin of both coronary arteries from the pulmonary artery.[31,37–39]

Myocardial bridging occurs when a segment of an epicardial coronary artery courses below the epicardial surface, which leads to compression of the artery during ventricular contraction. Traditionally, this has been regarded as a benign condition without adverse effect on myocardial perfusion. Indeed, early studies with exercise thallium imaging in patients with muscle bridging have failed to demonstrate associated ischemia in these patients.[12,40] More recent studies with intravascular ultrasound, however, have shown that bridged segments show a marked reduction in luminal area throughout ventricular systole that persists into diastole. Studies have also shown that coronary flow velocities are increased and flow reserve is reduced in arteries in which bridging is present.[41] Several case reports have highlighted the possible association between bridging and ischemia and/or infarction.[42,43]

   - *Transposition of the great arteries*

Patients with ccTGA often present in adulthood with symptoms of heart failure or more rarely of angina.[44] Many of these patients develop progressive systemic right ventricular dysfunction. A postulated mechanism is myocardial ischemia and/or infarction secondary to an imbalance in oxygen supply and demand as a result of ventricular hypertrophy.[45] Both reversible and fixed perfusion abnormalities have been demonstrated on single photon myocardial perfusion imaging in such patients, lending support to this hypothesis.[46,47] Furthermore, adenosine-induced hyperemic coronary flow and myocardial perfusion reserve (MPR) have been shown to be attenuated in these patients using dynamic PET with nitrogen-13-ammonia.[33]

A similar situation arises in patients with simple TGA after treatment with an atrial switch procedure.[5] Long-term follow-up studies with SPECT have shown a high incidence of reversible and fixed perfusion defects in such patients. The extent of myocardial perfusion abnormalities has been found to correlate well with the impairment in ventricular function.[4,48] For patients with TGA treated with an arterial switch operation, there is also evidence from SPECT that late perfusion abnormalities are present.[49] Dynamic PET studies have also demonstrated that adenosine-induced hyperemic coronary flow and MPR are significantly reduced in these patients, even in the absence of symptoms. A postulated mechanism for this is coronary obstruction secondary to coronary mobilization and reimplantation which is an integral part of the arterial switch operation.[34,50] This hypothesis has been disputed, however, by a study that showed a similar incidence of perfusion defects on SPECT after arterial switch operation and cardiopulmonary bypass for other procedures in children with CHD.[51]

- *Other CHD*

There is little published work on the evaluation of myocardial perfusion by nuclear imaging techniques in patients with other forms of CHD.

- *Kawasaki disease*

Although coronary aneurysms can be detected by echocardiography, the accurate assessment of stenosis requires invasive coronary angiography.[52] Despite the direct visualization of coronary artery lesions with angiography, this technique is of little value in the assessment of myocardial perfusion (Figure 15.3a and b; see color section). In particular, the relationship between visually assessed coronary artery lesions on angiography in Kawasaki disease and coronary flow reserve (CFR) has been shown to be variable. A study using intracoronary Doppler guidewire measurement of flow has demonstrated that CFR tends to be reduced in aneurysms of moderate to large size only.[53] The same study also showed that patients with perfusion abnormalities on thallium SPECT but angiographically smooth coronary arteries had reduced CFR. In this setting, therefore, noninvasive nuclear imaging techniques have an important role in the assessment of myocardial perfusion and the management of patients with Kawasaki disease.

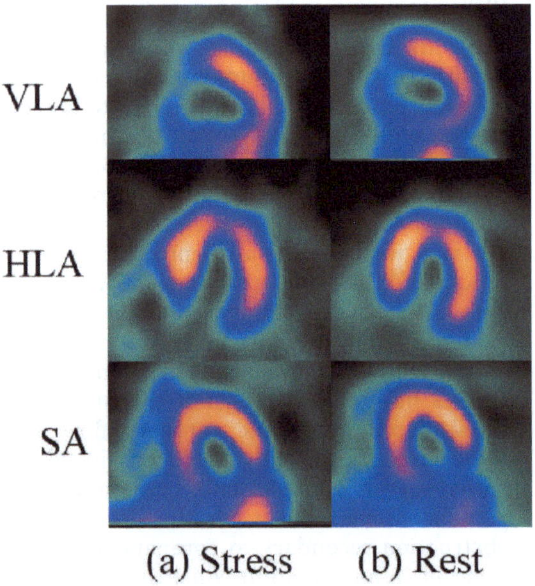

Figure 15.3b. Stress/rest technetium (Tc)-99m tetrofosmin myocardial perfusion SPECT from the patient in fig. 15.3a. The study was performed with intravenous adenosine at 140 μg/kg/min over 6 minutes. Image acquisition was performed under light sedation. The images after stress and rest injection of tetrofosmin show partial thickness infarction of the inferior wall. There is no scintigraphic evidence of residual myocardial ischemia. HLA, horizontal long axis; SA, short axis; VLA, vertical long axis.

In Kawasaki disease, both exercise and primary vasodilator stress have been shown to be safe and effective.[54–56] In young children, vasodilator stress may be easier to administer than exercise. Image acquisition parameters do not need to be changed, unless there is concomitant complex congenital defect and distorted cardiac anatomy. The diagnostic accuracy of SPECT in the detection of flow-limiting coronary stenosis in Kawasaki disease has been investigated by Fukuda et al.[55] In this study of 86 patients, a sensitivity of 90% and specificity of 100% for angiographic coronary stenosis ≥75% was demonstrated with dipyridamole-tetrofosmin SPECT. Another smaller study of 23 patients showed a sensitivity of 73% and specificity of 58% with exercise-thallium SPECT, although the angiographic "gold standard" for disease was that of coronary dilatation.[56] Serial monitoring of patients with nuclear imaging techniques may be useful to predict late progression in coronary stenosis and assist decision-making for angiography.[57,58] Furthermore, scintigraphic evaluation permits the functional assessment of demonstrated coronary aneurysms,[59] as well as documenting changes with therapy.[60] Some studies have showed a poor agreement between SPECT and coronary angiography, but this can be explained by the fact that the former assesses perfusion whereas the latter provides anatomic information.[61,62] This distinction is supported by evidence from dynamic PET studies in Kawasaki disease. Such studies have demonstrated that adenosine-induced absolute hyperemic coronary flow and MPR remain depressed in patients with previous Kawasaki disease even in the absence of angiographic coronary stenosis.[63,64]

There are also now data on the prognostic value of nuclear imaging techniques in patients with Kawasaki disease. In a prospective study of 90 patients, followed up for a mean of 8.8 years, the presence of thallium redistribution on SPET imaging was found to be the most significant independent predictor

($\chi^2 = 54.4$, $P < .0001$) and the best multivariate independent predictor (relative risk 57.8) of future cardiac events.[58] Patients with no redistribution (in other words, no ischemia) on thallium imaging had a low late cardiac event rate of 1.6% ± 1.6%.[65] This powerful prognostic value of SPECT imaging makes a strong case for its use in the management of all patients with Kawasaki disease.

5.4 The Role of Cardiovascular Magnetic Resonance Imaging

Cardiovascular magnetic resonance (CMR) is making increasingly significant contributions to clinical evaluation and research in the field of IHD. It is noninvasive, gives excellent access to all parts of the chest, is free of ionizing radiation, and is well suited for investigation of the right as well as the left ventricle.[66–68]

The majority of CMR studies are acquired during breathholds. Images are cardiac gated from the R wave of the electrocardiogram, with data collected over about 10 seconds. The resulting cine loop represents an averaged heart cycle, which means that image quality may be degraded if there is arrhythmia. Real-time imaging is also possible, but at a cost of temporal and spatial resolution. CMR is relatively expensive, and its availability remains limited to a few specialist centers. It is, however, the most versatile cardiac imaging modality, and allows several complementary approaches to investigation of ischemic and CHD.

5.4.1 Safety Issues

When used with appropriate vigilance, CMR is extremely safe. The most important contraindications are presence of a pacemaker or other implanted electrical device, the presence of a ferromagnetic clip in the brain, or suspicion of a steel fragment in the eye after injury. Otherwise, metallic implants in the chest, including prosthetic heart valves, stents, occlusion devices, and sternal wires, are regarded as safe, although they may cause local artifacts.

5.4.2 Ventricular Function

CMR has become the gold standard for visualization and measurement of regional and global function of both left and right ventricles. Selected long-axis cine acquisitions and a complete stack of short-axis cine acquisitions from the base of the ventricles to the apex are acquired for visual and quantitative assessment. These data are generally acquired in about 10 minutes, although methods are being developed for acquisition of 3D cine data for the measurement of the volumes and function of both ventricles in a single breathhold. Cine images using steady-state free precession give good contrast between blood and muscle which allows reasonably accurate tracing of cavity outlines. CMR can be a particularly helpful tool for the assessment of ventricular function and valvar regurgitation in patients with previous tetralogy of Fallot repair, atrial switch operation, ccTGA, or in patients with univentricular heart physiology.

5.4.3 Imaging of Myocardial Scarring and Viability

Over the last few years, CMR has become established as a technique for detecting the presence and distribution of myocardial scarring, and hence regional viability in IHD. The method, which is known as late gadolinium enhancement imaging, makes use of the property of intravenously injected gadolinium chelate, a paramagnetic contrast agent, to linger in scarred myocardial tissue after its concentration has begun to decrease in the bloodstream.[69,70] Imaging 5–20 minutes after injection allows the scarred tissue to be highlighted. An inversion recovery sequence is used which, with appropriate adjustment of parameters, allows healthy myocardium to appear dark, contrasting with the bright signal of scarred myocardium. The spatial resolution achieved by late gadolinium enhancement imaging is significantly better than that obtained by radionuclide techniques, allowing visualization of the thickness of scarring relative to the thickness of viable myocardial wall. This is important for viability and hibernation assessment in patients with left ventricular dysfunction and heart failure.[71] For a more detailed discussion on detection of viability and hibernation see also Chapter 13.

CMR can help to distinguish ischemic from cardiomyopathic causes of ventricular dysfunction. In ischemic disease, myocardial dysfunction tends to be regional, and any late gadolinium enhancement of infarcted tissue extends from subendocardial to full thickness in

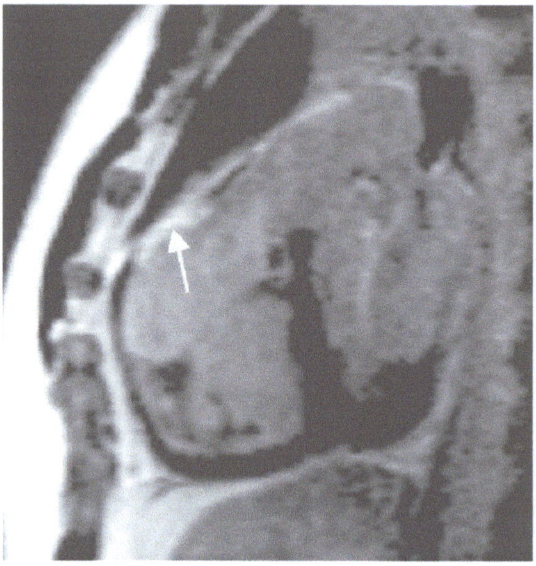

a

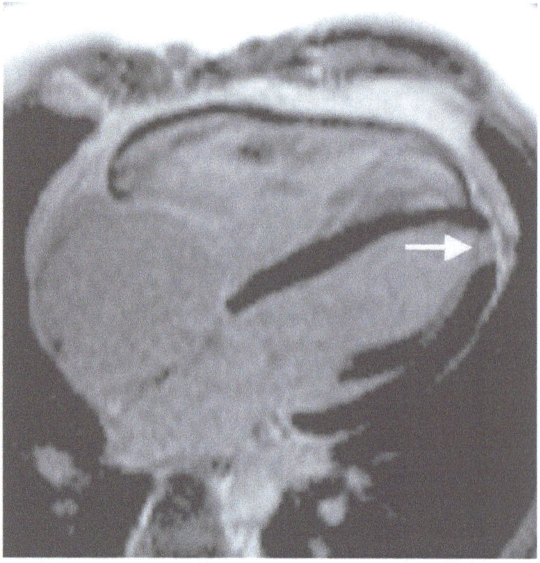

b

Figure 15.4. **a** Magnetic resonance imaging showing late gadolinium enhancement (see arrow) suggestive of scarring in the right ventricular outflow tract in a patient with tetralogy of Fallot. **b** Magnetic resonance imaging showing late gadolinium enhancement suggestive of previous surgical drain insertion through the left ventricular apex (as arrowed) on a ventricular four-chamber view.

a region supplied by an occluded coronary artery branch. In cardiomyopathy, however, dysfunction is generally more global, and if there is late gadolinium enhancement, it tends to be patchy and not in the subendocardial distribution typical of ischemia.[72,73]

The techniques of late Gadolinium enhancement imaging have been used for investigation of right as well as left ventricular scarring in patients with CHD particularly after surgery. In these patients scarring has been found to be common in a few distinct locations. These are often directly attributable to the interventions performed, for example, scarring of the wall of the partially resected infundibulum in patients after repair of tetralogy of Fallot (Figure 15.4a), or localized scarring of the left ventricular apex in patients who have had an apical vent (Figure 15.4b) at surgery. Less common but potentially more significant are occasional findings of more extensive left ventricular scarring in about 5% of patients after repair of Fallot's tetralogy,[74] and full-thickness scarring of regions of the anterior wall of the systemic right ventricle in about 15% of patients who had previously undergone Mustard or Senning procedures for TGA.[75] These types of scarring appear to have an adverse impact on ventricular function and may predispose to arrhythmias.

5.4.4 Stress Imaging

CMR imaging of ventricular function during pharmacologic stress, using dobutamine or adenosine,[76] or immediately after exercise using an appropriately designed ergometer[77] are feasible, and have been used in research and clinical practice. Lack of immediate patient contact during imaging, however, makes this approach slightly less safe and convenient than stress echocardiography, although visualization of both ventricles is likely to be better.

5.4.5 Perfusion

First-pass myocardial perfusion imaging after an intravenously injected bolus of gadolinium contrast agent is possible by CMR. The contrast agent is, however, not ideal as some of it passes from intravascular to extravascular spaces, and it may be technically difficult to acquire data on perfusion to all parts of the myocardium within the short period of the first pass. Nevertheless, in combination with the other approaches available to CMR, perfusion imaging in skilled hands can add information complementary to assessments of function and tissue characterization, and without ionizing radiation.[78,79] For a more detailed discussion see also Chapters 3 and 8.

5.4.6 CMR Angiography

Contrast-enhanced MR angiography is now the preferred method of choice in imaging patients with coarctation, branch pulmonary artery stenoses, and collateral vessels. Three-dimensional reconstruction of the obtained images appears superior to conventional catheterization and offers valuable data in the assessment of the patient before further surgical or transcatheter interventions.

However, coronary angiography by CMR remains challenging at the present time, because of the relatively small diameters and mobility of the coronary arteries. For assessment of coronary artery stenosis caused by atheromatous disease, CMR has been shown to be of use for exclusion of severe proximal multivessel disease at centers with appropriate expertise and resources,[80,81] but spatial resolution is not yet adequate for assessment of small coronary artery branches. The spatial resolution of CMR coronary angiography is slightly less good than that of computed tomography, and significantly less than that of invasive angiography. CMR is nevertheless a valuable approach for diagnosing or excluding anomalous coronary origins (Figure 15.2b), which are not uncommon in patients with CHD.[82,83] In the diagnosis and assessment of Kawasaki disease, CMR angiography can be used to visualize coronary artery aneurysms or stenosis,[84,85] and late gadolinium enhancement can be used to detect previous infarction.[86]

5.4.7 Future Prospects

Given the versatility of CMR, it is to be expected that further important and as yet unforeseen contributions to the understanding and investigation of IHD will be made in the coming years. Assessment of the coronary arteries not only by angiographic visualization of the lumen, but also by characterization of the arterial walls may become practicable by CMR. Furthermore, there is ground for further increase in the number of CMR-guided cardiac interventions in patients with CHD, whereas guided catheterization with simultaneous visualization of injected therapeutic material may contribute to delivery of stem cells or other agents to regions of diseased myocardium. Multislice CT is another possibility but at the time of writing there is limited information on its precise role in the patient population discussed here.

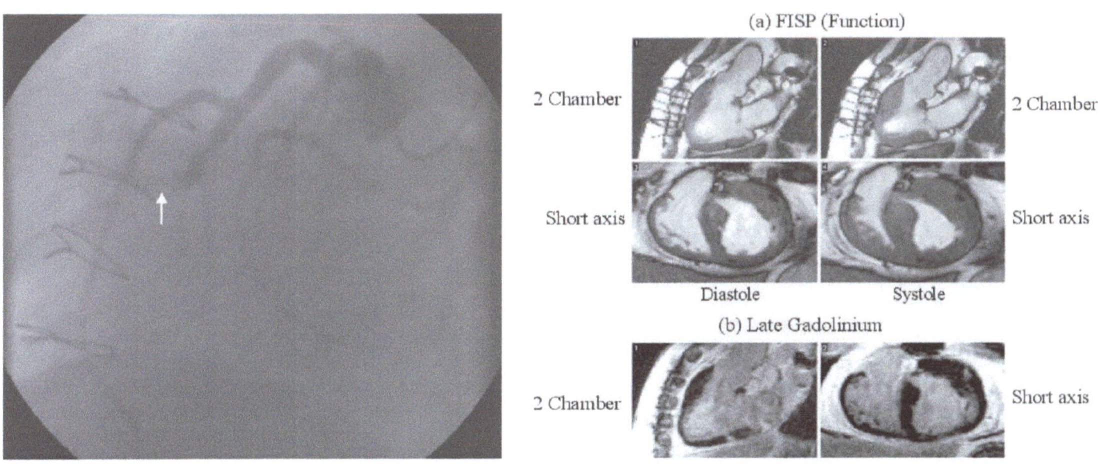

a b

Figure 15.5. **a** Coronary angiography. A 46-year-old man with complex congenitally corrected transposition of the great arteries (ccTGA) associated with dextrocardia, pulmonary stenosis, ASD, and VSD complained of atypical chest pain. He had previously undergone surgical closure of ASD and VSD, as well as insertion of a left ventricle to pulmonary artery conduit 13 years ago. Risk factors for atheromatous coronary artery disease (CAD) included previous smoking, dyslipidemia, and a family history of premature CAD. In view of his chest pain, he was referred for coronary angiography. Coronary angiography showing occlusion of a large left anterior descending (LAD) artery just distal to a coronary fistula with the left ventricular outflow tract (arrow) as shown. **b** Cardiac magnetic resonance imaging. Magnetic resonance imaging reveals reasonable biventricular function. There are small areas of late gadolinium enhancement in the inferior and anterolateral walls of the subpulmonary left ventricle (bottom panel). These may represent previous microinfarcts.

Table 15.2. Different imaging modalities

Imaging modality	Strengths	Limitations	Additional comments
Stress echo	– Safe, well established in normal population – Serial assessment – Assess contractility and regional wall motion especially for LV – Exercise or pharmacologic stress	– Occasional poor echo windows – RV wall motion and ischemia – Right-sided LV – Single ventricle	– Augment with tissue Doppler and longitudinal M-mode motion – Potential role – contrast echo and online live 3D – Data on Kawasaki Disease, Mustard patients available
Nuclear imaging (SPET and PET)	– Safe, well established in normal population – Perfusion defects not limited by cardiac position – Assess RV perfusion – Assess single ventricular perfusion	– Limitation in gamma camera resolution in grossly distorted heart – Axis and slice selection during stress/rest comparison	– Change acquisition arc in cardiac malposition – Published data on Kawasaki disease and patients with Mustard and congenitally corrected transposition of the great arteries
Cardiovascular magnetic resonance	– Excellent RV and LV resolution – Serial assessment – Pharmacologic stress possible – Assess regional wall motion – First-pass perfusion with gadolinium possible – Myocardial scarring seen with late gadolinium	– Expensive, not widely available – Contraindicated in patients with pacemakers, brain clips, etc. – Claustrophobia, need breathholding – Data averaged over 10 s, not real-time imaging – Image degradation in arrhythmias	– Very limited published data on stress CMR – Future: CMR coronary angiography and online 3D CMR

6. Conclusion

The role of noninvasive imaging in the detection of myocardial ischemia in the population with CHD is growing rapidly. The development of newer techniques from different imaging modalities will undoubtedly fuel and propel this area to greater growth in the next decade. A thorough understanding and working knowledge of each patient's underlying anatomy and physiology

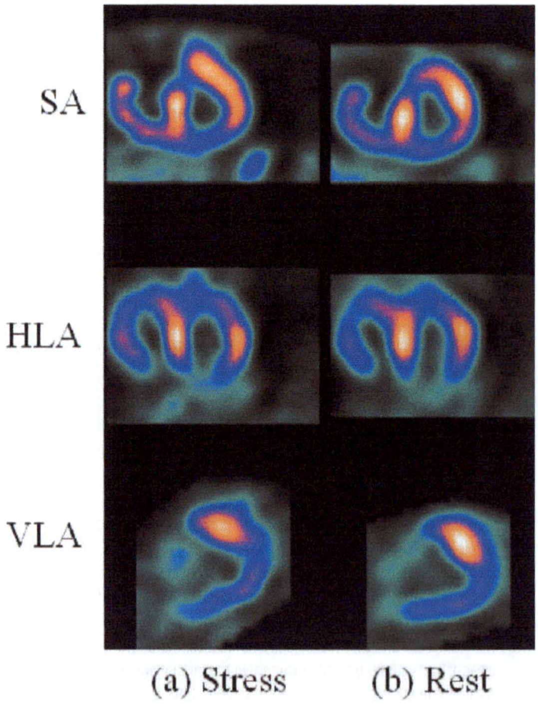

c

Figure 15.5c. (continued from page 301) Stress/rest Tc-99m tetrofosmin myocardial perfusion SPECT. Stress was performed with intravenous adenosine at 140 μg/kg/min over 6 minutes without exercise in view of resting bundle branch block. Image acquisition was altered to take into account his known dextrocardia. Tc-99m tetrofosmin myocardial perfusion SPECT images reveal hypertrophy of the systemic right ventricle, with fixed defects in the apex, anteroseptum, and inferior wall of the subpulmonary left ventricle. There was no scintigraphic evidence of myocardial ischemia. The patient was subsequently followed up with conservative medical therapy and aggressive risk-factor modification was continued. The assessment of myocardial perfusion in complex congenital heart disease is fraught with difficulties. At present, no single imaging modality can assess accurately the presence or absence of hemodynamically significant CAD in such cases. Our own approach is to evaluate the information obtained from a variety of complementary imaging techniques for each individual patient, in conjunction with the clinical details. HLA, horizontal long axis; SA, short axis; VLA, vertical long axis.

is essential to utilize each imaging modality to its maximum potential. Only then can the interpretation of each imaging study be accurately assessed and utilized. Different imaging modalities have their inherent strengths and limitations (Table 15.2). Often, one may have to use more than one imaging techniques (Figure 15.5; see color section) for the detection of myocardial ischemia and full appreciation of the anatomy and function of patients with complex CHD.

References

1. Wren C, O'Sullivan JJ. Survival with congenital heart disease and need for follow up in adult life. Heart 2001;85(4):438–443.
2. Child JS, Collins-Nakai RL, Alpert JS, et al. Task force 3: workforce description and educational requirements for the care of adults with congenital heart disease. J Am Coll Cardiol 2001;37(5):1183–1187.
3. Grown-up congenital heart (GUCH) disease: current needs and provision of service for adolescents and adults with congenital heart disease in the UK. Heart 2002;88(suppl 1):i1–14.
4. Millane T, Bernard EJ, Jaeggi E, et al. Role of ischemia and infarction in late right ventricular dysfunction after atrial repair of transposition of the great arteries. J Am Coll Cardiol 2000;35(6):1661–1668.
5. Hornung TS, Kilner PJ, Davlouros PA, Grothues F, Li W, Gatzoulis MA. Excessive right ventricular hypertrophic response in adults with the mustard procedure for transposition of the great arteries. Am J Cardiol 2002; 90(7):800–803.
6. Liberthson RR. Sudden death from cardiac causes in children and young adults. N Engl J Med 1996;334(16): 1039–1044.
7. Harpaz D, Rozenman Y, Medalion B, Geva Y. Anomalous origin of the left coronary artery from the pulmonary artery accompanied by mitral valve prolapse and regurgitation: surgical implication of dobutamine stress echocardiography. J Am Soc Echocardiogr 2004;17(1): 73–77.
8. Waller BF. Nonatherosclerotic coronary heart disease. In: Fuster V, Alexander RW, O'Rourke RA, eds. Hurst's the Heart. 11th ed. New York: McGraw-Hill; 2004.
9. Sorajja P, Ommen SR, Nishimura RA, Gersh BJ, Tajik AJ, Holmes DR. Myocardial bridging in adult patients with hypertrophic cardiomyopathy. J Am Coll Cardiol 2003; 42(5):889–894.
10. Polacek P, Kralove H. Relation of myocardial bridges and loops on the coronary arteries to coronary occulsions. Am Heart J 1961;61:44–52.
11. Mohlenkamp S, Hort W, Ge J, Erbel R. Update on myocardial bridging. Circulation 2002;106(20):2616–2622.
12. Greenspan M, Iskandrian AS, Catherwood E, Kimbiris D, Bemis CE, Segal BL. Myocardial bridging of the left anterior descending artery: evaluation using exercise thallium-201 myocardial scintigraphy. Cathet Cardiovasc Diagn 1980;6(2):173–180.
13. Jatene AD, Fontes VF, Paulista PP, et al. Anatomic correction of transposition of the great vessels. J Thorac Cardiovasc Surg 1976;72(3):364–370.
14. Bonhoeffer P, Bonnet D, Piechaud JF, et al. Coronary artery obstruction after the arterial switch operation for transposition of the great arteries in newborns. J Am Coll Cardiol 1997;29(1):202–206.
15. Tanel R, Wernovsky G, Landzberg M, Perry S, Burke R. Coronary artery abnormalities detected at cardiac catheterisation following the arterial switch operation for transposition of the great arteries. Am J Cardiol 1995;76:153–157.
16. Pretre R, Tamisier D, Bonhoeffer P, et al. Results of the arterial switch operation in neonates with transposed great arteries. Lancet 2001;357:1826–1830.
17. Tsuda E, Imakita M, Yagihara T, et al. Late death after arterial switch operation for transposition of the great arteries. Am Heart J 1992;124:1551–1557.
18. Hausdorf G, Kampmann C, Schneider M. Coronary angioplasty for coronary stenosis after the arterial switch procedure. Am J Cardiol 1995;76:621–623.
19. Tzifa A, Tulloh RMR. Coronary arterial complications before and after the arterial switch operation: is the future clear? Cardiol Young 2002;12:164–171.
20. Cohen M, Fuster V, Steele PM, Driscoll D, McGoon DC. Coarctation of the aorta. Long-term follow-up and prediction of outcome after surgical correction. Circulation 1989;80(4):840–845.
21. Kato H, Inoue O, Kawasaki T, Fujiwara H, Watanabe T, Toshima H. Adult coronary artery disease probably due to childhood Kawasaki disease. Lancet 1992;340(8828): 1127–1129.
22. Ogawa S, Fukazawa R, Ohkubo T, et al. Silent myocardial ischemia in Kawasaki disease: evaluation of percutaneous transluminal coronary angioplasty by dobutamine stress testing. Circulation 1997;96(10): 3384–3389.
23. Noto N, Ayusawa M, Karasawa K, et al. Dobutamine stress echocardiography for detection of coronary artery stenosis in children with Kawasaki disease. J Am Coll Cardiol 1996;27(5):1251–1256.
24. Henein MY, Dinarevic S, O'Sullivan CA, Gibson DG, Shinebourne EA. Exercise echocardiography in children with Kawasaki disease: ventricular long axis is selectively abnormal. Am J Cardiol 1998;81(11): 1356–1359.
25. Pahl E, Sehgal R, Chrystof D, et al. Feasibility of exercise stress echocardiography for the follow-up of children with coronary involvement secondary to Kawasaki disease. Circulation 1995;91(1):122–128.
26. Dahdah NS, Fournier A, Jaeggi E, et al. Segmental myocardial contractility versus perfusion in Kawasaki disease with coronary arterial aneurysm. Am J Cardiol 1999;83(1):48–51.
27. Li W, Hornung T, Francis D, et al. Relationship of biventricular function quantified by stress echocardiography to cardiopulmonary exercise capacity in adults with Mustard (atrial switch) procedure for transposition of the great arteries. Circulation 2004;110(11):1380–1386.
28. Redington AN, Rigby ML, Oldershaw P, Gibson DG, Shinebourne EA. Right ventricular function 10 years after the Mustard operation for transposition of the great arteries: analysis of size, shape, and wall motion. Br Heart J 1989;62(6):455–461.
29. Hiraishi S, Hirota H, Horiguchi Y, et al. Transthoracic Doppler assessment of coronary flow velocity reserve in

children with Kawasaki disease: comparison with coronary angiography and thallium-201 imaging. J Am Coll Cardiol 2002;40(10):1816–1824.
30. Taylor AJ, Rogan KM, Virmani R. Sudden cardiac death associated with isolated congenital coronary artery anomalies. J Am Coll Cardiol 1992;20(3):640–647.
31. Finley JP, Howman-Giles R, Gilday DL, Olley PM, Rowe RD. Thallium-201 myocardial imaging in anomalous left coronary artery arising from the pulmonary artery. Applications before and after medical and surgical treatment. Am J Cardiol 1978;42(4):675–680.
32. Rajfer SI, Oetgen WJ, Weeks KD Jr, Kaminski RJ, Rocchini AP. Thallium-201 scintigraphy after surgical repair of hemodynamically significant primary coronary artery anomalies. Chest 1982;81(6):687–692.
33. Hauser M, Bengel FM, Hager A, et al. Impaired myocardial blood flow and coronary flow reserve of the anatomical right systemic ventricle in patients with congenitally corrected transposition of the great arteries. Heart 2003;89(10):1231–1235.
34. Bengel FM, Hauser M, Duvernoy CS, et al. Myocardial blood flow and coronary flow reserve late after anatomical correction of transposition of the great arteries. J Am Coll Cardiol 1998;32(7):1955–1961.
35. Bjorkhem G, Evander E, White T, Lundstrom NR. Myocardial scintigraphy with 201thallium in pediatric cardiology: a review of 52 cases. Pediatr Cardiol 1990; 11(1):1–7.
36. Rapp AH, Hillis LD. Clinical consequences of anomalous coronary arteries. Coron Artery Dis 2001; 12(8):617–620.
37. Moodie DS, Cook SA, Gill CC, Napoli CA. Thallium-201 myocardial imaging in young adults with anomalous left coronary artery arising from the pulmonary artery. J Nucl Med 1980;21(11):1076–1079.
38. Gutgesell HP, Pinsky WW, DePuey EG. Thallium-201 myocardial perfusion imaging in infants and children. Value in distinguishing anomalous left coronary artery from congestive cardiomyopathy. Circulation 1980; 61(3):596–599.
39. Goldblatt E, Adams AP, Ross IK, Savage JP, Morris LL. Single-trunk anomalous origin of both coronary arteries from the pulmonary artery. Diagnosis and surgical management. J Thorac Cardiovasc Surg 1984;87(1): 59–65.
40. Voss H, Kupper W, Hanrath P, Mathey D, Montz R, Bucking J. [Clinical correlations, lactate extraction, coronary venous bloodflow and thallium-201 myocardial imaging in patients with isolated left anterior descending muscle bridges: normal variant or obstruction? (author's transl).] Z Kardiol 1980;69(5):347–352.
41. Klues HG, Schwarz ER, vom Dahl J, et al. Disturbed intracoronary hemodynamics in myocardial bridging: early normalization by intracoronary stent placement. Circulation 1997;96(9):2905–2913.
42. Agirbasli M, Martin GS, Stout JB, Jennings HS 3rd, Lea JWT, Dixon JH Jr. Myocardial bridge as a cause of thrombus formation and myocardial infarction in a young athlete. Clin Cardiol 1997;20(12):1032–1036.
43. Roul G, Sens P, Germain P, Bareiss P. Myocardial bridging as a cause of acute transient left heart dysfunction. Chest 1999;116(2):574–580.
44. Piran S, Veldtman G, Siu S, Webb GD, Liu PP. Heart failure and ventricular dysfunction in patients with single or systemic right ventricles. Circulation 2002; 105(10):1189–1194.
45. Connelly MS, Liu PP, Williams WG, Webb GD, Robertson P, McLaughlin PR. Congenitally corrected transposition of the great arteries in the adult: functional status and complications. J Am Coll Cardiol 1996;27(5): 1238–1243.
46. Bajwa N, Bianco JA, Stone CK. Thallium myocardial scintigraphy in congenitally-corrected transposition of the great arteries. J Nucl Med 1991;32(8):1611–1613.
47. Hornung TS, Bernard EJ, Celermajer DS, et al. Right ventricular dysfunction in congenitally corrected transposition of the great arteries. Am J Cardiol 1999;84(9):1116–1119, A10.
48. Lubiszewska B, Gosiewska E, Hoffman P, et al. Myocardial perfusion and function of the systemic right ventricle in patients after atrial switch procedure for complete transposition: long-term follow-up. J Am Coll Cardiol 2000;36(4):1365–1370.
49. Weindling SN, Wernovsky G, Colan SD, et al. Myocardial perfusion, function and exercise tolerance after the arterial switch operation. J Am Coll Cardiol 1994;23(2): 424–433.
50. Yates RW, Marsden PK, Badawi RD, et al. Evaluation of myocardial perfusion using positron emission tomography in infants following a neonatal switch operation. Pediatr Cardiol 2000;21:111–118.
51. Hayes AM, Baker EJ, Kakadeker A, et al. Influence of anatomic correction for transposition of the great arteries on myocardial perfusion: radionuclide imaging with technetium-99m 2-methoxy isobutyl isonitrile. J Am Coll Cardiol 1994;24(3):769–777.
52. Kato H, Ichinose E, Yoshioka F, et al. Fate of coronary aneurysms in Kawasaki disease: serial coronary angiography and long-term follow-up study. Am J Cardiol 1982;49(7):1758–1766.
53. Hamaoka K, Onouchi Z, Kamiya Y, Sakata K. Evaluation of coronary flow velocity dynamics and flow reserve in patients with Kawasaki disease by means of a Doppler guide wire. J Am Coll Cardiol 1998;31(4): 833–840.
54. Prabhu AS, Singh TP, Morrow WR, Muzik O, Di Carli MF. Safety and efficacy of intravenous adenosine for pharmacologic stress testing in children with aortic valve disease or Kawasaki disease. Am J Cardiol 1999; 83(2):284–286, A6.
55. Fukuda T, Ishibashi M, Yokoyama T, et al. Myocardial ischemia in Kawasaki disease: evaluation with dipyridamole stress technetium 99m tetrofosmin scintigraphy. J Nucl Cardiol 2002;9(6):632–637.
56. Jan SL, Hwang B, Fu YC, et al. Comparison of 201Tl SPET and treadmill exercise testing in patients with Kawasaki disease. Nucl Med Commun 2000;21(5): 431–435.
57. Spielmann RP, Nienaber CA, Hausdorf G, Montz R. Tomographic myocardial perfusion scintigraphy in children with Kawasaki disease. J Nucl Med 1987; 28(12):1839–1843.
58. Kondo C, Nakanishi T, Sonobe T, Tatara K, Momma K, Kusakabe K. Scintigraphic monitoring of coronary artery occlusion due to Kawasaki disease. Am J Cardiol 1993;71(8):681–685.
59. Hijazi ZM, Udelson JE, Snapper H, et al. Physiologic significance of chronic coronary aneurysms in patients with Kawasaki disease. J Am Coll Cardiol 1994; 24(7):1633–1638.
60. Nienaber CA, Spielmann RP, Hausdorf G. Dipyridamole-thallium-201 tomography documenting improved

myocardial perfusion with therapy in Kawasaki disease. Am Heart J 1988;116(6 pt 1):1575–1579.
61. Fukazawa M, Fukushige J, Takeuchi T, et al. Discordance between thallium-201 scintigraphy and coronary angiography in patients with Kawasaki disease: myocardial ischemia with normal coronary angiogram. Pediatr Cardiol 1993;14(2):67–74.
62. Fu YC, Kao CH, Hwang B, Jan SL, Chi CS. Discordance between dipyridamole stress Tc-99m sestamibi SPECT and coronary angiography in patients with Kawasaki disease. J Nucl Cardiol 2002;9(1):41–46.
63. Muzik O, Paridon SM, Singh TP, Morrow WR, Dayanikli F, Di Carli MF. Quantification of myocardial blood flow and flow reserve in children with a history of Kawasaki disease and normal coronary arteries using positron emission tomography. J Am Coll Cardiol 1996;28(3): 757–762.
64. Ohmochi Y, Onouchi Z, Oda Y, Hamaoka K. Assessment of effects of intravenous dipyridamole on regional myocardial perfusion in children with Kawasaki disease without angiographic evidence of coronary stenosis using positron emission tomography and H2(15)O. Coron Artery Dis 1995;6(7):555–559.
65. Miyagawa M, Mochizuki T, Murase K, et al. Prognostic value of dipyridamole-thallium myocardial scintigraphy in patients with Kawasaki disease. Circulation 1998; 98(10):990–996.
66. Manning WJ, Pennell DJ. Cardiovascular Magnetic Resonance. Edinburgh: Churchill Livingstone; 2002.
67. Mohiaddin RH. An Introduction to Cardiovascular Magnetic Resonance. London: Current Medical Literature; 2002.
68. Lardo AC, Fayed ZA, Chronos NAF, Fuster V. Cardiovascular Magnetic Resonance: Established and Emerging Applications. London: Martin Dunitz; 2003.
69. Kim RJ, Wu E, Rafael A, et al. The use of contrast-enhanced magnetic resonance imaging to identify reversible myocardial dysfunction. N Engl J Med 2000; 343(20):1445–1453.
70. Kim RJ, Shah DJ, Judd RM. How we perform delayed enhancement imaging. J Cardiovasc Magn Reson 2003; 5(3):505–514.
71. Rehwald WG, Fieno DS, Chen EL, Kim RJ, Judd RM. Myocardial magnetic resonance imaging contrast agent concentrations after reversible and irreversible ischemic injury. Circulation 2002;105(2):224–229.
72. Moon JC, McKenna WJ, McCrohon JA, Elliott PM, Smith GC, Pennell DJ. Toward clinical risk assessment in hypertrophic cardiomyopathy with gadolinium cardiovascular magnetic resonance. J Am Coll Cardiol 2003;41(9):1561–1567.
73. McCrohon JA, Moon JC, Prasad SK, et al. Differentiation of heart failure related to dilated cardiomyopathy and coronary artery disease using gadolinium-enhanced cardiovascular magnetic resonance. Circulation 2003;108(1):54–59.
74. Babu-Narayan SV, Kilner PJ, Moon JCC, Pennell DJ, Gatzoulis MA. Gadolinium cardiovascular magnetic resonance detection of myocardial fibrosis in adult patients after surgery for tetralogy of Fallot [abstract]. J Cardiovasc Magn Reson 2003;6(1):295.
75. Babu-Narayan SV, Goktekin O, Moon JC, et al. Late gadolinium enhancement cardiovascular magnetic resonance of the systemic right ventricle in adults with previous atrial redirection surgery for transposition of the great arteries. Circulation 2005;111(16): 2091–2098.
76. Nagel E, Lorenz C, Baer F, et al. Stress cardiovascular magnetic resonance: consensus panel report. J Cardiovasc Magn Reson 2001;3(3):267–281.
77. Roest AA, de Roos A, Lamb HJ, et al. Tetralogy of Fallot: postoperative delayed recovery of left ventricular stroke volume after physical exercise assessment with fast MR imaging. Radiology 2003;226(1):278–284.
78. Nagel E, al-Saadi N, Fleck E. Cardiovascular magnetic resonance: myocardial perfusion. Herz 2000;25(4): 409–416.
79. Wagner A, Mahrholdt H, Sechtem U, Kim RJ, Judd RM. MR imaging of myocardial perfusion and viability. Magn Reson Imaging Clin North Am 2003;11(1):49–66.
80. Danias PG, Stuber M, Botnar RM, et al. Coronary MR angiography clinical applications and potential for imaging coronary artery disease. Magn Reson Imaging Clin North Am 2003;11(1):81–99.
81. Kim WY, Danias PG, Stuber M, et al. Coronary magnetic resonance angiography for the detection of coronary stenoses. N Engl J Med 2001;345(26): 1863–1869.
82. Post JC, van Rossum AC, Bronzwaer JG, et al. Magnetic resonance angiography of anomalous coronary arteries. A new gold standard for delineating the proximal course? Circulation 1995;92(11):3163–3171.
83. McConnell MV, Stuber M, Manning WJ. Clinical role of coronary magnetic resonance angiography in the diagnosis of anomalous coronary arteries. J Cardiovasc Magn Reson 2000;2(3):217–224.
84. Mavrogeni S, Papadopoulos G, Douskou M, et al. Magnetic resonance angiography is equivalent to X-ray coronary angiography for the evaluation of coronary arteries in Kawasaki disease. J Am Coll Cardiol 2004; 43(4):649–652.
85. Greil GF, Stuber M, Botnar RM, et al. Coronary magnetic resonance angiography in adolescents and young adults with Kawasaki disease. Circulation 2002;105(8): 908–911.
86. Fujiwara M, Yamada TN, Ono Y, Yoshibayashi M, Kamiya T, Furukawa S. Magnetic resonance imaging of old myocardial infarction in young patients with a history of Kawasaki disease. Clin Cardiol 2001;24(3): 247–252.

Index

MIX
Papier aus verantwortungsvollen Quellen
Paper from responsible sources
FSC® C105338

If you have any concerns about our products,
you can contact us on
ProductSafety@springernature.com
In case Publisher is established outside the EU,
the EU authorized representative is:
Springer Nature Customer Service Center GmbH
Europaplatz 3, 69115 Heidelberg, Germany
Printed by Libri Plureos GmbH
in Hamburg, Germany